FAMILY NURSE PRACTITIONER

CERTIFICATION REVIEW

Edited by

Julie G. Stewart, DNP, MPH, MSN, FNP-BC, APRN
Associate Professor & Director of the FNP & DNP Programs
College of Nursing, Sacred Heart University
Fairfield, Connecticut

Nancy L. Dennert, MS, MSN, FNP-BC, CDE, BC-ADM
Clinical Assistant Professor
College of Nursing, Sacred Heart University
Fairfield, Connecticut

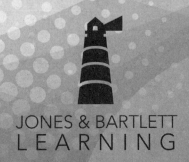

JONES & BARTLETT
LEARNING

World Headquarters
Jones & Bartlett Learning
5 Wall Street
Burlington, MA 01803
978-443-5000
info@jblearning.com
www.jblearning.com

Jones & Bartlett Learning books and products are available through most bookstores and online booksellers. To contact Jones & Bartlett Learning directly, call 800-832-0034, fax 978-443-8000, or visit our website, www.jblearning.com.

11064-7

Production Credits

VP, Executive Publisher: David D. Cella
Executive Editor: Amanda Martin
Acquisitions Editor: Teresa Reilly
Editorial Assistant: Lauren Vaughn
Director of Vendor Management: Amy Rose
Marketing Communications Manager: Katie Hennessy
Product Fulfillment Manager: Wendy Kilborn
Composition: S4Carlisle Publishing Services
Project Management: S4Carlisle Publishing Services
Cover Design: Kristin E. Parker
Rights & Media Specialist: Wes DeShano
Media Development Editor: Troy Liston
Cover Image: © Hluboki Dzianis/Shutterstock and
    © HAKKI ARSLAN/Shutterstock
Printing and Binding: Edwards Brothers Malloy
Cover Printing: Edwards Brothers Malloy

Library of Congress Cataloging-in-Publication Data
Names: Stewart, Julie G., author. | Dennert, Nancy L., author.
Title: Family nurse practitioner certification review/Julie G. Stewart and
    Nancy L. Dennert.
Description: First edition. | Burlington, Massachusetts: Jones & Bartlett Learning,
    [2017] | Includes index.
Identifiers: LCCN 2016005159 | ISBN 9781284081305
Subjects: | MESH: Family Nursing | Examination Questions
Classification: LCC RT55 | NLM WY 18.2 | DDC 610.73076—dc23
LC record available at http://lccn.loc.gov/2016005159

6048

Printed in the United States of America
21 20 19 18 17   10 9 8 7 6 5 4 3 2

Contents

Introduction

It is so exciting to be offering this certification review book to FNP students in preparation for their board examination and subsequent certification as a family nurse practitioner. We have incorporated questions that have topics from both the ANCC and AANP content outline. Each of the chapters was written by a colleague who works and/or specializes in that specific area. Therefore, we are able to provide you with the most current information and evidence-based practice. As FNP educators, we take pride in the fact that our students have had an exceptional pass rate that consistently exceeds the national percentage pass rate year after year. We are confident you will pass your certification exam if you apply yourself by studying each chapter's course materials and answering the practice questions that follow. Additionally, you will find that the first chapter contains vital information regarding test-taking strategies.

We are grateful to all the contributing authors, as well as our family and colleagues, for supporting our endeavor in writing this book.

Contributors

Pennie Sessler Branden, PhD, CNM, RN
Assistant Professor
College of Nursing
Sacred Heart University
Fairfield, CT

Kevin Chui, PT, DPT, PhD, GCS, OCS, CEEAA,
 FAAOMPT
Associate Professor
Department of Physical Therapy & Human
 Movement Science
Sacred Heart University
Fairfield, CT

Brandi Parker Cotton, PhD, MSN, PMHNP
Gateway Healthcare, Inc.
Pawtucket, RI

Maryanne Davidson, DNSc, APRN, CPNP
Associate Professor
Director, Undergraduate Nursing Program
College of Nursing
Sacred Heart University
Fairfield, CT

Nancy L. Dennert, MS, MSN, FNP-BC, CDE,
 BC-ADM
Clinical Assistant Professor
College of Nursing
Sacred Heart University
Fairfield, CT

Susan DeNisco, DNP, APRN, FNP-BC, CNE, CNL
Professor, Doctor of Nursing Practice Program
Executive Director, CHP Center for Community
 Health & Wellness
College of Nursing
Sacred Heart University
Fairfield, CT
Family Nurse Practitioner, St. Vincent's
 Medical Center
Bridgeport, CT

Heather Ferrillo, PhDc, MSN, APRN, FNP-BC, CNE
Clinical Assistant Professor
College of Nursing
Sacred Heart University
Fairfield, CT

Constance Glenn, MSN, APRN, FNP-BC, CNE
Clinical Assistant Professor
College of Nursing
Sacred Heart University
Fairfield, CT

Karen L. Gregory, DNP, APRN, CNS, RRT, AE-C
Advanced Practice Nurse
Oklahoma Allergy and Asthma Clinic
Oklahoma City, OK
Assistant Professor
Georgetown University School of Nursing and
 Health Studies
Washington, DC

Michelle Johnson, EdD, RN, CPNP-PC
Adjunct Faculty
College of Nursing
Sacred Heart University
Fairfield, CT

Julie A. Koch, DNP, RN, FNP-BC
Assistant Professor of Nursing
Assistant Dean of Graduate Nursing
Valparaiso University
College of Nursing and Health Professions
Valparaiso, IN

Judith Shannon Lynch, MS, MA, APRN-BC,
 FAANP
Assistant Clinical Professor
Yale University, School of Nursing
New Haven, CT

Kerry A. Milner, DNSc, RN
Associate Professor
College of Nursing
Sacred Heart University
Fairfield, CT

Lindsay A. Munden, DNP, RN, FNP-BC
Assistant Professor
Valparaiso University
Valparaiso, IN

Lynn Rapsilber, MSN, ANP-BC, APRN, FAANP, DNP(c)
Co-owner, NP Business Consultants, LLC
Connecticut GI
Torrington, CT

Sylvie Rosenbloom, DNP, APRN, FNP-BC, CDE
Adjunct Professor
College of Nursing
Sacred Heart University
Fairfield, CT
Nurse Practitioner
Stamford, CT

Rebecca Smart, MPH, MSN, APRN, NNP-BC, FNP-BC
Clinical Assistant Professor
College of Nursing
Sacred Heart University
Fairfield, CT

Julie G. Stewart, DNP, MPH, MSN, FNP-BC, APRN
Associate Professor
Director of FNP & DNP Programs
College of Nursing
Sacred Heart University
Fairfield, CT

Frank Tudini, PT, DSc, OCS, COMT, FAAOMPT
Clinical Assistant Professor
Department of Physical Therapy & Human
    Movement Science
Sacred Heart University
Fairfield, CT

Tina Walde, DNP, PMHNP
Psychiatric Mental Health Nurse Practitioner
Oregon Health & Science University
Portland, OR

Sherylyn Watson, PhD, MSN, RN, CNE
Clinical Assistant Professor
Assistant Dean of Nursing
College of Nursing
Sacred Heart University
Fairfield, CT

Stacie Zibel, DNP, APRN-BC, CDE
Family/Gerontological Nurse Practitioner
Newington Internal Medicine Primary Care
Newington, CT
Assistant Professor
Georgetown University School of Nursing and
    Health Studies
Washington, DC

1

Test-Taking Strategies for Nurse Practitioner Students

Sherylyn M. Watson, PhD, MSN, RN, CNE

As a nurse practitioner student, preparing for one of the national credentialing exams is a challenge that needs preparation and perseverance. Adequately preparing for the examination is similar to training for a marathon. With proper strategies, a systematic approach, and time, success is attainable!

Although all of the coursework and clinical experience have prepared the student for this exam, nurse practitioner (NP) students may find the national exam a new experience. Several best practices should help the NP student focus on the appropriate content and how to study. A number of common questions arise when beginning this process:

1. What areas should I concentrate on when studying?
2. What should I begin reviewing first?
3. What material, like textbooks, should I use in my review?
4. Should I review all class notes from the past 2–3 years?
5. How much time should I dedicate to studying?
6. Do I have to learn an entirely new way of studying for this exam?

This book was written to answer those questions and assist the NP student in preparing for the exam by offering a systematic approach to relevant content and outlining effective test-taking strategies. Use this book to review content you already learned and to fill in content gaps and take practice questions.

As you begin your marathon training, a few reminders will help you be successful:

1. Quality over Quantity—Quality studying means minimizing all distractions while studying. No cell phones, no studying on the beach, no drinking your favorite drink or snacking, and no listening to music or watching television. When taking the actual exam, the test-taker will not be allowed anything in their cubicles, so you should study under the same conditions. Second, study at your "best" time of the day.

   If you are a morning person, study during morning hours and plan to take your examination at the same time. If you are most alert during the afternoon, this is when you should study and plan your examination time. Studying after a long day of work or late in the evening are not ideal times, because you will have more reasons to be distracted

2. Practice Makes Perfect—Do as many questions as possible. Questions, questions, questions!
3. Believe in Yourself—You know the content and have been successful throughout your nurse practitioner program.

Where to Begin

Specific test-taking strategies assist the NP student in effectively preparing for the exam. Although there is always room for improvement, it is not recommended you change your approach to preparing for and taking the exam. You have been successful in reaching this point! Therefore, these same strategies will support your current knowledge, as well as offer you a path to improve your approaches and review the content.

1. Although you have been answering questions like these throughout your entire nurse practitioner program, recognizing how to approach these types of questions will be helpful. Employ simple strategies when answering *multiple-choice questions* that will assist you in differentiating between two answers or making an educated guess.

   - All information written in the question is critical to answering the question. If the question gives you the age, gender, or ethnicity of the patient or family, these items are relevant to the answer or they would not be added.

   - Ask yourself, "What is the question really asking?" Summarize this in your own words.

   - Identify key words. All the answer choices may be correct or reasonable; therefore, when reading the question stem the first time, look for key words. Specific ones that are important are: *immediate concern*, *first*, *best*, or *additional instructions*.

   - Answer the question objectively. Do not add information to the scenario. These questions were designed for nurse practitioner candidates across the nation; therefore, think about standard replies and not the atypical patient you may have seen in clinical practice.

   - Sometimes you may not know the answer due to a true knowledge deficit. Answer the best you can and move to the next question.

2. Have one *notebook* where you can write down content topics you need to review throughout your preparations.

3. Formulate a realistic, achievable *study plan*!

   An effective approach is to create a plan for 4–6 weeks, culminating with the taking of the actual exam. Marathons are not won by training for one day! Quality studying is more important than quantity; therefore, it is recommended that you study only 5 days a week. It is important to take 1–2 days off from studying to rest your mind; studying constantly is a mental workout and the resulting fatigue may undermine your efforts.

A typical plan looks like the following:

Day 1	• Answer 100 practice questions on a specific topic in one sitting. • Read the rationales. • Identify any knowledge deficit areas that need more review.
Day 2	• Answer 100 practice questions on a specific topic in one sitting. • Read the rationales. • Identify any knowledge deficit areas that need more review.
Day 3	• **"Content Day"**—Review content identified in your practice questions or in your coursework as "knowledge deficit."
Day 4	• Depending on how much content is identified in gap analysis, continue to study information that needs to be reviewed. • (or) Take a 100-question comprehensive examination. • Review the rationales. • Identify knowledge deficit areas that need more review.
Day 5	• Answer 100 practice questions on a specific topic in one sitting. • Read the rationales. • Identify knowledge deficit areas that need more review.

Important to Note

Take questions ALL in one sitting to mimic the exam. Do not underestimate how difficult this will be. There are many competing demands, thus sitting quietly for 2½ to 3 hours without a break is a challenge. Similar to training for a marathon, use your plan to increase the amount of questions in one sitting over 4 weeks. Since each exam will be either 165 questions (American Association of Nurse Practitioners) or 225 (American Nurses Credentialing Center, ANCC), the best strategy is to prepare to sit without any distractions for that amount of questions. For example, in week 1, start taking 100 questions in one sitting. Week 2, plan for 150 questions, and by week 4, plan to sit for 200 questions. By increasing in increments, and finishing as refreshed as you started, you will not answer questions incorrectly due to being distracted or tired.

4. Once an individualized plan is established, determine which type of test-taker you are in order to minimize answering questions inaccurately other than knowledge deficits.

   a. The first step is to take a 100-question practice exam. When reviewing the answers, complete a spreadsheet noting which questions you answered incorrectly and the reason why (Appendix A). The three reasons to use are: K—Knowledge Deficit, C—Changed Answer, M—Misread the Question.

   b. The second step is to analyze why you answered incorrectly.

   Did you answer any questions wrong because of "knowledge deficit"? If reviewing the rationale was sufficient in understanding the concept, then move on. If the rationale left you realizing you need to look up this content, write the topic down for further studying on "*content day.*" Always have a notebook ready to write down missed concepts so you can look them up later.

   Did you answer any questions wrong because of a "changed answer"? A recommendation is to reread the question stem again, looking for new and compelling information that would make you change your initial answer. Most people should not change their answer. Trust your instinct and thus your initial answer. Only after re-reading the question stem and perhaps finding a key word you initially missed should you change your answer. Trusting yourself and not changing answers takes practice; therefore, apply this strategy for two weeks before expecting to see marked improvement.

   Did you answer any questions wrong because of a "misread"? It is time to slow down. Perhaps you were distracted at that moment or rushing to finish. In either case, more than an occasional misread is a concern. A strategy to counteract this is to reread the stem of the question if you find yourself answering the question quickly. After picking the answer quickly, read the stem of the question to ensure that the answer fits. Typically, this issue can be resolved by taking questions for longer periods of time; this paces yourself and decreases distractions.

5. Now complete a visual assessment of your answer key. This is a mock one of only 40 questions, but it will help you understand how important a visual assessment can be in recognizing how you approach examinations.

1.	11.	21.	31. x
2. x	12.	22. x	32.
3. x	13.	23. x	33.
4.	14.	24.	34. x
5.	15.	25.	35. x
6.	16.	26.	36.
7. x	17.	27.	37.
8. x	18.	28. x	38.
9.	19.	29.	39. x
10.	20.	30.	40.

Were most questions wrong between 1 and 20? Typically, this occurs because of test anxiety. A strategy to counteract this is to begin each exam the same, creating a routine that can be mimicked for the actual examination. A proven strategy is to take 3 deep breaths prior to reading the first question. Say positive statements to yourself before beginning, such as "I know this material!" "I am prepared!" "Trust my initial instinct!" The key is to use the same exercise each time to settle your nerves and put your mind in the same setting as all of the other exams.

Were most questions wrong in the middle, between 40 and 60? Your mind may be wandering. To address this issue, check back in during the exam when you feel your mind drifting. Since you know you drift at a certain point, stop and close your eyes for 3–5 seconds. Stretching your neck and arms, closing your eyes, and counting to 10 are all small ways to recharge and refocus on the exam. Do NOT get up and take a break. On the day of the national exam, you cannot take a break; therefore, do not train yourself to stop every time you feel yourself getting distracted. Remember the "training for a marathon" analogy: Runners do not stop on mile 4 when they begin to get fatigued; they push on and refocus.

Were most questions at the end wrong; those between 80 and 100? Test takers know when the ending is near and sometimes lose focus to simply be done. The best approach is already what you agreed to do in your plan, extend the number of questions you take for each seating. If you start to get distracted and begin to rush around question 85, keep in mind that if you sit for 150 questions, #85 is still in the middle of the exam. Since we already know how long each exam will be, extend your exams to that many questions to practice sitting for that long a period of time and minimize rushing in the end. Also, when taking your practice questions, make sure to allow yourself enough time to finish completely. Using the formula of 1 minute for 1 question should give you a guideline of how long you will need to take the examination.

Were most of your answers wrong in pairs or triples? This indicates that although you answered a question and moved to the next, your mind remained on the preceding question. Allow yourself the full opportunity to answer the next question. Focus only on that: one question at a time. Here is an example of how you might stumble: Question #10 is difficult and you know the answer may be wrong, but you choose an answer and move on to question #11. Since you are still thinking about question #10, you haphazardly read question #11 and choose an answer without using your test training to find the correct answer. This happens subconsciously. The good news is that you can correct the problem. The goal is to clear your mind about the difficult preceding question in order to refocus on the next one. The physical act of clearing your mind works best. When you note a difficult question, answer the question and write the # of the question down on a blank piece of paper. Using this same example, write down #10. This physical act will stop your mind, clear it, and allow yourself to refocus for the next question. This strategy usually takes some practice before seeing improvement.

The following are some helpful reminders as you begin reviewing the content in each of these chapters and taking practice questions:

1. Do as many practice questions as possible.

2. Read the rationales carefully. They will help in understanding other concepts as well.

3. Review the content at the beginning of each chapter. If you are still struggling with understanding the information, then read your textbook or review class notes about that specific topic.

4. Sometimes you simply have to memorize certain information, such as lab values and medication classifications. Otherwise, learning the knowledge in order to apply the content to patients in different contexts is the best practice.

5. If you are a visual learner, draw out a patient with clinical features, diagnostic tests, and a treatment plan to help recall the information.

6. Keep thinking positive thoughts.

7. Properly preparing for the national examination will take some time; however, the successful outcome is worth the dedication and time investment!

Day Before the Examination

The goal is to be fresh for the next day. Therefore, it is important to relax your mind beforehand so you are not drained of energy. You need to save your strength and build up your endurance for the exam.

A few simple suggestions to consider when planning for this day include the following:

1. Limit your exposure to emotional situations with friends or family for the next two days that could distract you from focusing on yourself. Ask close relatives to not share any upsetting news with you this evening or tomorrow until the exam is over.

2. Avoid peers in the same situation because positive thinking is of the utmost importance. The day before the examination is not the time for you and a peer to compare how much prep time each of you dedicated to studying. Everyone takes examinations differently, and you have made your own concerted effort toward your preparation.

3. Double-check directions to the testing center, any IDs you need to bring, and what time you need to leave for the exam by taking into consideration traffic and construction on roads.

4. Eat well-balanced meals and go to bed early to get a good night's rest.

Day Of the Exam

1. Eat a well-balanced breakfast and reduce the amount of caffeine. Caffeine can make you alert, but too much caffeine can make some people lose focus and need to go to the restroom during the examination.

2. Do not take phone calls from people who may cause anxiety for you.

3. Think positive thoughts. Tell yourself you can do this: "I know this material! I am prepared! I will pass!"

4. As you sit in front of the exam, close your eyes and think of a safe place. Begin the exam just as you have practiced it over the past month.

Day After the Exam

1. Plan an activity that is fun, relaxing, and energy draining to keep your mind off the exam. You deserve this day!

Review Questions

1. An 8-year-old with a history of known allergies has been experiencing a non-productive cough for the past 9 days. On day 9, the child's temperature rose to 103.5 °F with an oxygen level of 92% on room air. Upon assessment, the child does not complain of ear or throat pain and has wheezes. The family nurse practitioner manages this patient by first:
   A. Ordering an immediate chest X-ray.
   B. Prescribing systemic antibiotics.
   C. Administering a bronchodilator via nebulizer.
   D. Referring the patient to a hospital for admission.

2. An elderly patient's family begs the nurse practitioner to start her on a medication to help with agitation, behavior problems, and sleep issues. The nurse practitioner counsels the family on the use of second-generation anti-psychotics. Which statement is true regarding these medications?
   A. "While they help with sedation, they have an increased cardiovascular risk."
   B. "These medications will help her sleep, but will lower her blood glucose levels."
   C. "While this will help with one problem, they place her at high risk for weight loss."
   D. "These medications will help her sleep, but we must monitor for suicidal ideations."

3. A 27-year-old male client with Hodgkin's lymphoma in the abdominal and pelvic regions is about to start radiation therapy. Which information is the most important for the nurse practitioner to address?
   A. Sperm production being permanently disrupted.
   B. Constipation that will be continuous throughout therapy.
   C. Baldness resulting from the radiation therapy will be permanent.
   D. The treatment will increase the risk for prostate cancer later in life.

4. What is the most common source for the hepatitis A infection?
   A. Needle sharing
   B. Consuming raw shellfish
   C. Contaminated water supplies
   D. Intimate person-to-person contact

5. The nurse practitioner is evaluating a pregnant woman who was bitten by a deer tick and will be receiving treatment. Which medication would not be appropriate to prescribe for this patient?
   A. Amoxicillin
   B. Azithromycin
   C. Doxycycline
   D. Cefuroxime axetil

6. An 18-year-old Chinese exchange student presents to student health for a well visit to follow up on his immunization record and the reading of his PPD result from 3 days ago. The PPD result is a 6-mm area of induration. What is the best initial intervention by the nurse practitioner?
   A. Order an immediate chest radiograph.
   B. Ask the student if he received BCG vaccine before.
   C. Prescribe isoniazid therapy immediately.
   D. Request the student to return in one month to repeat the PPD test.

7. The family nurse practitioner is reviewing results with a patient who has received a positive rapid human immune deficient virus (HIV) test. What would be the most appropriate response by the provider?
   A. "You will need a Western blot test to confirm a positive diagnosis of HIV."
   B. "You will need to have your CD4 count tested immediately."
   C. "You have acquired human immune deficiency virus (HIV)."
   D. "Rapid tests have false positives."

8. What is the common presentation between uncontrolled diabetes mellitus and human immune deficiency virus (HIV)?

    A. Pneumonia

    B. Vaginal candidiasis

    C. Retinopathy

    D. Gastric ulcer

9. Governing guidelines require that all patients seen in a primary care setting be routinely screened for domestic violence. During the screening, privacy and confidentiality are essential components. Which of the following statements made by the family nurse practitioner may help create a nonthreatening environment when asking the adult client?

    A. "I am going to ask you some questions that may make you uncomfortable, but it is important that you answer them honestly."

    B. "I see that there is a strong history of drug and alcohol abuse in your personal history. This places you at risk for domestic violence. Do you want to discuss this further?"

    C. "I noticed that you were seen several times this past year by other providers in this office for complaints of abdominal pains and headaches. These can be indicators of domestic violence. Should I review these records and we can discuss this?"

    D. "Since domestic violence is so prevalent, and it may be difficult for patients to bring up, I have started routinely screening all my patients."

10. The nurse practitioner evaluates a new patient who is an African American with hypertension who has been taking lisinopril (Prinivil). His current BP is 160/90. Which medication does the nurse practitioner prescribe to create a more effective treatment plan?

    A. Angiotensin-converting enzyme inhibitor

    B. Angiotensin II receptor blockers

    C. Calcium-channel blocker

    D. Beta-blocker

Answers and Rationales

1. C. This is the **first** decision. The key word in this question is *first*, because the nurse practitioner may do all of these actions, but the immediate issue is to improve breathing. Prescribing antibiotics without a source is not recommended. The differential diagnosis is pneumonia, thus requiring an order for a chest X-ray. The referral for a hospital admission is not necessary at this time, with the goal being to keep a child out of the hospital as long as possible. The other key word is the *age* of a child, because the decision tree would be different if the patient was an 88-year-old.

2. A. The key word is *true*. The learner needs to have knowledge about the medication prior to answering this question. This is an example of a question that if you do not know the answer, write it in your notebook to review the content. Also, to make an educated guess, elderly patients are at most risk for cardiovascular issues; therefore, this is a great concern for any elderly person. Do not read too much into the question and choose an answer based on thinking that perhaps the patient has diabetes mellitus or she is too thin. There is no indication that weight loss would be a bad issue for this patient. Be careful of adding your own subjectivity into the questions.

3. A. Although all of these answers are true, the key word that is most important identifies addressing an immediate and life-changing issue. The patient's age, which is noted in this question, clues you into the importance of it: having no future to produce a family, once undergoing radiation treatment, is extremely important. The nurse practitioner should address this immediately and suggest banking sperm for later use if desired, in order for the patient to have the future option of a family.

4. C. Although raw shellfish is a source of contracting hepatitis A, and the other two answers are other ways to transmit hepatitis B and C, the key words in this question are *most common*. This is an easy error to make by quickly answering the question after reading "raw shellfish" and not taking time to read the rest of the possible answers. The other strategy after choosing the answer is to reread the question if you are deciding between B and C and to pick up on the words *most common*. Another way to determine between B and C is to think about the entire world population and view this question in general terms, because eating raw shellfish does not happen in all cultures.

5. C. Although all of these antibiotics may be used in a treatment plan for Lyme disease, the key words in this question are *pregnant woman* and *not*. The inclusion of the pregnancy is important and should always be used when making the critical decision. In reading carefully, the stem of the question should have had you identifying the word *not*. If you missed them the first time, reread the question to see what the key words are, since all of these answers are associated with treatment of the disorder.

6. B. The key word in this question is *Chinese*. The CDC recommends anyone with a positive PPD, regardless of receiving the BCG vaccine, to be treated the same due to the false-positives. Since this student is in a high-risk category, the FNP must know what is positive for this group. The 6-mm induration would be read as negative. To account for the induration, asking about a history of receiving the BCG vaccine is the next step. An Interferon-Gamma Release Assay (IGRA) could be ordered to evaluate if the student has been infected with M. tuberculosis. The patient's ethnic background being Chinese was important; otherwise it would have been omitted in the question stem.

7. A. Requiring a Western blot test is important for a confirmed positive HIV diagnosis. The key words are *most appropriate*. The patient should not be told they are positive for HIV without a confirming diagnosis, and they should not be given false hope if the first test was false positive. The patient does not need an immediate CD4 count; however, this will be part of the comprehensive workup later if the Western blot is positive for HIV. Therefore, the word *immediate* in answer B rules out this answer as being correct.

8. B. Vaginal candidiasis is a shared clinical presentation because of the high glucose levels with uncontrolled diabetes and being immunocompromised. When answering this question, ask yourself if each one of these disorders is common (not atypical). That would rule out two of the answers. Retinopathy can occur with diabetes mellitus. Pneumonia can be associated with HIV/AIDS but not necessarily with DM, and gastric ulcers are not associated with either disease.

9. D. This is the most non-threatening answer that creates a non-judgmental atmosphere. The other answers are incorrect because the first answer would create an immediate defensive response since the NP is calling the client a liar before the question. B and C are incorrect because a judgment is being made about certain behaviors and placing blame on the client. When answering questions about statements that you should make to the client, repeat the answers out loud if you are unsure. Would anyone understand or accept that as a response? It is also helpful to think about a layperson who does not know anything medical and say those questions again. It is important not to think of yourself as the client because you already have a background in health care; therefore, *your* reactions would always be different than a regular person accessing health care.

10. C. Calcium-channel blockers work well with the African American population. The key word in this situation involves addressing the cultural aspect of the client in determining a correct answer.

Appendix 1A

1.	21.	41.	61.	81.
2.	22.	42.	62.	82.
3.	23.	43.	63.	83.
4.	24.	44.	64.	84.
5.	25.	45.	65.	85.
6.	26.	46.	66.	86.
7.	27.	47.	67.	87.
8.	28.	48.	68.	88.
9.	29.	49.	69.	89.
10.	30.	50.	70.	90.
11.	31.	51.	71.	91.
12.	32.	52.	72.	92.
13.	33.	53.	73.	93.
14.	34.	54.	74.	94.
15.	35.	55.	75.	95.
16.	36.	56.	76.	96.
17.	37.	57.	77.	97.
18.	38.	58.	78.	98.
19.	39.	59.	79.	99.
20.	40.	60.	80	100.

2

Principles of Family-Focused Clinical Practice

Adapted from Stewart & DeNisco, The Role of the Nurse Practitioner
Susan DeNisco, DNP, APRN, FNP-BC, CNE, CNL
Constance Glenn, MSN, APRN, FNP-BC, CNE

Introduction

Quality primary care must take into account the family from structural, developmental, and functional contexts. Family nurse practitioners (FNPs) interface with the patient at point of care and often neglect to consider the individual in the context of a family unit. By "family," it is meant to include the entire range of relationships, whether by blood or not, as well as marriages or other arrangements that comprise a patient's close social network. It is the FNP's moral and ethical obligation to consider the health of "families" over the life cycle. It is imperative to consider family backgrounds, structure, and level of function when caring for the individual patient. The information gleaned from the patient will have a significant impact on the health and well-being of the patient, and have the potential to impact the health of the family unit when the nurse practitioner collaborates with and involves families in the framework of the treatment plan.

Family Theory and Application to Clinical Practice

Nurse practitioners don't often think they are utilizing "theory" when taking a family history or conducting a review of systems in the examination room, but when studying the components of theory, the FNP is better able to understand its practical application in the clinical area. Family theory and family-focused clinical care serves as a basis for assessing the structure and development of families across the lifespan. At the macro system level, family theory is grounded in general systems theory, structural interactional theory, family interactional theory, and developmental theory, as well as other social sciences. At the microsystem level, families are assessed at the family systems, stress, and change levels. As a profession, nursing has emphasized the importance of "family" in nursing practice. Catch phrases such as "family health promotion," "family health care nursing," "family interviewing," and "family systems nursing," helped to define family-centered nursing care as an important part of practice. The propositions just outlined have been developed out of family social science theories and can be useful for practice. Figures 2-1 and 2-2 provide a summary of Family Theories that can be useful in clinical practice.

The FNP evaluates family structure and interaction to help individuals maximize their health given the actualities of their personal and family health histories, mental health histories, genetic predisposition, cultural and religious values, traditions, and

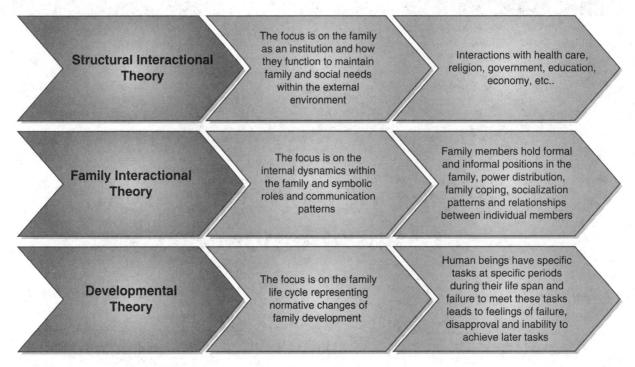

Figure 2-1 Macrosystem Family Theories

Data from Kaakinen, J. (2010). *Family Health Nursing: Theory, Practice and Research* (4th ed.). Philadelphia: Davis.

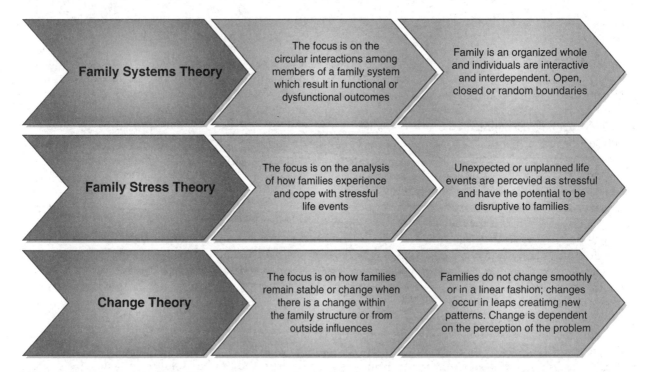

Figure 2-2 Microsystem Family Theories

Data from Kaakinen, J. (2010). *Family Health Nursing: Theory, Practice and Research* (4th ed.). Philadelphia: Davis.

socioeconomic status. The FNP must build family capacity, which is the extent to which the family needs, goals, strengths, capabilities, and aspirations can meet the family's ability to function to its fullest potential (Dunst & Trivette, 2009). It is the FNP's responsibility to assess the family's capacity to support the family's health and wellness, as well as prevent illness risks, treat medical conditions, and manage tertiary care needs. Table 2-1 represents the application of family theory to clinical practice.

Table 2-1	The Application of Family Theory to Clinical Practice

- Describe and explain family structure, dynamics, process, and change.
- Describe interpersonal structures and emotional dynamics within the family and the transmission of distress to individuals.
- The family is the liaison between the individual and culture.
- Describe the process of healthy individuation and differentiation of family members.
- Predict health and pathology within the family.
- Prescribe therapeutic strategies for dealing with family dysfunction, grief, and illness.
- Account for stability and change when viewed within the family's developmental life cycle.
- Build family capacity by helping the family recognize their needs, goals, strengths, capabilities, and aspirations.

Data from Denham, S. F. (2003). *Family Health: A Framework for Nursing*. Philadelphia: F.A.Davis.

Family Structure, Function and Roles

There are many clinical family assessment models that the nurse practitioner can use to assess family structure, function, and roles. Some of the popular models are:

- The Calgary Family Assessment (CFAM) (Wright & Leahey, 2009)
- The Family Assessment and Intervention Model (Kaakinen & Hanson, 2010)
- The Friedman Family Assessment Model (Friedman, 1998)

All three models may have different approaches in their theoretical underpinnings, scope, data collection methods (quantitative or qualitative), and unit of analysis, but have many similarities. Broadly, these assessment tools are available to expand the clinician's understanding and management of family-wide threats to both physiologic and psychological health. Box 2-1 explains the five key goals of family life.

Family Structure

There are many tools available to assess and treat families. The FNP may use a genogram or "family tree" or eco-map to gather much of the information regarding family structure. Family structure can be defined as the organizational framework that determines family membership and the way in which a family is organized according to roles, rules, power, and hierarchies. There is no typical family form in the 21st century. The FNP needs to expand his/her definition of the traditional nuclear family (or biological family of procreation) to include alternate forms of family life. The single or sole-parent family, blended families including step-children, grandparents raising grandchildren, communal families, and the lesbian, gay, bisexual, queer, inter-sexed, transgendered, or twin spirited (LGBQITT) couple or family (Wright & Leahey, 2009).

If the FNP is using a pictorial representation of the family structure such as the genogram or eco-map, the following components should be included in the interview data collection regarding family structure (Bomar, 2004). (McGoldrick, 2003) (McGoldrick M. C., 1999):

- Family constellation: who is in the immediate family, who lives in the house, how are the individuals related, relationship to extended family and boundaries.
- Family constellation changes: permanent (birth or death), temporary (illness, hospitalizations, co-parenting in divorced families, homelessness).
- Individual family members: age, gender, sexual orientation, ethnicity, race, health problems, occupation, educational level, and cultural/religious beliefs.
- Environmental: housing/ living situation.
- Social support: stress management, financial support, entitlements (i.e., Medicaid, WIC, food stamps, etc.).

BOX 2-1 Five KEY Goals of Family Life

1. Pass on culture (religion, ethnicity).
2. Socialize young people for the next generation (to be good citizens, to be able to cope in society through going to school).
3. Exist for sexual satisfaction and procreation.
4. Serve as a protective mechanism for family members against outside forces.
5. Provide closer human contact and relations.

Family Function

Family functioning can be defined as the processes by which the family operates as a whole, including communication patterns and manipulation of the environment for problem solving (Wright & Leahey, 2009). Each family possesses a distinctive operating system, and this can influence health care outcomes. Some specific areas to assess include:

- **Activities of Daily Living:** eating, sleeping, common tasks such as family participation in leisure activities and family rituals
- **Nutrition:** food insecurity
- **Communication Patterns:** how do family members communicate (is there one spokesperson when articulating health care issues)
- **Family perceptions:** what is the impact of illness on each family member, concerns for other family members, care seeking behaviors
- **Family members' mental health history:** psychiatric, substance, tobacco, and alcohol use
- **Problem-solving abilities:** family capacity, resources, and supports
- **Influence and power:** who is dominate, subordinate, controlling, abusive, guilt-inducing, the scapegoat, etc.

Family Development

The FNP must also consider the developmental life cycle for each family he/she encounters in the clinical setting. Families are shaped by people who share a past and future history together. As contemporary families move through time, there is a normative sequence by which families develop and change. McGoldrick and Carter (2003) have done extensive work on the family life cycle by describing the underlying factors that influence family development as the family expands and contracts by variables such as birth, death, marriage, divorce, adoption, poverty, catastrophic illness, etc. These events typically cause realignment of the family system to support the entry, exit, and developmental changes of family members through time. Major life-cycle transitions are marked by fundamental changes in the family system itself (second order changes) rather than rearrangements within the system (first order changes). McGoldrick and Carter (1999) have designed a classification system of normative stages that typical middle class American families go through across the life cycle. As these "normative" stages of the family life cycle are reviewed, the FNP must take into consideration societal influences and sweeping changes in the way the family functions. In this decade, it may be hard to conceptualize what is considered a typical family when there are gay and lesbian couples, sole-parent adoptions, dual-career families, grandparents raising grandchildren, co-habiting couples, military families, and foster families. In the Calgary Family Assessment Model, Wright and Leahey (2009) advise that the family developmental assessment include an overview of the stages, tasks, and attachments as well as common health issues important to each stage. Table 2-2 provides an overview of the stages, emotional tasks, and health issues of a two-parent nuclear family.

Table 2-2	The Family Life Cycle: "Traditional" Family Stages, Tasks, and Health Issues	
Stage	**Tasks**	**Health Issues**
Transitional Stage (Unattached Young Adult)	• Differentiation of self in relation to family of origin • "between families" • Development of intimate peer relationships • Establishment of self in a career and financial independence	*Anxiety, stress, body image disturbance, family planning*
Beginning a New Family	• The marriage of a couple marks the beginning of a new family • Establish a mutually satisfying marriage or coupling • "Couple identity" • Relating harmoniously to the kin network and including spouse • Planning a family	*Contraception, prenatal, counseling, sexual issues*

Table 2-2	The Family Life Cycle: "Traditional" Family Stages, Tasks, and Health Issues (*Continued*)	
Stage	**Tasks**	**Health Issues**
Child-bearing Families (Birth–30 months)	• Transition to parenthood (husband feels neglected, increase in arguments, tired all the time, social/sex life interrupted) • Integrating a new baby into the family • Changing roles in the family • Maintaining a satisfying relationship • Expanding relationships with extended family (grandparents, aunts, uncles, etc . . .)	*Well child care, immunizations, child development, family planning, day care*
Families with Preschool Children (2.5–5 y.o.)	• 3–5 family members • Family becoming more complex and differentiated • Tasks: meeting the family's need for space, privacy, adequate housing, safety • Integrating new child while meeting the demands of other kids • Maintaining healthy relationships with the family, marriage, extended family	*Prevention, bacterial/viral illness, accidents, falls, burns, lacerations, diminished marital satisfaction*
Families with School Age Children (6–13 y.o.)	• Maximum # of family members • Busy years; kids have own activities and interests (industry) • Parents are busy (generativity) • Parents feel pressure to have kids keep up with societal norms • Handicaps come to light; ADHD, vision, hearing, learning problems • Tasks: Promote school achievement and fostering healthy relationships with peers, preparing them for adolescence and letting go • Maintain satisfying marital relationships	*Meeting the physical and psychological health needs of all family members*
Families with Adolescents (13–19 y.o.)	• Most difficult, filled with turmoil • Balance of freedom and responsibility; teen becomes more mature and autonomous • If parents accept themselves (strengths and weaknesses), they have more acceptance for teenage child	*Accidents, drugs, alcohol birth control, social media influences, aging parent issues (i.e., CAD, HTN, DM)*
Families Launching Young Adults	• "Empty Nesters" • Stage varies in length from how many kids, how close in age, etc. . . . • Role transition problems for husband and wife; refocusing their marriage • Inclusion of new family members through marriage	*Emergence of chronic health problems, menopause, aging parents*
Middle-Aged Parents	• When last child leaves the house, ending with retirement or death of a spouse • 45–55 y.o. to 65 y.o. • Marital satisfaction and quality of life increase	*Chronic illnesses and death of aging parent, depression, anxiety, osteoporosis, hypertension, diabetes, hyperlipidemia, degenerative joint disease*
Families in Retirement and Old Age	• Retirement of both to death of spouse • Losses common to aging people: economic, housing, social, work, health	*Dementia, depression, functional and mobility issues, malnutrition*

Data from Wright, L. L. (2009). *Nurses and Families: A Guide to Family Assessment and Intervention* (5th ed.). Philadelphia: F.A. Davis.

Divorced Families

While the divorce rate fluctuates given geographic location, population, income, and educational status, single parent and divorced families are common in our society and have unique challenges. The term "divorce" invokes a series of images of bitter custody battles, financial hardship, broken families, vulnerable children, hostility, resentment, and failure to live up to commitments. While these images may be true of some divorces, research shows that most families will experience short-term, moderate effects post-divorce (Bowen, 2012; Demo, 2010). However, it is true that families experiencing divorce are under significant emotional pressure during the transition and must fulfill the same developmental tasks as the two-parent nuclear family, but without all the means.

Shortages in having time, money, and energy can cause single parents to experience self-doubt and often feel guilty for not meeting societal expectations of living in a two-parent family (Wright & Leahey, 2009). It is important for the FNP to assist the family experiencing a divorce to maintain homeostasis by selecting positive coping strategies as the family responds to stress and change. Table 2-3 depicts the Stages of the Divorce, Post-Divorce, and Remarriage Family Life Cycle.

Nontraditional Families

While societal perceptions of the "traditional family" may still be a certainty for some, this is clearly dependent on age, gender, education, religious beliefs, socioeconomic status, and geographic location. The reality is that less than 25% of U.S. households

Table 2-3	Stages, Tasks, and Health Issues of Divorce, Post-Divorce, and Remarriage		
	Stage	**Task**	**Health Issues**
Divorce	Decision to divorce	Accepting failure in the marriage	Weight loss, weight gain, stress, anxiety, grief reaction, depression, alcohol and substance abuse
	Planning the breakup of the marital and family system	Informing extended family about divorce Working cooperatively on custodial and financial arrangements	
	Separation	Realignment of relationships with extended family members Adapting to living apart Cooperative parental and financial support of children	
	Divorce	Emotional roller coaster Recovering from former hopes and dreams Takes 1–3 years for the family to reestablish itself	
Post-Divorce	Parenting issues	Maintaining financial responsibility to custodial family Supportive relationship and effective parenting for sake of the children Flexible visitation Rebuilding social networks	Grief reactions in children: denial, silence, bodily distress, hostility, guilt, panic, and confusion. Fear of abandonment: tantrums, whining and clinging, longing for noncustodial parent Regressive behaviors: bed wetting, use of pacifier, or favorite comfort item. Poor school performance Aggressive behaviors: anger at both parents. Stealing, lying
Remarriage	Entering into a new relationship	Emotional recovery from the loss of the first marriage Recommitment to marriage and to formation of a "new" family with foreseeable complications Readiness to deal with complexity in blending former families	

Table 2-3	Stages, Tasks, and Health Issues of Divorce, Post-Divorce, and Remarriage (*Continued*)	
Stage	**Task**	**Health Issues**
Planning the new marriage	Accepting self, new spouses, and children's fears about the remarriage and forming a blended family. Defining new family roles: setting boundaries, dealing with loyalty conflicts Maintaining former financial and co-parenting agreements Helping children adjust to membership into two-family systems Planning for inclusion of the ex-spouses' extended family in the children's lives	
Remarriage and redefining family	Acceptance of different family model Restructuring family boundaries to include new spouse/step-parent and his/her extended network Sharing memories and histories to enhance integration of set-family system Takes 2 to 3 years for step-parents and children to readjust	

Data from Wright, L. L. (2009). *Nurses and Families: A Guide to Family Assessment and Intervention* (5th ed.). Philadelphia: F.A. Davis.

are considered "traditional." In working with the families listed in the following, the FNP needs to help these families develop coping mechanisms and find community, legal, and financial resources to support them through issues of custody, as well as visitation social networks and employment benefits, and develop effective parenting. The FNP must gain expertise in assessments and interventions that address the unique needs of these families in order to help parents and children deal with social stress from being perceived as "different" by other children, or as "problematic and threatening" by other parents. The nontraditional family configurations are:

- Single-parent families
- Same-sex couple families
- Foster families
- Grandparents raising grandchildren

Family Interviews

Genogram and Eco-Map

The relationship between family history and health risks has long been recognized. Indeed, family history is a risk factor for many pediatric and adult-onset diseases and disorders. It represents genetic susceptibility, shared environment, common behaviors, and the interactions between and among their family members. The genogram and eco-map are tools that can assist the FNP to assess families as a whole system, and as individuals within the family system.

Genograms

A genogram is an assessment tool or clinical method of taking, storing, and processing family information for the benefit of the patient and the family. It is displayed as a graphic representation of family members and their relations over three generations (McGoldrick, 2008). The information collected for the genogram may include genetic, medical, social, behavioral, and cultural aspects of the family. Some key indications for the nurse practitioner to develop a family genogram are represented in Table 2-4.

Table 2-4	Key Indicators to Develop a Family Genogram

- Depression
- Somatic problems (e.g., headache, abdominal pain, chest pain)
- Frequent office visits
- Poor school or work attendance
- Behavioral problems
- Problems between family members
- Step-families with problems
- Obesity, smoking, alcohol, substance abuse
- Non-adherence to treatment regimen

Process of Developing the Genogram

The manner in which a genogram is taken is perhaps more important that what is elicited and the technique of recording. The diagramming of a family genogram must comply with the use of specific symbols to assure that the family and the nurse practitioner have the same understanding and interpretations of the meaning of the symbols. Authors may vary on symbols used for different nodal events, but all genograms are similar in terms of gathering information on family membership, structure, interaction patterns, and other important information. The genogram does not have to be completed in one session; in general, nurse practitioners working in a primary care setting will see patients and their families over time and data can be collected and added to as a continuous process.

See Boxes 2-2, 2-3, and 2-4 Family Genogram Interview Data: Factual Events, Expanded Events, and Relationships.

BOX 2-2   Family Genogram Interview Data: Factual Events

- Family Composition: Who is the immediate family and who has the identified health problem
- Who lives with the immediate family and how are they related
- Dates of births, miscarriages, abortions, and stillbirths
- Dates of any adoptions
- Dates and causes of deaths
- Major illnesses and dates
- Dates of marriages, separations, divorces, remarriages, retirement, relocations

---

BOX 2-3   Family Genogram Interview Data: Expanded Events

- Religion, ethnic factors, occupations, social class, education, military service
- Additional births, abortions and miscarriages, adoptions and infertility
- Congenital abnormalities, mental handicaps, learning problems
- Illnesses similar to presenting illness
- Cancer, heart disease, hypertension, asthma, hyperlipidemia, diabetes
- **Depression, alcoholism, substance abuse**
- Common causes of death in that family
- Family secrets
- Troubles with the law, incest

BOX 2-4   Family Genogram Interview Data: Relationships

Who is close to whom?

- Is there over-closeness,
- Are there favorites and/or "isolates"?

Relationships and alliances between:

- marriage partners
- siblings
- children and parents
- children and grandparents

Boundaries between family members:

- Permeable
- Loose
- Rigid

Power and patterns of avoidance

Patterns of friendships and relationships with work colleagues

Matters that cannot be talked about in the family

Understanding and Interpreting the Genogram

Discussion of the completed genogram can offer alternatives to the family for their current behaviors, and a chance to escape from repetitive family patterns if the family views this as helpful. Furthermore, a genogram will help the family make sense of unexplained fears and anxieties about family patterns and illness. One of the challenges for the FNP is to take the vast amount of information collected during the interview process and consolidate the data into categories that can be analyzed for repetitive relationship patterns between generations. Categorizing the data groups can assist in the identification of the most pertinent or priority family problem that needs immediate attention. Box 2-5 represents Family Genogram Red-Flag Themes for identification of problems and patterns that may impact family functioning and individual family members' well-being.

The Eco-Map

Similar to the genogram, the eco-map is a pictorial representation of the family's contact with the larger systems. These systems can include school, work environment, place of worship, health care agencies, social support agencies, courts, recreation, housing, friends, etc. The eco-map is used to clarify reciprocal relationships between family members and the broader community. It provides a way of assessing resources and strengths of family relationships with significant others, organizations, and institutions. The eco-map allows the FNP to view both the nurturing aspects of the families' world and the stress-producing connections. Often it shows deprivation of resources which can assist the nurse practitioner in developing an adequate plan of care for the family (Wright & Leahey, 2009).

BOX 2-5 Family Genogram Red-Flag Themes

- Repetitive patterns between generations (e.g., alcoholism, drug addiction, divorce, mental illness)
- Chronological coincidences (e.g., births, marriages, and deaths)
- Similarity of names, possible personality resemblances or identity in upbringing (e.g., family favorite, family scapegoat)
- Cultural, educational, ethnic, and religious backgrounds—**differences and similarities**
- Family patterns from husband's and wife's relations: similarities and differences
- Family secrets (e.g., abortions, adoptions, secret affairs)
- Significance of nicknames
- Over-closeness between generations (absence of **"boundaries"**)
- Poor or loose contact between the generations (e.g., cutoff)
- Inappropriate alliances
- Fighting and domestic abuse

Family Problem List

Following careful assessment of the individual in the context of the family unit, the FNP must develop a comprehensive prioritized problem list. The Problem Oriented Medical Record (POMR) and the "problem list" date back to the 1960s. It was developed by Dr. Lawrence Weed as a simple way to document and manage important health problems facing a patient (Holmes, 2011). Today, it still exists as an acceptable model of documentation in both paper and electronic medical records. The contents of the problem list may vary from one health care organization to the next and also on health care provider preference. In general, FNPs and other primary care providers agree that the problem list should contain the following general information:

- A list of chronic diseases or illnesses
- An ongoing or active problem that has been identified and is being addressed with the patient and/or family
- A summarization of the most important things about a patient and/or family

Primary care FNPs provide integrated, accessible health care services and are accountable for addressing a large majority of personal health care needs, developing a sustained partnership with patients, and practicing in the context of family and community (DeNisco & Barker, 2012). In caring for the individual patient in the context of the family unit, it is important for the nurse practitioner to maintain clear documentation of the family's health care needs. At minimum, the problem list should include the following elements: acute self-limiting problems, routine health maintenance issues, allergies, family planning, social problems, and chronic health problems.

Acute self-limiting problems are problems that may be acute or short term in matter. For example streptococcal pharyngitis is an example of an acute self-limiting problem. Nocturnal leg cramps, upper respiratory infection, and contact dermatitis are other problems that fall into this category. Routine health maintenance refers to health promotion and screening activities that are needed by the patient per age and risk factor analysis. This includes but is not limited to mammograms, annual physical examinations, pap smears, immunizations, well-child care, etc. . . . Allergies would include allergies to medications, food, and allergens present in the environment. Family planning would address the contraceptive needs of the family, including infertility issues. Social problems take into account toxic habits that the patient or family members may have (e.g., tobacco use, substance abuse, alcohol use). Chronic health problems include long-standing diagnoses that the health care provider is following (e.g., hypertension, type 2 diabetes, hyperlipidemia, asthma, migraine headaches, etc . . .). The other category is a net to catch all other problems that may be important to remember as you care for the patient. This may include family problems (death of a family member, mental health issues, school truancy), financial problems (unemployment, entitlements such as food stamps), sexual preferences, etc. . . . The usefulness of problem lists in the care of the individual patient and family is based on the ability of the FNP to articulate patient problems (when identified) and follow consistent guidelines that ensure the lists are current and useful. See Box 2-6 for an example of a family problem list.

BOX 2-6   Family Problem List

#1 ASLP (Acute Self-Limiting Problem)

#2 RHM (Routine Health Maintenance)

#3 Allergies

#4 Family planning

#5 Social

#6 Chronic health problems

#7 And other

Review Questions

1. In considering the impact of family on health care, the FNP is aware that:
   A. The family has a significant impact on the health and well-being of its individual members.
   B. Family is considered only in cases of chronic illness.
   C. Family members develop according to an established pattern.
   D. The family structure is a consistent and static phenomenon.

2. In order to avoid the three most common errors in family nursing, the FNP is aware it is important to:
   A. Give advice early in the intervention so that progress can be instituted.
   B. Take sides with the most communicative family member.
   C. Plan to create a context for change.
   D. Let the family know what the FNP sees as the most pressing problem.

3. In applying family theory to clinical practice, the FNP assists the family in recognizing their needs, goals, and strengths, as well as their capabilities and aspirations, which is called:
   A. Applying microsystem family theories.
   B. Building family capacity.
   C. Providing a foundation to change.
   D. Applying macrosystem family theories.

4. While the definition of the traditional family differs according to many factors, the FNP realizes that:
   A. The majority of families are 'traditional."
   B. Expertise in assessments and interventions for nontraditional families are not unique to these families.
   C. The social stress of being perceived as "different," problematic, or threatening does not exist today.
   D. Finding coping mechanisms and community resources to support nontraditional families through many challenging issues is needed to reduce stress.

5. In order to understand the practical application of family theory in the clinical area, it is important to consider that at the macrosystem level family theory is grounded in:
   A. General Systems Theory, Structural Interactional Theory, Family Interactional Theory, and Developmental Theory.
   B. General Systems Theory, Structural Interactional Theory, Family Interactional Theory, and Developmental Theory, but not those from the social sciences.
   C. General systems theory, Structural Interactional Theory, Family Interactional Theory, and Developmental Theory, Stress and Change Levels, and those borrowed from the social sciences.
   D. General Systems Theory, Structural Interactional Theory, Family Interactional Theory, and Stress and Change Theory.

6. Hector and Marianne have been married for 25 years. Their three children—ages 18, 20, and 21—live with them. This family is in the developmental stage called:
   A. Families Launching Young Adults.
   B. Families in Retirement and Old Age.
   C. Families with Adolescents.
   D. Middle-aged Parents.

7. When Hector and Marianne name their family members, the FNP includes all members of the family in the genogram who are:
   A. Individuals related by marriage.
   B. Individuals related by birth.
   C. Individuals adopted by them since they were married.
   D. All individuals that are named.

8. When initially meeting with Hector and Marianne to provide primary health care, the FNP realizes it is important to:
   A. Gather information about the family status.
   B. Consider only the developmental level of the patient.
   C. Question only the structure of the patient's family.
   D. Request information about the patient's family function, structure, and developmental context.

9. When questioning Hector about the reason for his visit, the FNP realizes:
   A. The main concern is if he perceives himself as healthy.
   B. Knowledge of his family unit will assist the FNP in determining his risk factors for future health.
   C. His individual health status has little impact on the health of the family unit.
   D. His current level of function is the main consideration.

10. A family assessment model aids the FNP in assessing the family structure and roles and expands the clinician's understanding and management of:
    A. Threats to physiological and psychological health.
    B. Family member relationships.
    C. Culture and religious spiritual issues.
    D. Therapeutic relationships.

11. In application of theory to clinical practice and understanding the importance of building family capacity, the FNP:
    A. Is mainly concerned about the presenting complaint of the patient.
    B. Evaluates chief socioeconomic status and genetic predisposition.
    C. Considers the history of mental health issues, as well as personal and family goals and strengths.
    D. Supports the family's ability to function to its fullest potential.

12. Marianne's elderly mother has suffered a stroke, so she will be moving into her home with Hector and their three children. In order to provide constant care at all times at home, their work schedules are realigned to accommodate this. This is an example of:
    A. Developmental Theory.
    B. Family Structure.
    C. Family Systems Theory.
    D. Structural Interactional Theory.

13. Each family possesses distinctive operating systems in family function that include:
    A. The developmental life cycle for each family member, as well as the family as a whole.
    B. Who is considered to be a family member.
    C. Family perceptions, problem-solving abilities, mental health history.
    D. The employment history of individuals within the family.

14. The FNP explains the purpose for drawing a genogram and eco-map is:
    A. To draw a map of the neighborhood of the patient and family.
    B. To provide an organizational framework used to assess the family structure and interests.
    C. To provide an organizational framework to understand who fits in the family.
    D. To provide a diagram of a typical family.

15. In considering the developmental life cycle for each family, the FNP considers:
    A. Only the developmental life cycle of the patient.
    B. The developmental life cycle of each family member.
    C. The developmental life cycle of the family as a whole.
    D. The developmental life cycle of those older than the patient.

16. The FNP recognizes that as the divorced family experiences progression through the stages, it is:

    A. Important to assist the family to maintain homeostasis with positive coping strategies.

    B. Important to assist the family to work on new relationships.

    C. Important to assist the family to realize divorce is now the "new norm."

    D. Important to assist the family to try reconciliation at all costs.

17. Graphic representation that also serves as an assessment tool of storing family information over three generations is called:

    A. A genogram.

    B. An eco-map.

    C. A key indicator.

    D. A genetic format.

18. It is important that the FNP use clear and specific symbols when recording a genogram or eco-map and post in the legend/key in order to: (select all that apply)

    A. Create an interesting diagram of the family.

    B. Ensure the same understanding of the interpretations between the family and clinician.

    C. Clearly depict the style of the diagram.

    D. Assure the information is transferrable to others.

19. Graphic representation that also serves as an assessment tool of family contact with larger systems is called:

    A. A genogram.

    B. An eco-map.

    C. A key indicator.

    D. A genetic format.

20. Following careful assessment of the patient, the FNP must develop or add to a comprehensive problem list, which includes:

    A. A list of chronic diseases and acute self-limiting problems.

    B. The educational level of the patient.

    C. The chief complaint of the patient.

    D. Any recent travel by the patient.

21. Acute self-limiting (ASL) problems include:

    A. Cardiac disease.

    B. Streptococcal pharyngitis.

    C. Routine health maintenance.

    D. Immunization status.

22. An example of routine health maintenance is:

    A. Cardiac disease.

    B. Streptococcal pharyngitis.

    C. Penicillin allergy.

    D. Immunization status.

23. Susan and Ace are two women who state that they have recently married due to the change in law that allows them to create a civil union. They are expecting a new baby and have biological children from prior heterosexual relationships. The correct developmental theory stage of this relationship is:

    A. Traditional.

    B. Single-Parent Families.

    C. Transitional Stage.

    D. Child-bearing Family.

24. Susan and Ace are the parents of a newborn daughter and two step-children (one biological from each mother) from previous relationships. When constructing a genogram, the FNP is careful to:

    A. Include all the children.

    B. Include only the newborn daughter.

    C. Include only the children from previous relationships.

    D. Not add children to the genogram.

25. Sharon and John have three children ages 6, 10, and 12. When the six-year-old has to be hospitalized due to an emergency illness, the grandparents and the ten- and twelve-year-old assume some of the duties of their parents in order to help out while the parents alternate spending time with their youngest child at the hospital and being home with the rest of the family. This is an example of:

    A. Developmental Theory.

    B. Family Structure.

    C. Family Systems Theory.

    D. Structural Interactional Theory.

26. When working with a family of divorce, the FNP assists the family in maintaining homeostasis by:

    A. Reminding the individuals to move forward.

    B. Selecting positive coping strategies as the family responds to stress and change.

    C. Reminding them to forget past issues of conflict.

    D. Expecting the process will be over once the divorce becomes legally final.

27. When interviewing the family for the genogram component of assessment, the FNP asks questions to determine: (select all that apply)

    A. Factual or objective events.

    B. Community involvement.

    C. Family composition.

    D. Family boundaries.

28. It is important to discuss and review the genogram with the family in order to:

    A. Help the family make sense of family patterns and risks.

    B. Offer suggestions of community resources to assist them.

    C. Create opportunity to explain who is in the family.

    D. Maintain order of the family unit.

29. In divorce, redefining the family is important in order to:

    A. Restructure family boundaries to include the new spouse/step-parent and the extended network.

    B. Separate the different families.

    C. Expect the immediate transfer for readjustment.

    D. Understand loyalties.

30. In order to successfully conclude or terminate clinical work with families, it is important to:

    A. Doubt the sustainability of progress and hope for the future.

    B. Expect that the family will carry forth with the information the FNP provided.

    C. Begin the process as soon as possible so that all concerns are addressed.

    D. Encourage the family to see progress as a result of their own efforts and hard work, not as a result of working with the clinician.

Answers and Rationales

1. A. Family has significant impact on the health and well-being of its individual members. While there are normative sequences of family development, there are many underlying factors that influence lifestyle transitions and the passage through those stages. Family structure may expand and/or contract by birth, death, divorce, marriage, etc.

2. C. Creating context for change is essential. Empathy, mindfulness, and empathetic responding are all needed to create a healing context for change. A. Incorrect: Offer advice, opinions, or recommendations only following a full and thorough assessment of the family's health needs and concerns. B. Incorrect: Aligning with one person or subgroup can make others feel disrespected, disempowered, and non-influential. D. Incorrect: While the clinician offers input, the family determines what their most pressing concerns are.

3. B. In applying family theory to clinical practice to assist this family in recognizing their needs, goals, and strengths, as well as their capabilities and aspirations to meet their ability to function to its fullest potential, the FNP is building family capacity.

4. D. In working with nontraditional families such as single-parent, same-sex couples, foster, and grand-parents raising grandchildren, the FNP needs to help these families develop coping mechanisms and find community, legal, and financial resources to support them through issues of custody, visitation social networks, employment benefits, and effective parenting. The FNP must gain expertise in assessments and interventions that address the unique needs of these families in order to help parents and children deal with social stress from being perceived as "different" by other children, or as "problematic and threatening" by other parents.

5. C. At the macrosystem level, family theory is grounded in general systems theory, structural interactional theory, family interactional theory, and developmental theory, as well as others borrowed from the social sciences. At the microsystem level, families are assessed at the family systems theory, family stress theory, and change theory levels.

6. A. They are in the developmental stage called: Families Launching Young Adults.

7. D. A family is whoever they say they are: all those named who comprise their social network. The geno-gram clearly defines the biological ties and potential health risks.

8. D. Quality primary care must take into account the family from structural, developmental, and functional contexts. The complete information may be taken over successive visits.

9. B. The impact of health issues on one family member can have a significant impact on the well-being of all the family members.

10. A. There are many clinical family assessment models that the nurse practitioner can use to assess family structure, function, and roles. Broadly, these assessment tools are available to expand the clinicians' understanding and management of family-wide threats to both physiological and psychological health.

11. D. In application of the theory to clinical practice, the FNP must build family capacity, which is the extent to which the family's needs, goals, strengths, capabilities, and aspirations can meet the family's ability to function to its fullest potential.

12. C. This is an example of Family Systems Theory. All parts of a system are interrelated and dependent to one another. When one part of a system becomes dysfunctional for any reason the rest of the system is affected. If one family member becomes dysfunctional, another family member may compensate and assume the duties or role of the dysfunctional family member.

13. C. Family function is defined as the process by which the family operates as a whole and includes communication patterns and manipulation of the environment for problem solving.

14. B. A genogram and eco-map are pictorial representations of the family structure. Family structure can be defined as the organizational framework that determines family membership and the way in which a family is organized according to roles, rules, power, and hierarchies.

15. B. According to Wright and Leahey (2013), the family developmental assessment includes an overview of the stages, tasks, and attachments, as well as common health issues important to each stage of each family member and to the family as a whole.

16. A. It is important for the FNP to assist the family experiencing a divorce to maintain homeostasis by selecting positive coping strategies as the family responds to stress and change.

17. A. A genogram is an assessment tool or clinical method of taking, storing, and processing family information for the benefit of the patient and the family. It is displayed as a graphic representation of family members and their relations over a minimum of three generations.

18. B and D. The diagramming of a family genogram must comply with the use of specific symbols to assure that the family and the nurse practitioner have the same understanding and interpretations of the meaning of the symbols. Authors may vary on symbols used for different nodal events, but all genograms are similar in terms of gathering information on family membership, structure, interaction patterns, and other important information.

19. B. The eco-map is used to clarify reciprocal relationships between family members and the broader community. It provides a way of assessing the resources and strengths of family relationships with significant others, organizations, and institutions. The eco-map allows the FNP to view both the nurturing aspects of the family's world and the stress-producing connections. Often, it shows deprivation of resources, which can assist the nurse practitioner in developing a plan of care for the family.

20. A. At minimum, the Problem List should include the elements of acute self-limiting problems (ACLPs), routine health maintenance issues (RHMs), allergies, family planning, social problems, and chronic health problems.

21. B. Acute self-limiting problems are problems that may be acute or short term in manner. For example, streptococcal pharyngitis is an example of an acute self-limiting problem.

22. D. Routine health maintenance refers to health promotion and screening activities that are needed by the patient per age, gender, and risk factor analysis.

23. D. Child-bearing families consist of transitioning to parenthood and integrating a new baby into the family, but, depending on the ages of the other two children, this may also be considered Families with School Age Children with a combination of health issues from each stage to consider as well.

24. A. Include all children because the genogram depicts three generations of family members, and the family consists of "who they say they are."

25. C. All parts of a system are interrelated and dependent to one another. When one part of a system becomes dysfunctional for any reason, the rest of the system is affected. If one family member becomes dysfunctional, another family member may compensate and assume the duties or role of the dysfunctional family member.

26. B. Selecting positive coping strategies as the family responds to stress and change.

27. A, C, and D. Community involvement is depicted in the eco-map.

28. A. Help the family make sense of family patterns and risks. B. Incorrect: That information would be included in the eco-map. C. Incorrect: Composition of the family is determined by the family members. D. Incorrect: All families experience fluctuation in order and composition through time.

29. A. Restructure family boundaries to include new spouse/step-parent and extended network.

30. D. Encourage the family to see progress as a result of their own efforts and hard work, not as a result of working with the clinician. A. Incorrect: The goal is to offer the family hope for the future and progress. B. Incorrect: Provide the family with needed contacts and needed information, confirming through written and verbal documentation that is understood. C. While it is unrealistic to expect that all concerns can always be resolved prior to conclusion of intervention, it is important to set goals that give the family hope and in which they can sense progress.

● ● ● **References**

Births, deaths, marriages, and divorces. (2012, September 27). Retrieved from United States Census Bureau: http://www.census.gov/compendia/statab/

Bomar, P. (2004). *Promoting health in families: Applying family research and theory to practice* (3rd ed.). Philadelphia: Saunders.

Bowen, M. (2012 , October 12). *Bowen theory.* Retrieved from The Bowen Center: http://www.thebowencenter.org/pages/theory.html

Bray, J., & Campbell, T. L. (2007). The family's influence on health. In R. Rakel (Ed.), *Textbook of family medicine* (pp. 25–34). Philadelphia: Elsevier.

DeNisco, S., & Barker, A. (2012). *Advanced practice nursing: Evolving roles for the transformation of the profession.* Sudbury: Jones and Bartlett.

Demo, D. F. (2010). *Beyond the average divorce.* Thousand Oaks, CA: Sage.

Denham, S. F. (2003). *Family health: A framework for nursing.* Philadelphia: F. A. Davis.

Drummond. J., Kysela, G. M., McDonald, L., & Query, B. (2002). The family adaptation model: Examination of dimensions and relations. *Canadian Journal of Nursing Research, 34*(1), 29–46.

Dunst, C. J., & Trivette, C. M. (2009). Capacity building family systems intervention practices. *Journal of Family Social Work, 12,* 119–143.

Friedman, M. (1998). *Family nursing* (4th ed.). Stamford: Appleton & Lange.

Holmes, C. (2011). The problem list beyond meaningful use: The problem with problem lists. *Journal of AHIMA* (February), 30–33.

Kaakinen, J., Gedaly-Duff, V., Coehlo, D. P., & Hanson, S. M. H. (2010). *Family health care nursing: Theory, practice and Research* (4th ed.). Philadelphia: Davis.

Loveland-Cherry, C. (2004). Family health promotion and health protection. In P. Bomar (Ed.), *Promoting health in families* (pp. 61–89). Philadelphia: Saunders.

McCubbin, M. A. (1993). Family stress theory and the development of nursing knowledge about family adaptation. In S. Feetham, S. Meister, J. Bell, & C. L. Gillis (Eds.), *The nursing of families* (pp. 46–58). New Bury Park: Sage.

McGoldrick, M., & Carter, B. (1999). *The expanded family life cycle: Individual, family, and social perspectives.* Allyn & Bacon.

McGoldrick, M., & Carter, B. (2003). The family life cycle. In F. Walsh (Ed.), *Normal family processes.* Guilford: Sage.

McGoldrick, M. S. (2008). *Genograms: Assessment and intervention.* New York: W. W. Norton & Company.

McKenry, P. (2000). *Families and change: Coping with stressful events and transitions* (2nd ed.). Thousand Oaks, CA: Sage.

Rakel, R. (2007). *Textbook of family medicine* (7th ed.). Philadelphia: Elsevier.

Wright, L. L., & Leahey, M. (2009). *Nurses and families: A guide to family assessment and intervention* (5th ed.). Philadelphia: F. A. Davis.

3

Health Assessment

Michelle Johnson, EdD, RN, CPNP-PC

Health assessment is not simply a synonym for physical exam. The two terms should not be used interchangeably. Although a physical exam is a component to health assessment, a physical exam alone is not the only component of health assessment. A thorough health assessment includes gaining knowledge about a patient's past and present medical history, gaining knowledge about past and present factors that can and do currently impact the patient's present and future health, and assessment of a patient's physical, mental, and sometimes spiritual health and well-being.

Chief Complaint

The chief complaint ideally should be exactly what the patient states he/she is at the office to be seen for in quotes. However oftentimes the FNP may summarize a lengthy list of reasons the patient came to be seen.

History of Present Illness

This portion of the interview and documentation must thoroughly cover the seven attributes of a symptom (or eight if using OLD CARTS mnemonic). It is one of the most important portions of the patient visit.

O = onset, L = location, D = duration, C = character, A = alleviating & aggravating factors, R = radiation, T = timing, S = setting. Be sure to include pertinent negatives as well as pertinent positives.

Another mnemonic often used is PQRST: P = provocation & palliation, Q = quality (of the pain such as stabbing, dull, etc.), R = region and radiation, S = severity (using a 0 [none] to 10 [worst] pain scale is most often used), and T = timing (how long has it been occurring, how long does it last, did it ever occur before).

Review of Systems (ROS)

Review of Systems information is gained by doing a thorough interview with the patient or reporting individual. The goal is to gain information related to the patient's past medical history and current medical condition. The ROS encompasses "EVER." For example, "Do you have a history of headaches?" This is not the same question as "Do you have a headache?" The purpose of the ROS is not to just gain information about the presenting symptoms, but also gain information about the patient's past medical history, as well as patterns of symptoms, which can lead to diagnoses, sometimes of conditions unrelated to the present visit, but that are nonetheless important.

General Survey

A general survey relates to what the FNP sees: What is the appearance of the patient? This relates to the patient's physical appearance, body structure, mobility, and behavior. Are they appropriate or congruent for the patient's stated age and gender? In addition, it is important to evaluate if they are appropriate for the current situation, including the setting and climate.

Genogram (Family History)

Completing a three-generation genogram or family tree can provide a lot of information about a patient's family. It is a quick and easy visual tool that can be used to assess familial patterns of disease.

Observation

Observation and inspection are essential components to health assessment and the physical exam. Before laying hands on a patient, it is important to observe him or her. The general survey, patient interview, and physical exam all involve observation. One must determine if what is seen correlates to what is heard and felt.

Variations Related to Age

There should be variations in the approach to health assessment based on the age of the patient. Although students are taught that the physical exam is a head to toe exam and students will work under that premise, the statement "head to toe" may not always be 100%. In small children, especially infants, it is important to work under the premise of going from least invasive to most invasive. It is vital to be as nonthreatening as possible. After observing the infant, assess the fontanels, and then move to the hands, finger grasp, ROM (range of motion), and then head lag, moving from outward (hands and arms) to inward (body). Be sure to make eye contact and talk to the child in a calm voice. Prenatal history is an important component to the child's overall health history.

For adolescents, ask if it is okay for the parent to stay in the room early in the process. For elderly patients, it is important to have them move/change positions as little as possible, performing the exam in the front (respiratory, cardiac, abdomen) before moving to the back. Make sure ROM and most neuro are saved for last, anything that involves movement. Additional questions may also be needed—for instance, be sure to ask questions that explore changes in ADL that may be caused by the aging process or chronic illness.

IPPA/IAPP

Inspection, percussion, palpation, and auscultation (IPPA)—remember the order—with the order changing to inspection, auscultation, percussion, and palpation (IAPP) for the abdomen. An orderly systematic exam is key, especially for novice and advanced beginners. Performing the exam in a routine manner will help in remembering the steps and create a systematic flow to the physical exam.

Documentation

The following are a couple of key things to note about documentation.

Mixing Data

Do not mix up data. *Subjective* data relates to what the patient says, while *objective* data relates to what the FNP sees. When writing a SOAP (subjective data, objective data, assessment, and plan) note, subjective data should only be presented under "S" and objective data under "O." In addition, the assessment or interpretation of findings should only be presented in your A.

Normal/WNL

What is normal? Avoid using this term. What is "normal" for one patient may not be "normal" for another. Document what is seen or what is found on the exam. Medical records, whether paper or electronic, are legal records, and should, as accurately as possible, reflect the history and physical findings. Vagueness or ambiguity can lead to misinformation and negatively impact patient care. So, use extreme caution when using terms like "normal" or "within normal limits."

Review Questions

1. Open-ended questions are more pertinent to:
   A. Review of systems.
   B. Past illness.
   C. Present illness.
   D. Family history.

2. Mary is a 62-year-old female established patient who presents to the clinic with complaints of intermittent diarrhea and nausea for the past week. The type of history taking most appropriate will be:
   A. Clinician-centered.
   B. A comprehensive health history.
   C. A detailed review of systems.
   D. Focused or problem-centered.

3. Jennifer is a 16-year-old female who comes to the clinic with complaints of a headache and stomachache for 4 days. To elicit the most information, it is best to ask as many _____ questions as possible.
   A. open-ended
   B. closed-ended
   C. guided
   D. direct

4. The patient is a 68-year-old Asian American female seeing the FNP for the first time. The female provider starts the interview by asking some basic questions like "What brings you here today?" Her responses are very brief and she nods frequently during the conversation. Understanding about Asian culture, the FNP knows that:
   A. The patient may expect you to already know what is wrong with them.
   B. Nodding reflects her full understanding of what is being said.
   C. The patient would prefer to see a male provider.
   D. Nodding reflects her agreement with the provider.

5. Some cultures consider direct eye contact impolite or aggressive. _____ may avoid eye contact with both male and female providers.
   A. Muslim-Arabs
   B. American Indians or Native Americans
   C. Hasidic Jews
   D. The Amish

6. When interviewing a patient, it is best to be:
   A. Standing above the patient.
   B. Sitting below the patient.
   C. At eye-level with the patient.
   D. 2 to 3 feet from the patient.

7. Note-taking during an interview:
   A. Can be threatening to patients when discussing sensitive issues.
   B. Should never be done and is always avoidable.
   C. Makes the patient feel you are paying attention to them and you are carefully noting their comments.
   D. Shifts the attention to the patient and gives them a sense of importance.

8. When using an interpreter, it is important to note that:
   A. The same or similar age is often preferred.
   B. The same gender is often preferred.
   C. A summary of the conversation is often relayed.
   D. Using children of the patient is best.

9. Johnny is a 2-year-old male who was diagnosed with sickle cell anemia shortly after birth. Prior to conducting a physical assessment, it is important to note which of the following can be a chronic manifestation of sickle cell anemia?
   A. Stroke
   B. Sepsis
   C. Priapism
   D. Jaundice

10. Mrs. Adam's note says that she has a lesion that is confluent in nature. On examination, the FNP would expect to find:
    A. Lesions that run together.
    B. Annual lesions that have grown together.
    C. Lesions arranged in a line along a nerve route.
    D. Lesions that are grouped or clustered together.

11. Assessing a patient's ability to think abstractly can be done in one of two ways:
    A. Asking them who the president of the United States is or five previous presidents.
    B. Ask the patient to count backward or give them a proverb and ask them to explain it.
    C. Give them a proverb and ask them to explain it, or ask them to explain how two words are alike.
    D. Give them two words and ask them to explain how they are different, or ask them to calculate several numbers.

12. It is important for clinicians to understand the terminology when assessing for alcohol and drug usage and possible addiction. A state of adaption in which exposure to a drug induces changes that result in a diminution of one or more of the drug's effects over time is the definition of:
    A. Alcoholism.
    B. Tolerance.
    C. Physical dependence.
    D. Addiction.

13. When assessing for domestic violence, a statement such as, "I routinely ask all my patients about domestic violence" should come:
    A. Prior to asking probing questions.
    B. Prior to asking in-depth questions.
    C. After asking in-depth questions.
    D. At the end of the overall interview.

14. Which statement is true about dying patients?
    A. Dying patients often want to talk about their illness at each encounter.
    B. Dying patients may experience Kübler-Ross's stages for death and dying in any sequence, and stages may overlap.
    C. Dying patients often want to discuss their condition with multiple people.
    D. Media often gives the dying patients a realistic view of the effectiveness of resuscitation.

15. When interviewing a patient, he says he doesn't have any energy. What are some general statements about the fatigue that will assist in asking further appropriate questions?

    A. Fatigue is a specific symptom with few causes.

    B. Fatigue is an abnormal response to stress.

    C. Fatigue can be a normal response to grief.

    D. Fatigue related to stress or hard work requires further investigation.

16. A 45-year-old man presented to the urgent care with a fever (oral temp 102.5). The FNP will want to ask questions related to:

    A. The timing of illness and associated symptoms.

    B. Recent travel and contacts.

    C. The recent ingestion of an anti-pyretic.

    D. All of the above.

    E. A and B.

17. The PQRSTU or PQRST mnemonic is a way to:

    A. Assess a patient's pain level or presenting symptom.

    B. Assess a patient's skin.

    C. Determine a patient's level of understanding of instructions.

    D. Assess a patient's family history.

18. A family tree can also be described as a:

    A. Family map.

    B. Genogram.

    C. Pedigree.

    D. B and C.

    E. All of the above.

19. The FNP is doing an interview of a 21-year-old male. In the assessment, the FNP asks the patient, "You don't smoke, do you?" This type of question is:

    A. An appropriate open-ended question.

    B. An appropriate close-ended question.

    C. An inappropriate leading question.

    D. An inappropriate open-ended question.

20. A 39-year-old female presents to the clinic for her annual GYN visit. During her interview, she uses unusual frequent and long pauses with speech that is slow and monotone. The patient is most likely:

    A. Distracted.

    B. Depressed.

    C. Anxious.

    D. Angry.

21. When assessing the patient for strabismus, an eye muscle problem such as esotropia or exotropia, the practitioner should select which of the following eye tests?

    A. An ophthalmoscope exam

    B. The cover-uncover test

    C. The confrontation visual field test

    D. The eye test for distance vision

22. A 37-year-old male arrives at the clinic for a work physical. The FNP places both hands on the patient's shoulders and asks him to shrug his shoulders. This tests which cranial nerve?

    A. IX

    B. XI

    C. IV

    D. VI

23. A 43-year-old female presents to the clinic with complaints of frequent headaches. While attempting to test her cranial nerve function, she is requested to: puff out her checks, close her eyes tightly, and clench her teeth. Which of the following cranial nerves was tested?

    A. V and VII

    B. III, IV, and VI

    C. III and V

    D. IV, V, and VI

24. Mr. Davis is a 42-year-old construction worker. He has come to the clinic complaining of decreased hearing over the last few months. Upon examination, the FNP notes that both his ear canals are occluded with dark brown cerumen. Hearing loss due to impacted cerumen is an example of:

    A. Otitis media.

    B. A conductive hearing loss.

    C. A sensorineural hearing loss.

    D. Otitis externa.

25. Boggy turbinates is usually associated with which condition?

    A. Allergic rhinitis

    B. Nasal polyps

    C. A deviated septum

    D. A foreign body in the nose

26. A 27-year-old patient is 27 weeks pregnant and has come to the clinic for her prenatal exam. The fundal height measures 21 centimeters. This may be a sign of:

    A. Too much amniotic fluid.

    B. Twin gestation.

    C. Slow fetal growth.

    D. An expected finding for gestational age.

27. While performing a 24-year-old female's GYN exam, it is observed that the cervix is friable. This condition is most commonly associated with what?

    A. Cervical cancer

    B. Pelvic Inflammatory Disease (PID)

    C. Trichomoniasis

    D. A and B

    E. All of the above

28. A patient is being assessed for range of motion. He is asked to move his arms in toward the center of his body. This movement is called what?

    A. Adduction

    B. Abduction

    C. Flexion

    D. Extension

29. A 57-year-old bank teller comes to the office complaining of fever, shortness of breath, and a productive cough with slightly brown sputum. She says she had a cold the last two weeks and her symptoms continue to get worse. She has been taking over-the-counter cold and flu medications without any improvement. She mentions a slight chest pain upon breathing deeply, and has a history of HTN and a grade II murmur. She denies alcohol or drug use. She smokes half a pack of cigarettes a day. Both her parents are living. Both have HTN and elevated cholesterol. She looks ill and her temperature is elevated (100.7). Her blood pressure is 140/87 and pulse 85. On auscultation, she has decreased air movement, and fine crackles are heard over the right lower lobe. There is dullness on percussion, and increased fremitus during palpation. What disorder of the thorax or lung best describes her symptoms?

    A. COPD

    B. Upper respiratory infection

    C. Pneumothorax

    D. Pneumonia

30. A 36-year-old man comes to the ER for examination after a motorcycle accident. It was reported that he landed on his left side on the handlebars. It is suspected that he may have some internal injuries. Which of the following is the best response regarding assessment of the spleen in this situation?

    A. It is normal for the spleen to be palpable.

    B. The spleen can be enlarged as a result of trauma.

    C. If an enlarged spleen is noted, palpate thoroughly to determine size.

    D. An enlarged spleen should not be palpated because it can rupture easily.

31. While assessing the carotid pulse of a 57-year-old male, the FNP notices that the pulse is bounding. This would be documented as what?

    A. A normal carotid pulse

    B. 2+

    C. WNL

    D. 3+

32. The finding in the previous question may be due to:

    A. A normal physiological reaction.

    B. Fluid overload.

    C. Dehydration.

    D. Hypotension.

33. When assessing heart sounds, auscultate in _____ areas. These include:

    A. 4; apical, pulmonic, tricuspid, mitral.

    B. 5; aortic, pulmonic, Erb's point, tricuspid, mitral.

    C. 5; apical, pulmonic, Erb's point, tricuspid, mitral.

    D. 3; pulmonic, tricuspid, apical.

34. It is not unusual for patients with GERD to have atypical respiratory symptoms. These may include all of the following except:

    A. Aspiration pneumonia.

    B. Wheezing.

    C. Rhonchi.

    D. Cough.

35. Jarrod is a 62-year-old male who presents to the ER with complaints of chest pain across the anterior chest that sometimes radiates to the shoulders, arms, and lower jaw. On a scale of 1–10 he reports the pain at a 9. He describes the pain as pressing, tight, and sharp. He states the pain may last 10–15 minutes and then subsides. Based on his presenting symptoms, which diagnosis would you immediately rule out?

    A. Dissecting aortic aneurysm

    B. Angina pectoris

    C. Myocardial infarction

    D. Pericarditis

36. When auscultating over a patient's left femoral arteries, the presence of a bruit is noted on the left side. The initial assessment is that it indicates:

    A. Venous disease.

    B. A history of MI.

    C. An aortic aneurysm.

    D. Partial occlusion of the left femoral artery.

37. Mark is a 73-year-old male who was diagnosed with COPD 4 years ago. While doing the exam, it is observed that he has a barrel chest. In the note, the documentation is that the AP ratio is:

    A. 2:1.

    B. 1:2.

    C. 1:1.

    D. normal.

38. Which is true of a fourth heart sound (S4)?

    A. It is caused by rapid deceleration of blood against the ventricular wall.

    B. It is abnormal or rare in trained athletes.

    C. It is heard in atrial fibrillation.

    D. It marks atrial contraction.

39. Abby is an 11-year-old girl who presents to the ER after having had a seizure at school. She has a history of epilepsy, and is currently awake but drowsy. She begins to complain of a headache. The FNP knows that this is:

    A. Common.

    B. Slightly unusual.

    C. Abnormal and requires follow up within the next 24 hours.

    D. Highly unusual and requires immediate intervention.

40. The next step in Abby's care would be to:

    A. Provide analgesics and continue to monitor her postictally.

    B. Provide analgesics and consider an MRI.

    C. Provide analgesics and refer her to a neurologist within 24 hours.

    D. Obtain an MRI immediately.

41. When assessing a patient with complaints of headaches, what is the single most important factor?

    A. Neuro exam

    B. Their history

    C. Prior treatment

    D. Location of pain

42. Parity is documented in terms of mnemonic TPAL, which stands for:

    A. term pregnancies, premature births, abortions (therapeutic), and live births.

    B. term deliveries, premature births, abortions (therapeutic), and living children.

    C. term pregnancies, premature births, abortions (spontaneous), and live births.

    D. term deliveries, preterm deliveries, abortions (spontaneous and therapeutic), and living children.

43. While assessing the neurologic status of a 63-year-old male who has a late-stage brain tumor, the FNP strokes up the lateral side of the sole of the foot and inward with a reflex hammer. The patient fans out his toes, and the big toe shows dorsiflexion. This would be documented as:

    A. A negative Babinski's reflex, which is normal for adults.

    B. A positive Babinski's reflex, which is abnormal for adults.

    C. A positive Babinski's reflex, which is normal for adults.

    D. A negative Babinski's reflex, which is abnormal for adults.

44. The FNP is assessing Tanner staging of the breast in a young woman. It is observed that projection of the areola and nipple forms a secondary mound above the level of the breast. Which Tanner stage would this be?

    A. IV

    B. III

    C. I

    D. II

45. Ellen is a 40-year-old woman with three children who presents to the clinic with complaints of painful periods. She is diagnosed with secondary dysmenorrhea. What assessment data is the best indicator that she has secondary dysmenorrhea versus primary dysmenorrhea?

    A. It occurs at the onset of menses.

    B. She has no signs or symptoms of uterine problems, such as uterine fibroids or PID.

    C. She has had a history of normal periods until one year ago.

    D. She has had three normal pregnancies.

46. Abraham is a 54-year-old male who presents to the office with a complaint of joint pain. Certain symptoms will help determine whether it is inflammatory or non-inflammatory in nature. Which one of the following factors is consistent with an inflammatory process?

    A. Tenderness

    B. Cool to the touch

    C. History of injury

    D. Redness

47. Trina is a 22-year-old woman who is 28 weeks pregnant. She presents to the clinic for her prenatal visit. She has complaints of occasional nosebleeds, some hair loss, a rash on her face, and she thinks her face has really gotten fat over the past two weeks. Which symptom is of the greatest concern?

    A. Nosebleeds

    B. Facial edema

    C. Generalized hair loss

    D. Rash on her face

48. A lesion that is a change in color, flat circumscribed, and less than 1 cm is generally a:

    A. Café au lait spot.

    B. Freckle.

    C. Mole.

    D. Mongolian spot.

49. A lesion that is encapsulated-fluid filled in a dermis or subcutaneous layer, elevating the skin, is what?
    A. Pustule
    B. Nodule
    C. Wheal
    D. Cyst
50. A fissure can be described as:
    A. Scooped out but shallow.
    B. A self-inflicted abrasion.
    C. An irregular shaped deep depression in the dermis.
    D. A linear crack with abrupt edges.

Answers and Rationales

1. C. Open-ended questions are especially pertinent to eliciting the patient's chief concerns and the History of the Present Illness.

2. D. For patients who seek care for specific complaints—for example, coughs or painful urination—a more limited interview tailored to that specific problem may be indicated. This is sometimes known as a focused or problem-oriented history.

3. A. Open-ended questions are best for getting information about chief complaints, but they are especially important when working with adolescent patients. Adolescents tend to be very brief with their answers and asking as many open-ended questions as possible will yield more details about their symptoms.

4. A. Some Asian Americans may expect providers to already know what is wrong with them. Nodding is not a reflection of agreement or understanding but their cultural value for interpersonal harmony.

5. B. American Indians/Native Americans may consider direct eye contact impolite or aggressive, regardless of the gender of the provider. They will often stare at the floor during conversations. For Muslim-Arabs and Hasidic Jews, eye contact may be dependent on the gender of the patient and the gender of the provider.

6. C. Ideally, the FNP should be at eye level, with the patient four to five feet from the patient. Avoid facing a patient across a desk.

7. A. Note-taking should be avoided whenever possible, but is sometimes necessary. It can, however, be threatening to a patient, especially when discussing sensitive issues. It can shift the attention away from the patient and make them feel unimportant.

8. B. Older interpreters are often preferred by patients. An interpreter of the same gender is often preferred. Avoid using children of the patient when at all possible. An interpreter should provide a line-by-line verbatim account of the conversation.

9. D. Jaundice can be a chronic manifestation of sickle cell anemia, whereas the other conditions may be an acute manifestation that can lead to chronic issues.

10. A. Confluent is defined as flowing together, blending as one, or merging together.

11. C. Interpreting proverbs measures one's ability to think abstractly, as does interpreting similarities and differences between words.

12. B. This is the definition for tolerance.

13. A. A normalizing statement should be at the beginning of the interview. First ask probing questions, then follow with more in-depth questions.

14. B. The patient may experience the stages of death and dying in any stage or sequence or combination thereof.

15. C. Fatigue can be a normal response to hard work, stress, or grief. If it is not related to such situations, it requires further investigation.

16. D. Each component is relevant assessment data; they relate to exposure, manifestation, and masking agents.

17. A. The PQRST method of assessing pain is a valuable tool to accurately describe, assess, and document a patient's pain (or other presenting symptoms).

18. D. A family tree may be referred to as a genogram or pedigree.

19. C. This type of question is leading, and leading questions imply that there is a right or wrong response, and if the person wants to please you, they will respond how they think you want them to respond.

20. B. Depressed: Unusually frequent and long pauses in speech that are slow and monotone are usually a sign of depression and need further investigation.

21. B. A cover test or cover-uncover test is an objective determination of the presence and amount of ocular deviation.

22. B. You are testing cranial nerve 11 (cranial nerve XI).

23. A. To test cranial nerve V, ask the patient to clinch their teeth. To test cranial nerve VII, have the patient puff out their cheeks and close their eyes tightly.

24. B. Conductive hearing loss occurs when there is a problem conducting sound waves anywhere along the route through the outer ear, tympanic membrane (eardrum), or middle ear (ossicles). This can be caused by obstruction.

25. A. Nasal turbinates that are swollen, pale, boggy, or bluish are a sign of allergic rhinitis.

26. C. After 16 weeks of gestation fundal height measurement often matches the number of weeks gestation. A smaller than expected measurement can be a sign of slow fetal growth.

27. B. In rare cases, a friable cervix is an early sign of cervical cancer. The most likely cause is HPV or chlamydia. Commonly, it is a sign associated with PID. It may also be due to trichomoniasis, but is more likely a result of chlamydia or PID.

28. A. Adduction is movement toward the mid-line of the body.

29. D. Pneumonia is usually associated with dyspnea, cough, and fever. On auscultation, there can be coarse or fine crackles heard over the affected lobe. Percussion over the affected area is dull and there is often an increase in fremitus.

30. D. If an enlarged spleen is palpated, do not continue to palpate and order an immediate ultrasound. An enlarged spleen is friable and can rupture easily with overpalpation.

31. D. A forceful pulse might be described as 3+ or even 4+ and is also described as bounding.

32. B. Increased carotid-pulse amplitude may be associated with fluid-volume overload or hypertension.

33. B. The clinician should listen in five locations, both with the bell and the diaphragm of the stethoscope. These are the aortic, pulmonic, Erb's point, tricuspid, and mitral areas.

34. C. Some patients with GERD may present with aspiration pneumonia, wheezing, or coughing.

35. A. All but dissecting. An aortic aneurysm may present with shoulder pain and is often described as a ripping or tearing pain. The pain is persistent.

36. D. A bruit occurs with turbulent blood flow, indicating partial occlusion of the artery.

37. C. In patients with COPD, it is common for them to present with a barrel chest. In a barrel chest, the AP ratio is usually 1:1.

38. D. The S3 gallop is caused by rapid deceleration of blood against the ventricular wall. S4 is heard with atrial contractions and is absent in atrial fibrillations for this reason. This is occasionally normal in trained athletes.

39. A. Peri-ictal headaches are common in children who have epilepsy.

40. A. Because peri-ictal headaches are common in children with epilepsy, no further diagnostic measures are necessary.

41. B. The patient's history is the single most important factor in the evaluation of a headache.

42. D. TPAL is the mnemonic for term deliveries, preterm deliveries, abortions (spontaneous and therapeutic), and living children.

43. B. The Babinski reflex occurs after the sole of the foot has been firmly stroked. The big toe then moves upward or toward the top surface of the foot. The other toes fan out. This appears in infants up to 2 years old but is seen as abnormal after that.

44. A. This would be a Tanner stage IV because there is elevation of the nipple and areola above the level of the surrounding breast tissue, as well as formation of a secondary mound.

45. C. Secondary dysmenorrhea is menstrual pain that develops later in women who have had normal periods. It is often related to problems in the uterus or other pelvic organs.

46. A. Tenderness implies an inflammatory process, along with increased temperature and tenderness.

47. B. Generalized hair loss, a hyperpigmented maxillary rash (chloasma), and nosebleeds are usually benign and common in pregnancy. Facial edema after the 24th week of gestation may indicate gestational hypertension.

48. B. A macule is a flat, discolored, circumscribed area of skin that is less than 1 cm in size. Examples of this include freckles, petechia, and flat nevi.

49. D. A cyst is a fluid-filled lesion that involves the dermis or subcutaneous layer of the skin and is encapsulated. None of the other lesions have all these characteristics.

50. D. A fissure is a linear crack that extends into the dermis with abrupt edges.

● ● ● **References**

Bickley, L. (2012). *Bates' guide to physical examination and history taking* (11th ed.). Philadelphia, PA: J.B. Lippincott.

Jarvis, C. (2012). *Physical examination & health assessment* (6th ed.). St. Louis, MO: Saunders, Elsevier.

4

Epidemiology and Population Health

Julie G. Stewart, DNP, MPH, MSN, FNP-BC, APRN
Nancy L. Dennert, MS, MSN, FNP-BC, CDE, BC-ADM

The health of an individual is the focus of the clinician. However, the FNP is charged with being educated on the health of communities, and indeed, in attempting to make a difference in global health initiatives. Nurse practitioners need to stay informed regarding global and national trends in all diseases, be on the lookout for patients with any forms of infectious diseases, and appropriately assess, treat, and report patients who need treatment. With the ability to develop trusted patient–FNP relationships and see patients finish appropriate treatment regimens, nurse practitioners can help mitigate the spread of infectious diseases and be alert to emerging illnesses within our own communities.

The FNP must remain current in what issues are contributing to health problems, and be actively engaged in health promotion and disease prevention efforts. Having a concrete knowledge base from which to intertwine concepts of epidemiology and clinical prevention with the population's health is vital for success in the role.

Epidemiology is derived from the following Greek words: *epi* (on, befall); *demos* (the people); and *logos* (the study of). It is the branch of medicine that covers the incidence, distribution, and attempts to control diseases and other factors relating to health.

According to the World Health Organization (WHO), "Epidemiology is the study of the distribution and determinants of health-related states or events (including disease), and the application of

this study to the control of diseases and other health problems" (WHO, 2015).

A population consists of a group of people who have some common characteristics. It can be large (such as an entire nation), or small (as in a neighborhood). Characteristics are not solely related to physical boundaries of where one may reside. A community may include members who share interpersonal and/or intrapersonal connections, known as a *Phenomenological community* (Maurer & Smith, 2009). We see that the types of characteristics held in common for a population subset/community can include age, gender, health behaviors, exposure to a virus, etc.

One method for identifying an unhealthy community is the lack of support for vulnerable populations that exist within the community. Including all members of the community in addressing poverty, providing adequate housing, healthy food, job opportunities, and proper air, water, and sanitation is vital to the health, development, and resilience of the population.

Population Health and *Healthy People 2020*

In 1979, the Department of Health and Human Services launched an initiative aimed at improving the health of the United States population. This effort was titled *Healthy People 2000*, which was followed by *Healthy People 2010*, and now *Healthy People 2020*. The agency amassed baseline data and then set goals on the prioritized health targets (Koh, 2010). *Healthy People 2020* not only keeps the past overarching goals from *Healthy People 2010*, which were to increase the quality of life and lifespan, and to decrease health disparities, but has supplemented those with: "promoting quality of life, healthy development, and healthy behaviors across life stages; and creating social and physical environments that promote good health" (Koh, 2010, p. 1656).

Morbidity rates tell us how fast a disease is occurring in a population. The proportion is what fraction of the population is affected by the disease, and the incidence rate is the number of new cases of the disease in a specific time period.

The *epidemiological triangle*. When considering the course of infectious diseases, this triad posits that infections result from the interaction of agent, host, and environment. Transmission occurs when the agent leaves its **reservoir** or host through a **portal of exit**, is conveyed by some **mode of transmission**, and enters through an appropriate **portal of entry** to infect a **susceptible host** (CDC, 2012).

Other important terms are epidemic, pandemic, and endemic. An *epidemic* is when there is an outbreak that is limited in time and locations.

A disease is said to be endemic if it remains present in an area for a long period of time. For example, malaria is endemic in tropical climates, and hepatitis B (HBV) is endemic in China and many Asian countries.

A *pandemic* is an epidemic extending to an entire country or a large part of the world. HIV/AIDS is an example of a global pandemic disease.

The natural history of a disease refers to the progression of that disease if there were no intervention or treatment to alter the disease process. For instance, from researching history, and unfortunately from data obtained through the Tuskegee study, there is much information about an infectious disease that has likely been around for well over a thousand years: syphilis.

The PRECEDE-PROCEED Model is another design for planning and evaluating population health programs (Green & Kreuter, 2005). PRECEDE stands for Predisposing, Reinforcing, and Enabling Constructs in Educational/environmental Diagnosis and Evaluation. PROCEED stands for Policy, Regulatory, and Organizational Constructs in Educational and Environmental Development. While this may seem overwhelming and complex, it is more easily understood as a roadmap for health promotion that includes the environment, as well as people's beliefs, abilities/skills, and behaviors (Crosby & Noar, 2011). It is an approach that utilizes the gathering of information for PRECEDE, which then acts as the framework for the PROCEED steps. It is a continuing process because the evaluation portion of PROCEED helps to inform and revise the steps in the PRECEDE portion of this model.

Measures of disease outbreaks:

- **RATES** tell us how fast the disease is occurring in a population.
- **PROPORTIONS** tell us what fraction of the population is affected.
- **INCIDENCE RATE** is the number of new cases of a disease in a specific time period.

Disease Registries

Syndromic surveillance is one mechanism that can be used to detect uncommon and unusual health

---

# of new cases of a disease occurring in the population during a specific time period

$$\frac{\text{\# of new cases of a disease occurring in the population during a specific time period}}{\text{\# of persons who are at risk of developing the disease during that time period}} \times 1000$$

Mortality rates can be used for the overall population, or be cause- or age-specific. Typically, mortality rates are going to increase with age increases (outside of suicide and homicide rates). For example, to calculate a mortality (death) rate, one would use the following:

$$\frac{\text{\# of deaths in the population during a specified time period}}{\text{\# of persons in the population during the specified time period}}$$

Figure 4-1 Incidence Rate per 1,000

Reproduced from Fos, P. (2011). Epidemiology foundations: The science of public health. San Fransisco: Jossey-Bass, pp. 80, 81, 90.

occurrences. This approach is based on an epidemiological perspective, and relies on the recognition of unusual patterns of illness. Biological terrorism is suspected if a set of health patterns appear that are out of the ordinary, such as the following:

- A cluster of diseases with similar clinical presentations and at a similar stage of illness
- A cluster of unexplained illnesses in a well-defined population
- An unusually severe disease or higher mortality than expected for a given agent
- A cluster of cases with an unusual mode of transmission
- Multiple or serial outbreaks
- A disease not typical for a specific age group
- A disease unusual for a season or region of the country
- Clusters of the same illness in various locations
- Clusters of morbidity or mortality in animals or livestock similar to humans

MRCs are designed to be prepared to assist and respond to both public health/medical and emergency preparedness/response events such as the following:

Public Health/Medical

- Surgeon General priorities (disease prevention, elimination of health disparities, health literacy)
- Disease detection
- Health promotion
- Health education
- Health clinic support and staffing

Emergency Preparedness/Response

- Mass dispensing/vaccinations
- Pandemic flu planning
- Preparedness campaigns
- Shelter operations/support
- First-responder rehab
- Mass casualty incident/emergency response
    (MRC Registration Criteria FAQs, 2011)

Primary Care Definition

Health care services

Integrated

Accessible

Clinicians

Accountable

Address majority of personal health care needs

Develop sustained partnership with patient

Practice within context of family and community

Concepts of Health

Normal state of functioning

Optimal state of well-being

Absence of disease

Health-illness-disease continuum

Perception of health

Multidimensional: health, person, environment, nursing

Health Belief Model (Nora Pender)

Behavioral expression of Health (Pender)

Affect, Attitudes, Actualization, Activity, Aspiration, Accomplishments

- Health focuses on capabilities rather than pathology
- Concepts common to nurse practitioner roles:
    a. Health promotion
    b. Health protection
    c. Disease prevention

Healthy People 2020

U.S. Department of Health and Human Services

Healthy People 2020 strives to identify nationwide health improvement priorities, such as:

- Increase public awareness and understanding of the determinants of health, disease, and disability and the opportunities for progress.
- Provide measurable objectives and goals that are applicable at the national, state, and local levels.
- Engage multiple sectors to take actions to strengthen policies and improve practices that are driven by the best available evidence and knowledge.
- Identify critical research, evaluation, and data collection needs.

Overarching Goals

- Attain high-quality, longer lives free of preventable disease, disability, injury, and premature death.
- Achieve health equity, eliminate disparities, and improve the health of all groups.

- Create social and physical environments that promote good health for all.
- Promote quality of life, healthy development, and healthy behaviors across all life stages.

Levels of Prevention

There exist three levels of prevention that focus on various aspects of prevention from avoiding disease altogether, early diagnosis of disease, and measures taken to prevent or limit disease progression.

Primary Prevention

The goal of primary prevention is to prevent a disease or injury before it occurs. This can be done by changing risky or unhealthy behaviors and increasing disease resistance to infectious diseases. Some examples of Primary Prevention are:

- Use of seat belts and helmets, and banning hazardous products.
- Provide education about healthy habits, such as quitting smoking, eating healthy meals, and exercising regularly.
- Immunizations against infectious diseases.

Secondary Prevention

The goal of secondary prevention is to reduce the impact of the disease or the injury that has already occurred. This is done by treating the disease as soon as possible to slow or halt the progression, encouraging strategies to prevent reoccurrence, and implementing programs to return people to their original health. Some examples of secondary prevention are:

- Screening tests to detect disease in the early stages, such as mammograms or Pap smears.
- A daily low dose of aspirin in appropriate populations to prevent MIs or strokes.
- Modifications in the workplace so that an injured worker may continue to safely do his or her job.

Tertiary Prevention

The goal of tertiary prevention is to decrease the impact of an ongoing illness or injury. This is done by helping the patient manage their chronic disease or permanent impairment to let them function as much as possible and improve their quality of life and life expectancy. Examples include:

- Chronic disease management programs such as diabetic programs, arthritis, or depression.
- Support groups that encourage members to share strategies to improve their quality of life.

- Vocational rehabilitation programs to assist workers in new jobs once they have recovered as much as possible.

Prevention Applied to Specific Diseases

- Coronary artery disease (MI)
- Stroke
- Alcohol and substance abuse
- Cancers
- Osteoporosis
- Sexually transmitted diseases
- Infectious diseases
- Chronic obstructive pulmonary disease
- Accidents
- Diabetes
- Glaucoma

Criteria for Screening

- Screening is to be distinguished from diagnostic evaluation.
- Screening presumes that the patient has no symptoms.
- Screening should be based on the patient's individual risk factor profile.

Characteristics of the Disease Targeted for Screening

- The targeted disease should be serious and sufficiently prevalent in the group being screened to justify the costs and risks of screening.
- The patient's risk of future morbidity and mortality must be reduced as a result of early detection of the condition.
- The screening maneuver itself must be acceptable to the patient.

Characteristics of the Screening Test

1. Sensitivity:

   A sensitive test will identify people who actually have the disease or the percent of positive test results.

   Sensitive tests show a positive result when an asymptomatic condition is truly present.

2. Specificity

   A specific screening test will reveal a negative result when the disease is absent.

A specific test can eliminate people that do not have the disease.

Nonspecific tests will yield many false positives.

Reasons for Diagnostic Testing

a. To make a diagnosis in a patient who is ill or has a new medical problem
b. To provide information for a patient that already has a known disease
c. To alerta patient who is at risk for subsequent diseases
d. To monitor ongoing treatment, and conduct surveillance tests
e. To determine, in part, the frequency with which patients should return to the outpatient setting

Guidelines for Ordering Diagnostic Tests

a. There should be a good reason for ordering a test.
b. Studies have shown that clinicians frequently order excessive, hard to justify tests (sedimentation rates, coagulations studies).
c. The old maxim is that if a test will not affect patient management, it should not be done.
d. Consider the costs involved and the probability of obtaining a result that will change the treatment.

Testing Considerations

a. Alternative management courses; including not testing or treating.
b. The importance of the diagnosis being entertained: If it is a significant diagnosis that should not be missed, then test even if the pretest probability is low.
c. The patient's values regarding the different interventions and outcomes.
d. Test costs, risks, and the degree of invasiveness.
e. Concurrent problems (i.e., patients with terminal or end-stage diseases should not have extensive workups for new problems).

Consider Test Outcome Probability

a. Estimate the pretest probability by history, physical, and previous test results.

b. For example, there is no reason to test every patient for HIV (being there is no predictive value of a positive test), since the result will be low for the general population.
c. Test a prison population for HIV. The disease prevalence is higher and there will be more true positive results.

Confirmatory Testing

a. All confirmatory testing should have a relatively high specificity to minimize false positive results.
b. Examples: Western blots for HIV, biopsies, cardiac catheterization.
c. Refer patients to specialists for confirmatory testing.

Exclusion Testing

a. Must be highly sensitive to minimize false negatives.
b. Often used in outpatient settings.
c. Chest x-ray (CXR) to R/O pneumonia (CXR is not sensitive for lung cancer, however).
d. An EKG is not sensitive for coronary artery disease.
e. Stool hemoccult is not sensitive for colon cancer.
f. Serum creatinine is not sensitive for kidney disease.

To increase the sensitivity of these tests:

a. Repeat the tests (hemoccult 3x).
b. Lengthen the test interval (24-hours: Holter monitor).
c. Enhance the test (use a CT scan for lung cancer).
d. May need to add other tests (e.g., culture and sensitivity for U/A with positive nitrates).

Test Panels

a. Order tests selectively.
b. Avoid general panels.
c. Consider what to do with abnormal results.
d. The clinician that orders the test is responsible for the test results.
e. Repeating the abnormal test is often the appropriate thing to do.

Guide to Clinical Preventative Services

1. Task forces that make recommendations based on current best evidence
   a. USPSTF, AAFP, ACS, Canadian Task Force
   b. USPSTF (www.epss.ahrq.gov)
2. Suggest criteria for screening.
3. Provide classification codes regarding the strength of recommendation and the quality of the evidence.
4. Recommendations range from conservative to aggressive.
5. Use Routine Health Maintenance flow sheets.
   - Task forces meet to make recommendations based on current best evidence and create suggested criteria for screening.
   - Classification Codes (Grades) are used regarding strength of recommendation and quality of the evidence.
   - Recommendations range from conservative to aggressive:
     - Grade A = Good Evidence: The USPSTF recommends the service. There is high certainty that the net benefit is substantial.
     - Grade B = Fair Evidence: The USPSTF recommends the service. There is high certainty that the net benefit is moderate, or there is moderate certainty that the net benefit is moderate to substantial.
     - Grade C = No recommendation: The USPSTF recommends against routinely providing the service. There may be considerations that support providing the service in an individual patient. There is at least moderate certainty that the net benefit is small.
     - Grade D = Recommends against in asymptomatic: The USPSTF recommends against the service. There is moderate or high certainty that the service has no net benefit or that the harms outweigh the benefits.
     - Grade I = Insufficient Evidence: The USPSTF concludes that the current evidence is insufficient to assess the balance of benefits and harms of the service. Evidence is lacking, of poor quality, or is conflicting, and the balance of benefits and harms cannot be determined.

Some Common Wellness Screening Recommendations in the Primary Care Setting: Adult

- Recommendation (**A**): Serum cholesterol screening at age 35 for a male (age 20–35 with risk) and age 45 for a female with no risk (age 20–45 with risk)
- Recommendation for ASA in men age 45–79 years when potential CVD risk outweighs the risk of GI hemorrhage. Grade (**A**)
  Recommend for ASA in women age 55–79 years when potential CVD benefit outweighs potential harm of GI hemorrhage. Grade (**A**)
- Recommendation for men: Screening for abdominal aortic aneurysm. Screen males age 65–75 years once with abdominal US if any history of smoking. Grade (**B**). Men ages 65–75 with no history of smoking: No recommendation for or against abdominal US. Grade (**C**)
- Recommendation (**B**): Screen for type 2 DM in asymptomatic adults with sustained B.P. > than 135/80. ADA recommends using fasting glucose and defines diabetes as fasting glucose > 126 with recommended confirmation screening. A screening interval of every 3 years is recommended for those that do not demonstrate a fasting glucose > 126.
- Screening for colorectal cancer with fecal occult blood annually, or sigmoidoscopy every 5 years or colonoscopy every 10 years for those age 50–75 years. Grade (**C**) recommendation for colorectal screening for adults 76–85. Grade (**D**) for adults > 85
- Screening for cervical cancer with Pap smear for women age 21–65: Grade (**A**)
- Screen women ages 30–65 using cytology and HPV every 5 years. Grade (**A**)
- Do not screen women with a Pap smear or HPV screening who are less than age 21 regardless of sexual history: Grade (**D**)
- Do not screen women over the age of 65 who have adequate prior screening and are not at high risk: Grade (**D**)
- Do not screen men for prostate cancer using a PSA-based screening: Grade (**D**)

Guidelines for children, adolescents, and special populations can be downloaded from the AHRQ website at http://www.ahrq.gov/professionals/clinicians-providers/guidelines-recommendations/guide/index.html.

Review Questions

1. Epidemiology is the area of health care that deals with:
    A. The physiological causes of disease and treatments to cure illness.
    B. The incidence, distribution, and efforts to control diseases and other factors relating to health.
    C. The incidence, prevalence, and attack rates of infectious diseases in a population.
    D. The holistic approach to disease prevention and social determinants of disease.

2. An example of a population that would be the BEST CHOICE to be studied related to a specific disease prevalence would be:
    A. A random sample of men and women arriving in an international airport.
    B. A group of adult dog owners (over 21 years old) who are members of a national dog organization.
    C. A sample of teenagers aged 15–18 years old attending public high schools in southwestern Connecticut.
    D. A convenience sample of families who shop at a local mall.

3. Aims to reduce health inequities among population groups is part of the definition of:
    A. Tertiary prevention.
    B. Secondary prevention.
    C. Epidemiologic case control research.
    D. Population health.

4. The three forms of observational research associated most often with epidemiologic research include:
    A. Randomized controlled trials, phenomenology, and case studies.
    B. Randomized controlled trials, cohorts, and true experiments.
    C. Cohort, cross-sectional, and case studies.
    D. Cohort, nested cases, and quasi-experimental.

5. An example of an epidemic would be the:
    A. Ebola outbreak in West Africa in 2014.
    B. Spanish influenza of 1918.
    C. Human Immunodeficiency Virus in this century.
    D. Smallpox in northeast America in 1633–34.

6. An epidemic becomes a pandemic problem when:
    A. More than 100 people get ill.
    B. An infectious disease moves from one state to another state.
    C. It lasts more than 6 months.
    D. It becomes a global problem.

7. Hepatitis B is endemic in which of the following areas or countries?
    A. Scandinavia
    B. China and Albania
    C. Canada
    D. Southwestern United States

8. Maternal mortality rates are calculated by:
    A. Counting deaths in women due to pregnancy or childbirth, divided by number of live births in the same time period.
    B. Counting maternal deaths in the first 5 years of life of a child, divided by the number of live births in the hypothetical cohort of newborns.

    C. Counting the number of live births in one year, divided by deaths in women due to pregnancy or child birth in a subset of months in that year.

    D. Counting the number of deaths of women in one year, divided by the number of deaths in women related to pregnancy or childbirth.

9. Morbidity refers to:

    A. The death rates in a population from a specific disease.

    B. Either the incidence rate, or the prevalence of a disease or medical condition.

    C. The absolute number of deaths from a disease in a specific population.

    D. Either the attack rates or deaths from a disease in a specific population.

10. (Number of New Cases) / (Person-Time at Risk) is a calculation formula for:

    A. Prevalence rates.

    B. Incidence rates.

    C. Mortality rates.

    D. Morbidity rates.

11. Globally, approximately 239,000 women had ovarian cancer in 2012. This statement reflects:

    A. A prevalence.

    B. An incidence.

    C. A disparity.

    D. Mortality.

12. Choose the correct term for the following statement. The _____ of developing invasive breast cancer in the next 10 years is 2.31%, or 1 in 43.

    A. Incidence

    B. Prevalence

    C. Probability

    D. Rate

13. A perfect test is one for which the result is always positive if you have the disease and always negative if you don't have the disease. This statement refers to:

    A. Health promotion.

    B. Metric testing.

    C. Health screenings.

    D. Risk stratification.

14. The time from the moment of exposure to an infectious agent until signs and symptoms of the disease appear is the definition for which of the following?

    A. Attack rate period

    B. Incubation period

    C. The natural history of a disease

    D. The pre-diagnostic span

15. You are reviewing a sample of screening tests for 100 people who eventually died from colon cancer and note that the vast majority had serum hemoglobin A1cs that were above normal. This association might indicate what type of correlational relationship?

    A. Positive *r*

    B. Negative *r*

    C. Positive *p*

    D. Negative *p*

16. An example of a good case-control study would be:
    A. A group of people who became ill with gastrointestinal symptoms after eating strawberries compared to a group of people who became ill with gastrointestinal symptoms who did not eat strawberries.
    B. A subset of teens who get screened for HPV and are found to be infected with HPV compared to teens who do not get screened for HPV.
    C. A population of adults with diabetes mellitus type II compared to a population of adults without diabetes mellitus type II.
    D. Children who have asthma who were breast fed as infants versus children with asthma who have pet allergies.

17. A study is looking at a group of patients and the time to an acute coronary event. This is known as:
    A. An attack rate.
    B. A proportion of probability.
    C. Survival analysis.
    D. The myocardial infarction risk factor span.

18. The Alzheimer's Prevention Registry and the Breast Cancer Surveillance Consortium are examples of:
    A. Disease registries.
    B. Support group agencies.
    C. Screening programs.
    D. Volunteer agencies.

19. The probability that the test says a person has the disease, when in fact they do have the disease, is known to be:
    A. Specificity.
    B. Sensitivity.
    C. Diagnostic.
    D. Probability.

20. The probability that the test says a person does not have the disease, when in fact they are disease-free, is known to be:
    A. Specificity.
    B. Sensitivity.
    C. Diagnostic.
    D. Probability.

21. There are seven agents of infectious disease. These include:
    A. Metazoa, protozoa, fungi, bacteria, rickettsia, viruses, prions.
    B. Metatarsus, fungi, HIV, Rocky Mountain Spotted Fever, bacteria, portioles.
    C. Protozoa, fungi, viruses, bacteria, coryza, parasites, myomata.
    D. Parasites, viruses, bacteria, influenza, tick-borne, fungi, jiroveci.

22. Diseases that have environmental reservoirs include:
    A. Jakob-Creutzfeldt, human immunodeficiency virus, and hepatitis B.
    B. Shigella, Lyme disease, and varicella.
    C. Croup, respiratory synctial virus, and anthrax.
    D. Histoplasmosis, botulism, and tetanus.

23. A patient with Type 2 Diabetes enrolls in a diabetes program that includes information on nutrition, exercise, and general wellness strategies. What type of prevention is this considered to be?

    A. Primary prevention
    B. Secondary prevention
    C. Tertiary prevention
    D. Type 2 diabetes prevention

24. Which of the following screening tests would be recommended for a 68-year-old male who smokes 1 pack of cigarettes a day for 20 years? (This is a 20 pack year history.)

    A. PSA testing
    B. ASA 81 mg daily
    C. CXR
    D. Abdominal ultrasound

25. Immunizations are considered to be what type of prevention?

    A. Primary
    B. Secondary
    C. Tertiary
    D. Immunizations are an active form of prevention.

26. A 67-year-old female comes to the wellness clinic for an annual gynecological exam and Pap smear. She has no history of abnormal Pap smears or any STIs. She states that she feels fine and has no concerns. She is in a monogamous relationship with her husband. It is appropriate at this time for the primary care provider (PCP) to inform the patient that:

    A. She should get a Pap smear and HPV screening now, and then again in five years.
    B. She should continue to get annual Pap smears, but she no longer needs HPV screening.
    C. She does not need any more gynecological exams since she has no history of any gynecological problems.
    D. She no longer needs to have a Pap smear.

27. A 45-year-old overweight male is having an annual physical exam. He has no complaints and states that he feels "healthy as a horse." The patient's BP is 140/92 in the office, and it is noted that at the last exam the patient's BP was 148/88 and the patient stated that he had "white coat syndrome." Screening guidelines for this patient include:

    A. PSA test.
    B. AAA ultrasound.
    C. Fasting plasma glucose.
    D. EKG.

28. A 58-year-old female hypertensive patient has been placed on ASA 81 mg by her PCP. This is considered to be:

    A. Primary prevention.
    B. Secondary prevention.
    C. Tertiary prevention.
    D. Active intervention.

29. The nurse practitioner orders a fasting glucose for a patient that is asymptomatic but has a strong family history of type 2 diabetes. The fasting glucose returns at 129. What would be the next best approach for the nurse practitioner?

    A. Explain to the patient that they have diabetes and need to begin a strict regimen of diet and exercise.
    B. Begin Metformin 500 mg once daily and repeat the fasting glucose in three months.
    C. Repeat the test prior to diagnosing the patient with diabetes.
    D. Refer the patient to a nutritionist.

30. A patient is having an annual physical. Statements that are made by the patient indicate that he may possibly have OSA. The FNP discusses with the patient that she would like to send him for a sleep study to confirm her suspicions. The patient states that no matter what anybody says "I would never wear one of those things over my face or nose, and I would not put anything in my mouth at night." The FNP notes that the patient would refuse any treatment even if he is found to have OSA. The FNP should then:

    A. Order the sleep study to confirm or refute her suspicions.

    B. Continue to educate the patient on the risks associated with OSA at each visit.

    C. Order home oxygen therapy and tell the patient to use it prn (*pro re nata*) at night if he develops any shortness or breath.

    D. Refer the patient to an otolaryngologist for follow-up.

Answers and Rationales

1. B. Epidemiology is the foundation of public health and is a data-driven science within health care.

2. C. This choice identifies a specific group of individuals and age-group within a specific geographical area, which will add strength to this study of disease prevalence.

3. D. A variety of definitions for population health are used. However, in general this refers to health outcomes within a group of individuals or the entire human population.

4. C. The three forms of observational research associated most often with epidemiologic research include: cohort, cross-sectional, and case studies. Epidemiological observational studies do not include any form of intervention.

5. A. An epidemic occurs when there are more cases of a disease than usually occurs in a specific population area.

6. D. Although definitions of pandemic vary, it typically includes a disease/illness that is traveling in wide geographic locations.

7. B. Hepatitis B has high prevalence rates defined as greater than 8% HbsAg in a country's population. This list is available from the Centers for Disease Control and World Health Organization.

8. A. The definition of maternal mortality rates is counting the deaths in women due to pregnancy or childbirth, divided by the number of live births in the same time period.

9. B. Morbidity refers to the incidence or prevalence of illness/disease in a population.

10. B. Incidence rates are a proportion of individuals who develop a disease/illness/condition during a specific time period.

11. A. Prevalence rates describe a proportion of individuals in a population at one point in time, or within a specific time frame, who have a particular disease/illness/condition.

12. C. The incidence proportion, risk, or probability of developing a disease within a specific time period is a form of morbidity frequency statistics. The absolute risk of developing a disease or illness can be expressed as a percentage.

13. C. A health screening is meant to detect individuals who are at high risk of, or have, a disease/illness by history, physical examination, or other testing procedures.

14. B. By definition, the time from the moment of exposure to an infectious agent until signs and symptoms of the disease appear is the incubation period.

15. A. A correlational study seeks to find a relationship between two variables. If one variable increases or decreases, does it have an effect on the other variable?

16. A. A case-control study is an observational study that determines how much exposure to a risk factor of interest has occurred in patients who have a disease or illness (cases) compared to those who do not (controls).

17. C. Survival analysis is a statistical method that looks at a time duration until an event (or series of events) occurs.

18. A. Disease registries are population-based and/or hospital-based databases of patients who are diagnosed with specific diseases.

19. B. By definition, the probability that the test says a person has the disease, when in fact they do have the disease, is known to be the sensitivity.

20. A. The probability that the test says a person does not have the disease, when in fact they are disease-free, is defined as specificity.

21. A. There are seven agents of infectious disease. These include: Metazoa, protozoa, fungi, bacteria, rickettsia, viruses, prions.

22. D. An environmental reservoir is an area where pathogens live and have the potential to be released and cause infection in humans.

23. C. The patient with type 2 diabetes has a chronic disease and therefore would benefit from strategies that help in disease management and improving the quality of life.

24. D. According to the USPSTF guidelines, all males over the age of 65 with a history of smoking (either current or past) should be screened once for an AAA. ASA 81 mg may be an appropriate recommendation but it is not a screening test.

25. A. Immunizations are a primary prevention strategy that aims to prevent a disease or injury before it occurs.

26. D. According to the USPSTF guidelines, the patient no longer needs a Pap smear since she has no previous history of any abnormal gynecological findings. Recommendation grade (D).

27. C. All adults with sustained hypertension should be screened for DM 2 per the USPSTF guidelines. Grade (B) recommendation.

28. B. Secondary prevention is designed to reduce the impact of the disease that has already occurred. The patient is at a higher risk of stroke due to her age and her comorbid condition. ASA 81 mg is an appropriate recommendation to prevent the occurrence of a stroke. Grade (B) recommendation.

29. C. Repeating an abnormal test is often the best appropriate approach and allows for confirmatory testing. If the patient had a fasting blood sugar > than 126 when the test was repeated, then A, B, or C would be the appropriate next steps.

30. B. A test should not be done if it will not have an effect on the management of the patient. (See guidelines for diagnostic testing.)

● ● ● **References**

Association for Prevention Teaching and Research. (January, 2009). Clinical prevention and population health curriculum framework. Retrieved from www.aptrweb.org/resource/. . ./revised_cpph_framework_2009.pdf

Centers for Disease Control and Prevention. (May, 2012). Principles of epidemiology in public health practice (3rd ed.). Available at http://www.cdc.gov/osels/scientific_edu/SS1978/Lesson1/Section10.html

Crosby, R., & Noar, S. (2011). What is a planning model? An introduction to PRECEDE-PROCEED. *Journal of Public Health Dentistry, 71.* doi: 10.1111/j.1752-7325.2011.00235.x

Curley, A. & Vitale, P. (Eds.) (2012). *Population-based nursing: Concepts and competencies for advanced practice.* New York: Springer Publishing.

Fos, P. (2011). *Epidemiology foundations: The science of public health.* San Francisco: Jossey-Bass.

Friis, R. H., & Sellers, A. T. (2004). *Epidemiology for public health practice* (3rd ed.). Sudbury, MA: Jones & Barlett.

Green, L., & Kreuter, M. K. (2005). *Health program planning: An educational and ecological approach* (4th ed.). New York: McGraw-Hill.

Institute of Medicine. (2012). Primary care and public health: Exploring integration to improve population health. Washington, DC: National Academy of Sciences. Retrieved from: http://www.iom.edu/Reports/2012/Primary-Care-and-Public-Health.aspx

Koh, Howard K. (2010). Perspective: Healthy people 2020. *The New England Journal of Medicine, 362,* 18, 1653–1656.

Macha, K., & McDonough, J. (2012). *Epidemiology for advanced nursing practice.* Sudbury, MA: Jones & Bartlett.

Maurer, F. A., & Smith, C. S. (2009). Community/public health nursing practice: Health for families and populations (4th ed.). St. Louis, MO: Saunders Elsevier.

USAID. (2012). MEASURE evaluation. Retrieved from: http://www.cpc.unc.edu/measure/tools/population-health-and-environment/population-health-and-environment-training-materials/PHE%20complete%20indicator%20matrix%20example.doc/view

U.S. Preventative Services Task Force. (2014). The guide to clinical preventive services 2014. Retrieved from http://www.ahrq.gov

World Health Organization. (2015). Epidemiology. Available at http://www.who.int/topics/epidemiology/en/

WHO/UNAIDS. (2011). Global HIV/AIDS response: Progress report 2011. Available at www.unaids.org/en/media/unaids/. . ./20111130_UA_Report_en.pdf

5

Head, Ears, Nose, Throat, and Eye

Judith Shannon Lynch, MS, MA, APRN-BC, FAANP

General Approach to Ear, Nose, and Throat Health Problems

- Always use proper equipment, including:
  - A pneumatic otoscope
  - Anterior rhinoscope
- Treat acute presentations with antibiotics ONLY after the appropriate history, physical examination, and testing are completed.
- Listen to the patient's story: This will give you important diagnostic clues.
- Do not rely on clinical data alone. Know your anatomical landmarks.

ENT Emergencies Must Be Referred Immediately. These Include:

- Epiglottitis—Inflammation of the epiglottis most often due to infection. It can rapidly result in airway obstruction. Attempting to examine the oral cavity or inserting a tongue blade to examine the pharynx may result in acute airway obstruction.
- Angioedema—Abrupt onset of nonpitting, nonpruritic edema with lesions on lips, periorbital area, extremities, abdominal viscera, and genitalia. There may be associated urticaria. This is caused by either mast-cell or non mast-cell mediated mechanisms and may lead to laryngeal edema.
- Malignant otitis externa—Potentially life-threatening infection involving the external auditory canal, temporal bone, and surrounding

structures. It has an aggressive course and can result in a high mortality rate.
- Ludwig's angina—Rapidly progressive gangrenous cellulitis of the soft tissues of the neck and the floor of the mouth. It may result in airway obstruction.
- Tympanic membrane perforation—NEVER try to remove cerumen if there is a suspicion or history of perforation.
- Peritonsillar abscess.
- Rhinosinusitis complications:
  - External facial edema
  - Erythema or cellulitis over a suspected sinus
  - Diplopia or difficulty with EOMs
  - Proptosis

Abnormal neurological signs: facial drooping, drooling

Disorders of Balance

The Peripheral Vestibular System

The human ear has two divisions:
- Hearing portion (cochlea)
- Balance portion (peripheral meaning outside the central nervous system). This contains a network of tubes (semicircular canals) and sacs (the vestibule). These structures are filled with a fluid (endolymph). The perilymph fluid fills spaces between the semicircular canals, the vestibule, and the bone. The inner ear is called the labyrinth due to its anatomic complexity.

As the head position changes, endolymph moves within the inner ear and bends tiny hairs of sensory cells inside the canals. This initiates nerve impulses that pass along the vestibule-cochlear nerve to the brain.

These impulses provide information to the brain about changes in head position.

The brain then sends commands to initiate ocular movement. This is what enables clarity of vision, and also commands travel to muscles allowing balance AS MOTION OCCURS.

Defining Vertigo

The initial question must be one that establishes the person's perception of the word "dizzy." Once a subjective statement is precise, this early clue will lead to appropriate assessment strategies. Knowledge of the four most common types of complaints will guide this evaluation:

- Type 1: VERTIGO is a definite ROTATIONAL sensation in which the person feels as if (s)he or the environment is rotating. This may begin spontaneously, is episodic, and, when severe, may be accompanied by nausea, vomiting, and ataxia. These problems are almost always due to a problem in the peripheral labyrinth.

- Type 2: PRESYNCOPE is a sensation of an impending loss of consciousness, often beginning with vision loss and a roaring tinnitus. This usually implies inadequate blood perfusion to the brain rather than a focal event. It is usually gradual in onset and often is indicative of a metabolic disorder such as hypoglycemia or a rapid change in blood pressure such as with postural hypotension.

- Type 3: DISEQUILIBRIUM is a sense of impaired balance and gait frequently due to impaired motor function control.

- Type 4: LIGHTHEADEDNESS is an ill-defined term often referred to as a sensation of "wooziness" or "feeling drunk" and is usually a diagnosis of exclusion. It occurs with psychiatric problems, hyperventilation, various encephalopathies, and as part of a geriatric syndrome that often reveals associations between vertigo and cardiovascular, neurological, psychological, and sensory disorders.

Peripheral Vertigo Pathophysiology

Spatial orientation is automatic but complex. Continued sensory monitoring assesses the position of the body in space in relation to the surrounding environment. The five sensory modalities constantly sample position and motion: vision, vestibular sensation, proprioception, touch and pressure, and hearing. Normally, the brain integrates input from each of these modalities, giving a comprehensive image of position and movement in space. When the orienting image is unreliable, proprioception becomes impaired and the result is a sensation of vertigo. This could be central (brain) vertigo or, more commonly, peripheral (inner ear, 8th cranial nerve).

- CENTRAL—least common type, usually caused by:
  - Ischemia—Common after a CVA
  - Demylelinative disorder—Multiple sclerosis, Parkinson's disease
  - Neoplasms—Rare cause. Even an acoustic neuroma (see SNHL) causes vertigo in only about 20% of cases.
  - Head trauma with concussion—Acute problem and observable
  - Autoimmune diseases—Vertigo is part of the complex of systems found in Lyme disease, syphilis, and systemic lupus erythematosus when the disease affects the central nervous system.
- PERIPHERAL:
  - Benign paroxysmal positional vertigo
  - Vestibular migraine
  - Ménière's disease
  - Head trauma, especially under 50 years of age
  - Otitis media, acute sinusitis, whiplash injury to the cervical spine, and degenerative changes associated with aging
  - High doses or long-term use of ototoxic antibiotics
  - Labyrinthitis, usually from a viral infection

Benign Paroxysmal Positional Vertigo (BPPV)

Definition

This is a disorder of the inner ear that produces vertigo with certain head movements due to debris collected within the cochlea. This debris is thought to be small crystals of calcium carbonate derived from structures called "otoliths" that have been damaged by head trauma, infection, or degeneration of the inner ear due to aging.

Incidence/Prevalence

BPPV is fairly common, with an estimated incidence of 107/100,000/year and a lifetime prevalence of 2.4%. It is usually not a pediatric problem but can affect adults of any age, especially the elderly population. The majority of cases occur for no determined etiology, with many people describing that they simply went to get out of bed and the room began to spin.

Etiology

- Idiopathic in more than 50% of cases.
- Viruses affecting the ear—Vestibular neuritis, TIAs, Ménière's disease
- Head trauma
- Degeneration of the vestibular system in the elderly patient

Risk Factors

- Aging
- Head injury
- Recent viral illness
- Occasionally following a surgical procedure—Combination of trauma to the inner ear during surgery and a prolonged period of supine positioning.
- Irrigating the ear with water can cause a transient vertigo with presyncopal/syncopal sequelae.

Historical Data

- Sudden onset
- Abrupt awakening with a spinning sensation while turning over in bed
- Nystagmus—Rapid oscillation of the eyeballs
- Transient—Episodic and lasting seconds to minutes
- Aggravated by head movements, changes in position, riding in a fast car or on an amusement park ride
- May be unilateral or bilateral
- Associated with nausea and vomiting
- Hearing loss, tinnitus, and aural fullness may be present
- Asymptomatic between episodes

Physical Assessment

- Orthostatic blood pressure readings
- Otoscopic examination of the middle ear
- Weber and Rinne testing—See acute otitis media/otitis media with effusion.
- Nasal and sinus evaluation to r/o sinus disease
- Cranial nerve assessment
- Cervical spine assessment to r/o degenerative disease and trauma
- Romberg, tandem walk, and march–in-place testing
- Hyperventilation testing if psychiatric disorder is suspected
- Assessment of the eyes:
  - Pupils—Especially following trauma
  - Extraocular movements testing for nystagmus
  - Vestibular testing. In primary care, the most common test is the Dix–Hallpike maneuver.

Diagnostic Studies

- Weber and Rinne testing will be normal in BPPV.
- Audiometric testing if available
- Dix-Hallpike—The patient is asked to turn his head. A rapid change in position from sitting to supine (with the head hanging over the edge of the examination table) will produce active rotary nystagmus when the head is turned so that the affected ear is facing the floor. This may be accompanied by nausea. A positive response is diagnostic for BPPV.
- Blood analysis is sometimes helpful. This would include:
  - Erythrocyte sedimentation rate to r/o inflammation.
  - Rheumatoid factor, Lyme titer, anti-nuclear antibodies, to r/o (rule out) auto-immune disorders.
  - Lipid profile to r/o possible fat emboli that can affect the 8th cranial nerve.
  - Rapid plasmin reagin to r/o undiagnosed syphilis.
  - Blood glucose, complete blood count, and thyroid-stimulating hormone to r/o metabolic problems.

Management

- Non-pharmacologic:
  - Supportive treatments:
    - Rest for 48–72 hours
    - Clear fluids when there is nausea and vomiting

- No driving
- A soft cervical collar
- Epley canalith repositioning maneuver may be performed. The patient is placed in the supine position with the head hanging position as earlier with the affected ear facing the floor. At 30-second intervals, specific head rotations permit the misplaced otolithic material to transit through the semicircular canal and be returned to the utricle, removing the cause of the problem. After the Epley is performed, the patient must be advised to:
  - Keep head erect for 48 hours
  - Avoid reaching for objects in high places, looking up suddenly, or bending over
  - Change position slowly

    The Epley maneuver eliminates vertigo in about 80% of patients after one treatment. There may be frequent vertigo recurrence over the next 6–10 weeks and the maneuver can be repeated a second time. Symptoms usually taper off gradually, with no episode matching the intensity of the original attack.

- Pharmacologic:
  - Diazepam 2–5 mg (benzodiazepine) administration bid can be used in the acute period as a muscle and central nervous system relaxant and antianxiety agent allowing the patient to rest.
  - Meclizine 12.5–25 mg (antihistamine) may be used as an alternative, but often makes the patient feel lightheaded and can mask the etiology of the disease.

Patient Education

- This is an anxiety-producing problem and the patient will need a complete explanation of the etiology and natural course of the disease.
- Emphasize no driving for self-protection and to avoid posing a danger to others.
- Discuss the self-limited nature of BPPV.
- Discuss fall risk, especially with the older patient.

Indications for Referral

- Refractory vertigo lasting more than 2 weeks, becoming more intense, or occurring with greater frequency.
- If a central etiology is suspected, make immediate referral to the appropriate health care provider.

- Physical therapy for vestibular therapy if peripheral vertigo becomes prolonged.

Expected Course

- Usually self-limited, with some less intense recurrence.
- Follow up in 7–10 days for reevaluation.

Other Peripheral Vertigo Etiologies

Vestibular Neuritis/Labyrinthitis
Definition
This affects the vestibular-cochlear nerve (8th cranial nerve) which has two branches. The cochlear branch transmits messages from the ear, and the vestibular branch transmits messages from the peripheral balance system. Neuritis affects the balance portion, resulting in vertigo but no change in hearing. Labyrinthitis occurs when an infection affects both branches, resulting in hearing changes as well as vertigo. Etiologies include:

- Bacterial infections, usually associated with untreated otitis media. It usually manifests in mild symptoms.
- Viral infections are more common and may be the result of a systemic viral illness (infectious mononucleosis, rubeola), herpes (varicella, zoster), influenza, hepatitis, Epstein–Barr.
- Symptoms:
  - Mild to severe
  - Subtle vertigo to violent spinning
  - Nausea, vomiting, unsteadiness, visual changes, impaired concentration
  - Tinnitus and hearing loss in labyrinthitis
- Treatment:
  1. Diphenhydramine, Meclizine, Phenergan, Ativan, Diazepam ONLY if other etiologies have been ruled out. These medications are used to suppress vertigo.
  2. Oral prednisone to reduce neural irritation
  3. Antibiotics if there is acute otitis media
  4. IV antibiotics with severe nausea and vomiting
  5. If treated promptly, many infections cause no permanent damage; sometimes permanent hearing loss results.
- Referral:

  *If you are unsure of etiology, refer immediately to otolaryngology!

Ménière's Disease
Definition
This is a chronic incurable vestibular disorder, a form of endolymphatic hydrops that produces a recurring set of symptoms due to abnormal amounts of fluid called endolymph collecting in the inner ear. Etiology is unknown. Theories include circulatory disease, allergies, auto-immune disorders, migraine headaches, and, possibly, genetics. An episode can be triggered by stress, overwork, fatigue, emotional distress, systemic illness, pressure changes, certain foods, and a large sodium intake.

- Symptoms:
  - Aura common and may include:
    - Balance disturbance
    - Vertigo
    - Headache
    - Increased aural pressure
    - Hearing loss increase
    - Tinnitus increase
    - Sensitivity to sound
    - Uneasy feeling
  - During an attack:
    - Spontaneous violent vertigo
    - Fluctuating hearing loss
    - Aural pressure
    - Roaring tinnitus
      ***These four symptoms MUST be present to make a diagnosis of Ménière's disease.
- Treatment—This is not treated in primary care and, if suspected, a referral to otolaryngology is necessary, especially to secure an audiologic evaluation during an attack.

Hearing Loss

Conductive Hearing Loss
Description
This occurs when there is a problem conducting sound waves anywhere along the channel from the ear canal through the tympanic membrane into the middle ear space. It may occur alone or with sensorineural hearing loss (mixed loss). It is usually temporary, fluctuating, and mild.

Incidence
More children in the Western world visit their provider because of middle ear disease than for any other health problem. Among groups of Aboriginal children, the incidence may be as high as 50–90%. Other populations known to have a high incidence are the Maori of New Zealand, Pacific Islanders, Native Americans, and the Canadian Inuit.

Otosclerosis is the most common cause of progressive hearing loss in young adults. All ages are affected and prevalence is equal among genders.

Etiology
- Malformation of the outer ear, ear canal, or middle ear structures (ossicles)
- Fluid in the middle ear from episodes of acute otitis media
- Nasal allergies
- Eustachian tube dysfunction
- Perforated tympanic membrane
- Benign tumors of the middle ear with ossicular erosion (cholesteatoma)
- Cerumen impaction
- Acute otitis externa
- Foreign body in ear canal
- Otosclerosis

Risk Factors
- Genetics—Otosclerosis (immobility of the ossicles of the middle ear)
- Middle ear disease—Recurrent acute otitis media
- Otitis media with effusion
- Nasal allergies
- Cerumen impaction
- Head trauma

Historical Data
- Patient usually complains of a unilateral hearing loss.
- Young children often have speech problems or language delay.
- Parents complain that children are not doing well in school.
- Patient will often have a long history of acute otitis media or otitis media with effusion.
- Often asymptomatic

Physical Assessment
Always Use a Pneumatic Otoscope to Assess Tympanic Mobility*
- Cerumen impaction or foreign body in ear canal
- Tympanic membrane may be perforated as a result of acute otitis media.

- Tympanic membrane may be dull and retracted or immobile due to the presence of fluid.
- Tympanometry (if available) will show negative pressure or the presence of fluid.
- Audiology (if available) shows the presence of an "air-bone gap," where hearing is superior when sound is transmitted in such a way that it bypasses the ossicles in the middle ear.
- Nasal exam will often show the presence of congestion and clear drainage.

Differential Diagnosis

- Sensorineural hearing loss
- Mixed hearing loss
- Congenital hearing loss
- Superior canal dehiscence—very rare—surgery required

Diagnostic Studies

- Assess hearing acuity to a whispered or spoken voice.
- Weber test—Place tuning fork in center of skull at hairline. Patient with normal hearing or with a symmetrical hearing loss localizes the tone either in the center of the head or equally in both ears. Patient with a unilateral conductive hearing loss localizes the tone in the diseased ear.
- Rinne test—If air conduction is better than bone conduction, the test is POSITIVE. This is the finding in normal hearing or sensorineural hearing loss. If bone conduction is better than air conduction, the test is NEGATIVE. This is found in conductive hearing loss. Ask the patient if the tuning fork placed in front of the ear is heard better than when placed in back of the ear upon the mastoid process without striking it again.

Complications

- Delayed speech
- Social problems
- Isolation from loss of communication, especially in the elderly
- Safety in the elderly
- Middle ear problems may progress to chronic problems—chronic otitis media.
- Otosclerosis may worsen during pregnancy.

- Untreated cholesteatoma can cause balance problems, facial nerve paralysis, meningitis, and brain abscesses.

Management

- Non-pharmacologic/pharmacologic:
  - Keep ear canals free of cerumen—Over-the-counter drops are available; discuss dangers of self-irrigation.
  - In cases of AOM, OME, see the AOM/OME section.
  - In cases of a perforated tympanic membrane, invoke strict water precautions. See the AOE section.
  - Surgical:
    - Head trauma
    - Cholesteatoma
    - Otosclerosis
    - Myringotomy tubes for protracted cases of otitis media with effusion
    - Hearing aids

Patient Education/Prevention

1. Avoid Q-tip, finger tip, and hair pin use in external auditory canal.
2. Prompt treatment of all episodes of acute otitis media
3. Use protective measures when flying to prevent Eustachian tube dysfunction.

Indications for Referral

- Any conductive hearing loss that does not respond after initial treatment
- Sensorineural hearing loss
- Sudden hearing loss
- Audiologist for hearing aid evaluation/hearing aid management
- Speech therapist if speech delay or impediment
- Neurotology if intracranial lesion suspected or surgery in middle ear is needed

Expected Course

- Temporary hearing problems are reversible when related to common health issues. Eustachian tube dysfunction, acute otitis media, cerumen impaction, foreign body in external auditory canal.
- Less common/surgical problems will have a longer and, sometimes a progressive, course.

Sensorineural Hearing Loss (SNHL)

Description

The dysfunction is in the inner ear (cochlea), the 8th cranial nerve, or both. In the elderly client, it is known as presbycusis.

Incidence/Prevalence

Roughly 1–3/1,000 children are born with profound hearing loss and 3–5/1,000 are born with mild to moderate hearing loss that may affect language. Prevalence of hearing loss requiring intervention from infants coming out of neonatal ICUs is 1–4%.

Prevalence of hearing loss in adolescence aged 12–19 years has increased in the U.S. over the past 10 years. Significant hearing loss (>25 decibels) has increased to 1 in 20 adolescents. SNHL contributes to the increasing incidence in this population. There is some evidence that adolescents may have a mid to high frequency hearing loss that is irreversible.

Globally, SNHL occurs in 9–27/1,000 children. No gender difference is known.

The incidence of SNHL increases with age.

Etiology

- Aging with degeneration of nerves leading from the cochlea to the brain
- Congenital syndromes
- Prenatal infections—Cytomegalovirus, herpes, rubella, toxoplasmosis
- Fetal exposure to teratogens—Thalidomide, retinoic acid
- Long-term exposure to environmental noise (occupational or recreational)
- Long-term playing of loud music at high decibels with/without earphones
- Smoking/second-hand smoke
- Infectious diseases
- Immunological responses
- Ménière's disease

Classification of Hearing Loss

The American National Standards Institute defines hearing loss in terms of decibels lost.

- Slight   16–25 dB
- Mild   26–40 dB
- Moderate   41–54 dB
- Moderately severe   55–70 dB
- Severe   71–90 dB
- Profound   greater than 90 dB

Risk Factors

- Increasing age
- Occupations with high levels of noise/no ear protection—Construction, factory work
- Genetics
- Prematurity, low birth weight, low Apgar score, Hyperbilirubinemia
- Childhood infections—Meningitis, mumps
- Ototoxic medications—Aminoglycosides, furesomide, aspirin
- Multisystem autoimmune disorders
  - Systemic lupus erythematous
  - Rheumatoid arthritis
  - Sjögren's syndrome
  - Ulcerative colitis
  - Sudden SNHL—Some evidence of a viral etiology causing irritation/damage to the 8th cranial nerve
  - Metabolic diseases—Diabetes mellitus
  - Infectious diseases—Syphilis
  - Trauma to temporal bone

Historical Data

- Patient may or may not be aware of a hearing loss. In presbycusis, it is a bilateral loss.
- Hears better in quiet settings—Ambient noise increases inability to hear.
- May be associated with tinnitus (noise in affected ears).
- May be associated with vertigo.
- Sudden SNHL—May be viral or an acoustic neuroma. This is a benign slow-growing tumor that develops on the 8th cranial nerve.

  *This demands an immediate referral to otolaryngology. Do not assume it is an otitis media with effusion unless you have evidence of fluid in the middle ear.**

- In childhood:
  - Problems in school
  - Falling grades

- Lack of attention to parental directions
- Language delay
  *All infants are screened for hearing loss before leaving the hospital after birth.

- Thorough history of any known autoimmune or infectious disease

Physical Assessment

- Patient may speak loudly.
- Otological exam is usually completely within normal limits.
- May fail whispered hearing screening.

Differential Diagnosis

*A note about presbycusis. It is usually bilateral, associated with advancing age and identified by a gradual hearing loss often associated with tinnitus and reduced hearing sensitivity and speech understanding in noisy environments.

- Conductive hearing loss
- Ménière's disease
- Ototoxicity
- Viral labyrinthitis

Diagnostic Studies

- Assess hearing acuity to whispered voice
- Weber test (see conductive hearing loss) will lateralize to unaffected ear
- Rinne test (see conductive hearing loss) air conduction > bone conduction bilaterally
- Laboratory testing if a known or suspected autoimmune disease
  - Sedimentation rate
  - Lyme titer
  - RPR titer
  - Rheumatoid factor
  - Antinuclear antibody titer
- Vestibular testing if associated vertigo (see vertigo)

Complications

- Isolation in the elderly client
- Safety in the elderly
- Loss of communication
- Long-term tinnitus
- Vertiginous disorders

Management

- Non-pharmacologic:
  - Ear protection is mandatory to prevent progressive SNHL.
  - Annual hearing tests for persons in occupations with loud noise exposure
  - Smoking cessation
  - Reduce volume on mobile devices—iPods, MP3 players
  - Hearing aids
  - Adaptive measures—Lip reading, sign language
- Pharmacologic:
  - Discontinue any ototoxic drugs
  - Sudden SNHL—may respond to systemic steroids—immediate referral
- Surgical:
  - Cochlear implants

Patient Education/Prevention

- Routine screening after age 65 years
- Mandatory newborn screening
- Audiological testing after any intracranial infection
- With children, help parents identify available community resources and refer family to a social worker for specialized assistance
- Hearing aids as soon as possible if necessary to increase possibility of normal speech in children, improved hearing in adults

Indications for Referral

- Otolaryngology if any hearing loss of unknown etiology or sudden SNHL
- Genetics if a congenital syndrome is suspected
- Speech therapy if needed
- Endocrinology if metabolic disease is suspected
- Rheumatologist if autoimmune disease is suspected
- Neurotology if acoustic neuroma is suspected

Expected Course

- Presbycusis and SNHL are usually progressive and irreversible
- Sudden SNHL may be reversed with immediate referral to otolaryngology

Acute Otitis Media (AOM)/Otitis Media with Effusion (OME)

Definition

AOM is an inflammation of the middle ear often associated with a viral upper respiratory infection. Organisms enter through the nasopharynx into the sterile middle ear creating purulent exudates and increased pressure.

Otitis media with effusion (OME) is the presence of an effusion in the middle ear without infection. It can follow an episode of AOM, especially in the pediatric population. In adults, it is associated with Eustachian tube dysfunction (ETD).

Incidence

AOM is the most common condition for which antibacterial agents are prescribed for children in the U.S. Current incidence is 634/1,000 children. It occurs most frequently between ages 6 months and 2 years and is rare in adults. It is most common in spring and autumn months.

OME—at least 90% children have at least one episode by age 10 years.

Etiology

AOM

- Follows viral upper respiratory illness causing Eustachian tube dysfunction.

- Viral—includes respiratory syncytial virus, parainfluenza, influenza, enteroviruses, adenoviruses.
- Bacterial causes:
  - Streptococcus pneumonia 40–50%
  - Hemophilus influenza 20–30%
  - Moraxella catarrhalis 10–15%
  - Staphylococcus aureus 2–4%

OME

- Residual middle ear fluid s/p AOM
- Eustachian tube dysfunction. The Eustachian tube runs from the middle ear to the nasopharynx (see Figure 5-1). In children, these tubes are short and horizontal, allowing them to become easily edematous or obstructed. Adults have longer Eustachian tubes at an angle and are less prone to dysfunction.
- Etiologies include:
  - Allergies
  - Upper respiratory infections and acute sinusitis
  - Excessive mucous and saliva produced during wheezing
  - Infected or hypertrophied adenoids
  - Tobacco smoke

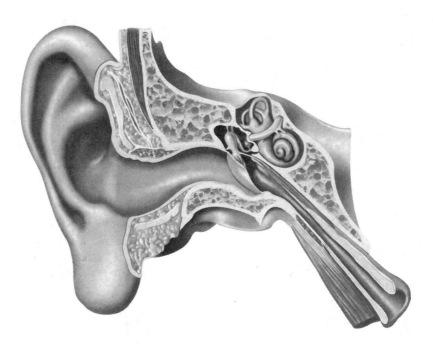

Figure 5-1 Eustachian Tube
© Leonello Calvetti/Science Photo Library/Getty

Risk Factors

AOM

- Day care (increased with more than six children present)
- Changes in altitude/climate
- Second-hand smoke
- Family history of AOM
- Bottle feeding in supine position
- Pacifier after age of 6 months
- Low socioeconomic status
- Poor nutrition
- Comorbid ENT problems—hypertrophied adenoids, cleft palate, allergies
- Immunocompromised
- Ethnicity—Native Americans, Eskimos, and Australian aborigines

OME

- Early onset of first episode of AOM (before 3 months of age)
- Nasal allergies
- Recurrent AOM episodes
- Second-hand smoke
- Adenoidal hypertrophy
- Environmental allergies

Historical Data

AOM

- Preverbal children
  - Tugging, rubbing, holding an ear with excessive crying, fever, or change in sleep or behavior pattern
- Older children
  - Rapid onset of otalgia
  - Fever common
  - Fullness in ear
  - Decreased hearing
  - Popping and crackling sensation in affected ear
  - Vomiting, diarrhea

OME

- Asymptomatic in infants and young children
- Decreased conductive hearing
- Usually no popping or crackling sensation in affected ear

- Sensation of pressure and fullness
- Pain may be present but dull.
- May feel lightheaded (adults)

Physical Assessment

ALWAYS use a pneumatic otoscope to assess tympanic membrane mobility and thoroughly assess the nose, pharynx, and neck. See Figure 5-2 for an illustration of tympanic membrane.

AOM

- Irritated or crying infant or child
- Bulging of the tympanic membrane with inability to identify landmarks
- Erythema of the tympanic membrane with increased vascular markings
- Decreased mobility of tympanic membrane
- May visualize purulent fluid behind the tympanic membrane
- Preauricular or cervical lymphadenopathy with tenderness on affected side
- A normal examination demands looking for comorbidity—acute sinusitis, TMJ dysfunction, dental problems

OME

- Retraction of the tympanic membrane with diffuse light reflex
- Tympanic membrane is dull and pale with frequent air bubbles present in the middle ear.
- Decreased tympanic membrane mobility

Differential Diagnosis

AOM

- Upper respiratory infection
- Crying causing erythema of tympanic membrane
- Referred pain from jaw, teeth, or nasopharynx—more common in adults
- Trauma
- Bullous myringitis—A blister on top of the tympanic membrane that may rupture causing an immediate cessation of otalgia and bloody discharge from the affected ear.

OME

- Hearing loss
- Eustachian tube dysfunction

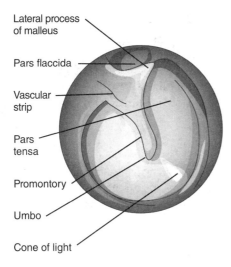

Lateral process of malleus

Pars flaccida

Vascular strip

Pars tensa

Promontory

Umbo

Cone of light

Figure 5-2 Tympanic Membrane

Diagnostic Studies

AOM/OME

- Pneumatic otoscopy. Attempt to remove any cerumen from the ear canal for better visibility but do **NOT** irrigate. Mobility is the key indicator as to whether there is fluid within the middle ear space.

Clinical Pearl

Water is the enemy of the ear and, if the tympanic membrane has perforated, you will introduce infection directly into the middle ear.

- Tympanometry can be used as an adjunct to pneumatic otoscopy but not a substitute. This is more often used to diagnose OME.
- Audiometry (if available) when hearing loss persists > 3 months or at any time with language delay, significant hearing loss, or learning problems.
- CBC if complicated or systemic infection is suspected.

Complications

AOM

- Permanent hearing loss (conductive)
- Speech difficulties and delay (children)
- Balance disturbances
- Tympanic membrane perforation
- Facial nerve paralysis
- Otic hydrocephalus

- Mastoiditis
- Cholesteatoma
- Tympanosclerosis
- Intracranial abscess
- Meningitis

OME

- Tympanic membrane atelectasis
- Atrophy of tympanic membrane
- Retraction pockets
- Conductive hearing loss
- Cholesteatoma
- Tympanosclerosis
- Fixation of the ossicles

Management

AOM

Non-pharmacologic:

- Fever control
- Warm water bottle to affected ear
- Pain control—Use of ibuprofen or acetaminophen in correct doses for age and weight

Pharmacologic:

- Either viruses or bacteria can cause AOM. Antibiotics will not help an infection caused by a virus. All children less than 6 months of age should, however, be treated with an antibiotic. Other reasons to prescribe an antibiotic may include:
  - Under age 2 years
  - Fever greater than 103 degrees F
  - Appears ill
  - No improvement in 24–48 hours
  - Initial antibiotics:
    - Amoxicillin—Do not use if child has taken medication within the past 30 days, has concurrent purulent conjunctivitis, or is allergic to penicillin.
    - Pediatric dosing:
      - Suspension 125, 200, 250, 400 mg/kg based on age and weight po bid or tid × 10 days
        - Under 3 months 20–30 mg/kg/day po divided q12 hours.

- Over 3 months 25–45 mg/kg/day po divided q12 hours.
- Ages 6–12 years 80–90 mg/kg/day po divided q8–12 hours.
- Adult dosing:
- Tablets 250, 500, 875 mg po bid (dependent on infection severity) × 10 days
  - 875 mg po bid × 10 days for serious infections
  - 500 mg po bid-tid for less severe infections
- Amoxicillin-clavulinic acid based on age and weight
- Pediatric dosing:
  - Suspension 250/125, 500/125, 875/125 mg po bid × 10 days
    - Under 3 months 30 mg/kg/day po divided q12 hours
    - Over 3 months 25–45 mg/kg/day po divided q12 hours
  - Adult dosing:
  - Tablets 250/125, 500/125, 875/125 mg po bid × 10 days
- Azithromycin based on age and weight × 10 days

  Use when patients are allergic to penicillin
- Pediatric dosing:
  - 100/5mL, 200/5mL
    - 10 mg/kg po × 1 day—then 5 mg/kg/day po q24 hours × 4 days
  - Adult dosing:
  - Tablets 250, 500, 600 mg
    - 500 mg po × 1 day—then 250 mg po × 4 days
- Other categories of antibiotics can be used if there is no positive response or worsening symptoms after 24–48 hours. These include:
  - Cephalosporins—Use caution with patients sensitive to penicillin because there is a cross-sensitivity greater than 10%.
  - Erythromycin-Sulfisoxazole—Do not use with sulfa allergy.
  - Trimethasone-sulfamethozazole—Do not use with sulfa allergy.

- Decongestants are not effective in AOM.
- Adverse reactions may include nausea, vomiting, diarrhea, rash, and, rarely a systemic allergic reaction. The medication should be promptly discontinued and your office notified.

OME

- Non-pharmacologic:
  - Watchful waiting—Most effusions resolve spontaneously. However, an OME persisting for more than 3 months has a spontaneous resolution rate of only 10–15%.
  - Chewing gum
  - Use Valsalva maneuver to facilitate opening of the Eustachian tubes
  - After 3 months, audiometric evaluation is mandatory (referral).
  - Appropriate management of nasal allergies if present (see Allergic Rhinitis)
- Pharmacologic:
  - Decongestants/antihistamines are NOT recommended because they are ineffective unless there is the presence of nasal allergies.
  - Mucolytics (Gauifenesin) are helpful in keeping the middle ear fluid from drying and becoming sticky (glue ear).
  - Intranasal steroids may be used if there is the presence of nasal allergies.
  - There is some evidence that systemic steroids are helpful in adults but are **NOT** recommended in children of any age.
  - Antibiotic therapy has largely been discontinued in cases of OME.
- Surgical
  - Myringotomy with tube placement
  - Adenoidectomy with myringotomy with/without tube placement

Patient Education

AOM

- Thorough explanation of medication prescribed, along with discussion of dosing, timing, and adverse events. Instructions on calling the office with signs of allergy.
- Comforting techniques
- Discourage second-hand smoke

- Discourage pacifier use if child is over 6 months of age.

OME

- Patience with resolution of symptoms. The patient will note popping and crackling sensations in the affected ear as fluid dries. This is a good sign that the effusion is resolving.
- If surgery becomes necessary, the patient will be referred to otolaryngology. You can explain to the parent(s) that this is a very common procedure consisting of the insertion of a tiny tube into the eardrum, keeping a small hole open that allows air to get in so fluids can drain easily. Usually, tubes fall out by themselves after a period of time unique to each patient.

Indications for Referral

AOM

- Cases of treatment failure following the use of a second- or third-line drug
- Multiple AOM episodes
- Signs of intratemporal or intracranial complications including:
  - Mastoiditis
  - Facial nerve paralysis
  - Intracranial abscess
  - Necrotizing OM
  - Otic hydrocephalus

OME

- Fluid persists more than 3 months
- Bilateral hearing loss
- Vertigo
- Retraction pocket
- Craniofacial abnormalities—Cleft palate, Down syndrome
- Eustachian tube dysfunction
- Suspected ossicular discontinuity or fixation
- Suspected middle ear anomaly
- Tympanic membrane perforation, nonresponsive to treatment within 48–72 hours

Expected Course

AOM

- Simple cases resolve in 7–10 days and should be reevaluated 2 weeks afterward.

OME

- Middle ear effusions commonly persist after course of treatment for AOM.
- Effusion is present in 60% of cases at 2 weeks, 40% at 4 weeks, 20% at 2 months, 10% at 3 months.
- Recheck can be in 2–8 weeks, depending on reliability of patient or parent.

Prevention

AOM/OME

Wash hands and toys.

- If possible, use a day care center with less than 6 children.
- Avoid pacifiers.
- Breastfeed. If bottle feeding, always hold baby in upright position.
- NO second-hand smoke
- Immunizations up to date. Pneumococcal vaccine prevents infections from bacteria that commonly cause AOM.
- Avoid overuse of antibiotics because this leads to antibiotic resistance.
- Avoiding AOM will reduce the risk of OME, especially in infants and children.

Otitis Externa

Definition

Generalized inflammation of the external ear canal, which may also involve the pinna or tympanic membrane.

Incidence

1/100–250. Most prevalent during the summer months. No gender difference.

Etiology

Primary etiology is from water trapped in the ear canal that allows bacteria that normally inhabits the skin and ear canal to multiply and infect the ear canal. Other causes include ears traumatized by Q-tip use, fungal infections, and various dermatological conditions including eczema, psoriasis, and seborrheic dermatitis.

Common bacterial causes:

- *Pseudomonas aeruginosa* (most common)
- *Proteus mirabilis*
- *Staphylococcus aureus*
- *Streptococcus pyogenes*

Common fungal causes:
- Aspergillus (most common)
- Candida albicans

Desired Outcome
- Clinical resolution is primary.
- Minimization of ineffective treatments
- Eradication of pathogens
- Minimization of recurrence, cost, complications, and adverse events
- Increased patient satisfaction
- Allowance of the continued use of hearing aids

Risk Factors
- Swimming
- Foreign body, especially in pediatric patients
- Cerumen impaction
- Hot humid weather
- Prolonged use of earplugs
- Hearing aid use
- Dermatological problems
- Diabetes mellitus
- Immunosuppression
- Q-tip use
- Inadequate drying of ears after showers
- Use of chemical irritants (hairsprays)
- Anatomic factors—Narrow ear canals
- Presence of tympanostomy tubes in middle ear

Historical Data
- Intense pruritus
- Otalgia—Usually unilateral, often severe
- Fever, lymphadenopathy—When virulent
- Erythema and edema of the ear canal—Rarely the tympanic membrane
- Exudate—Color varies from white to gray, yellow, or green
- Hearing loss if edema severe

Physical Assessment
ALWAYS do a thorough assessment of the nose, pharynx, and neck in addition to the otoscopic examination.
- Erythema of the ear canal
- Purulent discharge and debris
- Pain on movement of tragus or pinna

- Possible inflammation of periauricular lymph nodes
- Possible low-grade fever

Differential Diagnosis
- Tempomandibular joint dysfunction—Clinical Pearl: most common etiology for adult ear pain
- Perforated tympanic membrane
- Eruption of a wisdom tooth
- Foreign body
- Mastoiditis—Tenderness over mastoid bone is present

Diagnostic Studies
Culture may be indicated only in cases of treatment failure or underlying medical condition

Complications
- Osteomyelitis of temporal bone
- Cholesteatoma in middle ear
- Mastoiditis

Management
Non-pharmacologic:
- Do NOT irrigate the ear canal!
- If edema is present and debris is present in the ear canal to the extent that you cannot see into the canal, do NOT place the otoscope into the canal. This will cause severe pain. An attempt to remove debris GENTLY may be attempted with a curette.
- Wick placement is helpful with a greatly narrowed lumen to draw in ear drops; leave in place for 48–72 hours.
- Place hot water bottle on outer ear for analgesia.
- No swimming until complete resolution.

Pharmacologic:
- Pain medication—Opioids may be necessary for first 24–48 hours. Give small doses.
- Bacterial causes
  - TOPICAL otic antibiotics
    - Ofloxacin Otic gtts (drops); 3–5 gtts bid (two times a day) × 7 days
    - Ciprofloxacin and Dexamethasone Otic gtts 4 bid × 7 days—This is optimal because it contains both an antibiotic and a steroid.

■ Cortisporin Otic (Neomycin, hydrocortisone, colestin, thonzonium bromide)—Gtts 5 tid–qid (three times a day to four times a day) × 10 days. The quinolones have replaced these drops because they have better efficacy.

– If patient is immunocompromised, an oral antibiotic MAY be needed. Quinolones are the optimal drugs in adults.

- Fungal causes:
  – Acetic acid—Acidifying agent to inhibit fungal growth
  – Clortrimazole solution—Gtts 3–5 bid × 10 days
  – OTC Lotrimin solution can also be used.
  – Clinical Pearl: Fungal infections take much longer to resolve.

Patient Education

- Teach patient the correct use of ear drops.
- Emphasize that a wick should be in place for 48–72 hours and there may be some hearing loss in the affected ear.
- No water in ear canal—Teach earplug precautions for showers. (**Clinical Pearl:** Put dry cotton ball in ear canal and put Vaseline over cotton to waterproof ear canal.)
- Call if pain or edema increases, fever persists, or lymphadenopathy becomes more pronounced.
- Follow up should be in 72 hours when wick is removed and additional evaluation is made.
- If patient wears a hearing aid, remove for the first week of infection unless absolutely necessary.

Indications for Referral

- Presence of facial paralysis
- Erythema and edema over mastoid bone
- Granulation in ear canal
- Unresolved fever and lymphadenopathy following initial management
- Repeated episodes of otitis externa

Expected Course

- Simple cases resolve with initial treatment.
- Recurrent chronic problems require ongoing monitoring and preventive measures (ear plugs, use of acetic acid otic drops after swimming or showering).

Epistaxis

Definition

Epistaxis is defined as any bleeding from the nostril, nasal cavity, or nasopharynx due to the bursting of a vessel within the nose. Nosebleeds are rarely life-threatening and usually resolve spontaneously but may also be indicative of an underlying health problem. They are classified as anterior (90%) or posterior dependent on the site of bleeding. Posterior bleeds are an emergency and demand a specialist's attention.

Incidence

Approximately 60% of the population will be affected by epistaxis during their lifetime with 6% requiring medical attention. They are rare in children younger than 2 years of age.

Etiology

- Idiopathic
- Direct trauma to nose
- Nose picking
- Foreign body
- Nasal/sinus fracture
- Nasal septal perforation
- Cocaine abuse
- Infection
- Irritant inhalation
- Low humidity in winter months
- Vascular health issues—Aging vessels
- Hypertension
- Coagulation defects—Von Willebrand disease, leukemias, blood dyscrasias, platelet dysfunctions
- Medications:
  – Aspirin
  – Warfarin
  – Non-steroidal anti-inflammatories
  – Clopridogril and other newer anticoagulant medications
- Neoplasm—< 10%—consider in unilateral cases

Risk Factors

See section under Etiology.

Historical Data

Control of significant bleeding takes precedence over a lengthy history.

- Severity, frequency, duration, and laterality of the bleed
- Influence of exercise
- Occurs during sleep
- Associated with migraine headache
- Precipitating and aggravating factors
- Methods used to stop bleeding
- Foreign body (unilateral)
- Past history epistaxis
- Medical comorbid health issues:
  - Hypertension
  - Hepatic disease
  - Von Willebrand disease
  - Coagulation defects
- Medications:
  - Aspirin
  - Anticoagulants
  - Non-steroidal anti-inflammatories
- Positive family history
- Tobacco and alcohol history

Physical Assessment

- Vital signs—Elevated blood pressure (hypertension) or tachycardia (significant blood loss)
- Inspect skin for petechiae/bruising.
- Have patient gently blow nose to clear nasal cavity. Insert a nasal speculum into the cavity and spread naris vertically. Look for obvious bleeding sites on the septum that may be amenable to direct pressure/cautery.
- If bleeding is bilateral or if there is a constant dripping of blood in the posterior pharynx, consider a posterior bleed. These are more common in the elderly, can result in a significant hemorrhage, and may be associated with nausea or coffee-ground emesis.
- Massive epistaxis may be confused with hematemesis or hemoptysis.

Differential Diagnosis

- Hematemesis
- Hemoptysis
- Nasal cocaine use
- Isolated event, especially in children

Diagnostic Studies

- Only needed for recurrent or severe cases!
  - CBC, platelets, prothrombin time, bleeding time
  - Type and cross match
  - Partial prothombin time if on anti-coagulant
  - CT scan of head
  - Run toxicology screening if drug use is suspected.

Complications

- Nasal septal hematoma/perforation
- External nasal deformity
- Mucosal pressure necrosis
- Vasovagal episode
- Acute rhinosinusitis
- Aspiration

Management

Non-pharmacologic:

- Direct pressure to front of nose for up to 20 minutes
- Upright position
- Ice packs
- Nasal saline gel to anterior nose qd (four times a day) for moisturization and prevention of nasal dryness.
- Avoid trauma to nose—No picking or removing scab formations or blowing nose aggressively.
- For anterior bleeds that do not respond to pressure, place a cotton ball moistened with 1:1000 epinephrine or a vasoconstrictor nasal drop just inside the affected naris and apply pressure for 5–10 minutes. You can also cauterize with a silver nitrate stick applied to the bleeding site.
- For posterior bleeds, make immediate referral to ENT office.

Pharmacologic:

- Vasoconstrictors and topical anesthetics for bleeding cessation and analgesia
- Epinephrine
- Antibiotic ointment bid to affected site for 1 week
- Treatment of any underlying health issue

Patient Education

- Avoid blowing nose for 3–4 days, then gentle blowing only.

- Sleep in upright position.
- Apply antibiotic ointment to affected area bid for 1 week.
- Apply icepacks prn (*pro re nata*) to external nose.
- Avoid rubbing site with tissues, fingers.
- Report any new bleeding.

Indications for Referral
- Posterior bleed
- Recurrent epistaxis
- Hematology referral for intractable cases
- Appropriate provider for underlying health issues

Follow-up
- One week to reevaluate bleeding site and check on further episodes

Acute Rhinosinusitis

Definition
Rhinosinusitis (ARS) is the symptomatic inflammation of the paranasal sinuses and nasal cavity. When uncomplicated, there is no clinical evidence of inflammation outside the paranasal sinuses and nasal cavity at the time of diagnosis (neurologic, soft tissue). Chronic sinusitis is not managed in primary care and will not be covered here.

Classification
1. Acute—less than 4 weeks
2. Chronic—lasting more than 12 weeks
3. Bacterial—needing antibiotic therapy
4. Viral—no antibiotics needed
5. Recurrent—four or more annual episodes without persistent episodes in between

Incidence
- Twelve percent of U.S. population (1 in 8 adults) are diagnosed annually, accounting for 30 million diagnoses
- Most common in women between 45 and 64 years of age
- Accounts for more outpatient antibiotic prescriptions than any other illness—82% of visits
- Fifth most common diagnosis responsible for antibiotic therapy

- Direct cost of management exceeds 11 billion dollars/year.
- Additional expenses from lost productivity, reduced job effectiveness, and impaired quality of life

Etiology
- Multiple viruses—See upper respiratory infection.
- Streptococcus pneumonia 20–43%
- Hemophilus influenza 22–35%
- Moraxella catarrhalis 2–10%
- Streptococcus pyogenes and anaerobes 3–7%

Risk Factors
- Viral URI
- Allergy
- Trauma
- Early fall to early spring
- Deviated septum
- Nasal polyps
- Immune system disorder
- Cystic fibrosis
- Gastroesophageal reflux disease
- Exposure to smoke
- Tonsillar and adenoidal hypertrophy, hypertrophied nasal turbinates

Historical Data
The major challenge to correct diagnosis is to differentiate between viral and bacterial disease.
- Nasal drainage and congestion
- Facial pain and pressure, especially when unilateral and focused in the area of a specific sinus group
- Post nasal drip
- Hyposmia/anosmia
- Headache—pressure
- Fever
- Cough worse at night
- Fatigue
- Maxillary dental pain
- Aural fullness/pressure
- Predictive symptoms for bacterial disease include:
  - Worsening symptoms > 5–7 days
  - Persistent symptoms for > 10 days

– Persistent purulent drainage
– Unilateral dental pain
– Unilateral maxillary sinus tenderness
– Persistent fever

Physical Assessment

Always use a Nasal Speculum to Inspect the Inner Nasal Cavity!

- Vital signs to assess fever
- Otoscopic examination to look for otitis media
- Anterior rhinoscopy will show edema and erythema of the nasal mucosa and purulent discharge.
- Sinuses will be tender to palpation—Transillumination of limited/no value.
- Posterior pharynx will show purulent drainage.
- Lungs may be involved if there is comorbid asthma exacerbation.

Differential Diagnosis

- Viral URI
- Dental disease
- Trauma
- Foreign body
- Tension, migraine headache
- Allergy
- Immune disorders, HIV
- Cystic fibrosis

Diagnostic Studies

- No diagnostic test can differentiate between viral and bacterial rhinosinusitis.
- No labs are indicated in routine evaluations.
- Imaging value is limited and CT scans should be reserved for recurrent infections or failure to respond to medical therapy.

Complications

- Chronic rhinosinusitis
- Asthma exacerbation
- Meningitis when infection spreads to brain lining
- Brain abscess
- External facial edema, erythema, or cellulitis over an involved sinus
- Vision changes—Diploplia
- Impaired external ocular movements
- Proptosis
- Impaired cranial nerve function—Drooping face, inability to smile

Management

Non-pharmacologic:

- Hydration
- Steam inhalation
- Saline rinses
- Sleeping with head of bed elevated
- Avoiding tobacco smoke
- Avoiding caffeine, alcohol
- Warm facial packs—Sinus masks are valuable because they can be put in the refrigerator or microwave oven and can be used for the patient's comfort.

Pharmacologic:

- Analgesia:
  - Acetaminophen, especially in children
  - Aspirin
  - Non-steroidal anti-inflammatories
  - Opioids in severe cases only
- Decongestants may be used for a limited time to dry nasal secretions. Avoid promoting tolerance.
- If the patient is on an intranasal steroid for allergies, this may be continued.
- There is no indication for the use of oral corticosteroids.
- Antibiotic therapy

Only about 0.5–2.0% of viral rhinosinusitis are complicated by bacterial infection. In the first 3–4 days of illness, VRS cannot be differentiated from early onset ABRS. Only patients with severe symptoms are presumed to have a bacterial infection. Between 5–10 days of persistent symptoms are consistent with VRS OR may represent the beginning stages of ABRS. In this time period, however, a pattern of initial improvement followed by worsening is consistent with ABRS. Beyond 10 days, residual sinus mucus thickness induced by the virus may persist, but the probability of confirming a bacterial infection is about 60%.

Watchful waiting refers to deferring antibiotic therapy up to seven days after diagnosis and limiting management to supportive measures. Patients are candidates when follow-up is ensured and a system is in place that permits reevaluation. Antibiotics are started if symptoms worsen. This should be decided in concert with the patient after a thorough discussion takes place.

Initial antibiotic therapy:

Choice should be based on predicted effectiveness, cost, safety, and side-effect profile.

- High dose of Amoxicillin 875 mg po bid for 10–14 days
  - Children 6–12 years—Use suspension 80–90 mg/kg/day po divided q8–12 hours
- Amoxicillin-Clavulinic acid (XR)—1 gram po bid for 10 days
  - Children 6–12 years—use suspension 90 mg/6.4 mg/kg/day po divided q12 hours
- For penicillin-allergic patients:
  - Doxycycline 100 mg po bid for 10 days (adults only)
  - Respiratory quinolones—Initial treatment only for penicillin-resistant patients (adults only)
  - Children—Cefpodoximine proxetil, cefuroxamine axetil, cefdinir. Caution with cephalosporins because there is a cross-sensitivity with penicillin greater than 10%.
- Macrolides and sulfa drugs should not be used in the initial treatment due to the high prevalence of U.S. drug resistance, which may lead to treatment failure.

Treatment Failure After 7 Days

- High dose of Amoxicillin—Clavulinic acid—2 gms/day po q12 hours for 10 days
- Levofloxacin 750 mg po qd for 14 days
- Moxifloxacin 400 mg po qd for 14 days
- Children—azithromycin, clarithromycin. TMP/SMX have limited effectiveness and treatment failure is possible.

Oral cephalosporins and macrolides are predicted to offer inadequate coverage for *S. pneumoniae* or *H. influenzae*.

If the patient fails to respond after 3 weeks of antibiotics, consider a CT scan and referral to otolaryngology.

Patient Education

- Every URI is not a sinus infection. Encourage patients to use watchful waiting for 7 days. Explain the differences between a sinus infection and a URI.
- Discuss your area antibiotic drug-resistance rates.
- Supportive measures are as important as medications and will enhance treatment success.

- No smoking or exposure to smoke
- Stress importance of follow-up and contacting you with worsening symptoms.
- Report visual problems or neurological abnormalities immediately.

Indications for Referral

- No treatment success after 3 weeks of antibiotic therapy.
- Presence of chronic sinus disease.
- Anatomic abnormalities—Nasal septal deviation
- Presence of nasal polyps
- Allergy evaluation
- Visual problems
- Neurological impairment

Follow-up

- See patient in 2 weeks or sooner if there are worsening symptoms or a symptom recurrence after initial improvement.

Allergic Rhinitis

Definition

Allergic rhinitis is an inflammatory condition of the nasal mucosa caused by immunoglobulin E(IgE)-mediated early-phase and late-phase hypersensitivity responses, usually to inhalant allergens, similar to those in allergic asthma.

Incidence

- One of the most common diseases affecting adults. Affects 1 in 6 Americans and generates 2–5 billion dollars in direct health expenditures annually.
- Through loss of work and school, allergic rhinitis is responsible for 2–4 billion dollars in lost productivity each year.
- Most common chronic disease in children in the United States
- Fifth most common chronic disease in America
- Prevalence is equal between genders.
- Mean age of onset—8–11 years

Health Burden

- Impairs quality of life
- Poor quality of sleep

- Fatigue
- Poor concentration
- Decreased work and school performance
- Exacerbates asthma
- Major factor is asthma development
- Often comorbid with gastroesophageal reflux disease
- Peaks during adolescence and young adulthood and declines with age

Etiology

When AR patients are exposed to allergens, allergic reactions develop in two different patterns according to time sequence. One is the early reaction, in which sneezing and rhinorrhea develops in 30 minutes and disappears. The other is the late reaction, which shows nasal obstruction approximately 6 hours after exposure to allergens and subsides slowly. The early reaction is the response of mast cells to offending allergens (type I hypersensitivity). Stimulated mast cells induce nasal symptoms by secreting chemical mediators such as histamine, prostaglandins, and leukotrienes. In contrast to the early reaction, eosinophil chemotaxis is the main mechanism in the late reaction, which is caused by chemical mediators produced in the early reaction. Several inflammatory cells, eosinophils, mast cells, and T cells migrate to nasal mucosa, and break up and remodel normal nasal tissue. These processes result in nasal obstruction, which is the main symptom of AR patients.

Risk Factors

- Family history of atopy or allergy
- Asthma
- Pets in house
- Exposure to indoor allergens—Dust mites
- Eczema
- Small family size

Historical Data

- Ocular edema
- Ocular pruritus
- Ear fullness
- Scratchy throat
- Fatigue
- Nasal pruritus
- Nasal congestion
- Hyposmia
- Headache
- Lightheadedness
- Sneezing

Physical Assessment

- Allergic shiners—Circles under eyes
- Allergic salute—Transverse line on external nose from frequent rubbing
- Periorbital edema
- Conjunctivitis
- Pale boggy nasal mucosa
- Blue-tinged turbinates
- Serous otitis media
- Pharyngeal cobblestoning
- Post-nasal drainage
- Signs of coexisting asthma—Wheezing
- Skin—Signs of atopic dermatitis

Differential Diagnosis

- Upper respiratory infection
- Vasomotor rhinitis
- Atrophic rhinitis

Diagnostic Studies

- Allergy Testing
  - Skin Testing is the most specific screening method for detecting IgE antibodies. Should correlate with the patient's history. Not performed in primary care.
  - Blood testing (RAST or ELISA) is preferable when the patient has severe dermatological problems, is taking certain medications, or refuses skin testing. Often done with children. Can be ordered in primary care but you must know what to do with the results. Preferable to have it done in specialist office.

Complications

Poorly controlled symptoms of allergic rhinitis may contribute to sleep loss, secondary daytime fatigue, learning impairment, decreased overall cognitive functioning, decreased long-term productivity and decreased quality of life. Additionally, poorly controlled allergic rhinitis may also contribute to the development of other related disease processes, including acute and chronic sinusitis, the recurrence of nasal polyps, otitis media and otitis media with effusion, hearing impairment, abnormal craniofacial development, sleep apnea and related complications, aggravation of underlying asthma, and an increased propensity to develop asthma.

Management

There are four strategies to ensure the optimal management of allergic rhinitis:

1. Environmental Controls—Avoid all factors that cause symptoms. Keeping a symptom diary is very helpful.

2. Pharmacotherapy:
   - Second-generation antihistamines are the mainstay of pharmacologic management. These are over-the-counter medications that the patient may already be using before diagnosis. They have a rapid onset of action, relieve rhinorrhea, pruritus, and sneezing, and may reduce symptoms in the eyes and throat. They are generally considered ineffective for treating nasal congestion. Older antihistamines have inherent sedative side-effects that may affect cognition and motor function.

   - Topical antihistamines are effective but generally have a bitter taste.

   - Decongestants relieve the symptoms of nasal congestion by constricting the turbinate vessels. They can be used for a short time only because tolerance can occur and they have a serious side-effect profile. Limit use to the immediate attack phase and as an adjunct to treatment during a co-existing URI. Avoid topical decongestants (see URI). Stay away from combination antihistamine/decongestant products as much as possible.

   - Intranasal steroids are the first line of therapy when obstruction is a major component of the patient's rhinitis. They reduce congestion, sneezing, rhinorrhea, palatal pruritus, and coughing. Time to onset is longer than with antihistamines, but they can be given in concert with all antihistamines. These medications have been extensively studied and may be given in some cases to small children and pregnant women. They are safe and many are now over-the-counter.

   - Oral corticosteroids reduce the inflammatory component of allergic rhinitis. They reduce inflammatory cell infiltration in the superficial nasal mucosa, increase sympathetic vascular tone, reduce endothelial and epithelial permeability, decrease the response of mucous glands to cholinergic stimulation, and reduce nasal hyperreactivity. They should be used only when symptoms do not respond to first-line drugs. A short course is appropriate. Use a Medrol Dosepak (methylprednisolone) 4 mg in a tapered dose.

   - Mast cell stabilizers (cromolyn agents) are topical over-the-counter nonsteroid anti-inflammatory agents that block both the early and late phase nasal allergic response. They relieve sneezing, rhinorrhea, nasal congestion, and nasal pruritus. They are most effective when used 4–6 times/day, starting early relative to the allergen exposure and continued throughout the exposure period.

   - Anticholinergics can be tried if other medications are not effective. They are not well absorbed by the nasal mucosa and do not relieve nasal congestion, pruritus, or sneezing.

   - Leukotriene receptor antagonists should only be used in the patient who has established asthma comorbid with allergic rhinitis. These drugs are not routinely used in primary care.

3. Evaluate for immunotherapy in the following patients:
   - There is a long allergen season.
   - Patient has year-round symptoms.
   - Patient does not respond to medications.
   - Symptoms are worsening.
   - Presence of chronic or recurrent rhinosinusitis.
   - Presence of chronic or recurrent middle ear disease.

4. Patient education and follow-up—See the following.

Patient Education

- Education should begin at the time of diagnosis and be integrated into every step of clinical care.
- Teach risks of anaphylaxis
  - Faintness
  - Syncope
  - Difficulty breathing
  - Throat closing
  - Skin rash, hives
  - Trouble talking, swallowing
  - Chest tightness/pain
- Give instructions about use of an epinephrine auto-pen if necessary.
- Keep therapy simple.

- Number of medications:
  - Doses/day
  - Costs and insurance coverage policies
- Enlist family support
- Be open to alternative therapies as long as they are not harmful.
- Use educational materials to support your education.

Indications for Referral

- Patient does not respond to first-line medications and environmental control.
- Immunotherapy evaluation
- Chronic comorbid conditions—Asthma, rhinosinusitis, middle ear disease, gastroesophageal reflux disease
- Severe symptoms

Follow-up

- Three to four weeks after initial treatment plan of environmental controls and first-line medications
- This is a chronic disease needing frequent follow-up. Patient should be seen on a monthly basis until symptoms have decreased.

Other Forms of Rhinitis

Vasomotor Rhinitis

Sometimes known as non-allergic rhinitis, this is found in adults. It has an abrupt onset of nasal congestion and pronounced watery postnasal drip and sneezing and is thought to be caused by an environmental irritant. On examination, the turbinates are pale and edematous with no other findings. Treatment may be successful with a topical antihistamine or an intranasal steroid. Appropriate allergy testing must be performed before making this diagnosis.

Atrophic Rhinitis

This is found in older adults and the elderly. Symptoms include nasal congestion, thick postnasal discharge, frequent throat clearing, and a foul odor in the nose. The nasal mucosa will be dry and nonedematous with no other findings. This is caused by aging changes in the nasal cells. Treatment can be frustrating. Sinus rinses can be helpful and intranasal steroids can be used.

Acute Stomatitis

Definition

Stomatitis is an inflammation of the lining of any of the soft-tissue structures of the mouth, including the mucous lining of the cheeks, gums, tongue, lips, and roof or floor of the mouth. It is usually a painful condition, associated with redness, swelling, and occasional bleeding from the affected area. Halitosis may also accompany the condition.

Incidence

- Increased incidence with crowded living environments and in poor families
- Daycare attendance
- More common in children but may occur throughout the life span
- Increased incidence in:
  - Smokers
  - Denture wearers
- Most common:
  - Herpes stomatitis
  - Hand, foot, and mouth disease (Coxsackie Virus A16)
  - Recurrent aphthous ulcers (RAU)
- Prevalence can be throughout the year with coxsackie viruses more prevalent in the summer and autumn

Etiology

- Persistent irritation:
  - Poorly fitting oral appliances
  - Cheek biting
  - Jagged uneven teeth
  - Orthodontic appliances
  - Chronic mouth breathing leading to dry mouth
- Irritation and pain from drinking liquids too hot leading to burns
- Smoking, chewing tobacco
- Food allergies
- Immunosuppression
- Medications:
  - Antibiotics
  - Chemotherapy
  - Radiation therapy
  - Anti-epileptics
  - Drugs used to treat rheumatoid arthritis

- Medical conditions:
  - Herpes infections
  - Gonorrhea
  - Rubeola
  - Leukemias
  - HIV/AIDS
  - Vitamin C deficiency
  - Inflammatory bowel disease
  - Celiac disease
  - Behçet's disease—Causes blood vessel inflammation throughout the body and is marked by oral lesions.
  - Autoimmune diseases—Lupus, Crohn's disease
  - Aphthous stomatitis, also known as recurrent aphthous ulcers (RAU), is a specific type of stomatitis that presents with shallow, painful ulcers that are usually located on the lips, cheeks, gums, or roof or floor of the mouth.
    - These ulcers can range from pinpoint size to up to 1 in (2.5 cm) or more in diameter.
    - Though the causes of canker sores are unknown, nutritional deficiencies, especially of vitamin B12, folate, or iron are suspected.
    - Can be caused by emotional stress.
  - Generalized or contact stomatitis—Excessive use of alcohol, spices, hot food, or tobacco products. Sensitivity to mouthwashes, toothpastes, and lipstick can irritate the lining of the mouth.
  - Exposure to heavy metals—Mercury, lead, bismuth
  - Herpangina—Occurs during the summer and usually develops in children, occasionally occurring in newborns, adolescents, and young adults. It is one of many manifestations of a virus (enterovirus) and can occur in association with enteroviral exanthem, acute flaccid paralysis, aseptic meningitis, encephalitis, and other clinical syndromes.
  - Oral candidiasis is a type of stomatitis.

Risk Factors

- Poor oral hygiene
- Ill-fitting dentures
- Smoking
- Vitamin deficiency
- See Etiologies

Historical Data

- Burning sensation
- Intolerance to hot and cold temperatures and spicy foods
- Minimal to severe pain
- Fever, malaise
- Headache
- Recurrent aphthous ulcers:
  - Can be painful
  - Genetic predisposition
  - Usually lasts 5 to 10 days
  - Tends to recur
  - Are generally not associated with fever
- Herpes simplex:
  - Usually painful with a decreased ability to eat
  - May become dehydrated
  - Usually gone in 7 to 10 days
  - Sometimes associated with cold symptoms
  - Preceded by fever and irritability
- Herpangina
  - Sudden onset
  - Headache
  - Fatigue
  - Sore throat
  - Cervical pain

Physical Assessment

- Vital signs to assess fever
- Oral and cervical assessment:
  - Herpes simplex:
    - Lesions may be found on the lips, gingiva, and tongue
    - Vesicles that break down to friable greyish ulcers
    - Cervical lymphadenopathy
    - Poor oral intake
    - Drooling
  - Herpangina
    - High fever
    - Vomiting in young children
    - Back pain and headache in older children
    - Small vesicular or ulcerative lesions on the posterior oropharyngeal structures
    - Heals in 1–7 days

– Hand, foot, and mouth disease
  ▪ Mimics herpangina
  ▪ Addition of vesiculopapular lesions on the palms of the hand and soles of the feet
– Recurrent aphthous ulcers (RAU)
  ▪ Recurrent small, round, or ovoid ulcers with circumscribed margins, erythematous haloes, and yellow or gray floors

Differential Diagnosis

- Tonsillitis
- Pharyngitis
- Oral trauma
- Squamous-cell carcinoma
- Stevens–Johnson syndrome

RED FLAGS:

- Cutaneous bullae suggest Sjögren's syndrome, pemphigus vulgaris, or bullous pemphigoid. Prodrome of malaise, fever, conjunctivitis, and generalized macular target lesions suggests Sjögren's. Pemphigus vulgaris starts with oral lesions, then progresses to flaccid cutaneous bullae. Bullous pemphigoid has tense bullae on normal-appearing skin.

- Cutaneous vesicles are typical with varicella, or herpes zoster unilateral lesions in a band along a dermatome suggest herpes zoster. Diffuse, scattered vesicular and pustular lesions in different stages suggest varicella

- Kawasaki disease usually has a macular rash, desquamation of hands and feet, and conjunctivitis; it occurs in children, usually those < 5 yr. Oral findings include erythema of the lips and oral mucosa.

- Location of oral lesions may help identify the cause. Interdental ulcers occur with primary herpes simplex or acute necrotizing ulcerative gingivitis. Lesions on keratinized surfaces suggest herpes simplex, or physical injury. Physical injury typically has an irregular appearance and occurs near projections of teeth, dental appliances, or where biting or an errant toothbrush can injure the mucosa. An aspirin burn next to a tooth and pizza burn on the palate are common.

- Acute necrotizing ulcerative gingivitis shows inflammation and punched-out ulcers on the dental papillae and marginal gingivae. A severe variant called noma (gangrenous stomatitis) can cause full-thickness tissue destruction (sometimes involving the lips or cheek), typically in a debilitated patient. It begins as a gingival,

buccal, or palatal (midline lethal granuloma) ulcer that becomes necrotic and spreads rapidly. Tissue sloughing may occur.

- Isolated oral gonorrhea very rarely causes burning ulcers and erythema of the gingiva and tongue, as well as the more common pharyngitis. Primary syphilis chancres may appear in the mouth. Tertiary syphilis may cause oral gummas or a generalized glossitis and mucosal atrophy. The site of a gumma is the only time that squamous cell carcinoma develops on the dorsum of the tongue.

- A common sign of HIV becoming AIDS is hairy leukoplakia (vertical white lines on the lateral border of the tongue).

Diagnostic Studies

- Patients with acute stomatitis and no symptoms, signs, or risk factors for systemic illness probably require no testing.

- Diagnosis of recurrent aphthous ulcers (RAUs) is based on history and clinical features. No specific tests are available; however, to exclude the systemic disorders discussed earlier, the following tests may be helpful:
  – Complete blood cell count
  – Hemoglobin test
  – White blood cell count with differential
  – Red blood cell indices
  – Iron studies (usually an assay of serum ferritin levels)
  – Red blood cell folate assay
  – Serum vitamin B12 measurements
  – Serum antiendomysium antibody and transglutaminase assay (positive in celiac disease)

- Biopsy at the periphery of normal and abnormal tissue can be done for persistent lesions that do not have an obvious etiology.

Complications

- Herpetic keratoconjunctivitis, a secondary herpes infection in the eye, may develop. This is an emergency and can lead to blindness.

- Dehydration may develop if the patient refuses to eat and drink enough because of a sore mouth.

- Weight loss secondary to appetite loss

Management

Non-pharmacologic:

- Avoid hot beverages and foods as well as salty, spicy, and citrus-based foods.

- Gargle with cool water or suck on ice pops if the mouth burns.
- Apply ice directly on lesions.
- Drink more water.
- Rinse with salt water.
- Practice proper dental hygiene.
- Avoid smoking.

Pharmacologic:

- Acetaminophen or ibuprofen for fever and analgesia
- Systemic: (RAU)
  - Valacyclovir (*Valtrex*) is an antiviral that can be started at the first sign of symptoms in appropriate doses.
  - Amlexanox (*Aphthasol*) is an anti-inflammatory and anti-allergic agent widely used in Japan for many years. It has been developed as a 5% topical oral paste and is the only U.S. Food and Drug Administration–approved agent for the treatment of RAU. Treatment must be started as soon as symptoms occur. Paste is applied directly to lesions after brushing the teeth. It can be used 3–4 times daily for 10 days.
  - Levamisole hydrochloride (*Ergamisol*), an antihelminthic drug, reduces the frequency and duration of outbreaks when given at the onset of ulceration formation. Remissions may last for several months. This medication is contraindicated in both pregnancy and lactation, has an elevated neurotoxicity in the geriatric population, and has some serious side effects (possible bone marrow depression, agranulocytosis, taste disturbances).
  - Thalidomide has pronounced efficacy in healing oral lesions. The effects are only temporary, with recurrence after approximately 20 days of therapy. This drug has only limited use in the general population due to well-known risks to child-bearing women and must be reserved for only the most severe cases. It has been successfully used in HIV-positive patients who are particularly sensitive to RAU.
  - Oral corticosteroids may be used for relief in severe cases. Prednisone 40–60 mg/day for 4–7 days is usually effective. This must be followed by a 2-week taper.
- Topical
  - Coating the lesions with a protective ointment such as an antiviral agent (for example, acyclovir 5% ointment)
  - Lidocaine rinse
  - Sucralfate plus aluminum-magnesium antacid rinse

A 2-min rinse is done with 15 mL (1 tbsp) 2% viscous lidocaine q 3 h (every 3 hours) prn; patient expectorates when done (no rinsing with water and no swallowing unless the pharynx is involved). A soothing coating may be prepared with sucralfate (1-g pill dissolved in 15 mL water) plus 30 mL of aluminum-magnesium liquid antacid; the patient should rinse with or without swallowing.

If the inflammation is not caused by an infectious organism, the patient can:

- Rinse and expectorate after meals with dexamethasone elixir 0.5 mg/5 mL (1 tsp)
- Apply a paste of 0.1% triamcinolone in an oral emollient
- Chemical or physical cautery can ease the pain of localized lesions. Silver nitrate sticks are not as effective as low-power (2- to 3-watt), defocused, pulsed-mode CO_2 laser treatments, after which pain relief is immediate and lesions tend not to recur locally.
- Magic mouthwash for all types of stomatitis with local etiologies:
  - Diphenhydramine liquid: 100 mL
  - Dexamethasone: 0.5 mg/5 mL elixir 20 mL
  - Nystatin suspension: 60 mL
  - Tetracycline (from capsules): 1500 mg—Amoxicillin can also be used

Order 1 teaspoon 6 times/day for 7 days after and in between meals and at bedtime. The mixture is swished, gargled, and swallowed. This mixture of antihistamine, steroid, antifungal, and antibiotic liquid will treat any allergy or inflammation present in the oral cavity, as well as eliminate secondary fungal or bacterial infections. It will have no effect on the future recurrence rate. The diphenhydramine dosing must be age-appropriate. For children, omit the tetracycline and substitute amoxicillin/clavulanate 125 mg/75 mL.

Prevention/Patient Education

- Repair all broken teeth, rough fillings, and sharp-edged teeth. Maintain gentle dental hygiene and regular dental appointments.
- Limit use of antiseptic mouthwashes and exercise caution with toothpaste selection—many brands containing sodium lauryl sulfate (SLS) are irritating to mucosa.

- Keep a food diary to monitor the effects of oral intake. Once identified, an elimination trial of a particular food may be helpful.
- Take a daily multivitamin to decrease the possibility of nutritional deficiencies.
- Vitamin B12 may be helpful.
- Avoid hard crunchy foods and highly acidic drinks (tomato or orange; avoid juices).
- Reduce stress.
- Consider over-the-counter medications:
  - *Lactobacillus acidophilus* may prevent outbreaks if taken daily
  - Herbal remedies (chickweed, rockrose)
- Diluted hydrogen peroxide may be used as a mouthwash to remove debris that collects within ulcers.

Indications for Referral

Depending on the etiology, the following providers may be consulted:

- Immunology
- Allergy
- Gastroenterology
- Hematology
- Rheumatology
- Dermatology
- Dentist

Follow-up

- Simple cases will resolve in 1–2 weeks.
- See patient for reevaluation in 2 weeks—If lesions persist, consider using systemic medications or referral.

Oral Candidiasis

Definition

Oral candidiasis (thrush) is a yeast fungal infection of the genus *Candida* that develops on the mucous membranes of the mouth. It is most commonly caused by *Candida albicans*, but may also be caused by *Candida glabrata* or *Candida tropicalis*. *Candidosis* or *Moniliasis* refers to adult oral thrush, while "oral thrush" can refer to both adults and babies.

Oral candidiasis causes thick white or cream-colored deposits, most commonly on the tongue or inner cheeks. The lesions can be painful and may bleed slightly when they are scraped. The infected mucosa of the mouth may appear inflamed and red. Oral thrush can sometimes spread to the roof of the mouth and the back of the throat.

Incidence

The infection is not common in the general population. It is estimated that between 5% and 7% of babies less than one month old will develop oral candidiasis. The prevalence of oral candidiasis among AIDS patients is estimated to be between 9% and 31%, and studies have documented clinical evidence of oral candidiasis in nearly 20% of cancer patients.

Etiology

Tiny quantities of candida fungus exist in various parts of the body, including the digestive system, skin, and mouth, causing virtually no problems to healthy individuals. However, people on certain medications, reduced immune systems and certain conditions/illnesses are susceptible to oral candida, which can cause an exacerbation.

Risk Factors

- **People who wear dentures**—Especially if they are not kept clean, do not fit properly, or are not taken out before going to sleep.
- **Antibiotics**—People who are on antibiotics have a higher risk of developing oral thrush. Antibiotics may destroy the bacteria that prevent the Candida from reproducing out of control.
- **Excessive mouthwash use**—Individuals who overuse antibacterial mouthwashes may also destroy bacteria that keep Candida at bay, thus increasing the risk of developing oral candidiasis.
- **Oral or inhaled corticosteroids**—Long-term use can increase the risk of oral candidiasis.
- **Oral contraception**
- **Hypothyroidism**
- **Hormonal changes**—Pregnancy
- **Other therapies**—Medications, chemotherapies, and radiotherapies that cause dry mouth
- **Immunosuppression**—Cancer, HIV
- **Organ transplantation**
- **Diabetes**—Poorly controlled
- **Stress**
- **Malnutrition**
- **Prematurity**

Historical Data

- Redness or soreness in the affected areas
- White coating on tongue, palate, tonsils, posterior pharynx
- Difficulty swallowing
- Cracking at the corners of the mouth (angular cheilitis)
- Fever
- Inability to suck in infants
- Decreased appetite in adults

Physical Assessment

- There will be white surface plaques covering the mucosa of the oral cavity: tongue, buccal mucosa, palate, tonsils, and posterior pharynx. These are easily removed, leaving a raw friable surface.
- Angular cheilitis
- There may be cervical lymphadenopathy.

Differential Diagnosis

- Exudative pharyngitis
- Leukoplakia in adults
- Lichen planus
- Geographic tongue (normal variant)
- Herpes simplex erythema multiforme
- Pemphigus (rare)
- Baby formula, breast milk

Diagnostic Studies

- Clinical diagnosis through physical examination
- KOH preparation for microscopy for persistent cases
- Fungal cultures if first-line treatment fails

Complications

- Dehydration secondary to feeding problems in infants
- Weight loss secondary to appetite loss

Management

Non-pharmacologic:

- No mouthwash during treatment
- Bland diet until symptoms resolve
- Avoid tobacco smoke
- Soothing cool liquids
- Take medication regularly

Pharmacologic:

Topical Nystatin oral suspension 100,000 U/mL, 1 mL on each side of mouth qid (four times a day) × 7–14 days

- Adult dose: 4–6 mL qid
- Pediatric dose: 2 mL qid

Clotrimazole troches 10 mg 5x/day

Severe cases: Fluconazole 100–200 mg qd × 7–14 days

Pregnancy—Miconazole is safe.

Prevention/Patient Education

- Rinse mouth after meals.
- Brush teeth with a toothpaste that contains fluoride, and perform interdental cleaning (flossing) regularly.
- Regular dental visits
- Remove dentures every night, cleaning them with paste or soap and water before soaking them in a solution of water and denture-cleaning tablets.
- Brush gums, tongue, and inside of mouth with a soft brush twice a day if patient has dentures or no/few natural teeth.
- Avoid mouthwashes.
- Dental consult if dentures do not fit properly.
- **Stop smoking!**
- Rinse mouth with water and spit it out after using a corticosteroid inhaler, and use a spacer (a plastic cylinder that attaches to the inhaler) when using inhaler.
- Judicious use of antibiotics.
- Ensure that any underlying condition, such as diabetes, is well controlled.
- If there is an underlying health issue or treatment that could put you at high risk of developing oral thrush, your provider may recommend taking a course of antifungal medication to prevent this from happening.

Indications for Referral

- If patient is immunocompromised, refer to the appropriate provider in protracted cases.
- Esophageal infections
- Failure to respond to first-line treatment

Follow-up

- Simple cases resolve within 7–10 days.
- Immunocompromised patients and infants should be seen in one week to reevaluate symptoms and weight.

Pharyngitis and Tonsillitis

Definition

Acute pharyngitis is an inflammatory syndrome of the pharynx and/or tonsils caused by several different groups of microorganisms. Pharyngitis can be part of a generalized upper respiratory tract infection or a specific infection localized in the pharynx.

Most cases are caused by viruses and occur as part of common colds and influenza syndromes. Bacteria are also important etiologic agents, and, when identified properly, may be treated with antibiotics, resulting in decreased local symptoms and prevention of serious sequelae.

Incidence

- Acute pharyngitis is a common condition, occurring half as often in adults as in children aged 4 to 7, who average about five upper respiratory infections every year and one strep infection in 4 years.
- An estimated 12 million individuals are diagnosed with acute pharyngitis each year.
- Group A *Streptococcus* (GAS) infection is diagnosed in about 15% percent of all individuals seeking emergency room care for a painful throat. GAS pharyngitis is estimated to occur in 616 million individuals worldwide each year, with acute cases resulting in rheumatic heart disease in 6 million individuals.
- The incidence of acute pharyngitis is reported to be higher internationally, primarily due to higher rates of resistance of bacterial pharyngitis to antibiotics.
- GAS is most prevalent in late fall through early spring. It is quite contagious, and individuals in group work or living situations, such as long-term care centers, day care centers, schools, or hospitals, are at greatest risk of developing the infection.

Etiology

- Viral pharyngitis
  - Rhinovirus—More than 100 different serotypes of rhinovirus cause approximately 20% of cases of pharyngitis and 30–50% of common colds. These viruses enter the body through the ciliated epithelium that lines the nose, causing edema and hyperemia of the nasal mucous membranes. This condition leads to increased secretory activity of the mucous glands; swelling of the mucous membranes of the nasal cavity, Eustachian tubes, and pharynx; and narrowing of nasal passages, causing obstructive symptoms.
  - Epstein-Barr virus (EBV)—The cause of infectious mononucleosis, EBV usually spreads from adults to infants. Among young adults, EBV spreads through saliva and, rarely, through blood transfusion. In addition to edema and hyperemia of the tonsils and pharyngeal mucosa, an inflammatory exudate and nasopharyngeal lymphoid hyperplasia also develop. Pharyngitis or tonsillitis is present in about 82% of patients with infectious mononucleosis.
  - Adenovirus—Causes uncomplicated pharyngitis (most commonly caused by adenovirus types 1–3 and 5). Unlike rhinovirus infections, adenovirus directly invades the pharyngeal mucosa.
  - Herpes simplex virus (HSV) types 1 and 2—Cause gingivitis, stomatitis, and pharyngitis. Acute herpetic pharyngitis is the most common manifestation of the first episode of HSV-1 infection. After HSV enters the mucosal surface, it initiates replication and infects either sensory or autonomic nerve endings. The virus then spreads to other mucosal surfaces through migration of infectious virions via peripheral autonomic or sensory nerves. This mode of spread explains the high frequency of new lesions distant from the initial crop of vesicles characteristic of oral-labial HSV infection.
  - Influenza virus—Pharyngitis and sore throat develop in about 50% of the patients with influenza A and in a lesser proportion of patients with influenza B. Severe pharyngitis is particularly common in patients with type A. The influenza virus invades the respiratory epithelium, causing necrosis, which predisposes the patient to secondary bacterial infection. Transmission of influenza occurs by aerosolized droplets.
  - Parainfluenza virus—Caused by parainfluenza virus types 1–4 and usually manifests as the common cold syndrome. Parainfluenza virus type 1 infection occurs in epidemics, mainly in late fall or winter, while parainfluenza virus type 2 infection occurs sporadically. Parainfluenza virus type 3 infection occurs either epidemically or sporadically.
  - Enterovirus—The major groups that can cause pharyngitis are coxsackie and

echovirus. Although enteroviruses are primarily transmitted by the fecal-oral route, airborne transmission is important for certain serotypes. Enteroviral lesions in the oropharyngeal mucosa are usually a result of secondary infection of endothelial cells of small mucosal vessels, which occurs during viremia following enteroviral GI infection.

- Respiratory syncytial virus (RSV)—Transmission occurs by large-particle aerosols produced by coughing or sneezing. The pathogenesis of RSV infection remains unclear, although a number of theories exist. Immunologic mechanisms may contribute to the pathogenesis of the severe disease in infants and elderly patients.

- Cytomegalovirus (CMV)—Transmitted by sexual contact, in breast milk, via respiratory droplets among nursery or day care attendants, and by blood transfusion. Infection in the immunocompetent host rarely results in clinically apparent disease. Infrequently, immunocompetent hosts exhibit a mononucleosis-like syndrome with mild pharyngitis.

- Human immunodeficiency virus (HIV)—Pharyngitis develops in patients infected with human immunodeficiency virus as part of the acute retroviral syndrome, a mononucleosis-like syndrome that is the initial manifestation of HIV infection in one half to two thirds of recently infected individuals.

- Bacterial Pharyngitis
  - The most common and important bacterial cause of pharyngitis is Streptococcus pyogenes (group A *Streptococcus* [GAS]). 15–30% of pharyngitis cases in children and 5–10% of cases in adults are caused by GAS.
  - Bacteria other than GAS that may cause pharyngitis are:
    - Group C and G Streptococci—Like GAS, these pathogenic bacteria cause beta-hemolysis and form large colonies,
    - Gonorrhea—Infection with this pathogen is associated with oral-genital contact and is often asymptomatic.
    - *Chlamydia trachomatis*
    - *Mycoplasma pneumoniae*—This atypical bacterium is increasingly being identified as an etiologic agent of pharyngitis. *M. pneumoniae* pharyngitis may be associated with pulmonary findings.

- *Corenybacterium diptheriae*—Toxigenic strains of this gram-positive bacillus are common causes of croup. Young patients with *C. diphtheriae* pharyngitis often exhibit inspiratory stridor, sternal retraction, and a barking cough. In severe cases, a membrane formation may impair breathing. The incidence of *C. diphtheriae* pharyngitis in developed countries is low because of high immunization rates.

- Chronic etiologies:
  - Non-infectious irritation from post-nasal drip
  - Allergies
  - Gastroesophageal reflux disease
  - Smoking
  - Neoplasms

Risk Factors

Individuals living in crowded conditions:

- Long-term care centers
- Day care centers
- Schools
- Hospitals
- Age (younger patients are more vulnerable)
- GAS pharyngitis is most common in individuals aged 5–15 years, although adults may also acquire the disease. Streptococcal pharyngitis is very uncommon in children younger than 3 years, with the exception of children with risk factors such as a close contact or household contact with GAS infection.
- Cold and flu seasons
- Having close contact with someone who has an upper respiratory infection or acute pharyngitis
- Smoking or exposure to second-hand smoke
- Frequent episodes of rhinosinusitis
- Environmental allergies
- Exposure to chemical irritants
- Immunosuppression
  - HIV
  - Diabetes mellitus
- Stress
- Fatigue
- Poor nutrition
- Chemotherapy

Historical Data

Viral Pharyngitis:

- Upper respiratory infection—Throat symptoms can be in the form of soreness, scratchiness, or irritation.
- Adenovirus—Sore throat (more intense than that of a common cold), high fever, dysphagia, and red eyes.
- EBV (Infectious mononucleosis)—Most commonly observed in adolescents and young adults. Sore throat and fatigue are the most common symptoms. Pharyngeal symptoms are usually associated with other features of the disease (e.g., fatigue, skin rash, anorexia).
- Acute herpetic pharyngitis—Most commonly observed in children and young adults. Sore throat may be accompanied by sore mouth with associated gingivostomatitis. Other symptoms include fever, myalgia, malaise, inability to eat, and irritability.
- Influenza—Sore throat is the chief symptom in some patients with influenza. The onset of illness is usually abrupt, with myalgia, headache, fever, chills, and dry cough. The pharyngitis usually resolves in 3–4 days.
- Enteroviruses—An important cause of viral pharyngitis in childhood. This condition has a peak occurrence in late summer and early fall. Distinctive clinical syndromes include (1) herpangina caused by coxsackievirus A2–6; (2) acute lymphonodular pharyngitis caused by coxsackievirus A10; and (3) hand, foot, and mouth disease caused by coxsackievirus A5, 9, 10, and 16, and enterovirus 71. Children with hand, foot, and mouth disease have a low-grade fever (temperature, 100–102°F/38–39°C), sore throat, sore mouth, anorexia, malaise, and a rash on the hands and feet.
- RSV—Immunocompetent adults with RSV infection present with nasal discharge, sore throat, low-grade fever, and cough. Infants, elderly persons, and patients with chronic obstructive pulmonary disease (COPD) or congestive heart failure are more likely to develop lower respiratory tract involvement, which manifests as dyspnea, wheezing, and respiratory failure. Outbreaks of illness occur during the fall, winter, and early spring.
- CMV—Patients tend to be older than those with EBV infectious mononucleosis. Sore throat is less salient, but fever and malaise are prolonged and are more prominent than in EBV infectious mononucleosis.
- HIV—Patients with acute retroviral syndrome develop an acute sore throat similar to infectious mononucleosis. Sore throat is usually accompanied by other symptoms. Fever, sweats, malaise, lethargy, myalgias, anorexia, nausea, diarrhea, and skin rash are prominent symptoms.

Bacterial Pharyngitis

Signs and Symptoms:

- Sore throat, usually with sudden onset
- Odynophagia, dysphagia
- Headache
- Nausea, vomiting, and abdominal pain
- Low-grade fever, chills
- Myalgias
- Cervical pain, swollen glands
- Joint aches, stiffness
- Dyspnea

Acute Tonsillitis

- Throat pain, tenderness
- Erythematous tonsils
- A white or yellow coating on the tonsils
- Painful ulcers on the tonsils
- Headache
- Ear pain
- Hoarseness or loss of voice
- Loss of appetite
- Mouth breathing
- Cervical lymphadenopathy
- Fever, chills
- Halitosis

Physical Assessment

*The diagnosis of acute pharyngitis cannot be made on the basis of history and physical examination.

- Airway patency must be assessed and addressed first.
- Temperature: Fever is usually absent or low-grade in viral pharyngitis, but fever is not reliable to differentiate viral or bacterial etiologies.
- Hydration status: Oral intake usually is compromised because of odynophagia; therefore, various degrees of dehydration result.

- Head, ears, eyes, nose, and throat may include the following symptoms:
  - Conjunctivitis—In association with an adenovirus
  - Scleral icterus—Epstein–Barr virus
  - Rhinorrhea—A viral cause
  - Tonsillopharyngeal/palatal petechiae—GAS infections and infectious mononucleosis
  - Oropharyngeal vesicular lesions—Coxsackievirus and herpesvirus. Concomitant vesicles on the hands and feet—Coxsackievirus (hand, foot, and mouth disease)
- Lymphadenopathy: Tender anterior cervical nodes are consistent with streptococcal infection, whereas generalized adenopathy is consistent with infectious mononucleosis or the acute lymphoglandular syndrome of HIV infection.
- Cardiovascular: Murmurs should be documented in an acute episode of pharyngitis to monitor for potential rheumatic fever.
- Pulmonary: Pharyngitis and lower respiratory tract infections are more consistent with *M. pneumoniae* or *C. pneumoniae*, particularly when a persistent nonproductive cough is present.
- Abdomen: Hepatosplenomegaly can be found in an infectious mononucleosis infection.
- Skin: A sandpapery scarlatiniform rash is seen in GAS infections, and a maculopapular rash is seen with various viral infections and with infectious mononucleosis empirically treated with penicillin.

Differential Diagnosis
- Allergic rhinitis with postnasal drip
- Airway obstruction
- Bacteremia
- Meningitis
- Head and neck neoplasias
- Gastroesophageal reflux disease (GERD)
- Peritonsillar cellulitis
- Peritonsillar abscess
- Retropharyngeal abscess
- Scarlet fever
- Rheumatic fever
- Post streptococcal glomerulonephritis
- Thyroiditis

Diagnostic Studies
Laboratory Testing:
- GAS rapid antigen detection test
  - Antigens are specific, but sensitivities vary. Children with a negative antigen test should have a follow-up culture unless the antigen being used in the office has been shown to be as sensitive as a culture (50–80% sensitivity; > 95% specificity).
  - The use of a GAS rapid antigen detection test can decrease the use of unnecessary antibiotics in patients when used properly.
  - Adults do not need follow-up culture after a negative antigen test because of the low incidence of GAS in this population.
- Throat culture
  - This is the criterion standard for diagnosis of GAS infection (90–99% sensitive).
  - Patients can be treated up to 9 days after onset of symptoms to prevent acute rheumatic fever, so immediate antibiotic therapy is not crucial if patients can be easily contacted for follow-up should a culture become positive.
- The procedure for a throat swab is to vigorously rub a dry swab over the posterior pharynx and both tonsils, obtaining a sample of exudate.
- Monospot is up to 95% sensitive in children (less than 60% sensitivity in infants).
- Peripheral smear may show atypical lymphocytes in infectious mononucleosis.
- Perform a gonococcal culture as indicated by history.
- A complete blood count (CBC), erythrocyte sedimentation rate (ESR), and C-reactive protein have a low predictive value and usually are not indicated.
- Use a potassium hydroxide (KOH) wet mount if oral candida is suspected.

Imaging Studies
- Imaging studies generally are not indicated for uncomplicated viral or streptococcal pharyngitis.
- Lateral neck film should be taken in patients with a suspected epiglottitis or airway compromise.
- Soft tissue neck CT can be used if concern for abscess or deep-space infection exists; however, peritonsillar abscess is almost always a clinical diagnosis.

Complications

- Otitis media
- Rhinosinusitis
- Peritonsillar abscess—Needs **IMMEDIATE** referral to otolaryngology!
- Airway obstruction—Needs **IMMEDIATE** emergency room referral!

Management

Non-pharmacologic:

- Clear fluids
- Rest
- Warm salt water gargles
- Humidification
- Judicious use of lozenges

Pharmacologic:

The **Centor Criteria** are a set of criteria which may be used to identify the likelihood of a bacterial infection in adult patients complaining of a sore throat. They were developed as a method to quickly diagnose the presence of GAS or the diagnosis of strep pharyngitis in adult patients who presented to an emergency room complaining of a sore throat.

Patients are judged on four criteria, with one point added for each positive criterion:

- History of fever
- Tonsillar exudate
- Tender anterior cervical lymphadenopathy
- Absence of cough

The Modified Centor Criteria adds the patient's age to the criteria:

- Age < 15, add 1 point
- Age > 44, subtract 1 point

Scores may range from −1 to 5.
Guidelines for management:

- −1, 0 or 1 points—No antibiotic or throat culture necessary (risk of strep. infection < 10%)
- 2 or 3 points—Should receive a throat culture and treat with an antibiotic if culture is positive (risk of strep. infection 32% if 3 criteria, 15% if 2)
- 4 or 5 points—Treat empirically with an antibiotic (risk of strep. infection 56%)

Notes on antibiotic use:

- If culture shows *Streptococcus* other than Type A, it is not necessary to treat.
- Household contacts only treated if symptomatic.

Antibiotic Therapy: All Courses Should Last 10 Days.

First-line drugs for GAS:

- Penicillin VK:
  - Adults—500 mg po bid
  - Children—25–50 mg/kg/day divided bid–qid
- Amoxicillin
  - Adults—500 mg tid or 875 mg po bid depending on severity
  - Children—12.25–22.5 mg/kg/day divided bid

Treatment for Patients with Allergy to Penicillin:

- Azithromycin—Use in doses based on age and weight
  - Adults—500 mg po day one, followed by 250 mg po qd × 4 days
  - Children—Not recommended under 2 years of age. After 2 years, 12 mg/kg qd × 5 days
- Other alternatives include Erythromycin and Clarithromycin.

Second-line drugs include cephalosporins and quinolones (not to be used in children).

- Chlamydia/Mycoplasmal infection:
  - Adults: Doxycycline 100 mg po bid or Azithromycin 500 m po qd day one followed by 250 mf po qd × 4 days
  - Children—Erythromycin 30–50 mg/kg bid × 10 days

Gonorrhea:

- Ceftriaxone 125–250 mg IM

Acute Tonsillitis:

- Clindamycin—150–300 mg q 6 hours to 300–450 mg q 6 hours WITH
- Medrol Dosepak as directed to decrease edema

Patient Education

- Do NOT self-treat without a culture. Some patients save antibiotics and will begin a course before a visit. This makes cultures inaccurate and forces antibiotic treatment.
- Children may return to normal activities and school after fever is gone and they have been on an antibiotic for 24 hours.
- Call with persistent or worsening symptoms after 3–5 days of therapy.
- Discourage second-hand smoke.

- Judicious use of commercial mouthwashes and lozenges to prevent changes in good bacterial flora

Indications for Referral
- Immediate referrals:
  - Airway obstruction—Emergency room
  - Peritonsillar abscess/retropharyngeal abscess—Otolaryngology or emergency room

Follow-up
Necessary only with persistent symptoms OR with
- Infectious mononucleosis
- Allergies
- Gastroesophageal reflux disease
- Serious viral/bacterial infections
- See patient in 2 weeks.

Upper Respiratory Infections (URIs)

Definition
URIs are one of the most common illnesses, leading to more health provider visits and school and work absences than any other illness annually. They are caused by over 200 viruses that inflame the mucosal linings of the nose and throat. The majority of URIs are caused by a rhinovirus.

Incidence
During a one-year period, people in America will suffer 1 billion URIs. Most children will develop between 6–8 colds/year. Adults develop between 2–4 colds/year.

Etiology
- Rhinoviruses
- Coronavirus
- Adenovirus
- Enterovirus
- Respiratory syncytial virus

Risk Factors
- Day care in children and elderly
- School attendance
- Being indoors and close to others—Theaters, malls, churches, and classrooms
- Decreased humidity in the winter months, making nasal mucosa dry and vulnerable to infection
- Direct contact with an infected person or their objects—Toys, shaking hands, kissing and hugging
- Immunocompromised with less of an immune response to infection
- Comorbid health problems of the respiratory tract—COPD, asthma, allergies
- Tobacco smoke decreases ciliary function in the nasopharynx, allowing infections to take hold.

Historical Data
- Nasal congestion
- Clear yellow nasal discharge
- Irritated pharynx with dry cough
- Watery eyes
- Sneezing
- Sore throat
- Myalgias
- Mild headache
- May be a low-grade fever and chills
- Mild fatigue

Physical Assessment
- Edema and hyperemia of the nasal mucosa
- Clear-mucoid nasal drainage
- Pharyngeal erythema without edema
- Post-nasal drainage in posterior pharynx
- Cervical lymphadenopathy may be present

Differential Diagnosis
- Acute rhinosinusitis
- Allergic rhinitis
- Vasomotor rhinitis less frequent as an acute presentation
- Foreign body in nasal chamber—Usually unilateral congestion and drainage
- Nasal polyps

Diagnostic Studies
Studies are only indicated in persistent cases. URIs usually resolve spontaneously.

Complications
- Otitis media
- Acute/chronic rhinosinusitis

- Pneumonia, especially in the elderly and with patients with COPD or immunocompromised health issues
- Bacterial pharyngitis

Management

Non-pharmacologic:

- Increased clear fluids
- Rest
- Saline nasal spray
- Humidification

Pharmacologic:

- Analgesia for myalgias and headache. **DO NOT use Aspirin with children**—Associated with Reye's syndrome, a potentially fatal disorder. Tylenol or Ibuprofen may be used in appropriate doses.
- In children younger than 4 years, there is an FDA ban on the use of over-the-counter cough and cold medicines.
- Guaifenesin is a mucolytic that may be purchased over-the-counter. It thins mucous, making it easier to drain nasal and sinus passages.
- Oxymetazoline hydrochloride is an over-the-counter topical decongestant. It may be used ONLY for 72 hours because prolonged use may result in tolerance and increased nasal congestion called rhinitis mendicamentosa. Dose: 2 sprays bid for 3 days.
- Over-the-counter decongestants cause vasoconstriction, decrease blood supply to the nasal mucosa, and cause decreased mucosal edema. There are numerous medications available.

Clinical Pearl

Advise patients to use medications with only one active ingredient. Otherwise, there may be an increased side-effect profile, especially in the elderly. They should be used with caution in this age group, many of whom have hypertension and heart disease.

Patient Education

- Stress importance of hand washing to prevent spread of infection.
- Avoid large groups in the winter if there are comorbid health issues.
- Emphasize that antibiotics are not needed for a viral infection and that overuse is leading to antibiotic resistance.
- Avoid second-hand smoke.

Indications for Follow-up

- Fever greater than 100.4 °F
- Persistent symptoms lasting more than 10–14 days
- Worsening symptoms
- Severe headache, ear, or throat pain
- Referral is rarely necessary in the treatment of uncomplicated URI.

Expected Course

- Most symptoms will last 7–10 days and spontaneously resolve.
- Office follow-up is not usually necessary unless there are worsening symptoms.

Cervical Lymphadeopathy

Definition

Lymph nodes, in conjunction with the spleen, tonsils, adenoids, and Peyer patches, are highly organized centers of immune cells that filter antigen from extracellular fluid. They have a high degree of lymphocytes and antigen-presenting cells and are ideal organs for receiving antigens that gain access through the skin or GI tract. They have a considerable capacity for growth and change. Size depends upon the person's age, the location of the nodes, and antecedent immunological events. They are most noticeable in childhood and begin to atrophy during adolescence. Generalized lymphadenopathy is described as the enlargement of more than two noncontiguous lymph node groups. There are approximately 300 lymph nodes in the adult human neck.

Incidence/Prevalence

- Precise incidence unknown. Estimates in childhood range from 38–45%, and lymphadenopathy is one of the most common clinical presentations encountered in pediatrics.
- In the U.S., common viral and bacterial infections are overwhelmingly the most common causes. Infectious mononucleosis and cytomegalovirus are important.
- Significant morbidity and mortality are due to malignancies, autoimmune diseases, and HIV.
- Race and sex do not influence lymphadenopathy.
- Most common in young children whose immune systems are responding to new infections (about 33% neonates and infants).

Lymph Node Pathophysiology

Lymphadeopathy refers to a disease involving the reticuloendothelial system secondary to an increase in normal lymphocytes, and macrophages in response to an antigen. Most pediatric cases are due to benign self-limited diseases (viral infections). Other less common etiologies include nodal accumulation of inflammatory cells in response to an infection, neoplastic lymphocytes or macrophages, or metabolic-laden macrophages in storage diseases.

Cervical Lymphadenopathy Etiologies

- Infection
  - Viral
    - Upper respiratory infections
    - Rubella
    - Infectious mononucleosis
    - Roseola
    - HIV
    - Adenovirus
    - Herpes
    - Coxsackie
    - Cytomegalovirus
  - Bacterial
    - Typhoid fever
    - Syphilis
    - Plague
    - Tuberculosis
    - Cat scratch fever
    - Streptococcal pharyngitis
  - Localized
    - Otitis
    - Herpes stomatitis
    - Dental abscess (submaxillary and submental nodes)
- Malignancy
  - Leukemias
  - Lymphomas
  - Hodgkin's Disease
- Storage diseases—Gaucher's disease
- Drug reactions
- Epstein–Barr associated lymphoproliferative disease

- Autoimmune disorders
  - Rheumatoid arthritis
  - Sarcoidosis
  - Graft vs. host disease
- Kawasaki disease
- Tinea capitis, seborrheic dermatitis, insect bites, pediculosis (occipital nodes)
- Conjunctivitis, Chlamydia trachomatis, adenovirus, eyelid edema (oculoglandular syndrome affecting the preauricular nodes)

Infectious Mononucleosis

Description

Infectious mononucleosis (IM) is a clinical syndrome and represents the immunologic expression that occurs under a specific set of circumstances and in response to infection with the Epstein–Barr virus (EBV). These circumstances primarily relate to the age and immuncompetency of the patient when the infection is acquired.

Epidemiology

The incidence of IM in the U.S. is estimated at 45/100,000 patients. Global incidence is unknown but, in developing countries, 90–95% of children experience an asymptomatic infection.

Fatalities are usually the result of splenic rupture. Less common mortalities include secondary bacterial infections, hepatic failure, myocarditis, and airway obstruction. There are no known racial or ethnic predilections, and the only sex-related factor is that splenic rupture occurs more than 90% of the time in males.

The highest occurrence rate is in those aged 15–25 years—1–3% college students annually. In children under 4 years, the infection is usually asymptomatic. In elderly patients, the symptoms may be vague—Myalgias, fatigue, fever, malaise.

Etiology

EBV, or human herpesvirus 4, is a gammaherpesvirus that infects more than 95% of the world's population. The most common manifestation of primary infection with the organism is acute IM, a clinical syndrome that affects mostly adolescents and young adults. It is the most common etiologic agent of acute IM. Other etiologies with a similar presentation may include (less than 10%):

- Adenovirus
- Cytomegalovirus (CMV)

- Group A Beta-Hemolytic Streptococci
- Hepatitis A
- Human Herpes Virus
- HIV
- Rubella
- *Toxoplasmosis gondii*
- Non-infectious causes of heterophile negative IM–like syndromes
  - Medications—Sulfas
  - Malignancy—Lymphoma, leukemia

Risk Factors

- Being a college or high school student
- Kissing
- Blood transfusion

Historical Data

- Prodromal symptoms—1–2 weeks of fatigue, malaise, myalgias
- Low-grade fever persisting up to 4–5 weeks
- Pharyngitis is a cardinal symptom—Usually severe and exudative. ALWAYS do a throat culture to rule out streptococcus pharyngitis.
- Tonsillitis
- Lymphadenopathy is almost universal and lasts 1–2 weeks. Posterior cervical lymphadenopathy is most commonly found.
- Headache
- Papular Erythematous rash of upper extremities and/or trunk (5%). DO NOT use Amoxicillin in these patients due to the possibility of a similar rash!
- Petechiae
- Jaundice
- Abdominal pain should alert provider to possible splenic rupture.

Physical Assessment

- Temperature—Should be less than 102 °F.
- Pharyngitis
- Tonsillar edema and erythema with a grayish/greenish exudates
- Symmetrical enlargement of lymph nodes that are firm, mobile, and tender. There is no overlying erythema or warmth.
- Splenomegaly is present in most cases. Avoid a vigorous abdominal examination d/t possibility of splenic rupture.

- Hepatomegaly (10–30%)
- Periorbital edema in 15–35% patients
- Petechiae of palate, occurring at junction of hard and soft palate (33%).
- Jaundice

Differential Diagnoses

- Acute mumps
- Diptheria
- Herpes simplex
- Rubella
- Pharyngitis—Other viral etiologies, as well as bacterial
- Peritonsillar abscess
- HIV
- Retropharygeal abscess
- Roseola
- Scarlet fever
- Toxoplasmosis

Diagnostic Studies

- Throat culture to rule out streptococcus pharyngitis.
- Complete blood count with differential. White blood count is modestly elevated with lymphocytes greater than 50%.
- Liver function tests—Abnormal in over 90% cases.
  - Serum transaminase and alkaline phosphotase levels are modestly elevated.
  - Serum bilirubin increase in 40% of cases.
- Heterophile antibody test is the most common and specific test to confirm the diagnosis. The antibody is present in 40–60% of patients in the first week, and in 80–90% of cases by the third–fourth week.
- EBV specific antibody tests are indicated only in atypical presentations or in patients with persistent negative heterophile antibody testing despite a clinical picture consistent with EBV-related illness.

Management

Non-pharmacologic:

- Rest
- Increased clear fluids
- Avoid any contact sports for at least 4–6 weeks

Pharmacologic:

The use of oral corticosteroids in severe cases is recommended only if there is an increased risk of airway obstruction, thrombocytopenia, or autoimmune hemolytic anemia. Do not use routinely because these medications can affect cell-mediated immune response and will increase the risk of bacterial super infection.

Complications

- Splenic rupture
- Hepatitis
- Peritonsillar abscess
- Cardiac complications—Myocarditis
- Airway obstruction
- Central nervous system complications

Patient Education

- Discuss etiology and natural progression of the disease
- Discuss prognosis—IM is self-limited and will usually resolve within 3–4 weeks. In some cases, low-grade symptoms may persist beyond that time.
- Avoid participation in ANY contact sport or vigorous physical activity for at least one month to minimize the possibility of splenic rupture.
- Emphasize that there may be symptoms of depression that will usually be self-limited.

Indications for Referral

- Emergency care if any symptoms/signs of airway obstruction or splenic rupture.
- If a peritonsillar abscess is suspected, refer to otolaryngology.
- If cardiac or neurological symptoms are present, refer to the appropriate provider.

Expected Course

- Usually self-limited. Follow-up in 1–2 weeks to check resolution of symptoms.

Eye

Julie G. Stewart, DNP, MPH, MSN, FNP-BC, APRN

The FNP in primary care has a responsibility to assess vision when a patient presents with any complaint related to the eye and vision. In addition, it is vital to be aware of complaints that require prompt referral to an ophthalmologist or emergency department. Many eye issues require referral to and treatment by an ophthalmologist/specialist. See Figure 5-3 for a side-view illustration of an eyeball.

Useful Tips and Terms When Performing an Exam with an Opthalmoscope:

- Use the RIGHT hand for the RIGHT eye; left hand for left eye.
- Arteries are brighter red and narrower than veins.

Visual acuity: Assessed with the Snellen test. A patient with 20/20 vision can see at 20 feet what the "normal" patient can see at 20 feet.

Refractive Errors

- Hyperopia—Farsighted (near-vision blurred)
- Myopia—Nearsighted (far-vision blurred)
- Presbyopia—Hard to maintain clear focus in near vision; common over age 40 yrs.
  - Arcus senilis—Cloudy appearance of cornea with gray/white arc or circle around limbus related to lipid material; has no effect on vision.
  - Hordeolum—Stye (usually staph); painful, abrupt, localized mass with erythema in eyelid. Treat with warm compresses, topical bacitracin or erythro ophthalmic ointment. Refer to ophthalmologist if not better in 2 days.
  - Chalazion—Cyst or infection of a gland on an eyelid; painless—use warm compresses. Can be surgically removed.
  - Blepharitis—Staph infection or seborrheic dermatitis on edge of lid. Warm compresses, bacitracin or erythro ophthalmic ointment, scrub lashes.
  - Conjunctivitis—Most common eye disorder, "pink-eye," caused by
  - allergies (stringy, tearing), use antihistamines
  - bacterial (purulent), antibiotic eye drops such as levofloxacin, Ciprofloxacin, tobramycin, gentamycin, or viral (watery) infections. Symptomatic treatment.
  - Gonorrhea or Chlamydia has copious purulent discharge. Treat GC (gonococcal infections) with ceftriaxone 250 IM; Chlamydia treat with erythromycin ophthalmic ointment or oral Zithromax, etc.
  - Cataracts—Highest cause of treatable blindness! Clouding and opacification of lens of eye; painless, cloudy vision, halos around lights, difficult night vision. Refer to ophthalmologist.

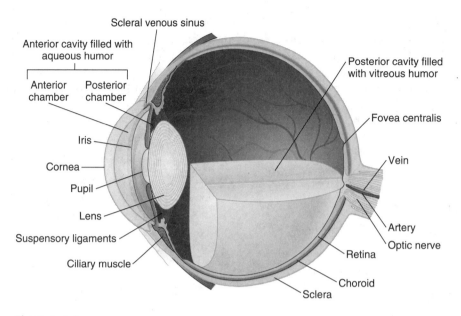

Scleral venous sinus

Anterior cavity filled with
aqueous humor

Anterior   Posterior
chamber   chamber

Posterior cavity filled
with vitreous humor

Iris

Fovea centralis

Cornea

Vein

Pupil

Lens

Suspensory ligaments

Artery

Ciliary muscle

Optic nerve

Retina

Choroid

Sclera

Figure 5-3 Eye

- Glaucoma—Chronic open-angle is slow, progressive optic nerve damage with increased intraocular pressure. Refer for treatment.

Primary closed-angle is acute elevated intraocular pressure associated with the closing of the filtration angle or obstruction of the circulation of aqueous humor. **Emergency referral!**

Any rapid onset of vision loss is an emergency and prompt evaluation by a specialist is required.

Eye Exam

1. Check vision using the Snellen chart for distance and small type (card, newspaper, etc.) for near vision. Test each eye independently.
2. Observe for symmetry of eyes, eyelids, and eyebrows. Cranial nerves (CN) 3 and 7 control eyelids. The sclera should be white, the conjunctiva light pink.
3. Check confrontation and perform cover/uncover test.
4. Check extraocular movements (CN 3, 4, 6) and accommodation.
5. Check for red reflections and pupillary reactions with light on ophthalmoscope.
6. With room darkened, perform eye exam finding blood vessel and follow to optic disk. Note any irregularities.

Conjunctivitis

Bacterial Conjunctivitis
Signs and Symptoms
- Normal visual acuity
- Yellowish discharge
- Painless

Treatment
- Antibiotic drops or ointment
- Do not wear contact lenses until healed

Allergic Conjunctivitis
Signs and Symptoms
- Normal visual acuity
- Mucous discharge
- Itchy but painless

Treatment
- Cool compresses
- Antihistamine drops or oral antihistamine
- Vasoconstrictor drops
- Mast cell stabilizer drops
- Steroid eye drops should be prescribed by specialist

Viral Conjunctivitis
Signs and Symptoms
- Minor pain
- Visual acuity may be reduced
- Teary discharge
- Not itchy
- History of recent upper respiratory infection
- Pre-auricular node

Treatment
- Lubricants (artificial tears)
- May need referral for steroid eye drops to reduce corneal infiltrates

Glaucoma (Referral)

Angle Closure Glaucoma
Anterior chamber angle is blocked by the iris so that aqueous fluid does not drain well.

Signs and Symptoms
- Visual acuity reduced
- Fixed ovoid pupil
- Clouded cornea
- Increased intraocular pressure

Treatment
- Make referral ASAP to specialist for the following:
  - Drops to lower the pressure in the eye
  - Laser iridotomy to improve aqueous release

    *Pupil dilating medication is contraindicated.

Open Angle Glaucoma (Most Common)
Anterior chamber angle is open but the trabecular meshwork does not drain aqueous fluid well. Can be congenital or steroid-induced.

Signs and Symptoms
- Painless, usually no symptoms
- Peripheral vision loss slowly over time
- Increased intraocular pressure
- Optic nerve cupping

Treatment
- Medications
- Usually eye drops
  - Beta-blockers
  - Prostaglandin analogues
  - Alpha-agonists
- Oral medication (carbonic anhydrase inhibitor)
- Surgical options

Corneal Issues

Corneal Abrasion
Signs and Symptoms
- Visual acuity reduced
- History of scratching the eye
- Normal pupil unless traumatic iritis
- Teary discharge
- Corneal florescence after instilling fluorescein drops in eye on Wood's lamp or slit lamp examination

Treatment
- Antibiotic drops or ointment

Corneal Foreign Body
Signs and Symptoms
- Visual acuity may be reduced
- History of getting something in the eye
- Usually normal pupil
- Tearing

Treatment (refer if not trained)
- Anesthetize cornea with topical anesthetic drops (i.e., Proparacaine).
- Remove foreign body with a sterile cotton swab.
- Use antibiotic drops or ointment.

Chalazion (Stye)

Sebaceous Cyst of Eyelid
Signs and Symptoms
- Inflamed eyelid lesion
- May have discharge

Treatment

- Warm compresses to eyelid four times a day.
- Can try antibiotic eye drops or ointment.
- Oral antibiotics typically not required.
- Make referral ASAP if there is restricted eye movement or a fixed dilated pupil, because these can be signs of orbital cellulitis.

Cataract (Opacity of the Lens)

Causes

- Congenital
- Disease-related
- Diabetes accelerates cataract formation
- Inflammatory disease (i.e., sarcoid)
- Senile (age-related) most common
- Medication related
- Prednisone can produce a posterior subcapsular cataract after three weeks of treatment.
- Psychotropic drugs can produce an anterior subcapsular cataract.
- In the early stages of a cataract
- Trauma

Signs and Symptoms

- Glare with night driving
- Lights appear to have starbursts
- Seen as a dark opacity in the media of the eye through an ophthalmoscope

Treatment

- In the early stages of cataracts, a change to the patient's prescription glasses may help initially. Ultimately, surgical removal of the lens with an IOL implant will be needed.
- Make referral for surgical removal of the lens, which is replaced with a piece of plastic called an intraocular implant (IOL).

Dry Eyes

Risk Factors

- Age-related
- Post-menopausal women
- Chemotherapy
- Diuretics
- Arthritis
- History of Lasik surgery

Signs and Symptoms

- Eye feels gritty or dry

Treatment

- Lubricants (artificial tears and ointments)
- Restasis—Cyclosporine eye drops to encourage tear production
- Punctal plugs

Diplopia (Double Vision)

Causes/Risk Factors

- Diabetes (small vessel damage in extraocular muscles)
- Thyroid disease
- Stroke
- Tumor of orbit or brain
- Trauma
- Subarachnoid hemorrhage

Signs or Symptoms

- Increased blood glucose
- Abnormal thyroid function tests
- Irregular extraocular movement
- Positive cover uncover test
- Single vision with one eye covered

Treatments

- Control underlying disease
- Surgical correction of tumor or trauma
- Prism glasses
- Make **immediate referral** if there is a fixed dilated pupil (sign of subarachnoid hemorrhage)

Presbyopia

- Age-related (over 40)
- Hardening of the lens of the eye

Signs and Symptoms

- Decreased near vision

Treatment

- Reading glasses

Herpes Simplex Keratitis (Type I Herpes Simplex)

Signs and Symptoms
- Visual acuity reduced
- Tearing
- Foreign body sensation
- Dendrite fluorescein pattern on Wood's lamp or slit lamp examination

Treatment
- Antiviral P.O. medication (i.e., Valtrex)
- Palliative lubricants (artificial tears and ointments)
- Steroids contraindicated
- **Referral**

Herpes Zoster Keratitis (Shingles)

Signs and Symptoms
- Visual acuity may be reduced.
- Lesions on half of face along nerve distribution
- Lesion at tip of the nose indicates ocular involvement.

Treatment
- Antiviral P.O. medication
- Palliative lubricants (artificial tears and ointments)
- Make referral to assess ocular involvement.

Macular Degeneration

Dry Macular Degeneration
Causes/Risk Factors
- Genetic
- Age-related (usually over 65)

Signs and Symptoms
- Central loss of vision slowly over time

Treatment
- None available. Antioxidants may be preventative.

Wet Macular Degeneration
Causes/Risk Factors
- Genetic
- Smoking
- Blood vessel proliferation in macula

Signs and Symptoms
- Sudden loss of central vision

Treatment
- Referral
- Laser to stop bleeding
- Smoking cessation
- Medication—Several options available by specialist.

Posterior Vitreous Detachment
(vitreous gel pulls away from retina)

Risk Factors
- Age-related (above age 40)
- Trauma

Signs and Symptoms
- New onset flashing lights
- New floaters

Treatment
- Make **referral** for a dilated eye exam to confirm diagnosis.

Retinal Detachment
(Separation of the retina from the underlying layers of the eye)

Causes
- High myopia (nearsightedness)
- Trauma
- Genetic—family history
- Retinal hole or tear
- Diabetes

Signs and Symptoms
- New onset flashing lights
- New onset floaters
- May have curtain coming down over the vision

Treatment
- Make **immediate referral** for a dilated eye exam to confirm diagnosis and treatment.

Retinopathy

Risk Factors
- Diabetes
- Hypertension

Treatment

- Referral
  - Control underlying disease.
  - Annual eye exams
  - Use laser on retina to slow vessel and hemorrhagic changes.
  - Medication—Make monthly injections into eye with anti-VEGF or anti-inflammatory agent.

Optic Neuritis

Definition
Inflammation of the optic nerve.

Causes
- May have had recent viral illness.
- Occurs frequently in multiple sclerosis.

Signs and Symptoms
- Decreased color vision in affected eye, especially red color vision
- Decreased pupillary reaction in affected eye
- Pain on eye movement
- Papillitis
- Central scotoma

Treatments
- Referral
  - Systemic steroids

Iritis

Definition
Inflammation of the iris.

Causes/Risk Factors
- Collagen vascular disease or rheumatologic disease (i.e., sarcoid, arthritis)
- Diabetes
- Lyme disease
- Trauma to eye

Signs and Symptoms
- Photophobic
- Pupil smaller in affected eye
- Visual acuity may be reduced
- Circum-limbal flush

Treatment
- Treat underlying disease.
- Make referral for steroid eye drops to reduce inflammation.

Visual Field Defects

Causes
- Stroke
- Pituitary or other brain tumor or aneurism
- Glaucoma

Treatment
- Make referral for complete examination and workup

Review Questions

1. The most common cause of bacterial pharyngitis is:
   A. Gonorrhea.
   B. Group C *Streptococcus*.
   C. Mycoplasma.
   D. Group A *Streptococcus*.

2. Risk factors for acute pharyngitis include all of the following EXCEPT:
   A. Age (older people are more vulnerable).
   B. Attendance at day care.
   C. Smoking.
   D. Allergies.

3. A new patient, aged 11 years, is suspected of having acute tonsillitis. The FNP would expect her to have which of the following symptoms?
   A. Oral lesions
   B. Tonsillar ulcers
   C. Dry cough
   D. Comorbid pulmonary disease

4. Treatment of the patient with acute tonsillitis will include all of the following EXCEPT:
   A. Assessment of airway obstruction.
   B. Judicious use of antibacterial mouthwash.
   C. Ofloxacin in appropriate dose.
   D. Warm salt water gargles.

5. The most common etiology for enlarged cervical lymph nodes is:
   A. Human immunodeficiency virus.
   B. Common viral and bacterial infections.
   C. Dental abscess.
   D. Rheumatoid arthritis and other autoimmune diseases.

6. Infectious mononucleosis is found most often in which age group?
   A. Pediatric
   B. Adolescent
   C. Adult
   D. Geriatric

7. After history and the physical exam, the FNP suspects a 22-year-old female has infectious mononucleosis. Of the following diagnostic studies that provide the most specific test, the result will be:
   A. A positive heterophile antibody test.
   B. A modest elevation of the white blood count.
   C. An elevated bilirubin.
   D. A decreased lymphocyte count.

8. The management plan for the patient with infectious mononucleosis will include:
   A. A course of systemic corticosteroids.
   B. Bed rest for 3–5 days.
   C. Avoidance of contact sports for 3–5 days.
   D. Increased clear fluids.

9. A 67-year-old male presents with a 72-hour history of sore throat associated with nasal congestion, clear rhinorrhea, and slight cough. This is most likely:

    A. Epstein-Barr virus.

    B. RSV.

    C. Bacterial pharyngitis.

    D. Viral pharyngitis.

10. A 10-year-old male presents with a 2-week history of nosebleeds from both sides of his nose. They usually stop with pressure but have been becoming more frequent. They generally last about 5 minutes. The mother is concerned that her son might have a significant health problem. The exam will most probably reveal:

    A. Hemoptysis.

    B. Hematemesis.

    C. Small sites of bleeding on the anterior nasal septum bilaterally.

    D. Dripping blood in the posterior pharynx.

11. A 72-year-old male presents with the acute onset of unilateral epistaxis. He has been unable to stop the bleeding, which is a steady drip from his right naris. He has been coughing up bright red blood. He has hypertension and no history of previous episodes. This is most likely caused by:

    A. A foreign body.

    B. A posterior bleed.

    C. An anterior bleed.

    D. Cocaine abuse.

12. The most common cause of an upper respiratory infection is:

    A. *Streptococcus.*

    B. Rhinovirus.

    C. RSV.

    D. Enterovirus.

13. Which of the following is NOT true about allergic rhinitis?

    A. Poor sleep quality

    B. Peaks during young adulthood

    C. Results in decreased school concentration

    D. May exacerbate asthma

14. After evaluating a 22-year-old female, the FNP diagnoses allergic rhinitis. What testing could be performed?

    A. Sinus films

    B. Sinus CT

    C. Blood testing for allergies

    D. Blood chemistries

15. What treatment will *initially* be prescribed?

    A. Oral antihistamine

    B. Leukotriene receptor antagonist

    C. Oral corticosteroid

    D. Topical decongestant

16. Upon evaluating a 73-year-old male for nasal congestion, a "bad smell" is noted in his nose. This patient may have:

    A. Allergic rhinitis.

    B. Vasomotor rhinitis.

    C. Atrophic rhinitis.

    D. An upper respiratory infection.

17. All of the following are risk factors for acute stomatitis EXCEPT:

    A. Day care attendance.

    B. Vitamin deficiency.

    C. Poverty.

    D. Intact dentures.

18. Common medical conditions that may have an oral presentation include:

    A. Vitamin A deficiency.

    B. Leukemias.

    C. HIV/AIDS.

    D. Celiac disease.

19. Oral apthous ulcers appear as:

    A. Vesicles that that break down to grayish ulcers.

    B. Small vesicles or ulcers only on the posterior pharyngeal wall.

    C. Small round or ovoid ulcers with circumscribed margins.

    D. Erythema of lips and oral mucosa.

20. First-line treatment for the patient with apthous ulcers would include:

    A. Oral corticosteroids.

    B. Thalidomide.

    C. Valacyclovir.

    D. Amlexanox.

21. The following is true of acute rhinosinusitis:

    A. An antibiotic is the only treatment.

    B. It is most common in adolescents and young adults.

    C. It is considered chronic if it lasts more than 2 months.

    D. The most common microbe involved is *S. Pneumoniae*.

22. Predictive symptoms that a viral rhinosinusitis has become infected with bacteria include:

    A. Worsening symptoms > 5–7 days.

    B. Bilateral dental pain.

    C. Persistent hyposmia.

    D. Persistent symptoms for > 7 days.

23. A 47-year-old female presents to the office with 3 days of nasal congestion with mucoid drainage, a dull frontal headache, and post nasal drip. She is concerned that she has a sinus infection. Treatment will include:

    A. High-dose Amoxicillin for 10 days.

    B. Watchful waiting with a backup of antibiotics if her symptoms worsen.

    C. Oral corticosteroids to decrease inflammation.

    D. Referral to a neurologist for a headache evaluation.

24. A patient that was seen a week ago and diagnosed with a common cold returns today with worsening nasal congestion and headaches and purulent post nasal drip. She has a low-grade fever. Her exam reveals purulent drainage in the posterior pharynx and an edematous erythematous nasal chamber. Treatment will include:

    A. High-dose Amoxicillin for 10–14 days.

    B. Referral to otolaryngology.

    C. Ordering a CT scan of the sinuses.

    D. Avelox 400 mg for 14 days.

25. The FNP is performing a risk assessment on a 9-month-old female infant with a history of two previous episodes of AOM. Which of the following is NOT a risk factor?

    A. Second-hand smoke

    B. Bottle feeding in upright position

    C. Day care with seven children

    D. Pacifier use

26. The tympanic membrane of a child with an otitis media with effusion will appear:

    A. Bulging.

    B. Erythematous.

    C. Retracted.

    D. With increased vascular markings.

27. A 5-month-old male infant has a documented acute otitis media. He appears ill with a fever of 103.2 degrees F. The mother is a reliable witness. The treatment plan would include:

    A. Observation of the patient to see if he improves over the next 24–48 hours.

    B. Sending him to the emergency room because he is so ill.

    C. Placing him on amoxicillin suspension at the appropriate dose if he has no known allergy.

    D. Explaining to the mother that no treatment is needed but he should be followed up in 2 weeks.

28. A 4-year-old female patient has otitis media with effusion following an initial episode of acute otitis media 2 months ago. She is experiencing no hearing loss and has no speech problems. Which of the following is the best next step?

    A. Tell the patient's parents that this is within normal limits for resolution and to make a follow-up appointment in 4 weeks.

    B. Refer her to an otolaryngologist.

    C. Place the patient on a decongestant or antihistamine.

    D. Use Augmentin in appropriate doses.

29. Prevention measures for AOM/OME include:

    A. Choosing a day care with less than 20 children.

    B. Making sure that an antibiotic is used with each episode.

    C. Allowing infants to bottle feed in the supine position only.

    D. Preventing exposure to second-hand smoke.

30. During examination of a 4-year-old male child, it is noted that the left tympanic membrane is dull and immobile. The FNP suspects that he has an associated hearing loss. This type of hearing loss is most likely:

    A. Sensorineural.

    B. Conductive.

    C. Congenital.

    D. Mixed.

31. The parent of a 7-year-old female child is doing poorly in school and her grades are falling. She is having problems concentrating and her mother is concerned about her ability to hear the teacher. She has a long history of acute and chronic ear infections. A conductive hearing loss is suspected. The FNP expects to find the following:

    A. A Weber test that lateralizes to the unaffected ear

    B. A Rinne test where air conduction = bone conduction

    C. An audiometric test from school showing an "air-bone gap"

    D. A tympanometry test showing no negative pressure

32. A 76-year-old male patient presents with a suspected hearing loss in both ears. He notes that it is impossible for him to hear anyone when dining in a restaurant and he is sure that his wife mumbles all the time. The most likely diagnosis is:

    A. Mixed hearing loss.

    B. Sensorineural hearing loss.

    C. Conductive hearing loss.

    D. Sudden SNHL.

33. A 29-year-old female patient presents with a 10-hour history of sudden hearing loss in her right ear, accompanied by tinnitus and an echo sensation in the affected ear. The FNP suspects a sudden SNHL. The most appropriate next step is to:

    A. Order a CT scan of her head.

    B. Reassure her that this is temporary and will respond to steroid ear drops.

    C. Immediately refer her to otolaryngology.

    D. Begin her on Amoxicillin because this is probably a conductive hearing loss with an effusion of the middle ear.

34. A 32-year-old male patient is being seen for the first time in the office. He states he has a new job on a construction site. The treatment plan for his hearing will include:

    A. Discussing the need for yearly hearing tests and daily ear protection.

    B. Referring him for a hearing aid evaluation.

    C. Discussing the need for him to stay away from the noisiest machines.

    D. Referring him for genetic counseling.

35. Presyncope is defined as:

    A. A sensation of uneasiness.

    B. A sense of spinning.

    C. A sense of pending loss of consciousness.

    D. A sense of impaired balance.

36. An adolescent male patient is being evaluated for "dizziness" following a concussion. The FNP suspects:

    A. BPPV.

    B. Ménière's disease.

    C. Labyrinthitis.

    D. A central vertigo secondary to the concussion.

37. Ms. Hamilton, a 23-year-old female patient, presents with an acute onset of vertigo worsened by head movement and changes in position. She has severe nausea and vomiting and is acutely ill. The most likely diagnosis is:

    A. BPPV.

    B. Ménière's disease.

    C. Labyrinthitis.

    D. Neuritis.

38. The diagnosis of BPPV will be aided by:
    A. A CBC with differential.
    B. The Dix–Hallpike Maneuver.
    C. A CT of the head.
    D. An MRI of the brain.

39. Treatment measures for BPPV include all of the following EXCEPT:
    A. No driving.
    B. Clear fluids for hydration with nausea and vomiting.
    C. An immediate return to daily activities with periods of rest.
    D. The Epley maneuver.

40. Risk factors for oral candidiasis include all of the following EXCEPT:
    A. Hyperthyroidism.
    B. Denture use.
    C. Birth control pills.
    D. Stress.

41. A 45-year-old female patient has been on Nystatin Oral Rinse for oral candidiasis for 2 weeks without any symptom relief. She is now having increasing dysphagia and losing weight. The FNP will:
    A. Change the medication to Clotrimazole trouches.
    B. Repeat the Nystatin regime for another course.
    C. Refer the patient to infectious disease.
    D. Begin an antibiotic.

42. Risk factors for developing acute otitis externa include all the following EXCEPT:
    A. Swimming in chlorinated pools.
    B. Swimming in lakes.
    C. Excessive ear cleaning with Q-tips.
    D. Frequent upper respiratory infections.

43. The bacteria most responsible for acute otitis externa is:
    A. *Staphylococcus Aureus.*
    B. *Aspergillus.*
    C. *Pseudomonas Aeruginosa.*
    D. *Proteus Mirabilis.*

44. The patient with acute otitis externa will complain of which of the following?
    A. Nasal congestion
    B. Intense pain in the occipital area
    C. Severe sore throat
    D. Intense pain and pruritus from the affected ear

45. Management of the patient with acute otitis externa includes:
    A. Application of a hot water bottle to relieve pain.
    B. Irrigation of the ear canal.
    C. To continue swimming and showering and making sure to dry the ear thoroughly afterward.
    D. Oral antibiotics for 10 days.

46. Indications for referral for acute otitis externa include:

    A. Green drainage from the ear.

    B. Presence of facial paralysis.

    C. Wick has become loose, resulting in it falling out of the ear canal.

    D. Fever and otalgia.

47. A 4-year-old boy is at the office for a pre-school physical exam. The FNP performs the cover/uncover test to evaluate for:

    A. Strabismus.

    B. Presbyopia.

    C. Chalazion.

    D. Butler's sign.

48. A 42-year-old female is at the clinic with a complaint of having difficulty focusing on the words in newspapers. The FNP will most likely find that this patient has:

    A. Presbyopia.

    B. Strabismus.

    C. Cataract.

    D. Macular degeneration.

49. A 19-year-old male presents to the health center with complaints of "really itchy eyes, and my eyes were like they were glued shut this morning. I had to use a lot of warm water to clear them." The FNP suspects:

    A. Viral conjunctivitis.

    B. Bacterial conjunctivitis.

    C. Allergic conjunctivitis.

    D. Blepharitis.

50. The FNP is performing a physical examination in a 65-year-old female. Arcus senilis is noted during the examination. The FNP is aware that this finding requires:

    A. Referral to an ophthalmologist for possible surgical intervention.

    B. Referral to a cardiologist for cardiac workup.

    C. No referral because this is a normal finding in this age group.

    D. No referral; however, this finding by itself indicates a need for a lipid profile.

51. A 22-year-old male presents to the walk-in center with the chief complaint of "painful eye swelling." Upon examination, the FNP notes the right eye has a hordeolum. The FNP treats this patient's problem by:

    A. Writing a prescription for Tobrex eye drops.

    B. Encouraging the patient to use clean warm soaks to the affected area for 15 minutes four times per day.

    C. Referring the patient to an eye surgeon for incision and drainage of the hordeolum.

    D. Applying a patch to keep the eye covered and avoid further irritation to the eyelid.

Answers and Rationales

1. D. *Streptococcus A* is by far the most common cause of acute pharyngitis.

2. A. Younger patients are more vulnerable due to immature immune systems.

3. B. There will be ulcers and/or exudate prominent on the affected tonsils. Pulmonary symptoms are common with RSV or mycoplasma pneumonia and oral lesions with acute stomatitis.

4. C. Ofloxacin is a quinolone and should never be used in pediatric cases.

5. B. Although all of the answers can cause cervical lymphadenopathy, viral and bacterial infections account for the majority of infections.

6. B. The highest recurrence rate is in those aged 15–25 years; 1–3% of college students experience IM annually.

7. A. The heterophile antibody test is the confirming test in IM. It is present in 40–60% patients in the first week and 78–90% of cases by weeks 3–4.

8. D. Increased fluids are an important supportive measure during the acute phase of IM. Increased activity levels increase the possibility of splenic rupture, and sports should be avoided for at least 4–6 weeks. Systemic corticosteroids are only used with complicated cases because they can affect cell-mediated immune response and may increase the risk of secondary bacterial infection.

9. D. Viral pharyngitis usually presents with associated respiratory symptoms. Patient is in the wrong age group for EB virus or RSV.

10. C. This is most likely an anterior bleed (90%) in children. The other answers are indicative of a posterior bleed.

11. B. This is most likely a posterior bleed because he has been coughing up bright red blood. A foreign body is unusual in this age group, as is cocaine abuse.

12. B. Rhinovirus is the most common cause of a URI. Bacteria can be a complication but is never the primary offending agent.

13. B. Allergic rhinitis peaks during adolescence.

14. C. Imaging is not recommended for the diagnosis of allergies. A RAST or ELISA test could be done to see what allergies are present.

15. A. Oral antihistamines are always the drug of choice to begin therapy.

16. C. Atrophic rhinitis is usually found in the elderly and is distinctive by its foul odor.

17. D. Only poorly fitting dentures increase the risk for acute stomatitis.

18. A. Vitamin B12 and folate deficiencies may present with oral lesions.

19. C. Vesicles that break down to grayish ulcers are usually herpes simplex. Small vesicles on the posterior pharyngeal wall are usually indicative of herpangina. Erythema of the lips and oral mucosa is found in Kawasaki disease.

20. C. Valtrex may be used for RAU as an initial systemic treatment. The other medications must be reserved for severe cases.

21. D. All rhinosinusitis begins as a virus and only a small amount become infected with bacteria. It is most common in women between 45 and 64 years of age. It is considered chronic after 12 weeks of symptoms.

22. A. Dental pain is usually unilateral, and hyposmia is not a cardinal symptom for a bacterial super infection. Persistent symptoms should last >10 days before bacterial infection is suspected.

23. B. Watchful waiting is the best treatment plan at this stage because she has not been sick long enough to establish a bacterial diagnosis, and antibiotics are not necessary with her history.

24. A. Amoxicillin is an initial choice for uncomplicated bacterial rhinosinusitis. It is too early to order a CT scan or make a referral.

25. B. Bottle feeding in the SUPINE position presents a risk for AOM.

26. C. A bulging erythematous tympanic membrane with hyperemia are signs of acute otitis media.

27. C. An infant under the age of 5 months should be treated with an antibiotic but does not need emergency care. The mother can report his progress by phone in 24–48 hours to ascertain efficacy of the antibiotic.

28. A. It is too soon to refer this patient because there is a 40% presence of effusion at 4 weeks. Decongestants, antihistamines, and antibiotics are not effective in OME.

29. D. The smaller the day care center, the less the risk; 20 children is too great a number. Antibiotics are not indicated in OME and infants should always be bottle-fed in the upright position.

30. B. Conductive hearing loss is most prevalent in children. The presence of a dull and immobile tympanic membrane suggests the presence of fluid behind the TM, which is associated with conductive hearing loss.

31. C. In conductive hearing loss, the Weber test lateralizes to the affected ear, and the Rinne test will show bone conduction greater than air conduction. The tympanogram will show negative pressure or immobility.

32. B. Presbycusis occurs in the elderly with bilateral SNHL and problems with ambient noise. Physical examination of the ear will be completely normal. If SNHL is sudden, the patient will complain of a sudden loss of hearing, usually unilateral, and often accompanied by tinnitus.

33. C. Sudden SNHL is an emergency and should be immediately referred to ENT. A conductive hearing loss is seldom sudden and may be bilateral.

34. A. Having a job in a noisy environment heightens the risk for SNHL. He should always be tested annually for changes in hearing. Many employers offer this as a benefit for their workers.

35. C. Vertigo is a sense of spinning. Disequilibrium is a sense of impaired balance. Lightheadedness is a sense of uneasiness.

36. D. Any complaint of dizziness following head trauma must be considered central until the evaluation is completed.

37. A. BPPV begins suddenly and is always exacerbated by head movements and position changes. In labyrinthitis, head motion is not usually a positive symptom. Ménière's disease must have the four symptoms of vertigo, aural pressure, roaring tinnitus, and hearing loss.

38. B. The Dix–Hallpike is a diagnostic for BPPV. No radiology is necessary in the acute phase.

39. C. The patient with BPPV must rest until symptoms begin to resolve.

40. A. Patients with hypothyroidism are at higher risk for oral candidiasis.

41. C. This patient is likely having a spread of fungal disease into the esophagus and needs a referral for specific testing.

42. D. Otitis externa occurs only in the ear canal itself. Upper respiratory infections occur in the nasal chamber and Eustachian tubes. These are separated from the external ear canal by the tympanic membrane.

43. C. *Pseudomonas Aeruginosa* is the offensive agent in 67% of cases.

44. D. The external ear canal inflammation will cause LOCAL pain. There may be a comorbid upper respiratory infection, but this is coincidental. A sore throat can cause ear pain, but it is usually a dull aching rather than a severe pain with and without palpation.

45. A. Pain relief is an important supportive measure in the acute phase, and intermittent heat will relieve some of the discomfort. NO water should be inserted into the external ear canal, and antibiotic drops are now the drug of choice for otitis externa.

46. B. The presence of facial paralysis indicates the possibility of neurological involvement and should be referred immediately. Drainage and pruritus are symptoms of an acute infection that can be managed in primary care. A loose wick usually means that the ear canal edema is lessening and it does not have to be replaced.

47. A. The cover/uncover test will detect any ocular deviation such as occurs in strabismus.

48. A. Presbyopia typically occurs between the ages of 40–50. Patients complain of difficulty focusing on near objects and fine print.

49. B. Bacterial conjunctivitis typically causes redness and pyogenic exudate, which causes crusting and a scratchy or gritty sensation that feels "itchy."

50. C. Arcus senilis is a common finding in the elderly, caused by lipid deposits. However, it is not caused by high cholesterol. No referral is required.

51. B. Unless the stye persists, no treatment other than cleansing with mild soap and water, and warm soaks to reduce discomfort are required. If it does not go away on its own, other treatments, including antibiotics, may be needed.

● ● ● **References**

Academy of Otolaryngology-Head and Surgery. (2015). Clinical practice guidelines on adult sinusitis. *Otolaryngology—Head and Neck Surgery, 152*(S2), S1–S45.

American Academy of Allergy Asthma and Immunology. (2000). *The allergy report.* AAAI, Volumes 1, 2.

American Academy of Otolaryngology-Head and Neck Surgery. (2015). Tonsillitis. Retrieved from http://entnet.org/content/tonsillitis

American Academy of Pediatrics, Joint Committee on Infant Hearing. (2007). Principles and guidelines for early hearing detection and intervention problems. *Pediatrics, 120*(4), 898–921.

Aung, K. (2015). Viral pharyngitis. *Medscape.* Retrieved from http://www.medscape.com/viewarticle/225362

Banotai, A. (2006). iPods, earphones, and hearing loss. *Advance for speech-language pathologists and audiologists.* 7–8, 14.

Barclay, L. (2006). Guidelines issued for acute otitis externa. Medscape Family Medicine. Retrieved from http://www.medscape.org/viewarticle/529042

Bennett, N. J. (2015). Pediatric mononucleosis and Epstein–Barr Virus infection. *Medscape.* Retrieved from http://www.emedicine.medscape.com/article963894

Bickley, L. (2012). *Bates guide to physical examination,* 11th edition. Lippincott, Williams, & Wilkins: Philadelphia

Blunt, E., & Reinisch, C. (2009). *Family nurse practitioner review manual.* ANCC Credentialing Knowledge Center. Chapters on ENT Health Problems.

Carillo-Marquez, C. (2015). Bacterial pharyngitis. *Medscape.* Retrieved from http://www.medscape.com/viewarticle/225243

Centers for Disease Control and Prevention. (2015). Fungal diseases. Retrieved from http://cdc.gov/fungal/diseases/candidiasis

Centers for Disease Control and Prevention. (2015). Influenza. Retrieved from http://www.cdc.gov/flu

Choby, B. (2009). Diagnosis and treatment of streptococcal pharyngitis. *Am Fam Physician, 79*(5), 383–390.

Dancer, J. (2006), Does smoking affect hearing? *Advance for speech pathologists and audiologists.* 9, 50.

Derlet, R. (2015). Influenza. *Medscape.* Retrieved from http://www.emedicine.medscape.com/article/219557

Garry, G. (2011). Otitis externa. *Medscape.* Retrieved from http://www.emedicine.medscape.com/article/84923

Goldberg, C. (2015). *A practical guide to clinical medicine.* The Regents University of California. Retrieved from https://meded.ucsd.edu/clinicalmed/eyes.htm

Hollier, A., & Hensley, R. (2011). Clinical Guidelines in Primary Care. Advanced Practice Education Associates. Chapters on ENT Health Problems.

Kanegaonkar, R. G., & Tysome, J. R. (Eds.) (2014). *Dizziness and vertigo: an introduction and practical guide.* Boca Raton, LA: CRC Press.

Kanwar, V. S. (2015). Lymphadenopathy workup. *Medscape.* Retrieved from http://www.emedicine.medscape.com/article/956340

Lieberthal, A. S., Carroll, A. E., Chonmaitree, T., et al. (2013). The diagnosis and management of acute otitis media. American Academy of Pediatrics: Clinical guidelines. *Pediatrics, 131*(3), e964–e999.

Lynch, J. (2002). How should I assess and manage a patient with acute vertigo? *Medscape* Retrieved from http://www.medscape.com/viewarticle/437103

Lynch, J. S. (2004). What are the new guidelines for classifying allergic rhinitis? *Medscape.* Retrieved from http://www.medscape.com/viewarticle/471274

Lynch, J. S. (2006). What offers the most effective relief for severe aphthous stomatitis? *Medscape.* Retrieved from http://www.medscape.com/viewarticle/532727

Lynch, J. S. (2008). How should I treat acute bacterial rhinosinusitis? *Medscape.* Retrieved from http://www.medscape,com/viewarticle/580928

Lynch, J. S. (2011). External otitis. *Medscape.* Ask the Expert. (archived)

Maloney, C. (2008). Screening and treatment of common ocular problems in adults. Workshop handout, CTAPRNS conference, CT.

Mayo Clinic. (2015). Influenza. Retrieved from http://mayoclinic.org/diseases-conditions/flu

Medical News Today. (2015). Oral candidiasis. Retrieved from http://medicalnewstoday.com/articles,178864.php

Murcheson, D. (2015). Stomatitis. Merck Manual. Retrieved from http://merckmanuals.com/professions/dental-disorders

National Health Service. (2015). Oral thrush. Retrieved from http://nhs.uk/conditions/oral-thrush

Nguyen, Q. A. (2015). Epistaxis clinical presentation. *Medscape*. Retrieved from http://www.medscape.com/article/863220-clinical

Omori, M. S. (2014). Mononucleosis in emergency medicine. *Medscape*. Retrieved from http://www.emedicine.medscape.com/article784513

Scadding, G. K. (2015). Optimal management of allergic rhinitis. *Arch Dis Child*, *100*(6), 576–582.

Scully, C. (2015). Aphthous ulcers. *Medscape*. Retrieved from http://www.medscape.com/viewarticle/867080

Seidman, M. D., Gurgel, R. K., Lin, S. Y., et al. (2015). Clinical practice guidelines: Allergic rhinitis. *Otolaryngology—Head and Neck Surgery*. 152(S1); S1–S43.

Shah, R. K. (2015). Hearing impairment. *Medscape*. Retrieved from http://www.emedicine.medscape.com/article/994159

Suh, J. D. (2011). Epistaxis. American Rhinologic Society. Retrieved from http://care.american-rhinologic.org/epistaxis

Vestibular Disorders Association. (2004). Vestibular neuritis and labyrinthitis: Infections of the inner ear. VEDA publication #F-9. 4/22/04.

Vestibular Disorders Association. BPPV is the most common vestibular disorder. Retrieved from http://vestibular.org/understanding-vestibular-disorders/types-vestibular-disorders/

Waseem M. (2015). Otitis media treatment and management. *Medscape*. Retrieved from http://www.emedicine.medscape.com/article/994656-treatment

Winters, M. (2007). Evidence-based diagnoses and management of ENT emergencies. *Medscape*. Retrieved from http://www.medscape.com/viewarticle/551650

6

Respiratory System

Karen L. Gregory, DNP, APRN, CNS, RRT, AE-C

Basic Anatomy of the Respiratory System

Functions of the respiratory system include gas exchange, acid–base balance, phonation, pulmonary defense, and metabolism. The respiratory system is comprised of the lungs, conducting airways, and the chest wall. Slightly above the clavicle is the apex of the lung. Bases of the lungs extend to the diaphragm. The right lung consists of three lobes and is positioned in a more horizontal plane, while the left lung has upper and lower lobes, separated by an oblique fissure.

Lung parenchyma is part of the conduction system and is involved in the gas exchange at the alveolar level. Pleura are a double layer extending along the mediastinum from the inferior pulmonary vein to the diaphragm, the major muscle of respiration. Visceral pleura cover the lungs and are contiguous with the parietal pleura. The visceral pleura form fissures that separate the lung lobes. The extrathoracic (superior) airway includes the supraglottic, glottic, and infraglottic regions. The intrathoracic (inferior) airway includes the trachea, the mainstem bronchi, and multiple bronchial generations. The actual exchange of gases occurs in the respiratory bronchioles, alveolar ducts and sacs, and alveoli. Lung compliance determines the rate and force of expiration, and the thoracic compliance determines the elastic load during inspiration (Levitzky, 2013). Structural changes to the thoracic cage due to aging cause a reduction in chest wall compliance.

Surfactant, a lipoprotein secreted by type II alveolar cells to reduce surface tension and prevent alveolar collapse, remains in the alveoli at the end of expiration. Pulmonary arteries carry deoxygenated blood that follow the respiratory passages and end in capillaries in alveolar walls. The bronchial arteries carry oxygenated blood to the tissue of the bronchial tree and alveoli.

Clinical Pearl

Adults and children differ in airway anatomy and physiology. At approximately 8 years old, the pediatric airway anatomy and physiology becomes similar to the adult airway.

Assessment of the Respiratory System

Medical History and Physical Examination

The medical history for the respiratory system is a structured assessment conducted to produce a comprehensive portrait of a patient's respiratory health and clinical problems. A comprehensive medical history and physical examination are essential to the diagnostic process. Subjective and objective clinical findings may lack sufficient evidence to allow a definitive conclusion requiring further objective criteria, including pulmonary function testing and imaging studies.

Systemic manifestations of comorbid conditions are vital information to elicit the appropriate treatment regimen to achieve control of the disease and improve clinical outcomes. Obtaining a thorough patient history using open-ended questions and active listening will lead to critical clues that best guide medical management. The respiratory examination includes inspection, palpation, percussion, and auscultation. **Tables** 6-1 and 6-2 provide the components of obtaining a comprehensive respiratory medical history and physical examination.

Table 6-1	Obtaining a Respiratory History	
Chief Complaint	Foundation of the history! Reason your patient is seeking care	
History of Present Illness	Presenting problem: Frequency of daytime and nocturnal symptoms. Frequency of reliever inhaler (albuterol or levoalbuterol) Cough—character; Is it secondary to mediations? Wheeze—dyspnea Shortness of breath exertion at rest; exercise tolerance and limitations Orthopnea Chest pain—character Systematic symptoms (night sweats, weight loss, fatigue) Chest pain	For each symptom describe: Onset Location/radiation Duration Character Aggravating factors Relieving factors Temporal/timing Severity (quantitative value) Important Questions: What questions or concerns? What does the patient want the provider to know or answer? Management of disease(s) Adherence to medical treatment regiment Environmental exposures Barriers to medical care
Other Subjective Data	Activities of Daily Living Functional Status Development Status	
Past Medical History	Systematical review for any conditions that have the potential for respiratory manifestations or atopic components. Environmental allergy evaluation (including allergy testing), food allergy, anaphylaxis, hospital or emergency room admissions, ICU admission and intubations or noninvasive ventilation Include comorbid conditions (gastroesophageal reflux disease, obesity, sleep apnea, allergic diseases, food allergy, anaphylaxis, urticaria/ angioedema, vocal cord dysfunction, diabetes mellitus, anxiety or depression) Recurrent respiratory infections Injuries/chest trauma/head injury Other chronic illnesses Childhood disease or illnesses	Management of disease Adherence to medical treatment regimen
Past Surgical History Past Diagnostic Studies	Tonsil and adenoidectomy Cardiac surgery Chest or sinus radiograph Pulmonary function testing Allergy testing Bronchoscopy or laryngoscopy Tuberculin and/or fungal skin testing	
Immunizations	Influenza (month/year) Pneumococcal (month/year) Adult immunizations Childhood immunizations	

Table 6-1	Obtaining a Respiratory History (*Continued*)	
Medications	Short-acting beta agonist Inhaled corticosteroids Inhaled corticosteroids/long-acting beta agonist Ipratropium bromide Prednisone Home oxygen Other Herbal therapy Over-the-counter therapy	Barriers to medication adherence Technique of respiratory devices Knowledge of medical treatment regimen
Allergies	Medications	Type and reaction
Family History	Three generations History of asthma, cystic fibrosis	
Social History	Home, work, and school environment Occupation Environmental hazards Use of protective devices Use of heater, air conditioner, humidifiers Exercise habits Diet/nutrition Low socioeconomic status or inner-city residence Past and present illicit drug use, tobacco or marijuana use, alcohol use Second- or third-hand tobacco smoke exposure Travel outside the United States	

Diseases of the Respiratory System

Asthma

Asthma is a heterogeneous disorder of the lungs affecting approximately 25 million persons in the United States (Global Initiative for Asthma, 2015). The pathophysiology of asthma is complex and involves underlying inflammation, airflow obstruction, and bronchial hyperresponsiveness. The National Asthma Education and Prevention Program Expert Panel Report 3 (EPR-3), Guidelines for the Diagnosis and Management of Asthma, defines asthma as "a common chronic disorder of the airways that is complex and characterized by variable and recurring symptoms, airflow obstruction, bronchial hyperresponsiveness, and underlying inflammation" (EPR-3, 2007). Immunohistopathologic features of asthma include inflammatory cell infiltration eosinophils, neutrophils, lymphocytes, epithelial cell injury and mast cell activation (EPR-3, 2007; GINA, 2015). The development of asthma appears to involve the interplay between host factors, primarily genetics and environmental exposures, which occur at a crucial time in the development of the immune system (EPR-3, 2007; GINA, 2015). Gene-by-environment interactions are important to the expression of asthma. Atopy, the genetic predisposition for the development

of an immunoglobulin E (IgE)-mediated response to common aeroallergens, is the strongest identifiable predisposing factor for developing asthma.

IgE is the antibody responsible for activation of allergic reactions and is important to the pathogenesis of allergic diseases and the development and persistence of inflammation. When IgE receptors are activated with an antigen, they release mediators that initiate acute bronchospasms and release proinflammatory cytokines affecting underlying airway inflammation. Mast cells, basophils, and eosinophils are central effector cells in allergic inflammation and innate and adaptive immunity. IgE attaches to cell surfaces via a specific high-affinity receptor.

The EPR-3 was developed by an expert panel commissioned by the NAEPP Coordinating Committee, overseen by the National Heart, Lung, and Blood Institute (NHLBI) of the National Institutes of Health. EPR-3 contains nine tables that are used to guide the stepwise approach to managing asthma. EPR-3 recognizes six steps in the stepwise approach for management. EPR3 guidelines recommendations focus on three age groups: children aged birth to 4 years, children aged 5 to 11 years, and patients aged 12 years or older. Asthma severity is classified as intermittent, mild persistent, moderate persistent, or severe persistent. Measures of asthma severity are based upon two

Table 6-2	Physical Examination		
Inspection	**Palpation**	**Percussion**	**Auscultation**

General appearance
Cough or audible wheeze
Use of accessory muscles
Pursed-lip breathing
Dyspnea
Nasal flaring
Inability to speak in
   complete sentences
Cyanosis
Shape of the chest
   (barrel chest)
Paradoxical chest
   movement
Nail clubbing
   (<160 degree)
	Trachea
	Use index finger to
	determine central
	alignment or
	   deviation
	Thoracic expansion
	Adult is 4 to 5 cm
	Symmetrical
	Tactile fremitus
		Diaphragmatic excursion
		Assessment of diaphragmatic excursion
		   provides a method for evaluating
		   the degree of muscle deterioration
		   in neuromuscular and respiratory diseases.
		Ask patient to breathe deeply and hold
		   breath. Percuss downward along scapular
		   line, just below the scapula on one side
		   until tone changes from resonant to dull.
		   Mark the location
		   on the skin.
		Allow patient to breathe normally 2
		   or 3 breaths, then ask the patient to exhale
		   completely and hold. Percuss upward,
		   starting just below the mark, observing for
		   dull to resonant.
		Measure distance.
		Repeat on the opposite side.
		Ask patient to resume breathing comfortably.
		EXPECTED: 3 to 5 cm
		(higher on right than left)
		Percussion—over all lobes of the
		   lungs, comparing right and left.
		Resonant sounds are low-pitched, hollow
		   sounds heard over normal
		   lung tissue.
		Flat or extremely dull sounds are normally
		   heard over solid areas.
		Dull sounds are normally heard over dense
		   areas such as the heart or
		   liver. Dullness replaces resonance
		   when fluid or solid tissue replaces
		   air-containing lung tissues, such as occurs
		   with pneumonia, pleural effusions, or
		   tumors.
		Hyperresonant sounds are louder and
		   lower pitched than resonant sounds and
		   are normally heard when percussing the
		   chests of children and very thin adults.
		   May also be heard when percussing lungs
		   hyperinflated with air.
		Tympanic sounds are hollow, high, drumlike
		   sounds. Tympany is normally heard over the
		   stomach, but is not
		   a normal chest sound. Tympanic
		   sounds heard over the chest indicate
		   excessive air in the chest, such as
		   may occur with pneumothorax.
			Normal Lungs Sounds
			Vesicular: I > E low-pitch
			   soft intensity; turbulent
			   flow of air throughout
			   the airways of non-
			   diseased lungs.
			Bronchovesicular: I =
			   E moderate pitch and
			   intensity, turbulent,
			   heard over bronchi
			Bronchial/Tracheal: I < E
			   high-pitched, loud, less
			   harsh, easily, heard in
			   central airways
			
			Adventitious Sounds
			Wheeze: continuous, high-
			   pitched, musical, usually
			   expiratory, but can be
			   inspiratory or both.
			   Sounds are produced
			   by air flowing through
			   narrowed bronchi.
			Rhonchi: low-pitched,
			   loud, often gurgling,
			   generally heard on
			   inspiration, snore-like
			   sounds, often clears with
			   cough. Characterized by
			   secretions within the
			   large airways; can be
			   heard in a wide variety
			   of pathologies.
			Crackles are discontinuous,
			   explosive, "popping"
			   sounds that originate
			   within the airways.

domains: impairment of function and future risk of exacerbations. Impairment is the frequency and intensity of symptoms and functional limitations the patient is experiencing or has recently experienced. Risk is defined as the likelihood of asthma exacerbations, the progressive decline in lung function or reduced lung growth for children, or risk of adverse effects from medications (EPR-3, 2007). The goal of asthma therapy should be to maintain long-term control of asthma with the least amount of medication, thereby exposing the patient to the least risk for adverse effects from pharmacologic therapy (EPR-3, 2007). Both documents build upon the recommendations of former guidelines, utilizing evidence-based review of the published literature to revise algorithms for practice.

Viral respiratory infections are one of the most important causes of asthma exacerbation and may also contribute to the development of asthma. Asthma tends to develop earlier in life and is associated with variable airflow limitation and hyperresponsiveness (EPR-3, 2007). Asthma that is uncontrolled can lead to airway remodeling involving almost all the elements of the airway in the bronchial tree (Shifen, Witt, Christie, & Castro, 2011).

Physical Examination Findings

A classic physical examination finding in asthma is wheezing that occurs intermittently in association with cough or dyspnea. Uncontrolled asthma or status asthmaticus can reveal tachycardia, tachypnea, use of suprasternal and other accessory respiratory muscles, or nasal flaring. Signs of severe or life-threatening asthma include tachycardia (heart rate > 120 beats per minute), tachypnea (respiratory rate > 30 breaths per minute), pulsus paradoxus > 18 mmHg, evidence of a hyperinflated chest, cyanosis, difficulty speaking, and silent chest. Prolonged expiratory phases may present as a result of airway narrowing. The expiratory prolongation is greater with more severe obstruction. Pulsus paradox is an exaggeration of normal physiology in which the systolic arterial pressure is > 10 mgHg during inspiration. A drop of > 25 mmHg reflects severe airflow obstruction. Mental status changes may be present and are generally secondary to hypoxia and hypercapnia, indicative of intubation. The nurse practitioner must identify those patients at risk for fatal asthma. These patients require intensive asthma education, monitoring, and care. **Table 6-3** describes patients at risk for fatal asthma.

Diagnostic Testing

The EPR-3 highlights the importance of correctly diagnosing asthma by determining the episodic symptoms of airflow obstruction present, which airflow obstruction or symptoms are at least partially reversible, and the exclusion of alternative diagnoses (EPR-3, 2007). Spirometry should be obtained at the initial assessment and at least every 1 to 2 years after treatment is initiated (EPR-3, 2007; GINA, 2015). Spirometry with evaluation

Table 6-3	Risk Factors for Asthma-Related Death

Previous severe exacerbation (e.g., intubation or ICU admission for asthma)

Two or more hospitalizations or > 3 ED visits in the past year

Use of > 2 canisters of SABA per month

Difficulty perceiving airway obstruction or the severity of worsening asthma

Low socioeconomic status or inner-city residence

Illicit drug use

Major psychosocial problems or psychiatric disease

Comorbid diseases (such as cardiovascular disease or other chronic lung disease)

Modified from National Heart Lung and Blood Institute. (2007). Expert Panel Report 3 (EPR-3): Guidelines for the diagnosis and management of asthma summary report 2007. Retrieved from http://www.nhlbi.nih.gov/health-pro/guidelines/current/asthma-guidelines.

of post-bronchodilator response, exhaled nitric oxide, and according to the history chest radiograph, allergy skin testing, and measurement of sputum eosinophils may be indicated. Chest radiograph remains the initial imaging evaluation in most individuals with symptoms of asthma. Chest radiography findings are most often normal, but may indicate hyperinflation. Pulse oximetry measurement is desirable in all patients with acute asthma to exclude hypoxemia. Exercise challenge is the standard method for assessing patients with exercise-induced bronchospasm. **Table 6-4** provides key indicators for diagnosing asthma according to the EPR-3 Guidelines. **Table 6-5** lists EPR-3 Guidelines recommendations for referral to an asthma specialist. After diagnosis is established, the severity of the asthma should be classified before initiating therapy (EPR-3 2007; GINA, 2015).

Treatment

Short-acting β-agonist (SABA) medications or reliever medications are the mainstay of asthma therapy and are recommended treatment at all levels of asthma severity. Short-acting β-agonists bind to the beta-2 adrenergic receptor, causing smooth muscle relaxation and bronchodilation of the airway. Short-acting β-agonist (albuterol) is used as a "reliever" medication and administered approximately 15 minutes before sports or exercise. Ipratropium bromide (Atrovent) is a short-acting muscarinic antagonist (SAMA) for the adjunctive treatment of moderate or severe asthma. Ipratropium blocks the effect of acetylcholine on airways, reduces vagal tone in the airway, and decreases mucus secretions, providing additional bronchodilation. Valved holding chambers are used with metered dose inhalers, except

Table 6-4	Key Indicators for Diagnosing Asthma

Consider a diagnosis of asthma and perform spirometry if any of these indicators are present:

The symptoms of dyspnea, cough, and/or wheezing, especially nocturnal, difficulty breathing, or chest tightness

With acute episodes: hyperinflation of thorax, decreased breath sounds, high-pitched wheezing, and use of accessory muscles

Symptoms worse in presence of exercise, viral infections, inhaled allergens, irritants, changes in weather, strong emotional expression, stress, menstrual cycles

Reversible airflow obstruction: FEV1 > 12% from baseline, or increase in FEV1 > 10% of predicted after inhalation of a bronchodilator, if able to perform spirometry

Alternative diagnoses are excluded.

Modified from National Heart Lung and Blood Institute. (2007). Expert Panel Report 3 (EPR-3): Guidelines for the diagnosis and management of asthma summary report 2007. Retrieved from http://www.nhlbi.nih.gov/health-pro/guidelines/current/asthma-guidelines.

Table 6-5	EPR-3 Guidelines: Recommendations for Referral to an Asthma Specialist

Patient has had a life-threatening asthma exacerbation.

Patient is not meeting the goals of asthma therapy after 3–6 months of treatment.

An earlier referral or consultation is appropriate if the physician concludes that the patient is unresponsive to therapy.

Signs and symptoms are atypical, or there are problems in differential diagnosis.

Other conditions complicate asthma or its diagnosis (e.g., sinusitis, nasal polyps, ABPA, severe rhinitis, vocal cord dysfunction (VCD), GERD, chronic obstructive pulmonary disease (COPD)).

Additional diagnostic testing is indicated (e.g., allergy skin testing, rhinoscopy, complete pulmonary function studies, provocative challenge, bronchoscopy).

Patient requires additional education and guidance on complications of therapy, problems with adherence, or allergen avoidance.

Patient is being considered for immunotherapy.

Patient requires step 4 care or higher (step 3 for children 0–4 years of age). Consider referral if patient requires step 3 care (step 2 for children 0–4 years of age).

Patient has required more than two bursts of oral corticosteroids in 1 year or has an exacerbation requiring hospitalization.

Patient requires confirmation of a history that suggests that an occupational or environmental inhalant or ingested substance is provoking or contributing to asthma.

Depending on the complexities of diagnosis, treatment, or the intervention required in the work environment, it may be appropriate in some cases for the specialist to manage the patient over a period of time or to co-manage with the primary care provider (PCP).

Reproduced from National Heart Lung and Blood Institute. (2007). Expert Panel Report 3 (EPR-3): Guidelines for the diagnosis and management of asthma summary report 2007. Retrieved from http://www.nhlbi.nih.gov/health-pro/guidelines/current/asthma-guidelines.

Aerospan and Respiclick, for better drug deposition in the lungs, avoiding drug in the oropharynx.

Inhaled corticosteroids are recommended by the EPR-3 Guidelines as the preferred drug for all three levels of persistent asthma. Patients who are symptomatic, despite inhaled corticosteroids, may benefit from combination ICS/LABA. Long-acting beta-agonists (LABAs) provide a longer duration of bronchodilation compared to SABAs, with a slower onset of action. Formoterol has a faster onset of action compared to salmeterol (Bellinger & Peters, 2015). Long-acting beta-agonists are contraindicated for treatment of acute symptoms or exacerbations or as monotherapy asthma (EPR-3, 2007; GINA, 2015). Leukotriene agonist (LTRA) inhibits the inflammatory actions of leukotrienes and is considered as add-on therapy in mild and moderate persistent asthma and possibly an alternative to ICS in mild persistent asthma (EPR-3, 2007). Montelukast is approved from age 6 months, and zafirlukast is approved for aged 7 years and older. Mast cell stabilizers (cromolyn sodium and nedocromil) are listed in the EPR-3 guidelines, but are no longer available in the United States. Methylxanthines (theophylline or aminophylline) inhibits the phosphodiestrerase, which leads to an increase in intracellular cAMP in airway smooth muscle, causing bronchodilation. Theophylline may be used as nonpreferred adjunctive therapy to ICS (EPR-3, 2007). A serum concentration between 5 and 12 ug/mL is generally recommended for chronic theophylline therapy. Close monitoring of serum concentration is necessary in patients with liver disease, congestive heart failure, pregnancy, and when certain drugs are being used, such as quinolone antibiotics, cimetidine, or macrolides. Medications used to treat asthma are described in Table 6-6.

Table 6-6	Medications Used for Asthma

Combined Medication (Inhaled Corticosteroid + Long-acting Beta2-agonist)
Symbicort—Budesonide/Formoterol—HFA 80 mcg/4.5 mcg or 160 mcg/4.5 mcg
Advair—Fluticasone/Salmeterol—DPI 100 mcg/50 mcg, 250 mcg/50 mcg, or 500 mcg/50 mcg
HFA 45 mcg/21 mcg, 115 mcg/21 mcg, or 230 mcg/21 mcg
Dulera—Mometasone/Formoterol—HFA 100 mcg/5 mcg or 200 mcg/5 mcg
Breo Ellipta Fluticasone Furoate/Vilanterol—100 mcg/25 mcg, 200 mcg/25 mcg

Inhaled Corticosteroid (ICS)
Flovent—Fluticasone—44 mcg, 110 mcg, 220 mcg
Fluticasone diskus 50 mcg, 100 mcg, 250 mcg
Pulmicort—Budesonide 90 mcg, 180 mcg
Aerospan—Flunisolide 80 mcg
Alvesco—Ciclesonide 80 mcg, 160 mcg
Qvar—Beclomethasone 40 mcg, 80 mcg
Asmanex Twisthaler Mometasone 110 mcg, 220 mcg

Short-acting Beta-agonist
Albuterol—Proventil HFA, Ventolin HFA, ProAir HFA Albuterol nebulizer solution
Levalbuterol—Xoponex HFA, Xoponex nebulizer solution

Long-acting Beta2-agonists
Salmeterol diskus Serevent
Formoterol Foradil
Arcapta Neohaler (approved for COPD only)
Leukotriene Modifiers Leukotriene Receptor Antagonists (LTRAs) Montelukast—4 mg granule packet, 4 mg or 5 mg
  chewable tablet 10 mg tablet
Zafirlukast—10 mg or 20 mg tablet
Albuterol and Ipatropium Bromide combination Combivent® metered dose inhaler or DuoNeb nebulized solution
List of short-acting anticholinergic Ipratropium Bromide
Atrovent MDI DPI nebulizer

List of long-acting Anticholinergics
Tiotropium   Spiriva DPI   (approved for COPD)
Combivent Respimat Ipratropium Bromide and Albuterol (approved for COPD)

Table 6-7	Chronic Bronchitis and Emphysema

Chronic bronchitis (blue bloaters)
Patients may be obese.
Frequent cough and expectoration are typical.
Use of accessory muscles of respiration is common.
Coarse rhonchi and wheezing may be heard on auscultation.
Patients may have signs of right heart failure (i.e., cor pulmonale), such as edema and cyanosis.
Because they share many of the same physical signs, COPD may be difficult to distinguish from congestive heart failure (CHF). One crude bedside test for distinguishing COPD from CHF is peak expiratory flow. If patients blow 150–200 mL or less, they are probably having a COPD exacerbation; higher flows indicate a probable CHF exacerbation.

Emphysema (pink puffers)
Patients may be very thin with a barrel chest.
They typically have little or no cough or expectoration.
Breathing may be assisted by pursed lips and use of accessory respiratory muscles; they may adopt the tripod sitting position.
The chest may be hyperresonant, and wheezing may be heard; heart sounds are very distant.
Overall appearance is more like classic COPD exacerbation.

Patients with uncontrolled moderate or severe persistent asthma, despite an appropriate medical treatment regimen, should be considered for omalizumab (Xolair). Candidates for omalizumab are patients who have uncontrolled moderate or severe persistent asthma, positive test results for perennial allergens, and an IgE level between 30 IU/mL and 700 IU/mL. Omalizumab is a humanized monoclonal antibody that binds to free IgE to form immune complexes which then inhibits IgE from binding to the mast cells and basophils. Another treatment for consideration in uncontrolled moderate or severe persistent asthma is bronchial thermoplasty, which is used to reduce airway smooth muscle mass in adults with uncontrolled moderate or severe persistent asthma.

Assessment of Control

Poor asthma control can increase future risks of asthma, including exacerbation, accelerated decrease in lung function, and side effects of treatment (EPR-3, 2007; GINA, 2015). The EPR-3 and GINA (2015) guidelines define the goals of asthma control as minimal or no symptoms during the day or night, full physical activity including exertion, prevention of exacerbations, maintenance of (near) normal pulmonary function, decreased use of reliever medication (SABA), and minimal or no adverse effects from medications. Reliable assessment of asthma control is essential to manage asthma effectively and to initiate or change pharmacotherapy.

Expert Panel Report 3 (EPR-3, 2007) recommends that regular follow-up visits be held at 1- to 6-month intervals, depending on the level of control. Asthma control should be assessed at every patient encounter using a standardized, validated self-administered questionnaire, such as the Asthma Control Test (ACT) and the Asthma Control Questionnaire (ACQ), or TRACK. These questionnaires are based on the appropriate age and are completed by patients and/or the parent or caregiver before the patient's encounter with the health care professional. Assessment of asthma control is identified according to the patient and/or parent or caregiver's perception and provides information for asthma management. An Asthma Action Plan is recommended for all patients with asthma.

When asthma is well controlled and maintained for at least 3 months, a step-down or reduction in pharmacologic therapy may be implemented (EPR-3, 2007). Close monitoring and review of the written asthma action plan, which includes the medications, and the patient's self-management behaviors for daily management and worsening asthma,

is imperative and asthma control can deteriorate at a highly variable rate and intensity.

The goal of asthma management is to achieve and maintain control of the disease, prevent exacerbations, and reduce the risk of morbidity and mortality, and reduce the economic and societal burdens of asthma. A short-acting beta agonist used more than twice a week (excluding pre-medicating before exercise or sports) indicates poor asthma control. Adherence to the prescribed medical treatment regimen must be evaluated at each patient encounter. Poor inhaler technique is a common problem among patients with asthma, and asthma control worsens as the number of mistakes in technique increases. Nurse practitioners should be competent in correct administering of all inhaled medication devices. Assessment and demonstration of prescribed inhaled medications must be performed with appropriate corrections made at each patient encounter. Evaluation of unscheduled medical utilization, oral prednisone requirements, and limitations to exercise or activities, and barriers to asthma care must be addressed at each patient encounter.

Asthma education is the cornerstone of achieving asthma control. Asthma education must be provided to every patient with asthma and their caregiver. Reinforcement of all components of asthma education should be integrated into all aspects of asthma care, including every patient encounter. Nurse practitioners have a unique opportunity to identify patients at risk, and provide enhanced care and asthma education for control, because they are at the front line of patient care (Rance, 2011).

Clinical Pearl

The characterization of the heterogeneity has recognized that asthma consists of multiple phenotypes. Phenotypes are the observable cluster of characteristics that define a disease and its subsets. Recognition of specific phenotypes may enhance our understanding of pathophysiology, treatment response, prognosis, and the underlying genetic origins for asthma.

Chronic Obstructive Pulmonary Disease (COPD)

Chronic Obstructive Pulmonary Disease is the third leading cause of death in the United States (CDC, 2014) and is the leading cause of morbidity and mortality worldwide (Hillas, Perlikos, Tsiligianni & Tzanakis, 2015). Characterized by the presence of progressive airflow limitation, COPD is associated with enhanced chronic inflammatory response in the airways to noxious particles or gases (Global Initiative for Chronic Obstructive Lung Disease, 2015). Tobacco use is the most prevalent cause of COPD in the United States (GOLD, 2015). Approximately 80 percent of COPD deaths are caused by tobacco use (American Lung Association, 2014; CDC, 2014).

COPD is subdivided into two major groups based on clinical symptoms: emphysema and chronic bronchitis. Emphysema is defined pathologically as an abnormal, permanent enlargement of the air spaces distal to the terminal bronchioles, accompanied by destruction of their walls and without obvious fibrosis (GOLD, 2015). Emphysema affects the structures distal to the terminal bronchiole. Destruction of alveoli due to emphysema can lead to loss of the associated areas of the pulmonary capillary bed and pruning of the distal vasculature. Emphysematous patients, often known as "pink puffers," have a cachectic appearance and frequently use accessory muscles. Bullae and avascularity in the peripheral third of the lung are also clinical findings in emphysema.

Chronic bronchitis is defined clinically as the presence of a chronic productive cough for 3 months during each of 2 consecutive years, with other causes of cough being excluded (GOLD, 2015). Chronic bronchitis patients, often known as "blue bloaters," tend to have chronic hypoxemia and hypercapnia, peripheral edema from cor pulmonale, and a chronic, productive cough with large amounts of sputum. Table 6-7 describes the symptoms of chronic bronchitis and emphysema.

The acute exacerbation of chronic bronchitis is identified by the worsening airflow and symptoms.

Symptoms of COPD include cough, wheezing, dyspnea, and increased sputum production. Acute exacerbation of COPD is a clinical diagnosis with presenting symptoms or worsening dyspnea, increased sputum production and sputum purulence. The Global Initiative for Chronic Obstructive Lung Disease (GOLD) Guidelines criteria bases severity of airflow obstruction on the percent predicate Forced Expiratory Volume in 1 second (FEV1) in the setting of the ratio of Forced Expiratory Volume in 1 second and Forced Vital Capacity (FVC) less than 70% (see Table 6-8). Severity is used to guide initial therapy and deteriorating risk of exacerbation and mortality. The COPD Assessment Test (CAT) is an 8-item questionnaire that is used to measure symptoms. A score ranging from 0 to 40 determines the prevalence of respiratory symptoms. The CAT assessment scores are available at http://www.catestonline.org.

Management and treatment of COPD should be based upon current GOLD guidelines. Short-acting bronchodilators (SABA) (beta-agonist, anticholinergic agent) are prescribed as needed for dyspnea. When intermittent short-acting bronchodilators are insufficient in achieving control of the symptoms, severe or very severe airflow obstruction, or two or more exacerbations in the previous year, a long-acting inhaled bronchodilator can be prescribed for twice daily dosing. Long-acting bronchodilators (LABAs) improve lung function, decrease symptoms, improve lung hyperinflation and physical activity, and reduce exacerbations. Inhaled corticosteroids are recommended as add-on therapy in combination with LABAs for severe and very severe COPD (GOLD, 2015). Inhaled corticosteroids are not recommended for monotherapy in COPD (GOLD, 2015).

The GOLD guidelines assign patients with COPD into four groups based on the degree of airflow restriction, symptom score, and the number of exacerbations in one year. Continuous oxygen therapy improves mortality rates in patients with severe hypoxemia and COPD. Patients with COPD have an incomplete response to albuterol and an absence of an abnormal bronchodilator response to a methacholine challenge test.

Close follow-up and education is imperative for patients with COPD. Adherence to the medical treatment regimen and correct usage of all medical devices is imperative to achieve and maintain disease control. Patients with COPD should receive the pneumococcal vaccine and an annual influenza vaccine according to the current Advisory Committee on Immunization Practices (ACIP) recommendations.

Comorbidities of COPD must be identified and appropriately managed. Comorbid depression and anxiety in COPD is associated with increased health care utilization and cost. Pulmonary rehabilitation should be considered in patients with COPD, especially those who remain symptomatic, despite an optimal medical treatment regimen. Pulmonary rehabilitation is an individualized program comprised of education, exercise training, psychosocial and behavioral intervention, and outcome assessment. The rehabilitation intervention is geared toward the unique problems and needs of each patient and is implemented by a multidisciplinary team of health care professionals. Pulmonary rehabilitation is an essential component of the comprehensive management of patients with COPD. Clinical outcome goals of COPD treatment are to relieve symptoms, reduce the impact of symptoms and physical limitations, and reduce further exacerbations.

Table 6-8	Classification of COPD Severity GOLD Guidelines, 2015

Classification of Severity of Airflow Limitations in COPD (Based on Post-Bronchodilator FEV1)
In patients with FEV1/FVC < 0.70

Gold 1:	Mild	FEV1 ≥ 80% predicted
Gold 2:	Moderate	50% ≤ FEV1 < 80% predicted
Gold 3:	Severe	30% ≤ FEV1 < 50% predicted
Gold 4:	Very Severe	FEV1 < 30% predicted

From the Global Strategy for Diagnosis, Management and Prevention of COPD 2015, ©

Table 6-9	Signs and Symptoms of Bacterial Pneumonia

Streptococcus Pneumoniae: Rust-Colored Sputum
Pseudomonas, Haemophilus, and pneumococcal species: may produce green sputum
Klebsiella species pneumonia: red currant-jelly sputum
Anaerobic infections: foul-smelling sputum

Signs of bacterial pneumonia
  Hyperthermia (fever, typically > 38 °C)[2] or hypothermia (< 35 °C)
  Tachypnea (>18 respirations/min)
  Use of accessory respiratory muscles
  Tachycardia (> 100 bpm) or bradycardia (< 60 bpm)
  Central cyanosis
  Altered mental status
Physical findings may include the following:
  Adventitious breath sounds—rales/crackles, rhonchi, or wheezes
  Decreased intensity of breath sounds
  Egophony
  Whispering pectoriloquy
  Dullness to percussion
  Tracheal deviation
  Lymphadenopathy
  Pleural friction rub

Clinical Pearls

Individuals with normal spirometric values may report respiratory symptoms, whereas individuals who have severe to very severe airflow obstruction by spirometry may report no symptoms.

Pneumonia

Pneumonia is a serious, life-threatening illness and is a leading cause of increased morbidity and mortality, and costly medical utilization (CDC, 2014). Pneumonia can result from viral or bacterial infections and is associated with acute inflammation of the pulmonary parenchyma and consolidation of the alveoli. Symptoms generally include cough, dyspnea, fever, chills, and pleuritic chest pain. Objective findings of pneumonia include fever, tachycardia, tachypnea, asynchronous breathing, and dull percussion notes over the consolidations, bronchophony, and vocal fremitus. Diagnostic tests may include chest radiology, complete blood cell (CBC) count, ultrasonography, sputum and blood cultures, or serology. Table 6-9 describes the signs and symptoms of bacterial pneumonia.

Bacteria are a common cause of lower respiratory tract infections. *Streptococcus pneumoniae* is the most common source of bacterial pneumonia (Mizgerd, 2008).

Antibiotic therapy is the mainstay of treatment of bacterial pneumonia. Despite the development of broad-spectrum antibiotics, lower respiratory tract bacterial infections continue to be a major cause of morbidity and mortality in both industrialized and developing countries. Patients who have bronchospasms with infection benefit from inhaled bronchodilators, administered by means of a nebulizer metered-dose inhaler.

Pneumonia in children less than 5 years old generally has an etiology of a virus. Viral infections tend to be resolved within 1 to 3 weeks with symptomatic treatment. Viral infections are the most common cause of pneumonia in children younger than 5 years old. Most cases of viral pneumonia are mild. They get better in about 1 to 3 weeks without treatment. Some cases are more serious and may require treatment in a hospital.

Community Acquired Pneumonia (CAP)

Community-acquired pneumonia (CAP) is an acute infection of the pulmonary parenchyma acquired in the community setting and is a common presenting condition seen in primary care. Most forms of CAP are treatable; the selection of antimicrobial agents is notably simplified if the pathogen is defined. *Streptococcus pneumoniae* is the primary pathogen causing CAP. Haemophilus influenza, Mycoplasma pneumoniae, Influenza A, Legionella species, and Chlamydophilia pneumoniae are other common etiology factors of CAP. Community-acquired pneumonia is diagnosed by clinical presentation, including pleuritic chest pain, cough, and fever, and by infiltrates seen on chest radiography. Chest radiography is the initial test, followed by blood cultures and a sputum culture for gram stain prior to antibiotic therapy. Malnutrition contributes to the increasing risks for CAP.

Physical examination findings may include crackles upon auscultation, dullness to percussion of the

Table 6-10	Community-Acquired Pneumonia (CAP)

Outpatient

No comorbidities/previously healthy. No risk factors for drug-resistant *S. pneumoniae*.
Azithromycin 500 mg PO one dose, then 250 mg PO daily for 4 d or extended-release 2 g PO as a single dose **or**
Clarithromycin 500 mg PO bid or extended-release 1000 mg PO q24h **or**
Doxycycline 100 mg PO bid

If received prior antibiotic within 3 months:
Azithromycin or clarithromycin **plus** amoxicillin 1 g PO q8h **or** amoxicillin-clavulanate 2 g PO q12h **or**
Respiratory fluoroquinolone (e.g., levofloxacin 750 mg PO daily **or** moxifloxacin 400 mg PO daily)

Comorbidities present (e.g., alcoholism, bronchiectasis/cystic fibrosis, COPD, IV drug user, post-influenza, asplenia, diabetes mellitus, lung/liver/renal diseases):
Levofloxacin 750 mg PO q24h **or**
Moxifloxacin 400 mg PO q24h **or**
Combination of a beta-lactam (amoxicillin 1 g PO q8h **or** amoxicillin-clavulanate 2 g PO q12h **or** ceftriaxone 1g IV/IM q24h **or** cefuroxime 500 mg PO BID) **plus** a macrolide (azithromycin **or** clarithromycin)
Duration of therapy: minimum of 5 days, should be afebrile for 48–72 hours, or until afebrile for 3 days; longer duration of therapy may be needed if initial therapy was not active against the identified pathogen, or if it was complicated by extrapulmonary infections.

chest, bronchial breath sounds, tactile fremitus, and egophony. Tachypnea may be present, but is more common in older patients with CAP. Infiltrate patterns are typically seen with viral or atypical pathogens on chest radiographs. Consolidation is seen on chest radiographs with *Streptococcus pneumoniae*. Table 6-10 describes the treatment regimen for CAP.

Mycoplasma pneumoniae (*M. pneumoniae*) is a common cause of community-acquired pneumonia, usually affecting young adults, school-aged children, military recruits, and those living or working in crowded places (Watkins & Lemonovich, 2011). Symptomatology includes cough, rhinorrhea, pharyngitis, headache, fever, diaphoretic, and chills. Treatment for *M. pneumonia* includes macrolides (azithromycin, clarithromycin, or erythromycin), doxycycline, and fluoroquinolones. People who live or work in crowded places like schools, homeless shelters, and prisons are at higher risk for this type of pneumonia. *Mycoplasma pneumoniae* symptoms are generally mild and respond well antibiotic therapy.

Clinical Pearl

Routine administration of the pneumococcal conjugate vaccine has resulted in an overall reduction in the rate of invasive disease and pneumonia.

Lung Cancer

A primary lung neoplasm is a malignancy arising from lung tissue. The World Health Organization distinguishes 12 types of pulmonary neoplasms. The major types of neoplasm are large cell carcinoma,

Table 6-11	Common Signs and Symptoms of Lung Cancer

Cough, wheezing, dyspnea
Hemoptysis, hoarseness dysphagia
Recurring infections such as bronchitis and pneumonia
Weight loss, fever, fatigue, anorexia

Metastatic signs and symptoms
Bone pain
Spinal cord impingement
Neurologic problems such as headache, weakness or numbness of limbs, dizziness, and seizures

small cell carcinoma, non-small-cell, squamous cell carcinoma, and adenocarcinoma. Approximately 85% of lung cancer cases are non-small-cell lung cancer (Baraschino et al., 2011). Cigarette smoking is responsible for approximately 90 percent of cases of lung cancer (American Lung Association, 2014). Smoking cessation or never smoking is the most important method to decreasing the morbidity and mortality associated with this disease.

Lung cancer is often insidious, producing no symptoms until the disease has advanced. Symptoms of cough, pain, or hemoptysis may be present in patients with hilar involvement, particularly when the metastases adjoin or invade the bronchi. Table 6-11 describes common signs and symptoms of lung cancer. Many patients with lung cancer have advanced disease when metastatic disease is present. Effective screening is imperative for high-risk patients because many patients are asymptomatic

Table 6-12	Staging of Tumors, Lymph Nodes, and Metastatic Involvement

T—describes the size of the primary tumor
N—describes the spread of cancer to regional lymph nodes
M—indicates whether the cancer has metastasized

Primary tumor (T) involvement is as follows:
Tx—Primary tumor cannot be assessed
T0—No evidence of tumor
Tis—Carcinoma in situ
T1, T2, T3, T4: size and/or extension of the primary tumor

Lymph node (N) involvement is as follows:
Nx—Regional nodes cannot be assessed
N0—No regional node metastasis
N1—Metastasis in ipsilateral peribronchial and/or
    ipsilateral hilar nodes and intrapulmonary nodes,
    including involvement by direct extension
N2—Metastasis in ipsilateral mediastinal and/or
    subcarinal node
N3—Metastasis in contralateral mediastinal, contralateral
    hilar, ipsilateral or contralateral scalene node, or
    supraclavicular node

Metastatic (M) involvement is as follows:
M0—No metastasis
M1—Distant metastasis

Modified from National Cancer Institute. (2015). Cancer staging. Retrieved from http://www.cancer.gov/about-cancer/diagnosis-staging/staging/staging-fact-sheet.

until the late stages. The prognosis remains poor, with approximately only 15% of lung cancer patients still living 5 years after their diagnosis.

Clinical features that suggest malignancy on initial evaluation include older age, current or past history of tobacco abuse, hemoptysis, and the presence of a previous malignancy. The histologic subtype, molecular markers, stage of lung cancer and the patient's performance status guide treatment decisions and influence the prognosis. Chest radiography should be performed in patients with signs and symptoms consistent with lung cancer, and computed tomography (CT) scans with contrast should be performed if an alternative diagnosis is not identified on the chest radiograph. Chest CT scans should extend through the adrenals since metastatic disease to these glands is usually asymptomatic. A CT scan with contrast, magnetic resonance imaging (MRI), or an ultrasound of the liver should be ordered if the chest CT, laboratory results, or clinical assessment suggests metastatic disease to this organ. Treatment options are based on the staging of the cancer and other factors, such as pulmonary function testing, clinical presentation, and objective findings. **Table** 6-12 describes the staging of tumors, lymph node, and metastatic involvement.

Clinical Pearls

Prevention of smoking and cessation of smoking offer the most important route to decreasing the morbidity and mortality associated with lung cancer.

Tuberculosis

Tuberculosis (TB) is a common infectious disease and a leading cause of morbidity and mortality worldwide, particularly in developing countries. Approximately 1.5 million persons worldwide die of TB each year and 9 million become infected (CDC, 2015). Tuberculosis is a leading cause of death in people who are infected with the human immunodeficiency virus (HIV). Pulmonary tuberculosis (TB) is caused by the bacterium *Mycobacterium tuberculosis* (*M. tuberculosis*). Although pulmonary specialists generally manage TB, primary care providers play an essential role and must understand and identify the signs and symptoms of the disease to ensure early referral and accurate diagnosis.

M. tuberculosis is transmitted via airborne droplets (droplet nuclei) expelled by cough, sneeze, or talking with pulmonary or laryngeal tuberculosis. Extrapulmonary tuberculosis can result from *M. tuberculosis* spreading to other organs, including bone, joints, meninges, lymphatics, or pleura. Extrapulmonary TB is a disease involving any part of the body other than lung parenchyma, including other structures within the thorax, such as the pleura, pericardium, and perihilar lymph nodes. Air currents in a room or building can carry infectious particles.

The fever is most often low grade at the onset and becomes marked with progression of disease. Fever is classically diurnal, with an afebrile period early in the morning and a gradually rising temperature throughout the day, reaching a peak in the late afternoon or evening. Night sweats and fever are more common among patients with advanced pulmonary TB. Cough may be absent or mild initially and may be nonproductive or productive of only scant sputum. Initially, it may be present only in the morning, when accumulated secretions during sleep are expectorated. As the disease progresses, cough becomes more continuous throughout the day and productive of yellow or yellow-green and occasionally blood-streaked sputum, which is rarely foul smelling. Symptomatic individuals are more likely to have smear-positive sputum. Frank hemoptysis, due to caseous sloughing or endobronchial erosion, typically occurs later in the disease and is rarely massive. Nocturnal coughing is associated with advanced disease, often with cavitation.

Table 6-13	Pulmonary Complications and Clinical Features of TB

Pneumothorax
Hemoptysis
Bronchiectasis
Extensive pulmonary destruction
Malignancy
Chronic pulmonary aspergillosis
Cough
Weight loss
Anorexia
Fever
Night sweats
Hemoptysis
Chest pain
(Also from acute pericarditis)
Fatigue

Dyspnea can occur in the setting of extensive parenchymal involvement, pleural effusions, or a pneumothorax. Pleuritic chest pain is not common but, when present, signifies inflammation abutting or invading the pleura, with or without an effusion. Rarely, this can progress to frank empyema. Bronchiectasis may develop following primary or reactivation TB and can be associated with hemoptysis. In the absence of treatment, patients may present with painful ulcers of the mouth, tongue, larynx, or gastrointestinal tract due to chronic expectoration and swallowing of highly infectious secretions. These findings are generally rare in the setting of antituberculous therapy. Anorexia, wasting, and malaise are common features of advanced disease. Table 6-13 describes the complications and clinical features of TB.

In primary pulmonary TB, the chest radiograph is often normal. Hilar changes could be seen as early as one week after skin test conversion and within two months in all cases. People living with HIV are more likely than others to become sick with TB if they are exposed and become infected. The risk of death from TB is also higher in HIV-infected persons. Untreated latent TB infections (see the following) may quickly progress to the TB disease in people living with HIV, because the immune system is already weakened.

Diagnosis

Mycobacterium tuberculosis (MTB) isolation from clinical specimens is the standard for TB diagnosis. False-positive culture rates are reported to be approximately 2% to 4%. Abnormal findings on chest radiographs may be suggestive of TB in a patient with respiratory symptoms, but is not diagnostic for the disease. The CXR may show infiltrates with cavitation in the upper and middle lobes of the lung. The elderly and patients with HIV may have cavitation less often and may have lower-lob infiltrates as a prominent finding.

Latent TB infection (LTBI) is the presence of Mycobacterium tuberculosis (MTB) in an individual without clinical, imaging, or microbiologic evidence of active disease. Treatment of latent infection is a key component for controlling TB. Approximately one-third of the world's population is predicted to have LTBI, based on the Mantoux test.

Treatment

The standard short-course anti-TB regimen of isoniazid (H), rifampicin (R), pyrazinamide (P), and ethambutol (E) (HREZ) has been proven to be effective (Koul, 2011). Aside from symptomatic and radiographic improvements, the disappearance of acid-fast bacilli (AFB) from sputum smears and the conversion of culture results for MTB are used to assess therapeutic responses.

Cough

Cough is one of the most common complaints that prompts a patient to seek health care. Patients may report cough as the only complaint, or the cough may be accompanied by other non-specific symptoms, such as pharyngalgia, malaise, or low-grade temperature. Cough reflex is a physiologic function that protects the pulmonary tract from aspiration, inhaled irritants, particulates, and pathogens (Chung & Pavord, 2008).

Cough can be characterized as (1) acute, less than 3 weeks; (2) subacute, lasting 3 to 8 weeks; or (3) chronic lasting more than 8 weeks. A detailed history must be performed in all patients, which include an assessment of health status, cough severity, chronic illnesses, use of tobacco, environmental irritants, and medications, including ACE-inhibitors (ACE-I)(Chung & Pavord, 2008) and oxymetazoline (Afrin).

Identification of the contributing factor and achieving the correct etiology is crucial to avoid overlooking a potentially life-threatening condition. Management of acute cough includes evaluation and treatment of the likely causes of cough, using diagnostic tests and appropriate empiric therapy. After discontinuing ACE-I, the cough generally resolves within one to four days, but can take up to four weeks. In chronic cough, a heightened cough reflex may be the primary etiology. If a cough does not subside within 3 weeks, a chest radiograph should be obtained to exclude tuberculosis, carcinoma, or other serious pulmonary diseases. Optimal management should comprise a combination of diagnostic testing and treatment trials based on the most probable aggravate. Vagal-mediated esophageal reflux stimulated by acid or nonacid volume reflux should be considered in patients with chronic cough. If postnasal drainage is suspected as a contributing factor of cough and there is no improvement after two to three weeks of empiric therapy, then evaluation of spirometry should be performed.

Inflammatory mediators in the lower airways are elevated in patients with cough variant asthma, GERD, and upper airway cough syndrome (UACS), also known as postnasal drip. If the cough persists, empirical treatment gastroesophageal reflux with a proton pump inhibitor, and with appropriate lifestyle and dietary modifications, should be considered. Expectorants, such as guaifenesin, may be therapeutic with the presence of excessive mucus production, by increasing the volume of mucus and facilitating the removal of secretions by ciliary transport and/or cough. Antitussives, such as codeine and dextromethorphan, have been shown to have limited or no efficacy in the treatment of chronic cough, and any beneficial effect is largely due to the placebo effect (Bolser, 2010). Cough suppression must be carefully managed in patients with asthma or COPD. Health care professionals should try to elucidate and identify the underlying cause to determine the appropriate treatment regimen. Chronic cough is a multifactorial symptom that may require referral to allergy and asthma, pulmonology, and/or gastrointestinal specialists for consultation. **Table 6-14** describes the causes of chronic cough.

Acute Bronchitis

Acute bronchitis is a self-limited infection with the primary symptom of cough lasting 10 to 20 days. Etiology of acute bronchitis is most often viral and is generally associated with an upper respiratory infection. Wheezing may be present, along with chest wall tenderness that is generally related to muscle strain from coughing. The appearance of the sputum cannot be used to distinguish between viral and bacterial bronchitis.

Acute bronchitis should be differentiated from other respiratory complications. Cough accompanied by fever, sputum production, and constitutional symptoms are typically complications of influenza or pneumonia. Antimicrobial agents are not recommended in most cases of acute bronchitis.

Table 6-14	Causes of Chronic Cough
Common
Asthma
Gastroesophageal reflux disease (GERD)
Upper airway inflammatory diseases (e.g., allergic rhinitis, sinusitis)
Chronic bronchitis
Upper airway cough syndrome
Bronchiectasis
Nonasthmatic eosinophilic bronchitis
Other Causes
Angiotensin-converting enzyme inhibitor
Bronchogenic carcinoma
Chronic aspiration
Congestive heart failure (CHF)
Interstitial lung disease
Neuromuscular disorders
Pertussis
Psychogenic cough
Sarcoidosis
Tracheoesophageal fistula
Tuberculosis

Symptomatic treatment may include nonsteroidal anti-inflammatory drugs or acetaminophen directed toward presenting symptoms. Bronchodilators can help to relieve the cough in people who show evidence of bronchospasm. Antitussives (dextromethorphan) may be carefully considered in patients age 6 years and older. There are no data to support the use of oral corticosteroids in patients with acute bronchitis and no asthma (Albert, 2010).

Clinical Pearls

Acute bronchitis is one of the most common causes of antibiotic abuse.

Respiratory Syncytial Virus

Respiratory syncytial virus (RSV) is a common cause of severe lower respiratory tract diseases, including bronchiolitis, pneumonia, and acute respiratory failure, generally seen in infants and young children (Caswell-Dawson & Muncie, 2011). An RSV infection begins with replication of the virus in the nasopharynx and spreads to the bronchiolar epithelium lining the small airways within the lungs. The viral process impairs normal pulmonary gas exchange, leading to ventilation-perfusion mismatch and subsequent hypoxemia. There is increasing evidence indicating severe pulmonary disease caused by RSV infection in infancy is associated with recurrent wheezing and development of asthma later in childhood.

The clinical manifestations of RSV can vary depending on the age and health status. The treatment of RSV infection is primarily supportive care, maintenance of hydration, and oxygenation. Beta-agonists and ipratropium bromide treatment for RSV is controversial. Despite many randomized, controlled trials, no consistent benefit of beta-agonist has been demonstrated. A brief trial of bronchodilators could be considered while monitoring symptoms, but treatment should be continued only if clinical improvement can be documented by objective findings.

Ribavirin, a broad-spectrum antiviral agent in vitro, is licensed by the United States Food and Drug Administration (FDA) for the aerosolized treatment of children with severe RSV disease. The recommended dose is 6 g of drug in 300 mL of distilled water via a small-particle aerosol generator (SPAG unit) over 12–20 hours per day for 3–7 days, depending on the clinical response. Palivizumab is a humanized monoclonal antibody specifically targeting one of the RSV proteins that has been approved for use in the United States in a very select patient population. Palivizumab prophylaxis for RSV should be limited to infants born before 29 weeks gestation and to infants with chronic illness, such as congenital heart disease or chronic lung disease (Barclay, 2014).

Household members should be immunized against influenza and practice good hand and cough hygiene. RSV preventative measures are an ideal priority for patients who are at the highest risk of complications. Symptomatic RSV infections may occur in adults, primarily in health care workers or caretakers of small children. Clinical symptoms are usually consistent with an upper respiratory tract infection and last approximately five days.

Clinical Pearl

RSV is an enveloped, nonsegmented, negative-stranded RNA virus and a member of the Paramyxoviridae family.

Review Questions

1. In a patient in status asthmaticus, the FNP would most likely identify which of the following on a chest radiograph?
   A. Atelectasis
   B. Effusion
   C. Hyperinflation
   D. Pleural opacities

2. Ipratropium is available in a pressurized metered-dose inhaler or solution for nebulization and:
   A. Has dose-related adverse effects including nausea, vomiting, seizures, and arrhythmias.
   B. Is a short-acting bronchodilator administered four times daily as maintenance therapy for COPD.
   C. Can increase the risk of bone mineral density and/or bone fractures.
   D. Increases the risk of oral candidiasis, hoarseness, and bruising of the skin.

3. Pulmonary tuberculosis is caused by what gram-positive, rod-shaped aerobic bacterium?
   A. *Lactobacillus*
   B. *Streptococcus*
   C. *Renibacterium*
   D. *Mycobacterium*

4. *M. tuberculosis is* spread by:
   A. Body fluids.
   B. Airborne droplets.
   C. Fomites.
   D. Ingestion of bacteria.

5. A 53-year-old male with a 45 pack-year smoking history presents to the nurse practitioner's office for a follow-up visit. This patient had a recent emergency department admission for exertional dyspnea that has progressed to dyspnea at rest and a cough for 1 month. The nurse practitioner received the chest radiograph report, which demonstrates a suspicious nodule in the right hilar region. The nurse practitioner suspects small cell lung cancer and understands that:
   A. Small-cell lung cancer differs from non-small-cell lung cancer because small-cell lung cancer grows slowly.
   B. Small-cell lung cancer responds well to chemotherapy and radiation therapy.
   C. Small-cell lung cancer is generally not associated with distinct paraneoplastic syndromes.
   D. Small-cell lung cancer metastasizes slowly.

6. HIV co-infection is the most potent immunosuppressive risk factor for which of the following?
   A. Distal acinar emphysema
   B. Active TB disease
   C. Diabetes mellitus
   D. Paraseptal emphysema

7. Screening for latent tuberculosis infection (LTBI) is recommended:
   A. In persons at risk of recent infection and patients infected with HIV.
   B. Groups with an increased flow of progression to active disease.
   C. Persons with nocturnal coughing.
   D. In persons whose CD4 cell count increases to counts of > 600 cells/μL.

8. According to the EPR-3 Guidelines, poor asthma control can increase future risks of asthma, including all of the following EXCEPT:

   A. Airway remodeling.

   B. Accelerated decrease in lung function.

   C. Generally no side effects of treatment.

   D. Fatal asthma.

9. *M. Pneumonia* empiric treatment for suspected mycoplasma pneumonia involves which of the following?

   A. Five-day course of oral azithromycin (500 mg for the first dose, then 250 mg daily for the next four days)

   B. Dexilant 60 mg 1 tablet twice daily for 14 days

   C. Treat symptomatically

   D. Palivizumab according to weight for 14 days

10. Which of the following is considered accurate for Respiratory Syntial Virus (RSV)?

    A. Order palivmar 250 mg twice daily for 14 days at the onset of RSV symptoms.

    B. RSV is a highly contagious infection, occurring most often during the late spring and summer months.

    C. Treat symptoms with Aspirin 100 mg/5 mL. Take 5 mL orally three times daily.

    D. Premature infants have the highest risk of RSV.

11. One of the most important initial steps for management of COPD is to:

    A. Obtain base-line arterial blood gases.

    B. Order supplemental oxygen therapy at 2 lpm.

    C. Reduce exposure to risk factors, including smoking cessation.

    D. Start low-dose prednisone daily for 14 to 21 days to reduce inflammation.

12. For patients with COPD, long-acting bronchodilators are recommended as:

    A. Regular maintenance therapy for patients with moderate to severe COPD.

    B. Only in combination with inhaled corticosteroid.

    C. Reliever therapy for acute exacerbations.

    D. An alternative route of administration to treat chronic cough.

13. The nurse practitioner orders a chest radiograph on a 28-year-old Caucasian female who presents to the office for uncontrolled asthma with symptoms of cough, wheezing throughout all lung fields, and shortness of breath. Which clinical finding on the chest radiograph is not suggestive of asthma?

    A. Bronchial thickening

    B. Nodules

    C. Hyperinflation

    D. Focal atelectasis

14. A 62-year-old African American male with mild COPD presents to the clinic with a chief complaint of cough. The nurse practitioner understands pharmacological treatment is based upon all EXCEPT:

    A. Adherence to medical treatment regimen.

    B. The CAT score, breathlessness, and wheezing.

    C. Diet.

    D. Airflow limitations.

15. A 3-year-old male presents to the clinic with his mother who complains of coughing, sneezing, rhinorrhea, low-grade fever, and mild sore throat. The nurse practitioner obtained a laboratory diagnosis of RSV that was made by analysis of respiratory secretions. The nurse practitioner understands that:

    A. RSV infection usually is a self-limited process, but it is associated with recurrent wheezing in some patients.

    B. Infection with respiratory syncytial virus requires direct admission to the emergency department.

    C. Adolescents are most severely affected by RSV.

    D. Ribavirin is considered to be contraindicated in pregnant women.

16. Vesicular breath sounds:

    A. Are soft and high-pitched, and are heard throughout the lung.

    B. Are loud, hollow, harsh sounds, and are heard best over the manubrium.

    C. Are low-pitched sounds that can be heard over the periphery of both lung fields.

    D. Have an expiratory phase that is longer than their inspiratory phase.

17. The standard short-course anti-TB regimen includes which of the following?

    A. Enablex, Myrbetriq, and Ditropan

    B. Isoniazid, rifampicin, pyrazinamide, and ethambutol

    C. Linezolid and Sutezolid

    D. Panobinostat, palbociclib, and lenvatinib.

18. Lower respiratory tract infections cause disease in the alveolar sacs, and may result in which of the following?

    A. Emphysema

    B. Gastroesophageal reflux disease (GERD)

    C. Bronchiectasis

    D. Pneumonia

19. Chest radiographs showing new consolidations or infiltrates would suggest which of the following?

    A. Emphysema

    B. Acute respiratory distress syndrome (ARDS)

    C. Interstitial pulmonary edema

    D. Pneumonia

20. A 48-year-old African American male comes to the FNP's office for a follow-up visit complaining of shortness of breath, coughing, and dyspnea on exertion. The FNP identifies the findings of COPD as:

    A. appearance of Kerley lines on chest X-ray.

    B. FEV1/FVC < 0.70.

    C. hypotension and tachycardia.

    D. low serum glucose level and elevated serum lactate level.

21. Pulmonary tuberculosis (TB) is a chronic bacterial infection:

    A. with high CD4 cell counts that are associated with more severe forms.

    B. caused by hMPV and transmitted through aerosolized droplets.

    C. and fever associated with it is classically diurnal, with an afebrile period early in the morning, reaching a peak in the late afternoon or evening.

    D. and hemoptysis generally decreases in the setting of active tuberculosis.

22. An 18-year-old female presents to a clinic complaining of increased coughing and wheezing once or twice daily the past 3 days. She reports she has had "cold-like" symptoms that started 5 or 6 days ago that she is treating with over-the-counter cough syrup. She has a diagnosis of mild persistent asthma, but is non-adherent to her medical treatment regimen. No nocturnal symptoms. Asthma Control Test score is 18. A spirometry reveals FVC 78%, FEV1 75%, FVC/FEV1 73%, FVC 20%, FEV1 18%, and FVC/FEV1 18% responses to bronchodilator. Upon physical examination, few scattered end-expiratory wheezes are heard throughout all lung fields bilaterally and all were clear bilaterally after nebulized albuterol. The nurse practitioner prescribes:

    A. Theophylline 200 mg once daily after the theophylline level is ordered and an asthma education consult.

    B. Fluticasone 40 mcg 2 puffs twice daily using an aerochamber, albuterol 2 puffs every 4 to 6 hours as needed, asthma education consult, and follow up in 4 weeks or sooner if needed.

    C. Fluticasone/salmeterol 500 mg/50 mcg 1 puff twice daily, albuterol 2 puffs every 4 to 6 hours as needed, asthma education consult, follow up in 1 week.

    D. A prednisone burst.

23. According to the National Asthma Education Prevention Program Expert Panel Report 3, the risk factors for fatal asthma include all but:

    A. Two or more hospitalizations in the past year for severe exacerbation requiring admission for asthma into an intensive care unit or intubation.

    B. Perceiving an airway obstruction or the severity of worsening.

    C. Asthma.

    D. Higher income with varying sociodemographic groups.

24. Clinical features that suggest malignancy on initial evaluation include:

    A. Older age, a current or past history of tobacco abuse, hemoptysis, and the presence of a previous malignancy.

    B. Presence of a precious malignancy, cough, fatigue.

    C. Tobacco use, hemoptysis, chest congestion, and shortness of breath.

    D. Persistent cough or wheezing with white or pink blood-tinged mucus, fatigue.

25. Wheezing heard only on inspiration is referred to as stridor and is associated with which of the following?

    A. A mechanical obstruction at the level of the trachea/upper airway

    B. Focal wheezing

    C. COPD

    D. Cystic fibrosis

26. The National Asthma Education and Prevention Program, Expert Panel Report 3, highlights the importance of correctly diagnosing asthma, by establishing which of the following?

    A. Episodic symptoms of airflow obstruction are present, airflow obstruction or symptoms are at least partially reversible, and exclusion of alternative diagnoses

    B. Coughing and wheezing greater than twice a week with a family history of asthma

    C. Symptoms of airflow obstruction are present more than twice a week, airflow obstruction or symptoms are reversible, and exclusion of alternative diagnosis

    D. Shortness of breath, chest tightness, chronic productive cough

27. Wheezing produced during inspiration and/or expiration:

    A. Contributes to the pathological features of gastroesopheal reflux disease

    B. Is associated with diffuse processes that affect all lobes of the lung and is often audible in all lung fields.

    C. Is seen in severe bronchoconstriction as the inspiratory phase of respiration becomes noticeably prolonged.

    D. Contributes to symptoms of post–nasal drainage.

28. A 20-year-old male presents to the clinic with a chief complaint of a productive cough. The nurse practitioner diagnoses acute bronchitis with a treatment plan of which of the following?

    A. Augmentin

    B. Antiviral therapy

    C. Symptomatic treatment including acetaminophen as needed*

    D. Chest X-ray, CBC with differentials

29. Which of the following is considered true regarding inhaled corticosteroids in the treatment of asthma?

    A. It's the drug of choice for persistent asthma.

    B. It is associated with an increased risk of fatal asthma.

    C. It is never used as monotherapy.

    D. It inhibits muscarinic cholinergic receptors.

30. Pulsus paradox greater than 25 mmHg reflects which of the following?

    A. Controlled asthma

    B. Severe airflow obstruction

    C. Hypoventilation

    D. Hypotension

31. According to the National Asthma Education and Prevention Expert Panel Report 3, leukotriene receptor antagonists:

    A. Are considered as add-on therapy in mild and moderate persistent asthma.

    B. Are alternatives to ICS in moderate persistent asthma.

    C. Block the effect of acetylcholine on airways.

    D. Reduce vagal tone in the airway.

32. When a normal lung transmits a palpable vibratory sensation to the chest wall, this is known as what?

    A. Whispered pectoriloquy

    B. Bronchophony

    C. Tactile fremitus

    D. Egophony

33. Christopher is a 76-year-old Caucasian male who presents to the outpatient clinic for a routine follow-up visit and is complaining of shortness of breath with mild exertion. He was diagnosed with lung cancer 8 months ago and is undergoing treatment. The nurse practitioner understands dyspnea could possibly be contributing to which of the following?

    A. Anxiety

    B. Cough

    C. Lymphangitic tumor spread

    D. Costochondritis

34. Stephanie is a 47-year-old female with a history of hypertension and cough for the past 3 to 4 weeks. Physical examination findings are unremarkable. The nurse practitioner believes the cough is most likely caused by which of the following?

    A. An upper respiratory infection

    B. ACE-I

    C. Bronchogenic carcinoma

    D. A psychogenic cough

35. J.R. presents to the clinic with a depression of his sternum. The FNP identifies this finding as which of the following?

    A. Flail chest

    B. Barrel chest

    C. Pectus carinatum

    D. Pectus excavatum

36. Upon examination of a 55-year-old man, the percussion note is lower-pitched, and is a louder and longer sound heard normally over the lungs during maximum inspiration and is identified as which of the following?

    A. Resonance

    B. Hyperresonance

    C. Dullness

    D. Flatness

37. Emily is a 30-year-old Hispanic female with uncontrolled severe persistent asthma. She requires albuterol at least once or twice daily and has had 3 bursts of oral prednisone the past 12 months. Emily owns a restaurant working 60 hours a week. The FNP would most likely:

    A. Refer to a pulmonology or allergy provider requesting an immediate consult, implement a medical treatment regimen according to EPR-3, and give an asthma education consultation.

    B. Order a fluticasone 220 mcg 4 puffs twice daily using a valved holding chamber, plus an asthma education consultation.

    C. Request an asthma education consult, increase inhaled corticosteroids, and request Emily decrease her workload.

    D. Prescribe 60 mg prednisone once daily for 7 days and have Emily return to the clinic in 7 days.

38. Haemophilus influenzae is one of the major bacterial pathogens of upper respiratory tract infections in children. A primary concern for the nurse practitioner is:

    A. *H. influenzae* resistance to isoniazid is problematic.

    B. *H. influenzae* resistance to β-lactam antibiotics is problematic.

    C. Treatment is contraindicated with oral corticosteroids.

    D. A vigorous treatment regimen increases the risk of adherence.

39. Upon physical examination, the FNP assesses dullness on percussion, increased tactile fremitus, and whispered pectoriloquy is heard clearly. These findings are consistent with which of the following?

    A. Asthma

    B. Atelectasis

    C. Consolidation

    D. Pneumothorax

40. Which of the following drugs does pharmacodynamic criteria suggest are more potent against *S. pneumoniae*?

    A. Rifapentine and Moxifloxacin

    B. Doxycycline and omalizumab

    C. Levofloxacin and adriamycin

    D. Moxifloxacin and gemifloxacin

41. The nurse practitioner understands chronic cough is a multifactorial symptom and may require:

    A. Antitussive treatment.

    B. Prednisone 40 mg once daily for 5 days to reduce the inflammatory response from cough.

    C. Referral to allergy and asthma, pulmonology, and/or gastrointestinal specialists.

    D. ACE-I.

42. The United States Preventative Services Task Force (USPSTF) recommends annual screening for lung cancer. Which of the following is NOT recommended?

    A. Low-dose computed tomography in adults aged 55 to 80 years who have a 30 pack-year smoking history

    B. Screen all persons that are current smokers or who have quit within the past 15 years.

    C. Screening should be discontinued once a person has not smoked for 5 years.

    D. Patients who develop a health problem that substantially limits life expectancy

43. The FNP understands N2 is defined as:

    A. Metastasis in ipsilateral peribronchial and/or ipsilateral hilar nodes and intrapulmonary nodes, including involvement by extension.

    B. Metastasis in contralateral mediastinal, contralateral hilar, ipsilateral or contralateral scalene node, or supraclavicular node.

    C. Distant metastasis.

    D. Metastasis in ipsilateral mediastinal and/or subcarinal node.

44. IgE is the antibody responsible for activation of allergic reactions and is:

    A. Important to the development and persistence of inflammation.

    B. A critical component of lung function.

    C. Important for selecting inhaled corticosteroid dosages.

    D. A tool for determining airway remodeling.

45. Measurements of fractional exhaled NO (FeNO) are:

    A. Useful for monitoring responses to asthma treatment because of the association between FeNO and the presence of inflammation in asthma.

    B. Identified as a pathogenesis of allergic diseases.

    C. Responsible for activation of allergic reactions.

    D. Important in promoting Th1 cytokines to avoid asthma exacerbations.

46. In patients with asthma, the nurse practitioner understands that:

    A. Beta-blockers can cause increased bronchial obstruction, airway reactivity, and resistance to the effects of inhaler or oral beta receptor agonists.

    B. Topical ophthalmic administration of nonselective beta-blockers are in patients with COPD and not asthma.

    C. Pulmonary function tests must be performed every 3 to 4 weeks for patients with asthma who are prescribed a beta-blocker.

    D. Significant respiratory symptoms occur only in patients with moderate and severe persistent asthma who are prescribed a beta-blocker.

47. Patients with chronic bronchitis tend to have complications of which of the following?

    A. Chronic hypoxemia and hypocapnia

    B. Peripheral edema from cor pulmonale

    C. Ocular swelling and post–nasal drainage

    D. Muscle wasting and chronic, productive cough with large amounts of sputum

48. Auscultatory findings characterized as low-pitched, loud, generally heard on inspiration, and often cleared with cough is known as what?

    A. Wheezing

    B. Crackles

    C. Vesicular

    D. Rhonchi

49. A 76-year-old male with COPD presents to a clinic. Pulmonary function testing reveals an FEV1 of 71%. According to the Global Initiative for Lung Disease, the classification of severity is which of the following?

    A. Mild

    B. Moderate

    C. Severe

    D. Very severe

50. Regarding ipratropium bromide, the therapeutic action of ipratropium bromide is:

    A. Activation of β1 receptors that degrades cycle monophosphate.

    B. the bronchodilatory affect due to activation of β1 receptors.

    C. inducing positive inotropic, chronotropic output of the cardiac muscle.

    D. that it promotes the degradation of cyclic guanosine monophosphate and the activation of beta$_2$-adrenergic receptors on airway smooth muscle.

51. Systemic manifestations of comorbid diseases have a significant influence on the management of asthma. The FNP understands comorbidities should be considered, especially with uncontrolled asthma, and that it includes all except which of the following?

    A. Gastroesophageal reflux disease

    B. Diabetes mellitus

    C. Allergic rhinitis

    D. Vocal cord dysfunction

Answers and Rationales

1. C. Chest radiography is indicated in patients who have an atypical presentation or in those who do not respond to therapy.

2. B. Ipratropium, a SAMA, is as effective or better in improving FEV1 as SABA without tachycardia side effects. SAMAs decrease function residual capacity and residual volume and effectively reduce hyperinflation.

3. D. The lungs are the major site for *Mycobacterium tuberculosis* for primary infection and disease.

4. B. The bacteria are spread from person to person in tiny microscopic droplets when a TB sufferer coughs, sneezes, speaks, sings, or laughs. Only people with active TB can spread the disease to others.

5. B. Small-cell lung cancer responds well to chemotherapy and radiation therapy. Small-cell lung cancer (also called oat cell cancer) and non-small-cell lung cancer are the two main types of lung cancer. Small-cell lung cancer accounts for approximately 15% of all cases of lung cancer. Small-cell lung cancer grows rapidly and spreads quickly. Small-cell lung cancer is frequently associated with distinct paraneoplastic syndromes.

6. B. People living with HIV are more likely than others to become sick with TB if they are exposed and become infected. According to the Center for Disease Control and Prevention, tuberculosis remains a serious threat in the United States, especially for people living with HIV. People living with HIV are more likely than others to become sick with TB.

7. A. According to the Center for Disease Control and Prevention, screening for latent tuberculosis infection (LTBI) is recommended for HIV-infected persons and those at risk of recent LTBI infection. The diagnosis of LTBI is based on information gathered from the medical history, a tuberculin skin test (TST) or interferon gamma release assay (IGRA) result, chest radiographs, physical examination, and in certain circumstances, sputum examinations. The presence of TB must be excluded before treatment for LTBI is initiated, because failure to do so may result in inadequate treatment and development of drug resistance. A TST reaction of ≥ 5 mm of induration is considered positive in patients with HIV.

8. C. Poor asthma control can increase future risks of asthma, including exacerbation, accelerated decrease in lung function, and side effects of treatment. Increased risk for fatal asthma includes poor asthma control.

9. C. CAP may be treated with monotherapy or combination therapy. Effective monotherapy antibiotics include: combination therapy, which usually consists of ceftriaxone plus doxycycline or azithromycin doxycycline, and respiratory quinolones. Immunocompromised hosts who present with CAP are treated in the same manner as otherwise healthy hosts but may require a longer duration of therapy.

10. D. Premature infants have the highest risk of RSV.

11. C. Smoking cessation is relevant especially for individuals with COPD because it is known from multiple studies that patients who quit smoking experience improvement in pulmonary functions, a decreased rate of a normal age-related decline in FEV1, decreased unscheduled medical utilization, and improved survival.

12. A. Long-acting bronchodilators (LABA) increase FEV1, decrease symptoms, improve lung hyperinflation, increase physical activity, and reduce exacerbations.

13. B. Hyperinflation, focal atelectasis, and bronchial thickening are clinical findings on chest X-ray of exacerbated asthma. Nodules are diagnostic of cancer.

14. D. Symptoms can be assessed with validated tools such as the CAT. Adherence is important and is improved with an individualized approach. Pharmacological treatment is also based on airflow limitations, symptoms, and exacerbations. Diet may be considered, but other options have a higher ranking.

15. A. RSV infection usually is a self-limited process, but it is associated with recurrent wheezing in some patients.

16. C. Vesicular breath sounds are soft, low-pitched sounds that can be heard over the periphery of both lung fields.

17. B. The standard short-course anti-TB regimen includes Isoniazid, rifampicin, pyrazinamide, and ethambutol.

18. D. Lower respiratory tract infections cause disease in the alveolar sacs, and the resulting infection is pneumonia. Pneumonia can result from viral or bacterial infections and is associated with acute inflammation of the pulmonary parenchyma and consolidation of the alveoli.

19. D. Infiltrates consist of fluid/exudate in alveolar spaces, indicating pneumonia. Exudate can consolidate and is the cause of lobar pneumonia.

20. B. Airflow obstruction is determined by spirometry, where the ratio of forced expiratory volume in the first second to forced vital capacity (FEV1/FVC) after bronchodilation is less than 0.70.

21. C. TB is a chronic bacterial infection, and fever is classically diurnal, with an afebrile period early in the morning, reaching a peak in the late afternoon or evening. Fever is most often low grade at onset and becomes marked with the progression of the disease. Fever is classically diurnal, with an afebrile period early in the morning and a gradually rising temperature throughout the day, reaching a peak in the late afternoon or evening. Night sweats and fever are more common among patients with advanced pulmonary TB.

22. B. Fluticasone 40 mcg 2 puffs twice daily using an aerochamber, albuterol 2 puffs every 4 to 6 hours as needed, asthma education consult, and follow up in 4 weeks or sooner if need. It is imperative to regain asthma control, which is achieved with implementing an inhaled corticosteroid. Albuterol is used to relieve symptoms. An individualized asthma education program is imperative for all patients with asthma. This patient must understand how to use a metered dose inhaler and understand signs and symptoms of worsening asthma. A Prednisone burst is not indicated at this time. Combination therapy would be considered if this patient was adherent on inhaled corticosteroids, with the presence of increased symptoms. Asthma Control Test is 18. Asthma control is 20 or greater. All patients with asthma must have an asthma action plan with appropriate follow-up care.

23. A. According to the EPR-3, risk factors for asthma-related death include: Previous severe exacerbation, two or more hospitalizations or > 3 ED visits in the past year, use of > 2 canisters of SABA per month, difficulty perceiving airway obstructions or the severity of worsening asthma, low socioeconomic status or inner-city residence, illicit drug use, major psychosocial problems or psychiatric disease, and comorbidities such as cardiovascular disease or other chronic lung disease.

24. A. Clinical features that suggest malignancy on initial evaluation include older age, current or past history of tobacco abuse, hemoptysis, and the presence of a previous malignancy.

25. A. Wheezing heard only on inspiration is referred to as stridor and is associated with mechanical obstruction at the level of the trachea/upper airway.

26. A. According to EPR-3, correctly diagnosing asthma is attained by establishing a history of episodic symptoms of airflow obstruction are present, airflow obstruction or symptoms are at least partially reversible, and the exclusion of alternative diagnoses.

27. B. Wheezing produced during inspiration and/or expiration is associated with diffuse processes that affect all lobes of the lung and is often audible in all lung fields.

28. C. Symptomatic treatment, including acetaminophen as needed. Symptomatic treatment may include nonsteroidal anti-inflammatory drugs or acetaminophen directed toward presenting symptoms. Bronchodilators can help relieve the cough in people who show evidence of bronchospasm. Other options are not consistent with the initial treatment of acute bronchitis.

29. A. EPR-3 recommends inhaled corticosteroids as the drug of choice in the treatment of persistent asthma.

30. B. Pulsus paradox is an exaggeration of normal physiology in which the systolic arterial pressure is > 10 mgHg during inspiration. A drop of > 25 mmHg reflects severe airflow obstruction.

31. A. According to EPR-3, the leukotriene receptor antagonist is considered an add-on therapy in mild and moderate persistent asthma.

32. C. A normal lung transmits a palpable vibratory sensation to the chest wall. This is known as tactile fremitus.

33. C. This is a lymphangitic tumor spread. Symptoms of cough, pain, or hemoptysis may be present in patients with hilar involvement, particularly when the metastases adjoin or invade the bronchi.

34. B. ACE-I is a contributing factor to cough. After discontinuing ACE-I, the cough generally resolves within one to four days, but may take up to four weeks.

35. D. Depression of the sternum is known as pectus excavatum (funnel chest).

36. B. Hyperresonance is described as a lower-pitched, louder and longer sound heard normally over the lungs during maximum inspiration.

37. A. According to the EPR-3 guidelines, this patient should be referred to a pulmonary or allergy service for an immediate consult. In the interim, the FNP should prescribe a medical treatment regimen according to EPR-3 and begin an asthma education consult.

38. B. *H. influenzae* resistance to β-lactam antibiotics is problematic.

39. C. Clinical findings of dullness on percussion, increased tactile fremitus, and whispered pectoriloquy being heard clearly is consistent with consolidation.

40. D. Moxifloxacin and gemifloxacin are more potent against *S. pneumoniae*.

41. C. Causes of chronic cough include post-nasal drip, GERD, and other issues. Referral for evaluation may be needed to further evaluate the patient and reduce/eliminate the cough.

42. C. According to the United States Preventative Services Task Force, annual screening for lung cancer is recommended using low-dose computed tomography in adults aged 55 to 80 years who have a 30 pack-year smoking history, currently smoke or have quit within the past 15 years, and patients who develop a health problem that substantially limits life expectancy.

43. D. According to the American Joint Committee on Cancer, N2 is classified as metastasis in ipsilateral, mediastinal, and/or subcarinal lymph node(s); NX Regional lymph nodes cannot be assessed; N0 no regional lymph node metastases; N1 Metastasis in ipsilateral peribronchial and/or ipsilateral hilar lymph nodes and intrapulmonary nodes, including involvement by direct extension; N3 Metastasis in contralateral mediastinal, contralateral hilar, ipsilateral or contralateral scalene, or supraclavicular lymph node(s).

44. A. IgE is the antibody responsible for activation of allergic reactions and is important to the development and persistence of inflammation.

45. A. Measurements of fractional exhaled NO (FeNO) is very useful for monitoring the response to asthma treatment because of the association between FeNO and the presence of inflammation in asthma. Many insurance companies pay for this tool, which is helpful in evaluating the current treatment regimen, response to treatment over a period of time, and possibly adherence.

46. A. Beta-blockers can cause increased bronchial obstruction, airway reactivity, and resistance to the effects of inhaled or oral beta receptor agonists in patients with asthma. Topical ophthalmic administration of nonselective beta-blockers for the treatment of glaucoma can lead to exacerbated asthma but not exacerbated COPD. Pulmonary function testing is not indicated every 3 to 4 weeks in patients taking beta-blockers. Adverse reactions can occur in intermittent asthma, mild persistent, moderate persistent asthma, and severe persistent asthma.

47. B. Peripheral edema from cor pulmonale is a complication of chronic bronchitis.

48. D. Rhonchi is described as low-pitched and loud, generally heard on inspiration, and often cleared with cough. It is important to ask the patient to cough and then repeat auscultation of the lungs.

49. B. According to the GOLD, 2015 Guidelines:
Classification of Severity of Airflow Limitations in COPD
    In patients with FEV1/FVC < 0.70

Gold 1:	Mild	FEV1 ≥ 80% predicted
Gold 2:	Moderate	50% ≤ FEV1 < 80% predicted
Gold 3:	Severe	30% ≤ FEV1 < 50% predicted
Gold 4:	Very Severe	FEV1 < 30% predicted

50. D. Ipratropium bromide promotes the degradation of cyclic guanosine monophosphate and activation of beta$_2$-adrenergic receptors on airway smooth muscle.

51. D. Several comorbidities of asthma include gastroesophageal reflux disease, diabetes mellitus, and allergic rhinitis. Vocal cord dysfunction can mimic asthma.

• • • References

Albert, R. H. (2010). Diagnosis and treatment of acute bronchitis. *American Family Physician.* 82(11); 1345–1350.

American Lung Association. (2014). *Chronic obstructive pulmonary disease (COPD) fact sheet.* Retrieved from http://www.lung.org/lungdisease/copd/resources/facts-figures/COPD-Fact-Sheet.html?referrer=https://www.google.com/

Barclay, L. (2014). Palivizumab RSV prophylaxis guidelines updated. American Academy of Pediatrics. Available at http://www.medscape.com/viewarticle/828957.

Bareschino, M. A., Schettino, C., Rossi, A., Maione, P., Sacco, P. C., Zeppa, R., & Gridelli, C. (2011). Treatment of advanced non small cell lung cancer. *Journal of Thoracic Disease, 3,*122–133. doi: 10.3978/j.issn.2072-1439.2010.12.08

Bellinger, C. R., & Peters S. P. (2015). Outpatient chronic obstructive pulmonary disease management: Going for the GOLD. *Journal of Allergy and Clinical Immunology: In Practice, 3*(4), 471–478.

Bolser, D. C. (2010). Pharmacologic management of cough. *Otolaryngology Clinic of North America, 43*(1), 147–155.

Canning, B. J. (2010). Afferent nerves regulating the cough reflex: Mechanisms and mediators of cough in disease. *Otolaryngology Clinic North America*, 43(1), 15–vii. doi:10.1016/j.otc.2009.11.012. http://www.ncbi.nlm.nih.gov/pmc/articles/PMC2882535/pdf/nihms188187.pdf

Caswell-Dawson, M., & Muncie, H. L. (2011). Respiratory syncytial virus infection in children. *American Family Physician, 83*(2), 141–146.

Centers for Disease Control and Prevention (CDC). (2014). Morbidity and Mortality Weekly Report (MMWR). CDC national health report: Leading causes of morbidity and mortality and associated behavioral risk and protective factors—United States, 2005–2013. Retrieved from http://www.cdc.gov/mmwr/preview/mmwrhtml/su6304a2.htm

Centers for Disease Control and Prevention (CDC). (2014). 2014 Surgeon General's report: The health consequences of smoking—50 years of progress. Retrieved from http://www.cdc.gov/tobacco/data_statistics/sgr/50th-anniversary/index.htm

Centers for Disease Control and Prevention (CDC). (2014). Vaccines and immunizations: Pneumococcal. Retrieved from http://www.cdc.gov/vaccines/pubs/surv-manual/chpt11-pneumo.html

Centers for Disease Control and Prevention (CDC). (2015). Tuberculosis. Retrieved from http://www.cdc.gov/tb/

Chung, K. F., & Pavord, I. D. (2008). Prevalence, pathogenesis, and cause of chronic cough. *Lancet, 371,* 1364–1374.

Global Initiative for Asthma. (2015). Global strategy for asthma management and prevention. Retrieved from http://www.ginasthma.org/download.asp

Global Initiative for Chronic Obstructive Lung Disease. (2015). Global strategy for the diagnosis, management, and prevention of chronic obstruction lung disease. Updated 2015. Retrieved from http://www.goldcopd.org

Hillas, G., Perlikos, F., Tsiligianni, I., & Tzanakis N. (2015). Managing comorbidities in COPD. *International Journal of COPD, 10,* 95–109.

Koul, A. (2011). The challenge of new drug discovery for tuberculosis. *Nature, 469,* 483–490 (2011) doi:10.1038/nature09657.

Levitzky, M. G. (2013). Function and structure of the respiratory system. In *Pulmonary Physiology* (8th ed.). New York, NY: McGraw-Hill.

Mizgerd, J. P. (2008). Acute lower respiratory tract infection. *New England Journal of Medicine, 358,* 716–727.

National Heart Lung and Blood Institute. (2007). Expert Panel Report 3 (EPR-3): Guidelines for the diagnosis and management of asthma summary report 2007. Retrieved from http://www.nhlbi.nih.gov/health-pro/guidelines/current/asthma-guidelines

Price, D. B., Yawn, B. P., & Jones, R. C. M. (2010). Improving the differential diagnosis of chronic obstructive pulmonary disease in primary care. *Mayo Clinical Proceedings, 85*(12), 1122–1129.

Rance, K. (2011). Helping patients attain and maintain asthma control: Reviewing the role of the nurse practitioner. *Journal of Multidisciplinary Healthcare, 4,* 299–309.

Shifen, A., Witt, C., Christie, C., & Castro, M. (2011). Mechanisms of remodeling in asthmatic airways. *Journal of Allergy.* Retrieved from http://www.hindawi.com/journals/ja/2012/316049/

Watkins, R. R., & Lemonovich, T. L. (2011). Diagnosis and management of community-acquired pneumonia in adults. *American Family Physician, 83*(11), 1299–1306.

Cardiovascular Disorders in Primary Care

Heather Ferrillo, PhDc, MSN, APRN, FNP-BC, CNE

Murmurs

Basics of auscultating murmurs:

- Auscultate the patient supine, in the left lateral position and leaning forward.
- Auscultate with both the bell and the diaphragm.
  - Right sternal border—second intercostal space (aortic area)
  - Left sternal border—second intercostal space (pulmonic area)
  - Along the left sternal border at each intercostal space
  - Lower left sternal border—(tricuspid area)
  - Apex—(mitral area)
- Murmurs should be characterized by
  - Timing (systolic or diastolic)
  - Location (where the loudest)
  - Changes with position
  - Characteristic (i.e., crescendo-decrescendo)
  - Intensity of the murmur (1 to 6 for systolic, 1 to 4 for diastolic)
- Identification of murmurs
- Systolic
  - Innocent/physiologic murmur
  - Mitral regurgitation
  - Tricuspid regurgitation

- VSD
- Aortic stenosis
- Hypertrophic cardiomyopathy
- Pulmonic stenosis
- Diastolic—Diastolic murmurs are always pathologic
  - Aortic regurgitation
  - Mitral stenosis

Source: Bickley, 2013.

Valvular Disorders

Aortic Stenosis

- Most common Causes: bicuspid valve (congenital), calcification, RHD
- Manifestations
  - Angina
  - Syncope
  - Heart failure
  - Decreased BP
  - Narrowed pulse pressure
- Diagnosis
  - Murmur (see above)
  - Echocardiogram
  - Cardiac catheterization

- Treatment
  - Valve replacement when severe and symptomatic

Mitral Regurgitation

- Most common causes: Mitral Valve Prolapse (MVP) and Rheumatic Heart Disease (RHD)
- Manifestations
  - Few until severe, then heart failure (HF) results
- Diagnosis
  - Murmur
  - Echocardiogram
- Treatment
  - Medical management with BP (blood pressure) control and serial EKG until LV failure
  - Mitral valve repair or replacement

Aortic Regurgitation

- Common causes: Congenital (bicuspid valve) or acquired (RHD hypertension [HTN], endocarditis), significant portion are idiopathic
- Manifestations:
  - Widened pulse pressure
  - Heart failure symptoms
- Complications
  - Arrhythmias
  - Endocarditis
- Diagnosis
  - Murmur
  - Echocardiogram
- Treatment
  - Serial echocardiograms
  - Medical management with vasodilators until significant dysfunction, then valve replacement

MVP Mitral Valve Prolapse

- Common causes: Myxomatous degeneration of the valve, genetic link
- Manifestations
  - Mostly asymptomatic
  - Tachycardia
  - Palpitations
  - Lightheadedness
  - Atypical chest pain
  - Lethargy

- Complications
  - Mitral regurgitation
  - Atrial fibrillation
  - Rare endocarditis, stroke, and sudden death
- Diagnosis
  - Murmur of MR (mitral regurgitation) and mid-systolic click
  - Echocardiogram
- Treatment
  - Beta blocker may control symptoms
  - If patient presents with mitral regurgitation then they will need afterload reduction, diuresis, anticoagulation

Source: McCance and Heuther, 2014.

Subacute Bacterial Endocarditis Prophylaxis

Guidelines revised in 2007 to reflect the small likelihood of developing SBE (subacute bacterial endocarditis) post-dental procedure, rate of success in preventing SBE with premedication, and the increased incidence of antibiotic resistance.

Prophylaxis is warranted for procedure of the respiratory, skin, and MS tract in eligible patients, but not GI or GU procedures.

Diagnosis requiring SBE prophylaxis for dental procedures (not recommended in others)

- Prosthetic heart valves
- History of bacterial endocarditis
- Congenital heart disease (specific types)
- Heart transplant with valvulopathy

Recommended agents (given 30 to 60 min prior to procedure)

- First line
  - Amoxicillin 2 grams
- For PCN allergic patient
  - Clindamycin 600 mg
  - Azithromycin or clarithromycin 500 mg

Source: Wilson et al., 2007.

Heart Failure

- Heart failure is a state of decreased cardiac output due to the failure of the ventricles to pump sufficient blood to meet the demands of the body.
- Can be left or right or biventricular
- Causes
  - Right-sided (failure of right ventricle)

- Most common is a disorder that increases pulmonary pressures
  - COPD
  - Pulmonary embolism
- Left ventricular failure
- RV infarct (least common)
  - Left-sided (failure of the left ventricle) (systolic or diastolic)
    - Most common is LV infarct
    - HTN
    - Aortic stenosis
- Manifestations
  - Forward effects (both sides) due to decreased cardiac output
    - Fatigue
    - Shortness of breath with exertions
    - Decreased peripheral perfusions
  - Right-sided (backward effects due to fluid buildup)
    - Jugular venous distention
    - Peripheral edema
    - Ascites
    - Hepatosplenomegaly
  - Left-sided
    - Crackles in the lungs
    - DOE (dyspnea on exertion)
    - PND (paroxysmal nocturnal dyspnea)
    - Orthopnea
    - Pulmonary edema

- Diminished EF (ejection fraction on echocardiogram), normal is 55% +/− 10
  - Diastolic—Nonspecific
    - Dyspnea
    - Exercise intolerance
    - Fatigue
- Diagnostics: For recommendations for noninvasive cardiac imaging.
  - Right-sided
    - Echocardiogram—Increased pulmonary pressures, dilated RV
  - Left-sided
    - Echocardiogram—Left ventricular size and function, LVH, valvular disorders
    - MUGA (multi-gated acquisition scan)—Nuclear determination of ejection fraction
    - Nuclear stress test—Determine infarct, ischemia, dilation of LV, ejection fraction
    - Grading/classification (2 scales)—Treatment based on both systems
  - Grading is not dynamic. Cannot go backward in categories.
- NYHA classification is dynamic and changes depending on the current functional ability of the patient. Good indicator for treatment success

Treatment

Figure 7-1 identifies the treatments based on the stages.

Table 7-1	Grading and Classification
Class	**Objective Assessment**
A	No objective evidence of cardiovascular disease. No symptoms and no limitation in ordinary physical activity.
B	Objective evidence of minimal cardiovascular disease. Mild symptoms and slight limitation during ordinary activity. Comfortable at rest.
C	Objective evidence of moderately severe cardiovascular disease. Marked limitation in activity due to symptoms, even during less-than-ordinary activity. Comfortable only at rest.
D	Objective evidence of severe cardiovascular disease. Severe limitations. Experience symptoms even while at rest.

Reproduced from American Heart Association. (2015). Classes of heart failure. Retrieved from www.heart.org.

Table 7-2	Patient Symptoms
Class	**Patient Symptoms**
I	No limitation of physical activity. Ordinary physical activity does not cause undue fatigue, palpitation, dyspnea (shortness of breath).
II	Slight limitation of physical activity. Comfortable at rest. Ordinary physical activity results in fatigue, palpitation, dyspnea (shortness of breath).
III	Marked limitation of physical activity. Comfortable at rest. Less than ordinary activity causes fatigue, palpitation, or dyspnea.
IV	Unable to carry on any physical activity without discomfort. Symptoms of heart failure at rest. If any physical activity is undertaken, discomfort increases.

Reproduced from American Heart Association. (2015). Classes of heart failure. Retrieved from www.heart.org.

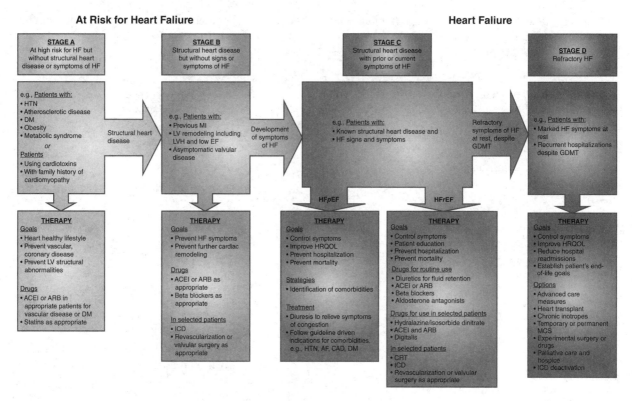

Figure 7-1 Stages in the Development of HF and Recommended Therapy by Stage
Reprinted with permission. Circulation. 2013;128:e240–e327. ©2013, American Heart Association, Inc.

HTN JNC 8

Overview

- HTN is one of the most preventable causes of morbidity and mortality.

- Most current guidelines are JNC 8 and focus on the decrease of morbidity and mortality through the diagnosis and management of HTN.

- Focuses on adults 18 years and older.

- Studies included only those that reported effects on hard outcomes including CV disease, MI, heart failure, stroke, coronary revascularization, and end-stage renal disease.

Goals for Treatment

- General population age >60 – 150/90
  - If treatment results in lower than goal and tolerated well, no adjustment needed.
- General population age <60 – 140/90
- Population with chronic kidney disease (CKD) – 140/90
- Population with diabetes – 140/90

Treatment Recommendations – The diagnosis of hypertension is based on two separate blood pressure readings obtained at two separate visits.

- General, nonblack population (including diabetics)
  - Thiazide diuretic
  - Calcium channel blocker
  - Angiotensin-converting-enzyme inhibitor (ACEI)
  - Angiotensin receptor blocker (ARB)
    - Per ADA (American Diabetes Association), ACEI or ARB preferred in diabetics for renal protection.
- General, black population (including diabetics)
  - Thiazide diuretics
  - Calcium channel blockers
    - Per ADA, addition of ACEI or ARB should be considered for renal protection.
- Population greater than 18 with CKD (regardless of race or diabetic status)
  - ACEI
  - ARB

- Therapeutic lifestyle changes
  - In conjunction with pharmacologic therapy
    - Diet (sodium restriction)
    - Weight control
    - Exercise
- Evaluate for presence of target organ damage
  - EKG—LVH (left ventricular hypertrophy)
  - Renal function
  - Ophthalmologic exam
- Consider secondary causes as indicated
  - Check medication list
  - Renal artery stenosis
  - Endocrine disorders—Thyroid, Cushing's, pheocromocytoma

Follow-up

- If not to goal within 1 month:
  - Increase dose or
  - Add a second agent from list of preferred agents
- If not controlled with two drugs:
  - Add third drug from recommended list
  - Do not use ACE and ARB together (contraindicated)
- If not controlled with three drugs or class of drug contraindicated:
  - Other antihypertensive classes can be considered
  - Consider referral to hypertensive specialist

Cholesterol Management

Based on the current (2013) ACC/AHA Guidelines on the Treatment of Blood Cholesterol.

Goals

- Lowering cholesterol lowers ASCVD (atherosclerotic cardiovascular disease) risk.
- Relationship between LDL and coronary and atherosclerotic disease.

Assessment

- Presence of clinical ASCVD
  - Acute coronary syndrome
  - History of MI
  - Stable or unstable angina
  - Coronary or other arterial revascularization
  - Stroke
  - TIA
  - Peripheral arterial disease

- Calculated 10-year risk of ASCVD using Pooled Cohort Equation
- Secondary causes of elevated LDL (Stone et al., 2014)
  - Diet
    - Saturated fats
    - Weight gain
  - Drugs
    - Diuretics
    - Steroids
    - Amiodarone
    - Cyclosporine
  - Diseases
    - Biliary obstruction
    - Nephrotic syndrome
    - Hypothyroidism
    - Obesity
    - Pregnancy
- Secondary causes of elevated triglycerides (Stone et al., 2014)
  - Diet
    - Weight gain
    - Very-low-fat diets
    - High intake refined carbs
    - Excessive alcohol
  - Drugs
    - Estrogens
    - Glucocorticoids
    - Bile acid sequestrants
    - Protease inhibitors
    - Tamoxifen
    - Beta blockers
    - Thiazides
  - Diseases
    - Nephrotic syndrome
    - Chronic renal failure
    - Poorly controlled DM
    - Hypothyroidism
    - Obesity
    - Pregnancy

Treatment Guidelines (Stone et al., 2014)

- Lifestyle changes
  - Heart-healthy diet
  - Exercise

- Avoidance of tobacco
- Healthy weight
- Focus is on LDL cholesterol
- Triglyceride is priority if >500
- Evidence supports the use of fixed-dose statins
  - High-, moderate-, and low-intensity statins. Refer to Figure 7-2 for recommendations regarding the initiation of statin therapy.
- Four major statin benefit groups
  - Secondary prevention in people with clinical ASCVD
  - Primary prevention in people with elevation of LDL-C ≥190 mg/dL
  - Primary prevention in people with DM 40–75 years old with LDL-C 70 to 189 mg/dL
  - Primary prevention in people without DM but with estimated 10-year ASCVD risk ≥7.5%, 40 to 75 years old and with LDL-C 70 to 189

Follow-up (See Figure 7-3 for Recommendations for Monitoring Statin Therapy)

- Monitoring for success of treatment
  - Initial fasting lipid panel
  - Second panel in 4–12 weeks to assess adherence
  - Then every 3–12 months as clinically warranted
  - Monitor for adherence and intolerance if less than anticipated therapeutic response.
  - Evaluate need for increased intensity of statin

- Safety and monitoring
  - Consider decreasing statin dose if 2 consecutive LDL < 40
  - Doses of simvastatin 80 mg may be harmful.
  - Monitor for new onset DM in patients on statin therapy.
  - Closely monitor patients on multiple drugs, especially those that interfere with metabolism of statin.
  - For patients presenting with confusional state or memory impairment, evaluate for nonstatin cause as well as adverse statin effects.
- Management of muscle symptoms:
  - Obtain a good baseline prior to initiating statin to avoid unnecessary discontinuation of statin.
  - Unexplained severe muscle symptoms
  - Discontinue statin.
  - Evaluate for rhabdomyolysis
    - CK (serum creatine kinase)
    - Urine
  - Mild to moderate symptoms
    - Discontinue statin until evaluation.
    - Evaluate for conditions that may increase risk.
    - If symptoms resolve, reinstitute statin therapy to establish causal relationship.
    - If causal relationship, discontinue statin and use low dose of different statin when symptoms resolve.

Table 7-3	High-, Moderate-, and Low-Intensity Statin Therapy (Used in the RCTs; Reviewed by the Expert Panel)	
High-Intensity Statin Therapy	**Moderate-Intensity Statin Therapy**	**Low-Intensity Statin Therapy**
Daily dose lowers LDL-C, on average, by approximately ≥ 50%	Daily dose lowers LDL-C, on average, by approximately 30% to < 50%	Daily dose lowers LDL-C, on average, by < 30%
Atorvastatin (40†)–80 mg **Rosuvastatin 20 (40) mg**	**Atorvastatin 10 (20) mg** **Rosuvastatin (5) 10 mg** **Simvastatin 20–40 mg‡** **Pravastatin 40 (80) mg** **Lovastatin 40 mg** *Fluvastatin XL 80 mg* **Fluvastatin 40 mg BID** *Pitavastatin 2–4 mg*	*Simvastatin 10 mg* **Pravastatin 10–20 mg** **Lovastatin 20 mg** *Fluvastatin 20–40 mg* *Pitavastatin 1 mg*

Reproduced from Stone, N. J., Robinson, J. G., Lichtenstein, A. H., Merz, C. N. B., Blum, C. B., Eckel, R. H., . . . Wilson, P. W. F. et al. (2014). 2013 ACC/AHA Guideline on the Treatment of Blood Cholesterol to Reduce Atherosclerotic Cardiovascular Risk in Adults: A Report of the American College of Cardiology/American Heart Association Task Force on Practice Guidelines. Circulation, 129(25 suppl 2), S1–S45. http://doi.org/10.1161/01.cir.0000437738.63853.7a

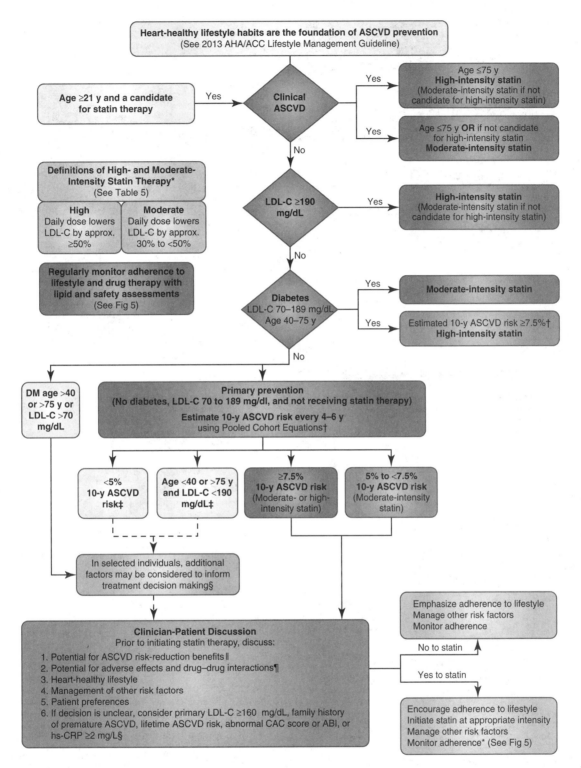

Figure 7-2 Summary of Statin Initiation Recommendations

Reproduced from Stone, N. J., Robinson, J. G., Lichtenstein, A. H., Merz, C. N. B., Blum, C. B., Eckel, R. H., . . . Wilson, P. W. F. (2014). 2013 ACC/AHA Guideline on the Treatment of Blood Cholesterol to Reduce Atherosclerotic Cardiovascular Risk in Adults: A Report of the American College of Cardiology/American Heart Association Task Force on Practice Guidelines. Circulation, 129(25 suppl 2), S1–S45. http://doi.org/10.1161/01.cir.0000437738.63853.7a

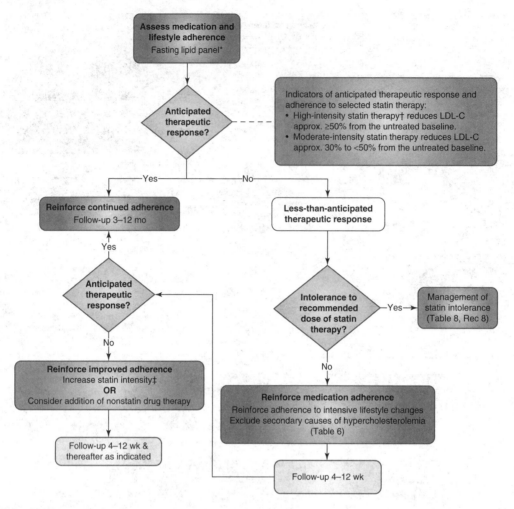

Figure 7-3 Statin Therapy Monitoring

Reproduced from Stone, N. J., Robinson, J. G., Lichtenstein, A. H., Merz, C. N. B., Blum, C. B., Eckel, R. H., . . . Wilson, P. W. F. (2014). 2013 ACC/AHA Guideline on the Treatment of Blood Cholesterol to Reduce Atherosclerotic Cardiovascular Risk in Adults: A Report of the American College of Cardiology/American Heart Association Task Force on Practice Guidelines. Circulation, 129(25 suppl 2), S1–S45. http://doi.org/10.1161/01.cir.0000437738.63853.7a

- Once low dose is tolerated, gradually increase dose.
- If after 2 months without statin symptoms do not resolve or elevated CK does not resolve, consider other cause of symptoms.
- If persistent symptoms determined to be from other condition, resume statin therapy at original dose.

Evaluation of Chest Pain

Pathogenesis
- Cardiac
- Musculoskeletal
- Neurologic
- GI
- Pleural
- Psychogenic

Assessment
- Location of the pain:
  - Ischemic pain is diffuse and usually difficult to localize
  - Levine sign (fist in center of chest) + predictive value
- Quality of the pain: Not often "pain"
  - Myocardial ischemia usually squeezing, tight, fullness, knot, ache, heavy weight, toothache, bra too tight

- Quantity/severity of the pain: Rate intensity on 0–10 pain scale (not useful in ACS)
- Radiation:
  - Myocardial ischemia can radiate to neck, jaw, teeth, throat, shoulder (radiation to BOTH arms is very predictive of MI).
  - Pain radiating to right shoulder with epigastric pain indicative of cholecystitis.
  - Pain that radiates between scapulae may be aortic dissection.
  - Pericarditis pain usually radiates to one or both trapezius ridges.
- Timing: including onset, duration, and frequency (quick and sharp, recurring or one-time, duration of each episode).
  - Gradual onset associated with myocardial ischemia
  - Abrupt with great intensity is more often dissection or PE
  - Myocardial ischemia more often in the morning (increased sympathetic tone r/t circadian rhythm)
  - Chest pain that only lasts for a few seconds or that is constant over weeks is most likely not due to ischemia.
- Setting where/when the pain occurs:
  - At rest—non-ischemic of unstable angina
  - With exertion—indicative of ischemia
  - With stressful situation—consider ischemia or psychogenic cause
- Aggravating factors:
  - Occurs with eating more suggestive of GI, although postprandial chest pain could be ischemic.
  - Provoked by exercise more likely cardiac.
  - Cold, stress, meals, intercourse can aggravate cardiac ischemia.
  - Worsens with swallowing = esophageal
- Alleviating factors:
  - Pain that goes away or is lessened with sublingual nitroglycerin
    - Cardiac
    - Esophageal
  - Improves with change of body position = musculoskeletal origin likely
  - Pain that abates with cessation of physical activity frequently is of cardiac origin.
  - Pain that improves with sitting upright and leaning forward = pericarditis likely

- Associated symptoms:
  - Dyspnea, especially in diabetics; more atypical presentation of ischemia
  - Elderly most often present with fatigue, confusion, dyspnea with chest pain
  - Cough—Include infection, CHF (congestive heart failure), PE (pulmonary embolism), neoplasm in differentials
  - Syncope—Patients with ACS (acute coronary symptoms) may have presyncope but syncope raises suspicion of aortic dissection, pulmonary embolism, or ruptured abdominal aortic aneurysm.
  - Belching, bad taste, dysphagia, consistent with esophageal disease
  - Vomiting common in MI in addition to PUD (peptic ulcer disease), cholecystitis, pancreatitis, DKA (diabetic ketoacidosis)
  - Diaphoresis more common in MI (myocardial infarction)
  - Palpitations – Ventricular ectopy
  - New onset of atrial fibrillation with chest pain, consider pulmonary embolism
- Past medical history:
  - Any prior history of CAD (coronary artery disease), PCI (percutaneous coronary intervention), CABG (coronary artery bypass graft), peripheral vascular disease
  - PUD (peptic ulcer disease), GERD (gastroesophageal reflux disease), gallstones
  - Panic disorder
  - Bronchospasm
  - Neoplasm
- Cardiac risk factors:
  - Age (40+) in men
  - Postmenopausal state for women
  - Hypertension (risk for MI and aortic dissection)
  - Dyslipidemia
  - Family history
  - Diabetes
  - Abdominal aortic aneurysm, CVA (Cerebrovascular accident), PVD (peripheral vascular disease), RAS
  - Obesity
  - Metabolic syndrome
  - Cigarette use (prior or current use)
  - Stress

- Sedentary lifestyle
- Cocaine use
- Assessment/differential diagnosis
  - Life-threatening conditions:
    - ACS
    - Stress induced cardiomyopathy
    - Tension pneumothorax
    - Gastric perforation
    - Aortic dissection
    - Pulmonary embolus
  - Other cardiac and non-ischemic conditions
    - CHF
    - Chronic stable angina
    - New arrhythmia
    - HTN
    - Infectious/bacterial process (i.e., pericarditis, myocarditis)
    - Musculoskeletal pain
    - Anxiety
    - GERD
- Diagnostics:
  - EKG—Compare to old:
    - Arrhythmias (atrial/ventricular)
    - ST-T abnormalities (depression/elevation)
    - New LBBB (left bundle branch block)
    - Cannot interpret with baseline LBBB, paced rhythm, LVH with strain
  - CXR
    - CHF
    - Infiltrates
    - Widened mediastinum
  - Blood work – Troponins, CBC (complete blood count), TFTS (thyroid function tests), BMP (basic metabolic panel)
  - Echocardiogram
  - Stress test
  - Cardiac cath
  - Endoscopy

Coronary Artery Disease
Pathogenesis
- MI—Complete occlusion of coronary artery
- Angina—Partial occlusion of coronary artery; supply versus demand problem
  - Stable—Occurs with exertion or other precipitating event

- Unstable—Occurs at rest
- Vasospastic—Not related to activity, often at night

Treatment
- Acute MI
  - Call 911
  - Aspirin—Chew 4 of 81 mg
  - SL nitroglycerin
  - Oxygen
  - Early revascularization shows most benefit and less mortality
- Ongoing care
  - Percutaneous angioplasty with stenting
  - Coronary artery bypass grafting
  - Meds
    - ASA
    - Beta-blockers—Mortality benefit and prevention of second MI
    - ACE inhibitors—Prevents remodeling
    - For significant, persistent LV dysfunction: HF management and consider defibrillator
- Angina
  - Revascularization via PTCA or CABG if feasible
  - Meds
    - ASA
    - Nitroglycerin for acute angina attacks
    - 1 tab SL q 5 min × 3, if no relief, go to ER
    - Long-acting nitrates
    - Calcium channel blockers

Atrial Fibrillation (January et al., 2014)

Definitions
- Paroxysmal
  - Episode lasting less than 7 days
  - Episodes may reoccur spontaneously
- Persistent
  - Continuous AFib > 7 days
- Permanent
  - Decision by patient and clinician to not pursue further rhythm control
- Nonvalvular AFib
  - AFib in the absence of rheumatic mitral stenosis, mechanical heart valve or valve repair

Pathophysiology

- Multiple pathways and mechanisms of AF are possible.

Assessment

- CHADS Score – Quantifies risk of thrombo-embolic event
  - CHF – 1 point
  - Hypertension – 1 point
  - Age ≥ 75 y – 1 point
  - DM – 1 point
  - Stroke/TIA/thrombotic event (doubled) – 2 points
- Assess for reversible causes
  - Thyroid disease
  - Anemia
  - Heart failure
  - OSA

Treatment (based on *AHA/ACC/HRS Guidelines for the Management of AFib*)

- Antithrombotic therapy
  - Indications
    - Should be shared decision based on risks of stroke and bleeding
    - Decisions regarding antithrombotic therapy should be made regardless of whether the AFib is paroxysmal, persistent, or permanent and regardless of whether rhythm or rate control strategies are utilized.
    - Patients with AF and heart valve, warfarin is recommended.
    - Nonvalvular AF with previous stroke/TIA or CHADS score ≥2—antithrombotic therapy recommended (warfarin, dabigatran, rivaroxaban, or apixaban)
    - Nonvalvular AFib with CHADS score of 1—Options for no antithrombotic therapy, thrombotic therapy or aspirin
    - Nonvalvular AFib with CHADS score of 0—Reasonable to omit antithrombotic therapy
    - Patients with atrial flutter should be treated with antithrombotic therapy using the same considerations
- Rate control
  - Control of ventricular rate to resting HR of 80 bpm
  - Resting HR less than 110 bpm is reasonable in the absence of symptoms and with normal ventricular function
  - Beta-blockers or nondihydropyridine calcium channel blockers
  - Symptoms during exercise should be evaluated to ensure HR control with exercise
- Rhythm control
  - Referral to cardiologist warranted
  - Options
    - Cardioversion
    - Antiarrhythmic therapy
    - Ablation

Prevention

- Data suggests the use of ACE or ARB is useful for prevention of AFib in patients with ventricular dysfunction.
- ACE or ARB therapy may be warranted to prevent AFib in the presence of HTN.
- Statin therapy may be useful in preventing AFib after coronary artery surgery.

Source: January et al., 2014.

Peripheral Vascular Disease—Atherosclerosis (PAD)

- Disease in arteries outside the heart
- Increased incidence with diabetes
- Most common sites
  - Abdominal aorta
  - Carotid arteries
  - Femoral and iliac arteries

Signs and Symptoms

- Increasing fatigue and weakness in the legs
- Intermittent claudication
  - Muscle ischemia
  - Sensory impairment—Tingling, burning, numbness
  - Peripheral pulses distal to occlusion become weak.
  - Appearance of the skin of the feet and legs:
    - Marked pallor or cyanosis
    - Skin dry and hairless
    - Toenails thick and hard

Treatment

- Revascularization
- Blood sugar control in DM

- Weight loss
- Cholesterol management
- Platelet inhibitors
- Cessation of smoking
- Increase activity and exercise—Ambulation through pain increases collateral development
- Maintain dependent position for legs—Improves arterial perfusion

Peripheral Vascular Disease—Venous Disorders

- Venous Insufficiency
  - Assessment:
    - Edema
    - Skin friable, weeping, open wounds
    - Chronic skin changes include brown and thick skin from hemosiderin deposits
    - Diminished pulses only if edema is affecting arterial circulation
  - Management
    - Leg position—Elevated
    - Monitor for s/s of infection
    - Compression—Need to rule out arterial involvement first
- DVT
  - Assessment
    - Maybe asymptomatic
    - Heaviness in extremities—Dull ache
    - Unilateral edema
    - Redness, warmth if superficial vein involved
    - Risk factors
      - Virchow's triad
        - Stasis
          - Immobility
        - Hypercoagulable state
          - Cancer
          - Pregnancy
          - Clotting disorders
        - Intimal changes
          - Inflammation
          - Trauma
  - Diagnostic
    - Doppler ultrasound of extremity
    - D-Dimer—Not specific
    - CT scan if inconclusive
    - Workup for clotting disorders if no apparent cause

- Complications
  - Goal is to avoid pulmonary embolism.
  - Can have chronic venous insufficiency as sequela.
- Management (Patel, 2015)
  - Anticoagulation—First episode 3–6 months, recurrent 1 year
    - LMWH or unfractionated heparin with bridge to warfarin
    - Other anticoagulants:
      - Rivaroxaban
      - Apixaban
      - Dabigatran
  - Bed rest—Controversial
    - Studies show no increase in PE with ambulation
    - Recommendation is early ambulation (day 2 after initiation of anticoagulation)
  - Invasive treatments
    - Thrombectomy (if extensive and flow limiting)
    - Placement of IVC filter
      - High risk for PE
      - Not candidate for anticoagulation
      - Risk of reoccurrence
  - Evaluate for familial clotting disorders if no obvious reason for DVT or in presence of recurrence

Varicose Veins

Risk Factors

- Prolonged standing
- Obesity
- Pregnancy
- Family history
- Weightlifting

Assessment

- Complaints of aching and fullness
- Presence of engorged, tortuous superficial leg veins
- Edema may be present if venous flow is limited

Management

- Elevation
- Exercise
- Compression
- Weight loss
- Avoid restrictive clothing
- Surgical intervention if symptoms warrant

Review Questions

1. A 62-year-old male patient presents with complaints of dyspnea on exertion, presyncope, and mild exertional chest pain. Exam reveals a harsh 3/6 late peaking systolic murmur loudest at the right sternal border that radiates to the carotids. Which disorder is suspected?
    A. Mitral valve prolapse
    B. Hypertrophic cardiomyopathy
    C. Aortic stenosis
    D. Mitral regurgitation

2. A patient with a history of Type 2 Diabetes and coronary disease has the following lipid panel: LDL 128, HDL 30, and Trig 208. What should the first-line treatment be?
    A. Lifestyle modification with diet and exercise
    B. Atorvastatin 20 mg daily
    C. Atorvastatin 80 mg daily
    D. Fenofibrate

3. The FNP is performing a routine physical exam on a 60-year-old male who is a new patient and has been lost to medical follow-up for 20 years. The patient denies any past medical history and has a family history of hypertension and CAD. BP today is 158/92. What would be the appropriate next step?
    A. Start Lisinopril 10 mg daily
    B. Have the patient return in 2 weeks
    C. Start HCTZ 12.5 mg daily
    D. Teach the patient lifestyle modification and have him return in 1 year for a follow-up.

4. A patient with a history of systolic heart failure presents for routine follow-up. His medication list consists of an ACE inhibitor, aspirin, and a statin. Which medication should be added for decreased mortality?
    A. Carvedilol
    B. Furosemide
    C. Digoxin
    D. ARB

5. A 45-year-old male presents with chest tightness with exertion that resolves with rest. He has a past medical history of HTN and high cholesterol. Which diagnostic test would be first line in identifying the likely etiology of these symptoms?
    A. EKG
    B. Exercise stress test
    C. Cardiac catheterization
    D. Troponin levels

6. A patient with a history of a mitral valve prolapse and an allergy to PCN asks about dental care. What does the patient need to know?
    A. No prophylaxis is needed in MVP.
    B. Take clindamycin 600 mg BID for 3 days before the treatment.
    C. Take amoxicillin 2 gms one hour prior to treatment.
    D. You should not have dental care if you have MVP.

7. A patient presents for a routine physical exam and the nurse practitioner identifies that the patient has a 2/4 diastolic murmur located at the midaxillary line. What would be the next step in the treatment plan?
    A. Assure the patient that it is likely a physiologic murmur.
    B. Order an echocardiogram.
    C. Order a stress test.
    D. Educate the patient on identification of symptoms of aortic stenosis.

8. During the routine physical exam of a new 30-year-old male patient, he states his father died of sudden cardiac death at the age of 40. What diagnostic test would be an essential part of the treatment plan?

    A. Echocardiogram

    B. Lipid panel

    C. Genetic testing

    D. Chest x-ray

9. A 38-year-old woman presents to the office with complaints of chest pain that started this morning. The pain is described as sharp and worsening on inspiration. The patient's HR is 108 and BP 100/70. What question is important to ask in order to support the most likely diagnosis in this patient?

    A. Does the patient have a family history of coronary disease?

    B. What is her normal blood pressure?

    C. What medications is the patient on?

    D. Is she a diabetic?

10. On a routine visit, a 78-year-old gentleman is found to be in atrial fibrillation on an EKG. The patient has a history of CAD and CHF and is asymptomatic. What is the most important thing to include in the patient's treatment plan?

    A. Immediate cardioversion

    B. Anticoagulation

    C. Beta-blocker therapy

    D. Stress test

11. While doing a cardiovascular exam on a patient, the FNP identifies that the PMI is 11 cm lateral to the midsternal border. What is the appropriate next step?

    A. Document the findings as this is normal.

    B. Get an EKG.

    C. Refer patient directly to a cardiologist.

    D. Start the patient on an ACE inhibitor.

12. In an adult, the finding of an S3 on cardiac auscultation may indicate what?

    A. Normal heart function

    B. Heart failure

    C. LVH

    D. Anemia

13. What should be included as part of the plan in a patient with heart failure who is taking an ACE inhibitor, a beta-blocker, and aldactone?

    A. Monitor potassium and renal function.

    B. Echocardiograms every 3 months.

    C. Encourage a diet high in bananas, orange juice, and salmon.

    D. Discontinuation of all other diuretics.

14. A 45-year-old obese female with a history of type 2 diabetes asks if she could start an aerobic exercise plan. How should the nurse practitioner respond?

    A. "Absolutely, you may begin immediately."

    B. "You should have a stress test before you begin intense exercise."

    C. "Aerobic exercise is not safe in a patient with diabetes."

    D. "Once your blood sugar is under control, you can start exercising."

15. A 65-year-old male patient with a history of DM is diagnosed with HTN. Which medication should the patient be started on first line?
    A. Ace inhibitor
    B. Calcium channel blocker
    C. Diuretic
    D. Beta-blocker

16. Therapeutic lifestyle changes are recommended for a patient with elevated cholesterol levels. Patient education should include:
    A. Weight training three times a week
    B. Low-sodium diet
    C. High-fiber diet
    D. Very-low-fat diet

17. What is the term used to determine a valve that is not able to open completely to allow the flow of blood through or out of the heart?
    A. Regurgitant
    B. Incompetent
    C. Prolapse
    D. Stenosis

18. What heart sound is characteristic of mitral valve prolapse?
    A. A diastolic murmur
    B. A midsystolic click
    C. S4 heart sound
    D. No findings are often the case.

19. Which condition requires prophylaxis prior to dental work to prevent bacterial endocarditis?
    A. Mitral valve prolapse
    B. Previous episode of endocarditis
    C. Mitral valve repair
    D. Presence of a pacemaker

20. What is the main goal for treatment of HTN?
    A. Maintain cerebral perfusion
    B. Prevent target organ damage
    C. Lower lipids
    D. Prevent obesity

21. A patient presents to the office with JVD, hepatomegaly, and bilateral 2+ pitting edema. The patient denies shortness of breath and lungs are clear to auscultation (CTA). What underlying problem is suspected in this patient?
    A. COPD
    B. Recent LV MI
    C. Anemia
    D. DVT

22. A patient presents with complaints of a "fast heartbeat." An EKG reveals sinus tachycardia 110 bpm. What would be the next appropriate step?
    A. Start a beta-blocker to lower the heart rate.
    B. Determine the underlying cause of the tachycardia.
    C. Discuss anxiety treatments.
    D. Explain to the patient that this is a normal variant.

23. A patient presents for follow-up of systolic heart failure with an ejection fraction of 30%. His meds consist of a beta-blocker, an ACE-inhibitor, and baby aspirin. He is NYHA class I. What should be included in the plan of care?

    A. Add aldactone 12.5 mg daily.

    B. Refer to a cardiologist for an implantable defibrillator.

    C. Discontinue aspirin.

    D. Limit activity.

24. A patient presents with a DVT and has no evident risk factors for the disorder. What would the FNP do next?

    A. Continue anticoagulation indefinitely since there is no known cause.

    B. Evaluate the presence of familial clotting disorders.

    C. Plan for insertion of an IVC filter.

    D. Since the patient does not have risk factors, there is no need for anticoagulation.

25. A 55-year-old patient with DM presents to the office with complaints of chest tightness intermittently over the past 2 months. The discomfort occurs with exertion or stress and is relieved with rest. The EKG is unchanged from previous. What should the FNP do next?

    A. Order an NSAID for musculoskeletal chest pain.

    B. Order an exercise stress test for the presence of coronary artery disease.

    C. Send the patient to the ER immediately.

    D. Repeat the EKG in 2 weeks to see if there are any further changes.

26. A patient with known PAD presents to the office with complaints of increasing leg pain at rest. What does the NP think may be occurring?

    A. Progression of the arterial disease

    B. Development of a DVT

    C. Normal PAD symptoms

    D. A clotting disorder

27. A 42-year-old female presents to the office with bulging and painful superficial leg veins. What would predispose this patient to the disorder that is suspected?

    A. A desk job

    B. Obesity

    C. HTN

    D. High cholesterol

28. What antihypertensive has been shown to be most effective in African Americans, as well as in decreasing stroke risk?

    A. Beta-blockers

    B. ACE inhibitors

    C. Calcium channel blockers

    D. ARBs

29. In evaluating a patient with chest pain, it is noted that the pain is resolved with sublingual nitroglycerin. What does this information indicate?

    A. The pain is ischemic in nature.

    B. The patient's blood pressure is too high.

    C. The pain may be ischemic or esophageal in nature.

    D. No further workup is necessary.

30. A 75-year-old patient with a history of HTN presents with dyspnea on exertion and palpations over the past 2 weeks. An EKG shows atrial fibrillation with a heart rate of 115 bpm. What would the treatment plan include?

    A. Anticoagulation and rate control

    B. Initiation of an antiarrhythmic drug

    C. Immediate hospitalization

    D. Immediate stress test

Answers and Rationales

1. C. The hallmark symptoms of aortic stenosis are exertional chest pain, dyspnea, and syncope. The typical murmur is a systolic murmur loudest at the aortic area radiating to the carotid. The severity of AS is related to how late it peaks and whether it obliterates the second heart sound. Loudness does not correlate with severity.

2. C. A patient with known coronary disease and DM is at high risk for a cardiac event. Per the ACC/AHA cholesterol management guidelines, the patient will need high-dose statin therapy such as Atorvastatin 80 as first-line treatment. Atorvastatin will also lower the triglycerides and raise the HDL somewhat in this patient.

3. B. In order to diagnose HTN, 2 measurements must be made on different occasions. Per JNC 8 guidelines, the BP is considered elevated and will need medication if it is elevated when he returns. Either Lisinopril or HCTZ will be appropriate as first-line treatment.

4. A. Patients with systolic heart failure should be on certain beta-blockers for their mortality benefits. Carvedilol and sustained-release Metoprolol are indicated for this. Other BB (beta blockers) do not have the mortality data and should not be used in heart failure. Lasix and digoxin are effective in symptom management in HF, but do not have mortality benefits. ARBs do have mortality data, but are not indicated if a patient is already on an ACE inhibitor. ARBs are used as an alternative to ACE inhibitors in HF.

5. B. The patient is likely experiencing stable angina, which is characterized by exertional chest pain resolved with rest. The patient has risk factors such as gender, HTN, and high cholesterol. An exercise stress test is the first-line test for diagnosing coronary artery disease; a cardiac catheterization is an invasive test that would be ordered as confirmatory if the stress test were positive. An EKG or troponins will only be helpful in the setting of current chest pain, a previous MI, or a current MI.

6. A. The most current guidelines for bacterial endocarditis prophylaxis do not include MVP as a condition that warrants prophylaxis. Based on the old guidelines, MVP was treated with prophylaxis and patients may be used to this. The NP should educate the patient on new guidelines. The correct dosage of prophylaxis in an eligible patient with a PCN allergy would be clindamycin 600 mg 30 to 60 min prior to dental care.

7. B. A diastolic murmur is never physiologic and should be evaluated by echo to determine the cause. A stress test will not give information on the etiology of the murmur.

8. A. Patients with a family history of early sudden cardiac death should be evaluated for hypertrophic cardiomyopathy. An echocardiogram is the most accurate means to identify this condition.

9. C. The patient presents with typical signs and symptoms of a pulmonary embolism. In a young patient, the most likely culprit would be the use of oral contraceptives which could be ascertained with a medication history.

10. B. A patient with AFib of unknown duration is not a candidate for immediate cardioversion without identifying if there is a clot present in the LA. A CHADS score should be calculated to determine the patient's risk of stroke and the need for anticoagulation. This patient's score is a 3 (age over 75, history of CHF, and history of HTN). A CHADS score greater than 2 indicates a high risk of CVA and that the patient needs to be anticoagulated. A stress test would not be indicated until the patient's rates were identified as controlled (via Holter) and beta-blockers are only indicated if a patient has a fast ventricular rate, which is not indicated in this scenario.

11. B. A PMI greater than 11 cm from the midsternal border is considered displaced and abnormal. It likely represents LVH, which can be seen by EKG. The patient will likely need an echo and then an ACE inhibitor, but the EKG would be the first thing that needs to be done. A cardiology referral is not immediately necessary.

12. B. A third heart sound is pathologic in adults. The most likely causes are heart failure, diminished contractility of the ventricle, mitral regurgitation, or tricuspid regurgitation (Bickley, 2013).

13. A. Patients with renal dysfunction are at risk for hyperkalemia on aldactone. Ace inhibitors also increase potassium levels. Therefore, renal function and potassium should be closely monitored, and

consideration made for discontinuation of aldactone in patients with renal insufficiency. Patients should follow a low-potassium diet. Echocardiograms are not warranted every 3 months, and aldactone dosage in heart failure is aimed at neurohormonal effects and is not sufficient enough to cause diuresis. Loop diuretics are still warranted for fluid management.

14. B. Patients with type 2 DM have the same risk of an MI as a patient with a previous MI. In addition, neuropathy from diabetes can mask the typical angina symptoms. A patient with DM should have a screening stress test before beginning an intense exercise program.

15. A. Diabetic patients with HTN should be treated with an ACE inhibitor or ARBs for renal protection, as well as for blood pressure control.

16. C. Therapeutic lifestyle changes for high cholesterol include changing to a low-saturated-fat and high-fiber diet. Maintaining a healthy weight is important, but very-low-fat diets can be counterproductive in cholesterol management. A low-sodium diet is helpful for HTN and heart failure but not for high cholesterol. Exercise should consist of aerobic exercise, not necessarily weight training.

17. D. A valve that cannot open fully is stenotic. The most common valve to develop stenosis is the aortic valve. A valve that does not close completely is termed regurgitant or incompetent.

18. B. The most common finding in MVP is a midsystolic click. If the patient has developed MR, a systolic murmur will also be noted. A diastolic murmur is usually found in aortic regurgitation or mitral stenosis.

19. B. According to the updated guidelines, prophylaxis is only warranted in high-risk conditions. Previous endocarditis is considered high risk for developing IE (infectious endocarditis) again. Mitral valve prolapse is no longer an indication. Valve replacement would be an indication, but not repair of a valve. A pacemaker or ICD does not necessitate SBE prophylaxis.

20. B. The goal of treating HTN is to prevent target organ damage. Avoiding hypotension will maintain perfusion. Lipid levels and obesity are not affected by HTN, but both are comorbidities that can contribute to cardiovascular complications.

21. A. The patient is exhibiting signs of right-sided heart failure (cor pulmonale) without left-sided involvement. The most common underlying cause of right-sided heart failure is increased pulmonary artery pressure from chronic lung disease. A recent MI would cause left-sided failure, and anemia would cause high-output failure. Manifestations of a DVT would include unilateral edema and not hepatomegaly and JVD.

22. B. Sinus tach is a sign of an underlying cause, and treatment is focused on finding and treating the cause. Beta-blockers would suppress and mask the underlying cause.

23. B. Patients with ejection fractions of less than 35% are at risk for sudden cardiac death from ventricular arrhythmias. Prophylactic placement of ICDs is indicated in this population. Aldactone is only indicated in class II and IV HF.

24. B. Without obvious risk factors or cause for the DVT, the provider should evaluate the patient for the presence of familial clotting disorders. Once the presence or absence of these disorders are identified, the time frame for anticoagulation can be determined.

25. B. Chest discomfort in a patient with risk factors that is exertional is likely ischemic in nature. A stress test will determine the presence of coronary artery disease. With stable angina, the EKG will be normal at rest and does not indicate that the pain is not cardiac in nature. Since the patient is exhibiting stable angina, a trip to the ER is not necessary at this time.

26. A. Patients with PAD experience intermittent claudication. Progression to rest pain means that the disease is worsening. A DVT often does not cause significant pain.

27. B. The symptoms described likely indicate varicose veins. Predisposing factors include standing for long periods of time, obesity, pregnancy, and family history.

28. C. African Americans have been shown to have a decreased risk of stroke with the use of calcium channel blockers compared to other antihypertensives. CCB are also effective in lowering BP in this population. ACE inhibitors should not be used first line unless other compelling evidence requires their use.

29. C. The fact that pain is relieved with nitroglycerin does not necessarily point to an ischemic cause for the pain. Nitroglycerin can also be effective at relieving the pain or esophageal spasm. Further assessment and workup is essential to determining the actual cause of this pain.

30. A. The patient has likely had AFib with rapid response for the past two weeks. The patient needs to be started on anticoagulation, and rate controlled to decrease his symptoms. The patient does not need to be sent to the hospital unless he is unstable. An antiarrhythmic drug would not be first line. A stress test would be indicated once the rate was controlled, but if done without rate control, it would likely cause worsening symptoms.

● ● ● References

American Heart Association. (2015). Classes of heart failure. Retrieved from http://www.heart.org/HEARTORG/Conditions/HeartFailure/AboutHeartFailure/Classes-of-Heart-Failure_UCM_306328_Article.jsp#.Vu6lcxEUWpo

Bickley, L. S. (2013). *Bates Guide to Physical Examination and History Taking*. Philadelphia: Lippincott, Williams and Wilkins.

James P. A., Oparil S., Carter B. L., et al. (2014). 2014 evidence-based guideline for the management of high blood pressure in adults: Report from the panel members appointed to the eighth joint national committee (jnc 8). *JAMA, 311*(5), 507–520. http://doi.org/10.1001/jama.2013.284427

January, C. T., Wann, L. S., Alpert, J. S., Calkins, H., Cigarroa, J. E., Cleveland, J. C., . . . Yancy, C. W. (2014). 2014 AHA/ACC/HRS guideline for the management of patients with atrial fibrillation: executive summary a report of the American College of Cardiology/American Heart Association Task Force on practice guidelines and the Heart Rhythm Society. *Circulation, 130*(23), 2071–2104. http://doi.org/10.1161/CIR.0000000000000040

McCance, K. L. & Huether, S. E. (2014). *Pathophysiology: The Biological Basis for Disease in Adults and Children*. St. Louis: Elsevier.

Patel, K. (2015). *Deep Venous Thrombosis Treatment & Management: Approach Considerations, General Principles of Anticoagulation, Heparin Use in Deep Venous Thrombosis*. Retrieved from http://emedicine.medscape.com/article/1911303-treatment

Stone, N. J., Robinson, J. G., Lichtenstein, A. H., Merz, C. N. B., Blum, C. B., Eckel, R. H., . . . Wilson, P. W. F. (2014). 2013 ACC/AHA guideline on the treatment of blood cholesterol to reduce atherosclerotic cardiovascular risk in adults a report of the American College of Cardiology/American Heart Association Task Force on practice guidelines. *Circulation, 129*(25 suppl 2), S1–S45. http://doi.org/10.1161/01.cir.0000437738.63853.7a

Wilson, W., Taubert, K. A., Gewitz, M., Lockhart, P. B., Baddour, L. M., Levison, M., . . . Prevention of Infective Endocarditis: Guidelines from the American Heart Association: A Guideline From the American Heart Association Rheumatic Fever, Endocarditis, and Kawasaki Disease Committee, Council on Cardiovascular Disease in the Young, and the Council on Clinical Cardiology, Council on Cardiovascular Surgery and Anesthesia, and the Quality of Care and Outcomes Research Interdisciplinary Working Group. *Circulation, 116*(15), 1736–1754. http://doi.org/10.1161/CIRCULATIONAHA.106.183095

VanMeter, K. C., & Huber, R. J. (2014). *Gould's Pathophysiology for the Health Professions*. St. Louis: Elsevier.

Yancy, C. W., Jessup, M., Bozkurt, B., Butler, J., Casey, D. E., Drazner, M. H., . . . Wilkoff, B. L. (2013). 2013 ACCF/AHA Guideline for the Management of Heart Failure: Executive Summary. A Report of the American College of Cardiology Foundation/American Heart Association Task Force on Practice Guidelines. Circulation, 128(16), 1810–1852. http://doi.org/10.1161/CIR.0b013e31829e8807

Gastrointestinal System

Sylvie Rosenbloom, DNP, APRN, FNP-BC, CDE
Julie G. Stewart, DNP, MPH, MSN, FNP-BC, APRN

Patients who present with abdominal pain require prompt and comprehensive evaluation. Obtaining an appropriate history and an accurate physical examination is key to rapid referral in acute situations. Acute abdominal pain may be related to obstruction, vascular injury, peritoneal irritation, etc., and may require immediate surgical intervention. Patients who present with fever, chills, and rebound tenderness should be sent to the closest emergency department for evaluation. Most often, in outpatient settings the FNP will encounter a wide variety of non-acute abdominal complaints that may or may not require consultation and/or referral. An accurate history of abdominal discomfort or pain must ascertain the eight attributes of a symptom:

- Onset
- Location
- Duration
- Character
- Aggravating/relieving
- Radiation
- Timing
- Severity

Physical Examination

1. Inspection: Examine abdomen and report any scars, rashes, striae, symmetry, contour, masses, pulsations, peristalsis, hernias, and skin discoloration. Divide the abdomen into four quadrants and know the location of the abdominal organs.

2. Auscultation: Done before palpation. Listen over all four quadrants for bowel sounds and for bruits over the aorta, iliac, renal, and femoral arteries.

3. Percussion: Note areas of dullness indicative of solid or fluid-filled masses rather than air. Percuss for the liver span and spleen to assess for organomegaly.

4. Palpation: Start with light palpation in non-tender areas and then move on to deep palpation to assess for organomegaly or masses.

5. Rectal Examination: Examine perianal area for hemorrhoids. Insert gloved finger into the anus and note sphincter tone, assess for internal hemorrhoids, fissures, masses, and tenderness.

Special Maneuvers

- Rebound tenderness: Increased pain intensity when quickly releasing the abdomen during palpation. Rebound pain is indicative of peritonitis, an inflammation of the peritoneal cavity.

- Rovsing's sign: Can be indicative of appendicitis. Pain to the right lower quadrant (RLQ) when the left lower quadrant (LLQ) is palpated.

- Obturator sign: With the knee slightly bent, have the patient rotate the hip inwardly, thus stretching the obturator internus muscle. Pain may signify appendicitis.

- Psoas sign: Have patient lift his leg while your hand is placed on the thigh, creating resistance. In appendicitis, the psoas contraction produces pain.
- Murphy's sign: As the patient takes a deep breath, palpate under the rib cage. Pain may be elicited in cholecystitis.
- Cullen's sign: Periumbilical ecchymosis associated with retroperitoneal bleeding.
- Hepatojugular reflux: As firm pressure is applied in the epigastrium, observe the neck for an elevation in jugular venous pressure (JVP). Note the drop in JVP as you release the abdomen.
- Scratch test: Position the diaphragm of your stethoscope over the liver and scratch with your finger or tongue depressor parallel to the costal margin until the intensity of the sound drops off, indicating the liver edge.
- Shifting dullness: This assesses for ascites. With the patient lying on their side, percuss for dullness on the dependent side of the abdomen.

Liver Enzymes

- Liver enzymes often provide information for the clinician about how well the liver is functioning.
- Gamma glutamic transpeptidase (GGT)—Marker of liver cell function; used to detect alcohol-induced liver disease; can also be elevated in patients with marked jaundice.
- Alanine aminotransferase (ALT)—Specific indicator for liver function (think A, L = liver, T)
- Aspartate aminotransferase (AST)—Can also be found in muscle, brain, kidneys, pancreas, lung.
- If both the ALT and AST are elevated, it is very likely there is liver inflammation and damage. Levels over 500 likely indicate some form of drug-related injury, viral hepatitis, or ischemia.

Other tests that may indicate issues with liver function include Alkaline Phosphatase (indicate bile flow issues and/or bone diseases). In true liver disease, the liver will have true function issues such as alteration in prothrombin time (elevated), albumin (low), and inability to break down bilirubin, which leads to jaundice as the bilirubin levels rise.

The ratio of AST/ALT may be >2 in alcoholic liver disease, if >1 may be fatty liver disease.

Cholecystitis

The patient complains of RUQ (right upper quadrant) or epigastric pain (can radiate to right shoulder), fever, and often has mild leukocytosis. Nausea and vomiting may also be present. Jaundice may be seen if there is obstruction of the common bile duct (elevated gamma-glutamyl transferase [GGT]). Pain most often occurs one hour after ingestion of a fatty meal and is often seen in overweight females. Risk factors include obesity, elevated cholesterol, pregnancy, rapid weight loss, female gender, and being over the age of 50.

A positive Murphy's sign may be a strong indicator of choleycystitis. Ultrasonography is often performed to assess for the presence of cholelithiasis. A more sensitive and specific imaging study called cholescinctigraphy (HIDA scan) can also be performed to confirm the diagnosis. Laboratory studies include: CBC (elevated WBC); ALT; AST, which may be over 300 IU/L; and amylase and lipase (both may be elevated). The GGT can be elevated when the bile duct is obstructed and jaundice develops.

Differential Diagnoses

- Acute pancreatitis
- Acute hepatitis
- Peptic ulcer disease
- Right-sided pneumonia
- Abdominal abscess
- Fitz-Hugh–Curtis disease (perihepatitis caused by gonococcal infection)

Treatment

- Low-fat diet, clear liquids, pain management, and surgical referral for gallbladder removal.

Follow-up

- Teach patients to avoid fatty meals.

Constipation

The passing of bowel movements that is less frequent than usual or the passing of stool that is dry/harder than usual defines constipation. It can be chronic or acute. Constipation is a common complaint among all individuals but more frequently with older adults. It is often the result of inactivity and inadequate water and fiber intake. It can also be seen in individuals resisting the urge of having a bowel movement.

Differential Diagnosis

- Colon cancer
- Diabetes
- Diverticulosis
- Parkinson's disease
- Bowel obstruction

Triggers

- Medical conditions: hypothyroidism, stress, chronic kidney failure, pregnancy
- Medications: narcotics, beta-blockers, antihistamines, muscle relaxants, diuretics, iron preparations, and tricyclic antidepressants

Management

- Dietary changes: increased fiber and fluids; low-fat diet
- Behavioral approaches such as biofeedback may help decrease involuntary pelvic muscle contractions and those of the external anal sphincter during bowel movements.
- Medications:
  - Fiber: The recommended daily allowance of fiber is 20–35g/day. Can be taken in natural (food) or supplements.
  - Bulk-forming laxatives such as Metamucil, Citrucel, FiberCon, Benefiber. They work by absorbing water in the colon and increasing fecal mass and softening the consistency of stools.
  - Osmotic laxatives such as Miralax (polyethylene glycol) and lactulose work by pulling in water in the intestine.
  - Stimulant laxatives, such as senna or bisacodyl, work by changing the intestinal wall's electrolyte transport, thereby increasing intestinal motility.
  - Surfactants (stool softeners) such as Colace help to decrease the stool's surface tension, thereby increasing the water absorption of the stool.

Complications

- Bowel obstruction
- Chronic constipation
- Hemorrhoids
- Anal fissures
- Hernia
- Laxative dependency

Treatment and Follow-up

- Prompt medical attention should be given to the individual who complains that she/he has not had a bowel movement in 5 or more days.
- Patient education with regard to therapeutic lifestyle changes, such as increasing activity, water, and fiber intake.
- Advise patient to try to defecate after meals, especially in the morning when bowel motility is optimal.

Gastroesophageal Reflux Disease (GERD)

Gastroesophageal reflux disease occurs when the gastric stomach contents ascend to the esophagus and cause symptoms such as burning, discomfort, or pain. It can lead to erosive esophagitis. Chronic GERD can damage the esophageal epithelium leading to Barrett's Esophagus, a precancerous condition, and esophageal cancer. Patient with five or more years of GERD symptoms should be referred to a gastroenterologist.

Triggers

- Many medications and foods and/or beverages can decrease the lower esophageal sphincter control. Drugs: theophylline, dopamine, diazepam, calcium-channel blockers, and NSAIDs. Foods/beverages: caffeine, alcohol, fatty foods, peppermint, spicy and acidic foods/drinks.
- Obesity
- Overeating
- Gassy foods
- Tight clothing (increases intra-abdominal pressure)
- Tobacco
- Lying position shortly after a meal

Clinical Manifestations

Heartburn after a meal is the most common symptom. It is often relieved with antacids. The patient may also experience burping, regurgitation, waking up with acid or bad taste in the mouth. The increased reflux of acidity to the throat most often occurs at night and can lead to coughing, wheezing, hoarseness, and aspiration.

Diagnostic Studies

The diagnosis of GERD is most often made by history. However, an upper endoscopy with possible biopsy may be performed if the patient experiences dysphagia, odynophagia, gastrointestinal bleeding, anemia, weight loss, or recurrent vomiting.

Treatment and Follow-up

- Weight loss
- Avoidance of triggers
- Avoid eating before bedtime
- Elevate the head of the bed
- Medications:
  - Antacids: Usually taken after meals, they will provide 1–2 hours of relief. Examples: *Calcium carbonate* antacids, such as Tums, also provide an additional source of calcium. *Antacids with alginic acid*, such as Gaviscon, which forms a barrier at the top of the stomach contents, thus decreasing stomach acid reflux to the esophagus. *Antacids with simethicone*, such as Maalox and Mylanta, which reduce gas in the stomach and prevent reflux from ascending to the esophagus.
  - H$_2$ blockers, such as ranitidine and famotidine, work by decreasing acid production in the stomach.
  - Proton-pump inhibitors, such as omeprazole, pantoprazole, rabeprazole, esomeprazole, and lansoprazole work by blocking acid production in the stomach.

Peptic Ulcer Disease (PUD)

Peptic ulcer disease is a lesion affecting the lining of the stomach or duodenum (more common). If untreated, PUD can lead to hemorrhage and perforation. *Helicobacter pylori* infection should be ruled out, as well as chronic use of NSAIDs.

Clinical Manifestations

Up to 70% of patients with PUD will be asymptomatic. Hematemesis (bright red or coffee ground–like) or melena (dark tarry stool) can occur and lead to bleeding, anemia, and hypovolemia. If untreated, this can result in the patient becoming hemodynamically compromised (hypovolemic shock). Epigastric pain is common: gastric ulcer disease causes pain when eating and duodenal ulcer pain is more common on an empty stomach and may awake the patient late at night. The pain is often described as burning or gnawing and may radiate to the back. Associated symptoms may include burping, bloating, nausea, and anorexia.

Diagnostic Studies

- Stool for guaiac (low sensitivity for upper GI bleed)
- *H. Pylori* testing:
  - Urea breath test: A labeled carbon isotope is given by mouth to the patient, allowing the tagged CO released by the *H. pylori* bacteria to be detected. Test sensitivity and specificity are about 88–95% and 95–100%, respectively.
  - Stool antigen test: Detects the presence of *H. pylori* in the stool. Sensitivity is 94% and specificity is 86%.
  - Serologic test: Blood test to detect immunoglubolin g (IgG). Sensitivity is 90–100% and specificity is 76–96%.
- Upper endoscopy with biopsy is the gold standard.
- Barium swallow (less often done)
- CBC to rule out anemia

Treatment

- Triple Therapy: Proton pump inhibitor (PPI) (omeprazole 20 mg BID, lansoprazole 30 mg BID, esomeprazole 40 mg QD, pantoprazole 40 mg QD, rabeprazole 20 mg BID) **plus** clarithromycin 500 mg bid (first-line) or metronidazole 500 mg bid (when clarithromycin resistance increasing) **plus** amoxicillin 1000 mg bid or metronidazole (if not used above) carries a 20% failure rate.
- Quadruple Therapy (for 10 days): omeprazole 20 mg bid **plus** bismuth subsalicylate 140 mg tabs—3 caps tid (three times a day) **plus** Metronidazole 250 mg qid (four times a day) (or levofloxacin) **plus** tetracycline 125 mg qid carries a 93% eradication rate.

Follow-up

Confirmation of eradication after treatment is highly recommended. (See testing methods mentioned earlier.)

Gastroenteritis

Acute viral gastroenteritis is defined as an increase in bowel movements or the passing of watery/loose stool usually accompanied by nausea, vomiting, abdominal pain, and fever. Both vomiting and diarrhea are usually present; however, at times they can occur alone.

Etiology

- Norovirus
- Rotavirus
- Enteric adenovirus
- Astrovirus

Clinical Manifestations

- Nausea/vomiting
- Diarrhea
- Abdominal pain
- Fever
- Red flags: dehydration, fluid/electrolyte imbalances, rectal bleeding/bloody stools, severe abdominal pain, antibiotic use within the last three to six months, pregnancy, elderly, immune-compromised individuals, and prolonged symptoms (over one week).

Differential Diagnosis

- Other infectious or non-infectious causes of diarrhea
- *Clostridium difficile* infection in patients with recent hospitalization or antibiotic usage
- Protozoal infection such as giardia or cryptosporidium in patients with recent travel
- Inflammatory bowel disease
- Irritable bowel syndrome
- Malabsorption syndrome
- Laxative abuse

Treatment and Follow-up

- Acute viral gastroenteritis is usually self-limiting and no treatment is recommended.
- Fluids and electrolyte replacements in volume-depleted patients.
- Small frequent bland meals, such as the B.R.A.T. diet (banana, rice, apple sauce, and toast)—Resume diet slowly as tolerated.
- Avoid greasy or spicy foods, caffeine, alcohol, and nicotine.
- Avoid NSAIDs because they may further irritate the gastric mucosa.
- Discuss hand hygiene.
- Anti-motility agents, such as loperamide (Imodium-AD), and anti-emetic medications, such as ondansetron (Zofran) or prochlorperazine, may be used cautiously.

- Hospitalization may be required in the very young or elderly patients, or if signs of volume depletion/electrolyte imbalances.

Appendicitis

Inflammation resulting from the accumulation of fecaliths in the vermiform appendix located at the base of the cecum. It is most frequently seen between 20 to 30 years of age. If left untreated, peritonitis can ensue. Most frequent cause of emergent abdominal surgery.

Clinical Manifestations

- Abdominal pain: Can be periumbilical or epigastric initially, and then may shift toward the RLQ region. Pain is usually worsened with moving, coughing, and walking (peritoneal irritation). Rebound tenderness in a common finding. Positive Rosving's, heel strike, psoas, and obturator signs.
- Anorexia
- Nausea, vomiting (later signs), diarrhea may be present
- Fever
- Leukocytosis: (10,000–16,000 cells/mm^3) with a shift to the left (neutrophilia/bandemia)

Diagnostic Testing

- Ultrasonography and abdominal CT. Abdominal x-rays do not aid in the diagnosis of appendicitis.

Differential Diagnosis

- Gynecologic: Pelvic inflammatory disease, ectopic pregnancy, ovarian tumor, ovarian torsion, mittelschmerz, endometriosis
- Gastrointestinal: Irritable bowel syndrome, inflammatory bowel disease, colitis, diverticulitis
- Renal: Nephrolithiasis, pyelonephritis

Treatment and Follow-up

- Urgent surgical referral for appendectomy

Diverticulitis

When uncomplicated, acute diverticulitis is usually self-limiting and does not involve abscess, perforation, and/or peritonitis. When the latter are involved, prompt referral and hospitalization are required. This acute stage involves further diagnostic testing, such as CT scans, to rule out other causes of acute abdominal pain.

Clinical Manifestations

- LLQ pain
- Nausea/vomiting
- Low-grade fever
- Diarrhea

  When acute: Signs of acute abdomen ensue, such as positive Rosving's sign, rebound tenderness, "board" like abdomen. CBC with leukocytosis, neutrophilia, and a left shift. (Bands usually indicate severe bacterial infection.) Referral to emergency department for evaluation and possible hospital admission.

Differential Diagnosis

- Gynecologic: Pelvic inflammatory disease, ectopic pregnancy, ovarian tumor, ovarian torsion, mittleschmerz, endometriosis
- Gastrointestinal: Constipation, inflammatory bowel disease, colitis
- Renal: Nephrolithiasis, pyelonephritis, UTI

Treatment and Follow-up

- Antibiotic therapy (mild/outpatient setting):
  - Ciprofloxacin 750 mg po bid (by mouth, two times a day) **or** levofloxacin 750 mg po qd **or** moxifloxacin 400 mg po qd (by mouth, four times a day) **or** bactrim DS po bid + metronidazole 500 mg po tid (by mouth, three times a day)
  - Monotherapy: Amoxicillin-clavulanate 825/125 mg po bid
- Anti-inflammatory agents such as mesalamine may be utilized
- Dietary: Clear-liquid diet during acute illness. When resolved, the patient should increase po fluid intake, increase dietary fiber (20–35 g/day). There is no longer a recommendation to avoid seeds, nuts, and corn.

Guidelines for Outpatient Management

1. Compliance with medical regimen
2. Able to tolerate po intake
3. Abdominal pain is not severe.
4. No fever/or low-grade fever
5. No or minimal comorbidities
6. Able to return for follow-up
7. Support system available

Colon Cancer

Cancer of the lower intestinal tract. It ranks as the third most common cause of death in the United States for both males and females. It is more common in Blacks and in patients of higher socioeconomic status. Median age at diagnosis: 69 years of age.

Clinical Manifestations

Most often dependent upon the location and stage of the disease:

- Change in bowel habit
- Hematochezia
- Iron deficiency anemia—Usually from unknown etiology
- Abdominal pain
- Tenesmus, bright red blood per rectum, rectal pain, and changes in stool caliber can be seen with rectal cancer.

Differential Diagnosis

- Diverticulitis
- Ulcerative colitis
- Crohn's disease
- Appendicitis
- Thrombosed hemorrhoids

Treatment and Follow-up

- Treatment will be dependent upon staging of the disease, but often includes surgery, chemotherapy, and radiation. The patient will then undergo routine colonoscopy, often yearly at first.
- Screening:
  - Should begin at age 50 in asymptomatic individuals or those without a family history.
  - American Cancer Society recommends:
    - To detect colon cancer: Yearly fecal occult blood testing or fecal immunochemical testing (FIT) or stool DNA test every three years. If these tests are positive, then a colonoscopy should be performed.
    - To detect polyps and cancer: Flexible sigmoidoscopy every five years, colonoscopy every 10 years, double contrast barium

enema or CT colonography (virtual colonoscopy) every five years.

- In patients with a strong family history of polyposis, first degree relative with colon cancer, patients are referred, and colonoscopies are done q3–5 years.

- In patients with colon cancer, a colonoscopy will be performed one year after resection.

- American Cancer Society recommends the following screening options for those with average risk should begin at age 50:

  The below are mainly to detect polyps and cancer

  - Flexible sigmoidoscopy every 5 years
  - Colonoscopy every 10 years
  - Double-contrast barium enema every 5 years
  - CT colonography (virtual colonoscopy) every 5 years

  Tests that mainly detect cancer:

  - Guaiac-based fecal occult blood test (gFOBT) every year
  - Fecal immunochemical test (FIT) every year
  - Stool DNA test (sDNA) every 3 years*

Hepatitis

Liver inflammation arising from autoimmune disorder (rare) or viral infection.

History

- Ask about alcohol use/abuse (CAGE questionnaire), IV drug use
- Tactfully obtain the patient's sexual history
- Ask about usage of potentially hepatotoxic medications (acetaminophen) or environmental toxins
- Assess for potential high-risk work environments, such as HIV or sexually transmitted infection (STI) clinics

Clinical Manifestations

- Jaundice
- Fatigue
- Anorexia, nausea, vomiting, diarrhea
- Abdominal pain
- Headache
- Fever
- Dark-colored urine and pale-looking stool

Liver Function Tests (LFTs)

- Serum aspartate aminotransferase (AST)—Also known as glutamic oxaloacetic transaminase (SGOT)
  - Normal: 0–45 mg/dL
  - Found in liver, heart muscle, skeletal muscle, kidney, and liver
  - Low specificity for liver injury because it is found in other organs and can be elevated in other conditions, such as acute myocardial infarction
- Serum alanine aminotransferase (ALT)—Also known as serum glutamic pyruvic transaminase (SGPT)
  - Normal: 0–40 mg/dL
  - Found mainly in the liver. An elevated value signifies liver inflammation.
  - ALT is a more specific marker of hepatic inflammation than AST.
- AST/ALT (aspartate aminotransferase/alanine aminotransferase) ratio (SGOT/SGPT ratio)
  - A ratio ≥2.0 is often found with alcohol abuse
- Alkaline phosphatase
  - Enzyme found in bone, liver, gallbladder, kidneys, GI tract, and placenta
  - Enzyme elevation is often seen during children's growth spurts, healing fractures, malignancy, and osteomalacia.
- Serum Gamma-Glutamyl Transpeptidase (GGT)
  - Normal: 0–51 IU/L
  - Indicator of alcohol abuse
  - Elevated in liver disease and acute pancreatitis
  - Can be affected by other drugs: alcohol, phenytoin, and phenobarbital can increase GGT levels, whereas birth control pills and clofibrate can decrease GGT levels.

Hepatitis A

Causative agent is RNA Picornavirus, which is single serotype worldwide. The virus is transmitted via fecal or oral route and has an incubation period of 15–20 days. Highest incidence rates are between the ages of 5–14 years old. Hepatitis A is an acute condition (as opposed to hepatitis B, which is chronic) and may lead to fulminant hepatitis. Antibodies

Table 8-1	Interpretation of the Hepatitis B Serologic Panel	
Tests	**Results**	**Interpretation**
HBsAg	Negative	Susceptible
anti-HBc	Negative	
anti-HBs	Negative	
HBsAg	Negative	Immune due to natural infection
anti-HBc	Positive	
anti-HBs	Positive	
HBsAg	Negative	Immune due to hepatitis B vaccination*
anti-HBc	Negative	
anti-HBs	Positive	
HBsAg	Positive	Acutely infected
anti-HBc	Positive	
IgM anti-HBc	Positive	
anti-HBs	Negative	
HBsAg	Positive	Chronically infected
anti-HBc	Positive	
IgM anti-HBc	Negative	
anti-HBs	Negative	
HBsAg	Negative	Four interpretations possible¶
anti-HBc	Positive	
anti-HBs	Negative	

HBsAg: hepatitis B surface antigen; anti-HBc: hepatitis B core antibody; anti-HBs: hepatitis B surface antibody; IgM: immunoglobulin M; HBV: hepatitis B virus.

* Antibody response (anti-HBs) can be measured quantitatively or qualitatively. A protective antibody response is reported quantitatively as 10 or more milliinternational units (≥10 milliint. unit/mL) or qualitatively as positive. Post-vaccination testing should be completed one to two months after the third vaccine dose for results to be meaningful.

¶ Four interpretations:

1. Might be recovering from acute HBV infection.
2. Might be distantly immune and test not sensitive enough to detect very low level of anti-HBs in serum.
3. Might be susceptible with a false positive anti-HBc.
4. Might be undetectable level of HBsAg present in the serum and the person is actually chronically infected.

Modified from Centers for Disease Control and Prevention. (2015). Interpretation of Hepatitis B serologic test results. Retrieved from http://www.cdc.gov/hepatitis/HBV/PDFs/SerologicChartv8.pdf.

resulting from infection will provide lifelong immunity. Hepatitis A vaccination is available.

Hepatitis B

A small DNA virus of the *Hepadnaviridae* family is the causative agent of hepatitis B. This virus has an inner core and an outer shell and has an incubation period of 60–90 days. Its mode of transmission is through blood and mucosal tissues exposed to blood or other bodily fluids (sexual contact), via drug use (parenteral), as well as perinatal (mother to child). Chronic infection can occur in 10% of infected adults, 30–50% of exposed children, and 90% of infants exposed to the virus. Oftentimes, hepatitis B–infected patients will also have a hepatitis D co-infection. Vaccination is encouraged. See Table 8-1 for interpretation of hepatitis B serologic panel.

Hepatitis C

Hepatitis C is transmitted through blood products, especially with blood transfusions or organ transplants prior to 1992 or transfusion of clotting factors prior to 1987. It is often seen in IV drug users. Hepatitis C infection is four times more likely to occur in IV drug users than HIV infection.

Sexual transmission has been known to occur, especially in individuals with multiple partners or with males having intercourse with other males. Hepatitis C has an incubation period of six to seven weeks and up to 85% of infected individuals will become chronically infected. Factors associated with increased progression and severity are as follows:

- Age > 40 years at time of infection
- HIV co-infection
- Chronic HBV co-infection
- Increased alcohol intake
- Male gender

There are no vaccinations available against hepatitis C. However, current therapies have shown great success rates in treating and curing hepatitis C infections. A patient with chronic hepatitis C should be vaccinated against hepatitis A & B if not immune.

Non-Alcoholic Steatohepatitis (NASH)

Commonly known as non-alcoholic fatty liver disease (NAFLD). Individuals with NASH have an increased risk of cardiovascular disease, diabetes, cirrhosis, and liver-related deaths. Liver biopsy is done to confirm diagnosis.

Risk Factors

- Obesity, especially in individuals with increased waist circumference
- Diabetes mellitus
- Hypertriglyceridemia
- Elevated LFTs (twice the upper limit of normal)

Treatment and Follow-up

- Encourage obese patients to lose weight
- Optimization of cardiovascular risk factors. Patients with NASH often have multiple cardiovascular risk factors and will benefit from therapeutic lifestyle changes to decrease their cardiovascular risk factors.
- Avoid alcohol and hepatotoxic medications.
- Patients with NASH should undergo screening for hepatocellular carcinoma.
- Patients should be referred to a hepatologist.
- Use of insulin-sensitizing agents, such as Metformin (Glucophage) and thiazolidinediones (in individuals with diabetes mellitus).

Irritable Bowel Syndrome (IBS)

Condition characterized by recurrent abdominal pain lasting at least three days per month and is associated with two or more of the following: abdominal pain improved with bowel movement, onset associated with diarrhea or constipation (stool frequency), onset associated with change in stool appearance. Cramping, flatulence, and bloating may also be present. Additional testing may be needed to rule out other potential malignant causes. Triggers can be foods (chocolate, spices, fats, carbonated beverages, alcohol), stress, or hormones. There is an increased prevalence of IBS in females (about twice as many as men), age under 40, family history and psychiatric disorders (anxiety, depression, personality disorder, history of childhood sexual abuse, or domestic abuse in women).

Differential Diagnosis

- Crohn's disease
- Inflammatory bowel disease
- Lactose intolerance
- Gluten intolerance
- Malignancy

Management

- Dietary modification:
  - A diet low in fermentable oligo-, di-, and monosaccharides and polyols (FODMAPs); in certain cases, avoidance of lactose and gluten
  - Avoidance of gas producing foods
  - Adequate fiber intake
- Food allergy testing may be needed
- Physical activity
- Medical management:
  - Constipation—Fiber, osmotic laxative such as lactulose or polyethylene glycol (Miralax), Lubiprostone, Linaclotide
  - Diarrhea: Antidiarrheal agent such as loperamide, Eluxadoline, and bile sequestrants (cholestyramine, colestipol, colesevelam) can be utilized if antidiarrheals are ineffective.
  - Antispasmodic agents (dicyclomine, hyoscyamine) as needed to provide short-term relief of abdominal pain
  - Psychiatric disorders should be treated with antidepressant or anxiolytics as needed.

– The role of probiotic is uncertain, but improvements in symptoms have been seen.

Follow-up

- Teach patients to keep food/symptoms diary to help identify potential triggers and to avoid these triggers.
- Teach patients about FODMAPs foods.
- Teach patients to seek medical attention if there is rectal bleeding, weight loss, or abdominal pain that progresses or occurs at night.

Inflammatory Bowel Disease

ULCERATIVE COLITIS (UC): Chronic inflammatory illness leading to ulcerations of the colon mucosa. It can occur anywhere from the rectum to the colon. It is more common between the ages of 20 and 40. In UC, the primary lesions are continuous (no skip lesions) and usually involve only the mucosa of the GI tract. The disease is usually most severe in the rectum and sigmoid colon. In severe inflammatory cases, the small erosions can lead to ulcers and abscess formation can ensue. Up to 10% of persons affected with UC can present with extraintestinal manifestations such as episcleritis, arthritis, erythema nodosum, fatty liver, and autoimmune diseases. Chronic complications can lead to strictures. Patients with UC have an increased risk of venous and arterial thromboembolism and colon cancer.

- Risk factors: Family history or Jewish descent. More prevalent in Caucasians and in Northern Europeans. Less common in smokers.
- Etiology: Unknown, but diet, genetics, infections, and immunologic causes are known to be associated with the disease.

Clinical Manifestations

- Characterized by periods of exacerbation and remission
- Diarrhea and bloody stool (common)
- Abdominal pain (occasional)
- Fever
- Weight loss
- Fatigue
- Tenesmus (sudden urge to move bowels)
- Characterized by remissions and exacerbations

Differential Diagnosis

- Crohn's disease
- Colitis (infectious, radiation, medication associated, especially NSAIDs)

Diagnostic Testing

- Stool cultures for *Clostridium difficile, Salmonella, Shigella, Campylobacter, Yersinia* and *E. coli O157:H7*
- Stool for ova and parasites
- Giardia stool antigen
- Serologic testing for STIs such as *Neisseria* gonorrhea, HSV, *Treponema pallidum*
- CBC, electrolytes, albumin, ESR, CRP
- Endoscopy and biopsy

Treatment and Follow-up

- The severity of UC needs to be assessed, and prompt referral given to GI when UC is moderate or severe.
- Mild UC: Topical 5-aminosalicylic acids, mesalamine, steroids such as beclomethasone, enemas, or oral prednisone.
- Moderate–severe UC (usually managed by gastroenterologist): Anti-TNF antibodies, cyclosporine, tacrolimus. In severe cases, surgery may be needed.
- Symptomatic treatment: In mild UC, loperamide can be given for diarrhea, and anticholinergic preparations, such as dycomine and hycosamine, can be given for abdominal discomfort.
- Immunizations: Routine immunizations are highly recommended because the patient is more susceptible to infectious conditions.
- Colon cancer screening: Patients with UC have an increased risk for colorectal cancer and should be screened. (See American Cancer Society recommendations mentioned earlier.)
- Pap smear: Women with UC have an increased risk of dysplasia.
- Skin cancer screening: Patients with UC have an increased risk of nonmelanoma skin cancers.
- Osteoporosis screening: Patients have in increased risk of osteoporosis, especially with increased corticosteroid use.
- Laboratory screening: Routine labs should be done to monitor for development of electrolyte imbalances that can ensue from severe diarrhea and CBC to monitor for anemia.

Complications

- Severe bleeding
- Toxic megacolon
- Perforations and strictures requiring prompt referral for surgery
- Development of colorectal cancer and cervical dysplasia

Crohn's Disease

Idiopathic inflammatory gastrointestinal disorder that can affect all portions of the GI tract from the mouth to the anus. The disease begins in the submucosa of the intestine and then extends to the intestinal wall, involving both the intestinal mucosa and serosa. The most commonly affected sites are the distal small intestine and proximal large colon, with the ileocolon being the most frequently involved site. Crohn's disease (CD) tends to affect the GI tract in some segments but not others, a pattern called "skip lesions." Patients may develop extraintestinal symptoms such as arthritis, eye involvement (uveitis, episcleritis, iritis), skin disorders (erythema nodosum), cholangitis, secondary amyloidosis, renal lithiasis, increased incidence of venous and arterial thromboembolism, osteoporosis, and vitamin B12 deficiency. It is slightly more prevalent in females than men and tends to develop under the age of 40. As many as 20–40% may require a colectomy.

- Risk factors: Smoking, Jewish descent, family history.
- Etiology: Genetic mutation

Clinical Manifestations

- Can be difficult to differentiate from UC.
- Abdominal pain and diarrhea (common)
- Blood stool (less common)
- Fever, fatigue, and weight loss may be present
- Abdominal mass, steatorrhea, malabsorption syndrome (common)
- Characterized by remissions and exacerbations

Differential Diagnosis

- Ulcerative colitis
- Colitis (infectious, radiation, diversion, medication associated, especially NSAIDs)
- Rectal ulcer
- Lactose intolerance

Diagnostic Testing

- Laboratory testing: CBC, blood chemistry including blood glucose, electrolytes, kidney and liver function tests, ESR, CRP, vitamin B12 levels and iron studies
- Stool culture for *Clostridium difficile*, ova, and parasites
- Colonoscopy is the preferred study for examination of the colon.
- Barium enemas can also be used if colonoscopy is not indicated.
- MRI are utilized for assessment of perianal fistulas.

Treatment and Follow-up

- Moderate or severe disease will require hospital admission and prompt referral.
- For mild disease, CD without systemic symptoms are treated with glucocorticoids, immunomodulator, and biologic therapies, utilizing either a "step-up" or "top-down" approach.

Complications

- Severe bleeding
- Toxic megacolon
- Abscesses, perforations, fistulae, obstructions, and strictures that may require prompt referral for surgery
- Development of colorectal cancer and cervical dysplasia

Hemorrhoids

These are normal vascular structures located in the anal canal. They are the result of arteriovenous connective tissues draining in the superior and inferior hemorrhoidal veins. Hemorrhoids can be classified as external (found distally to the dentate line), internal (situated proximally to the dentate line), or mixed (found both distally and proximally to the dentate line). Internal hemorrhoids can be classified depending on the degree of prolapse from the anal canal:

Grade I: May bulge into the lumen but do not prolapse distally to the dentate line. Can visualize with the anoscope.

Grade II: Can prolapse out of the anal canal with straining and defecation, but reduces spontaneously.

Grade III: Also prolapses out of the anal canal with straining/defecation but needs to be manually reduced.

Grade IV: Hemorrhoids cannot be reduced and may strangulate.

Prompt referral is recommended in patients with bright red blood per rectum, orthostatic changes, or in any patients with symptoms suggestive of malignancy (anemia, changes in bowel habits, or stool caliber or consistency. Patients with colon cancer or familial polyposis should also be referred for colonoscopy.

Clinical Manifestations

- Pruritus
- Rectal bleeding—Stool is usually bright red; can be copious amounts. May lead to anemia, or other associated symptoms such as weakness, dizziness, fatigue, exercise intolerance, headaches.
- Prolapse
- Anal swelling
- Rectal pain resulting from thrombosis
- Mild fecal incontinence, wetness, fullness feeling in perianal area

Differential Diagnosis

- Malignancy, chronic infection or inflammation (usually associated with systemic symptoms such as night sweats, fever, weight loss, and abdominal pain)
- Colorectal cancer or polyps
- Inflammatory bowel disease

Diagnostic Testing

- Perineal/anal inspection
- Digital rectal exam
- Anoscopy
- Colonoscopy
- Laboratory testing to rule out anemia or iron deficiency if complaints of bleeding or bleeding present during physical examination.

Treatment

- Initial approach: Conservative medical management aimed at prevention and symptomatic treatment.
  - Constipation: Increase PO fiber and fluid intake to decrease risks of constipation/

straining, including the use of bulk forming laxatives such as methylcellulose (Citrucel), polycarbophil (FiberCon, Konsyl), psyllium (Metamucil), wheat dextrin (Benefiber).

- Pain relievers and anti-pruritus: Benzocaine 5–20% rectal ointment (Americaine), dibucaine 1% rectal ointment (Nupercainal), pramoxine 1% rectal foam, ointment or wipes (Proctofoam, Pramox).
- Pain relievers and anti-inflammatory: hydrocortisone rectal creams 1–2.5% (Anusol–HC, Preparation H, Proctosol), hydrocortisone rectal suppository 25–30 mg (Anusol-HC).
- Stool softeners: Ducosate sodium (Colace)
- Pain associated with anal sphincter spasm: Nitroglycerin 0.2–0.5% ointment, phenylephrine 0.25% (Preparation-H, Rectacaine)

Follow-up

- Teach patient importance of prevention and avoidance of constipation/straining.

Perianal Fissures

Perianal/anal fissures are the result of increased anal pressure, and may be acute or chronic. They are usually caused by anal trauma (hard stool) or can be the result of an underlying medical/surgical condition, often attributed to symptomatic hemorrhoids. They can be primary (local trauma) or secondary (malignancy or resulting from IBD) depending on their etiology. Most commonly seen in middle-aged adults and infants.

All patients with rectal bleeding should have a sigmoidoscopy or colonoscopy, especially with a family history of colorectal cancers.

Clinical Manifestations

- Tearing pain, worse with bowel movements
- Burning
- Bright rectal bleeding, usually only small amount on toilet paper or on stool surface.
- Perianal pruritus or irritation
- On exam: Anal fissures are most commonly located in the posterior anal midline. May be superficial excoriation, shallow laceration, or deep wound that extends into the external sphincter.

Differential Diagnosis

- Perianal ulcers/sores
- Anorectal fistula

Treatment

- Referral to proctologist
- Conservative: Local wound care such as sitz bath, relief of constipation
- Medical management (more severe cases):
  - Topical vasodilators: Nifedipine or nitroglycerin cream/ointment
  - Stool softeners/laxative (bulk-forming) to relieve constipation

  - Topical analgesics without Xylocaine (see previous)
- With more chronic cases, botulinum toxin type A injection or lateral sphincterotomy may be considered.

Follow-up

- Increase fiber and fluid intake to avoid constipation
- Laxatives (see earlier)
- Keep anal area dry by wiping with soft cotton
- Used moistened wipes/cloths

Review Questions

1. One pharmacological intervention for a patient with diabetes or pre-diabetes with NASH is:

    A. Tenofovir.

    B. Acetylsalicylic Acid.

    C. Gabapentin.

    D. Metformin.

2. Of the following options, which two are factors that may lead to faster progression of hepatitis C (HCV) disease?

    A. Female gender, comorbid cardiovascular disease

    B. Male gender, comorbid HIV infection

    C. Male gender, comorbid pulmonary disease

    D. Female gender, comorbid irritable bowel syndrome

The next three questions are related to the 33-year-old patient described below:

3. A 33-year-old male patient is new to the FNP's practice. During the health history, he mentions he was told he had hepatitis. He is unsure which type of hepatitis and asks what it is. The FNP tells him that hepatitis is:

    A. Fibrosis of the liver.

    B. Infection of the liver.

    C. Cirrhosis of the liver.

    D. Inflammation of the liver.

4. The FNP is ordering bloodwork for this new patient. To evaluate which hepatitis the patient was previously diagnosed with, the **initial** laboratory testing will include:

    A. HAV viral load, HDV IgG.

    B. HCV Ag, HBV eAg, HAV viral load.

    C. HAV total Ab, HCV Ab, HBV sAg and HBsAb.

    D. HCV IgG, HAV IgG, HBV viral load.

5. The 33-year-old male patient's labs return. What do these results indicate?

    HBsAg = positive

    HBsAb = negative

    IgM HbcAB = negative

    HAV Ab total = positive

    HCV Ab = nonreactive

    A. Acute hepatitis C infection, past hepatitis A infection

    B. Chronic hepatitis B infection, acute hepatitis A infection

    C. Past hepatitis A infection, chronic hepatitis B infection

    D. Past hepatitis B infection, past hepatitis A infection

6. Which type of hepatitis is most commonly caused by contaminated foods?

    A. HBV

    B. HCV

    C. HDV

    D. HAV

7. A 50-year-old female patient thinks she may have gotten hepatitis C from a previous sexual partner. She asks what the signs and symptoms of acute infection are. The FNP responds listing which of the below options?

    A. Nausea, vomiting, bloody diarrhea

    B. Fever, fatigue, body aches

    C. Sweating, dyspepsia, tachycardia

    D. Vomiting, headache, diarrhea

8. Peter is a 50-year-old African American male who is HCV+ from IVDU (intravenous drug users) many years ago. He has not used street drugs for over 15 years and works long hours as a train conductor. He is asking about his routine health maintenance in regard to HCV. Which of the following yearly exams are recommended by the FNP?

    A. CT scan, liver biopsy, HCV viral load, and liver enzymes

    B. Liver ultrasound, liver enzymes, AFP, HCV viral load

    C. Liver biopsy, liver ultrasound, liver enzymes, CBC

    D. HCV viral load, genotype, and CT scan

9. A 62-year-old female patient comes to the FNP's office with complaints of constipation for the past few months. She has tried to increase her intake of water and fiber without much success. A yearly physical exam and colonoscopy were negative for any significant findings 6 months prior to this visit. Which of the following options would be most appropriate for the next step?

    A. Recommend daily Dulcolax use as an addition to the fiber and water.

    B. Recommend an increase in exercise, such as walking, and daily Miralax use for 2 weeks, then have her return for evaluation in one month.

    C. Recommend daily Fleet enema use upon arising in addition to current approach. Refer to GI specialist if no improvement.

    D. Recommend CT scan of abdomen to rule out malignancy.

The next three questions are based on the 42-year-old female patient described below. Vital signs are within normal limits. The patient's BMI (body mass index) is 31.

10. A 42-year-old female patient has a chief complaint of intermittent abdominal pain for about 2 months. The pain is generally in the right upper quadrant and is described as "stabbing," ranging from a 4–9 on the 1-to-10 pain scale. Nothing seems to help it go away but it only lasts about 20–30 minutes. Which of the following details should the FNP obtain next?

    A. Duration of pain, alleviating factors, family history

    B. Social history, sexual history, predisposing factors

    C. Alcohol intake, pain severity, radiation of pain

    D. Radiation of pain, predisposing factors, associated symptoms

11. Upon further interview, it is uncovered that the patient often includes fried foods and ice cream in her diet. When discussing the past 24-hour food intake, she recalls she felt nauseated and had slight RUQ discomfort after eating a fatty meal the night before. Which of the following signs is most likely to be found on physical exam?

    A. Cullen's sign

    B. Rosvig's sign

    C. Murphy's sign

    D. Psoa's sign

12. The FNP orders an abdominal ultrasound for this 42-year-old female patient as well as a complete metabolic panel and complete blood count. What other bloodwork should be ordered?

    A. Homocysteine and amylase

    B. Hbg A1c and amylase

    C. Amylase and lipase

    D. Lipase and homocysteine

13. A 50-year-old male with a BMI of 29 comes in for an annual physical exam. Upon review of systems, he mentions he has a lot of heartburn and is taking over-the-counter omeprazole twice a day. He also takes Tums throughout the day. When deciding whether to refer this patient to a gastroenterologist as the next step, what should the FNP take into consideration?

    A. How long the patient has had this problem

    B. How often he is taking the medications

    C. The severity of his symptoms

    D. His age

14. Which of the following medications can cause lower control of the esophageal sphincter?

    A. Ibuprofen

    B. Pseudoephedrine

    C. Furosemide

    D. ACE inhibitors

15. The FNP is treating a patient for an *H. pylori* infection. The patient has a penicillin allergy. Which regimen would be the best choice for this patient?

    A. Omeprazole 20 mg bid, clarithromycin 500 mg bid, and metronidazole 500 mg bid

    B. Lansoprazole 30 mg bid, amoxicillin 1 gm bid, and metronidazole 500 mg bid

    C. Omeprazole 20 mg daily, metronidazole 1 gm bid, and clarithromycin 1 gm bid

    D. Lansoprazole 30 mg bid, metronidazole 500 mg daily, tetracycline 500 mg daily

16. An 80-year-old male patient comes to the clinic with complaints of diarrhea for 2 days. The FNP notes that the patient had been hospitalized 2 weeks ago for pneumonia. What is the most appropriate next question to ask the patient?

    A. What type of antibiotic were you given in the hospital?

    B. How many days were you hospitalized?

    C. How many times per day are you passing stool?

    D. What over-the-counter medications are you taking for the diarrhea?

17. A patient with generalized lower abdominal pain and nausea is being evaluated. The patient has a low-grade fever (100.4 degrees F). Which of the following signs if found upon physical examination would suggest appendicitis?

    A. Mittleschmerz

    B. Psoas

    C. Murphy's

    D. Kernig

18. The correct sequence for physical examination of the abdomen is:

    A. Inspection, auscultation, percussion, palpation

    B. Inspection, percussion, auscultation, palpation

    C. Auscultation, inspection, percussion, palpation

    D. Auscultation, inspection, palpation, percussion

19. Crohn's disease differs from ulcerative colitis because:

    A. Crohn's disease causes more severe abdominal cramping.

    B. Crohn's may affect any part of the gastrointestinal GI tract. Ulcerative colitis is limited to the large intestine.

    C. Ulcerative colitis symptoms tend to flare up more often around menses.

    D. Ulcerative colitis is a chronic condition, whereas Crohn's disease may occur once and no further flare-ups happen.

20. A 52-year-old male patient is in the office for a physical examination. He has not been seen in three years. The FNP discusses three screening options for detecting colon cancer with the patient. These options include:

    A. Yearly fecal immunochemical testing (FIT), colonoscopy every 10 years, FIT every year along with flexible sigmoidoscopy every 5 years

    B. Colonoscopy every 5 years, FIT annually

    C. Annual FIT along with flexible sigmoidoscopy or colonoscopy every 3 years

    D. Yearly colonoscopy and FIT for those with genetic predisposition to colon cancer

21. A positive Murphy's sign occurs when:

    A. The diaphragm releases the inflamed gall bladder during percussion.

    B. The intestines push against the diaphragm.

    C. The diaphragm moves the inflamed gall bladder into the palpating hand.

    D. The colon moves the diaphragm against the costovertebral column.

22. A 28-year-old man with a long-standing history of IV drug use presents with malaise, nausea, fatigue, and "yellow eyes" for the past week. After ordering diagnostic tests, you confirm the diagnosis of acute hepatitis B. Anticipated laboratory results include:

    A. Positive hepatitis B surface antibody (HBsAB).

    B. Eosinophilia.

    C. Lymphopenia.

    D. Positive hepatitis B surface antigen HBsAG.

23. Which of the following is true concerning the hepatitis B vaccine?

    A. The vaccine contains live hepatitis B virus.

    B. The nurse practitioner should consider post-vaccination HBsAB titers for those at the highest risk of infection.

    C. The vaccine is contraindicated in the presence of HIV infection.

    D. Post-vaccine arthralgias are often reported.

24. Serologic features of acute hepatitis B are:

    A. HBsAg reactive, and high titer of immunoglobulin M(IgM).

    B. HBsAg reactive and high titer of immunoglobin G (IgG).

    C. HBeAg and HBsAg negative.

    D. IgM anti-HBc- (high titer) HBsAg-nonreactive.

25. Monitoring for hepatocellular carcinoma in a patient with chronic hepatitis B or C often includes the periodic evaluation of which of the following?

    A. Erythrocyte sedimentation rate

    B. HBsAB

    C. Alpha-fetoprotein

    D. Serum creatinine level

26. An acute febrile illness with jaundice, anorexia, malaise, and an incubation period of 45–150 days; having a chronic and an acute form; and transmitted by parenteral, transmitted by sexual activity, and perinatal routes *best* describes which of the following?

    A. Hepatitis A
    B. Hepatitis B
    C. Hepatitis C
    D. Hepatitis D

27. Which of the following laboratory studies is used to determine if a client has hepatitis A?

    A. Serum protein
    B. Protein electrophoresis
    C. Antibody testing
    D. Immunoglobulin levels

28. Which factor(s) is (are) predicative of the severity of chronic liver disease in a patient with chronic hepatitis C?

    A. Female gender, < 30 y.o.
    B. Genotype, viral load, and daily alcohol use
    C. Acquisition of the virus through IV drug use, and a history of hepatitis A infection
    D. Frequent use of aspirin
    E. ALT, AST levels

29. What is the *most common* source for hepatitis A infection?

    A. Needle sharing
    B. Raw shellfish
    C. Contaminated water supplies
    D. Intimate person-to-person contact

30. When answering questions about the hepatitis A vaccine, the FNP responds that it:

    A. Should be offered to patients with chronic hepatitis C.
    B. Should be offered to those who have traveled to western Europe
    C. Usually is a required immunization for all health care workers.
    D. Is protective after a single vaccine dose.

31. Diarrhea is often generally associated with:

    A. Infectious gastroenteritis, inflammatory bowel disease, and diverticulitis.
    B. Diseases of the colon or rectum.
    C. Fever and abdominal pain in sexually transmitted diseases.
    D. Dysuria and flank pain in urinary tract infections.

32. Effective treatment of *H. pylori* can be expected to result in the following:

    A. Treatment of the initial episode, which may recur with stress.
    B. Provide a protective mucosal barrier to gastric acid.
    C. The need to repeat triple therapy if symptoms persist.
    D. Eradication of the bacteria.

33. Potential complications of gastroesophageal reflux disease (GERD) include:

    A. Esophageal ulcers, Barrett's esophagitis, and esophageal stricture.
    B. Gastric ulcers, esophageal dilatation, and stricture of the lower esophageal sphincter.
    C. Peptic ulcers, esophageal ulcers, and gastric distension.
    D. Aspiration pneumonia, gastric ulcers, and esophageal bleeding.

Questions 34–37 pertain to the following case:

A 67-year-old male presents to the office with a chief complaint of a chronic cough ×3 years that has gotten worse in the past 2 months. The cough keeps him awake at night, is nonproductive, and he denies any wheezing, fever, chills, hemoptysis, dyspnea or shortness of breath, night sweats, or tuberculosis (TB) contacts. He has a history of chronic obstructive lung disease (COPD) and stopped smoking 10 years ago. Current medications include effective treatment of COPD with inhaled Advair (fluticasone propionate/salmeterol). He states he rarely needs to use a "rescue" treatment. He also states that he has a history of a hiatal hernia; however, it has "never been a problem" except for occasional indigestion. The patient states he enjoys a daily bourbon drink with dinner. Physical exam is essentially negative, with the exception of a BMI of 32, and respiratory exam reveals slight bibasilar crackles, which do not clear with cough, but no rales, rhonchi, and wheezes. Oropharynx is pink, and there is no evidence of ulcerations, lesions, or excessive mucus; nares are pink and are not inflamed or boggy.

34. With the information you now have, what is your differential diagnosis?
    A. Lung cancer, chronic bronchitis, and gastroesophageal reflux disease (GERD)
    B. Postnasal drip, tuberculosis, and upper respiratory infection
    C. COPD, esophageal reflux, and allergic rhinitis
    D. TB, pneumonia, postnasal drip, and GERD

35. Which of the following diagnostics would be *most* helpful in initial clinical decision making?
    A. PA and lateral chest x-ray, endoscopy
    B. Pulmonary function tests, CBC and SED rate
    C. Sputum smear and culture for acid-fast bacilli
    D. CBC, SED rate, Mono spot

The patient is diagnosed with GERD. Despite the implementation of lifestyle changes and antacids, he does not have significant relief. Omeprazole 20 mg is prescribed QD (every day) with the expectation that he will return for follow-up in 6 weeks. He returns 6 weeks later and continues to be symptomatic with the nocturnal cough.

36. The next step in management would include:
    A. Proton-pump inhibitors bid and reinforcement of lifestyle modifications.
    B. Antacids, inhaled steroids, and small frequent meals.
    C. Surgical consult, antacids, and nasal inhaled steroids.
    D. Colonoscopy, surgical consult, and H_2 receptor antagonist QD.

37. Patient education issues that need to be addressed with the goal of improved patient outcome include:
    A. Reinforce smoking cessation, weight reduction, avoidance of alcohol and caffeine.
    B. Eating no later than midnight, portion control or dietary restrictions, cough suppressants at bedtime.
    C. Elevate the head of the bed on blocks, prn (*pro re nata*) antacids, bland high-fat diet.
    D. Encourage bland snacks, use H_2 blockers, maintain weight restrictions.

38. Biliary colic may radiate to the:
    A. Infrascapular area.
    B. Right shoulder.
    C. Neck and left arm.
    D. Periumbilical area.

39. A 55-year-old schoolteacher with type 2 diabetes presents to your office with complaints of low-grade fever for 3 days and cramping right upper quadrant pain, radiating to the right scapula. Laboratory diagnostics indicate:

WBC	13,000	(NL 4.5–11,000)
SGOT (AST)	55	(NL 5–40)
SGPT (ALT)	65	(NL 5–55)
BUN	25	(NL 6–25)
Alk. Phos.	140	(NL 35–110)
Amylase	130	(NL 20–90)

Physical exam reveals epigastric tenderness, guarding, and a positive Murphy's sign. The FNP suspects:
   A. Acute cholecystitis.
   B. Acute appendicitis.
   C. Hepatitis.
   D. Peptic ulcer disease.

40. The most important contributing factor to the development of a peptic ulcer is:
   A. Eating spicy/acidic foods.
   B. Use of nonsteroidals (NSAIDs).
   C. Stress.
   D. Drinking alcohol.

41. A 25-year-old nursing student has just returned from a mission trip to Central America with traveler's diarrhea. Which antibiotic should the nurse practitioner order if the symptoms do not improve?
   A. Ampicillin
   B. Tetracycline
   C. Ciprofloxacin
   D. Zithromax

42. All the following are risk factors associated with long-term use of PPIs EXCEPT:
   A. Pneumonia.
   B. COPD.
   C. Anemia.
   D. Clostridium difficile.

43. A 19-year-old male comes to the college health center complaining of a "bulge" on the right side of his groin, which is not painful, but is "uncomfortable." Upon examination, the FNP is unable to reduce the inguinal hernia found in the right groin area. The best next step to manage this problem by the FNP is:
   A. Nothing. It will reduce eventually without any intervention.
   B. Immediate referral to a local emergency room. Call the patient's parents with this information.
   C. Instruct the patient to avoid any weightlifting and sports, and use supportive undergarments to hold the hernia in place.
   D. Instruct the patient to avoid any heavy lifting, and to go to the emergency department with any severe pain. Also let the patient know you are calling in a referral for consultation with a general surgeon today.

44. A 78-year-old male patient walks in to the office complaining of feeling lightheaded for a few hours. He appears pale and anxious. Past medical history includes controlled atrial fibrillation, hypertension, and hyperlipidemia. The patient's vital signs are: Temp. 98.2 degrees F, BP 100/58, heart rate 92, resp. rate 16, O_2 sat 94%. Which one of the following findings on physical exam are most concerning?

    A. Obturator sign
    B. Cohen's sign
    C. Jackob's sign
    D. Cullen's sign

45. A recently divorced 59-year-old female patient comes to the clinic with complaints of new onset diarrhea and alternating constipation over the past 3 months, occasional blood in stool, and unintentional 5 pound weight loss over the past 6 weeks. This patient's BMI is 30, vital signs are all within normal limits. Her social history includes smoking ½ ppd (pack per day) for 20 years, as well as one glass of wine per day, and she works as a receptionist. The physical examination is unremarkable. What are the best choices for the top 3 differential diagnoses?

    A. Diverticulitis, colon cancer, intestinal parasites
    B. Colon cancer, appendicitis, malaria
    C. Duodenal ulcer, peptic ulcer, Crohn's disease
    D. Intestinal parasites, irritable bowel disease, cytomegalovirus

46. For the above 59-year-old female patient, which of the following genetic disorders increases her risk for colon cancer?

    A. Murphy's syndrome
    B. BRCA 1 gene mutation
    C. FLAP syndrome
    D. Lynch syndrome

47. What is the best initial diagnostic test to find out if a patient actually has colon cancer?

    A. Colonoscopy and biopsy
    B. PET scan
    C. Abdominal ultrasound
    D. Fecal occult blood sample

48. Pain related to acute appendicitis can cause tenderness where?

    A. Curley's area
    B. McDowell's point
    C. Russell's site
    D. McBurney's point

49. A 72-year-old male presents to the office with severe abdominal pain that radiates to the back and genital area. The FNP knows that this may indicate which of the following conditions requiring immediate intervention?

    A. Inguinal hernia
    B. Lower lobe pneumonia with effusion
    C. Acute choleycystitis
    D. Dissection or rupture of abdominal aortic aneurysm

50. A 19-year-old male football player has suffered an injury during the game. The patient is pale, anxious, and complains of left upper quadrant abdominal pain radiating to the left shoulder. The FNP recognizes that this most likely indicates:

    A. A ruptured spleen.
    B. Acute pancreatitis.
    C. Right-sided pneumothorax.
    D. Testicular torsion

Answers and Rationales

· ·

1. D. One pharmacological intervention for a patient with diabetes or pre-diabetes with NASH is Metformin.

2. B. Of the following options, which two are factors that may lead to faster progression of HCV disease? Male gender, comorbid HIV infection.

The next three questions are related to the 33-year-old patient described in the question:

3. D. A 33-year-old male patient is new to the FNP's practice. During the health history he mentions he was told he had hepatitis. He is unsure which type of hepatitis and asks what it is. The FNP tells him that hepatitis is: Inflammation of the liver.

4. C. The FNP is ordering bloodwork for this new patient. To evaluate which hepatitis the patient was previously diagnosed with the **initial** laboratory testing will include: HAV total Ab, HCV Ab, HBV sAg and HBsAb.

5. C. Past hepatitis A infection, chronic hepatitis B infection.

6. D. The type of hepatitis most commonly caused by contaminated foods is HAV.

7. B. A 50-year-old female patient thinks she may have gotten hepatitis C from a previous sexual partner. She asks what the signs and symptoms of acute infection are. The FNP responds, listing fever, fatigue, body aches.

8. B. Peter is a 50-year-old AA male who is HCV+ from IVDU many years ago. He has not used street drugs for over 15 years and works long hours as a train conductor. He is asking about his routine health maintenance in regard to HCV. The FNP says that the following yearly exams are recommended: Liver ultrasound, liver enzymes, AFP, HCV viral load.

9. B. A 62-year-old female patient comes to the FNP's office with complaints of constipation for the past few months. She has tried to increase her intake of water and fiber without much success. A yearly physical exam and colonoscopy was negative for any significant findings 6 months prior to this visit. Which of the following options would be the most appropriate for the next step?

    Recommend an increase in exercise, such as walking, and daily Miralax use for 2 weeks.

    Have patient return for evaluation in one month.

The next three questions are based on the 42-year-old female patient. Vital signs are within normal limits. The patient's BMI is 31.

10. D. Radiation of pain, predisposing factors, associated symptoms.

11. C. Upon further interview it is uncovered that the patient often includes fried foods and ice cream in her diet. When discussing the past 24–hour-food intake, she recalls she felt nauseated and had slight RUQ (right upper quadrant) discomfort after eating a fatty meal the night before. Which of the following signs is most likely to be found on physical exam?

    Murphy's sign.

12. C. Amylase and lipase.

13. A. A 50-year-old male with a BMI of 29 comes in for an annual physical exam. Upon review of systems he mentions he has a lot of heartburn and is taking over-the-counter omeprazole twice a day. He also takes Tums throughout the day. When deciding whether to refer this patient to a gastroenterologist as the next step, what should the FNP take into consideration?

    How long the patient has had this problem.

14. A. Which of the following medications can cause lower control of the esophageal sphincter?

    Ibuprofen

15. A. The FNP is treating a patient for H. pylori infection. The patient has a penicillin allergy. Which regimen would be the best choice for this patient?

    Omeprazole 20 mg bid, clarithromycin 500 mg bid, and metronidazole 500 mg bid.

16. C. An 80-year-old male patient comes to the clinic with complaints of diarrhea for 2 days. The FNP notes that the patient had been hospitalized 2 weeks ago for pneumonia. What is the most appropriate next question to ask the patient?

    How many times per day are you passing stool? Individual perception of constipation or diarrhea can vary greatly.

17. B. A patient with generalized lower abdominal pain and nausea is being evaluated. The patient has a low grade fever (100.4 f). Which of the following signs if found upon physical examination would suggest appendicitis?

    Psoas

18. A. The correct sequence for physical examination of the abdomen is

    Inspection, auscultation, percussion, palpation.

19. B. Crohn's disease differs from ulcerative colitis because:

    Crohn's may affect any part of the gastrointestinal GI tract. Ulcerative colitis is limited to the large intestine.

20. A. A 52-year-old male patient is in the office for a physical examination. He has not been seen in three years. The FNP discusses three screening options for detecting colon cancer with the patient. These options include:

    Yearly fecal immunochemical testing (FIT), colonoscopy every 10 years, FIT every year along with flexible sigmoidoscopy every 5 years.

21. C. A positive Murphy's sign occurs when:

    The diaphragm moves the inflamed gall bladder into the palpating hand.

22. D. A 28-year-old man with a long standing history of IV drug use presents with malaise, nausea, fatigue, and "yellow eyes" for the past week. After ordering diagnostic tests, you confirm the diagnosis of acute hepatitis B. Anticipated laboratory results include:

    Positive hepatitis B surface antigen HBsAG.

23. B. Which of the following is true concerning the hepatitis B vaccine?

    The nurse practitioner should consider post vaccination HBsAB titers for those at the highest risk of infection.

24. A. Serologic features of acute hepatitis B are:

    HBsAg reactive, and high titer of immunoglobulin M(IgM).

25. C. Monitoring for hepatocellular carcinoma in a patient with chronic hepatitis B or C often includes periodic evaluation of:

    Alpha-fetoprotein (AFP). AFP is made by a fetus' liver and is found in low levels in adults unless they have certain cancers, in particular hepatocellular cancer.

26. B. An acute febrile illness with jaundice, anorexia, malaise, and incubation period of 45–150 days; having a chronic and an acute form; and transmitted by parenteral, transmitted by sexual activity, and perinatal routes **best describes:**

    hepatitis B. HDV can co-occur with HBV, hepatitis A is typically food/water borne and is not chronic, HCV is not commonly spread via heterosexual transmission in a monogamous relationship.

27. C. Which of the following laboratory studies is used to determine if a client had hepatitis A?

    Antibody testing.

28. C. Which factor(s) is (are) predicative of the severity of chronic liver disease in a patient with chronic hepatitis C?

    Genotype, viral load, and daily alcohol use. Male gender and HIV co-infection are risk factors for more progressive, severe HCV disease.

29. C. The *most common* source for hepatitis A Infection is:

    Contaminated water supplies.

30. A. When answering questions about hepatitis A vaccine, the nurse practitioner responds that it:

    Should be offered to patients with chronic hepatitis C. Patients with HCV infection need to be protected against other liver damaging infections such as HAV and HBV.

31. A. Diarrhea is often generally associated with:

    Infectious gastroenteritis, inflammatory bowel disease, diverticulitis.

32. D. Effective treatment of *H. pylori* can be expected to result in the following:

    Eradication of the bacteria.

33. A. Potential complications of gastroesophageal reflux disease (GERD) include:

    Esophageal ulcers, Barrett's esophagitis, esophageal stricture.

Questions 34–37 pertain to the following case:

A 67-year-old male presents to the office with the chief complaint of a chronic cough ×3 years that has gotten worse in the past 2 months. The cough keeps him awake at night, is nonproductive, and he denies any wheezing, fever, chills, hemoptysis, dyspnea or shortness of breath, night sweats, or tuberculosis (TB) contacts. He has a history of chronic obstructive lung disease (COPD) and stopped smoking 10 years ago. Current medications include effective treatment of COPD with inhaled Advair (fluticasone propionate/salmeterol). He states he rarely needs to use a "rescue" treatment. He states that he has a history of a hiatus hernia; however, it has "never been a problem," except for occasional indigestion. The patient states he enjoys a daily bourbon drink with dinner.

Physical exam is essentially negative, with the exception that the patient has a BMI of 32, and respiratory exam reveals slight bibasilar crackles, which do not clear with cough, but no rales, rhonchi, wheezes. Oropharynx is pink, and there is no evidence of ulcerations, lesions, or excessive mucus; nares are pink and are not inflamed or boggy.

34. A. With the information you now have, what is your differential diagnosis? Lung cancer, chronic bronchitis, gastroesophageal reflux disease (GERD).

35. A. Which of the following diagnostics would be most helpful in initial clinical decision making: PA and lateral chest x-ray, endoscopy. The CXR will rule out pneumonia, pleural effusion, and/or congestive heart failure, although it should not be used to assess for lung cancer. The endoscopy will evaluate for any erythema or ulcers related to GERD.

The patient is diagnosed with GERD; despite the implementation of lifestyle changes and antacids, he does not have significant relief. Omeprazole 20 mg is prescribed QD with the expectation that he will return for follow-up in 6 weeks. He returns 6 weeks later and continues to symptomatic with the nocturnal cough.

36. A. The next step in management would include: Proton-pump inhibitors BID and reinforcement of lifestyle modifications.

37. A. Patient education issues that need to be addressed with the goal of improved patient outcome include: Reinforce smoking cessation, weight reduction, avoidance of alcohol and caffeine.

38. A. Biliary colic may radiate to the infrascapular area.

39. A. A 55-year-old schoolteacher with type 2 diabetes presents to your office with complaints of low-grade fever for 3 days and cramping right upper quadrant pain, radiating to the right scapula. Laboratory diagnostics indicate:

WBC	13,000	(NL 4.5–11,000)
SGOT (AST)	55	(NL 5–40)
SGPT (ALT)	65	(NL 5–55)
BUN	25	(NL 6–25)
Alk. Phos.	140	(NL 35–110)
Amylase	130	(NL 20–90)

Physical exam reveals epigastric tenderness, guarding, and a positive Murphy's sign. The FNP suspects: Acute cholecystitis. Mild elevation of white blood cells, liver enzymes, and amylase are found in patients with choleycystitis.

40. B. The most important contributing factor to the development of peptic ulcer is:

Use of nonsteroidals (NSAIDs). Overuse of NSAIDS or infection with *H. Pylori* are risk factors for the development of peptic ulcer disease.

41. C. A 25-year-old. nursing student has just returned from a mission trip to Central America with traveler's diarrhea. Which antibiotic should the nurse practitioner order if the symptoms do not improve? Ciprofloxacin. In otherwise healthy patients with mild diarrhea of short duration, antibiotics are not required.

42. B. All the following are risk factors associated with long term use of PPIs EXCEPT:

COPD.

43. D. A 19-year-old male comes to the college health center complaining of a "bulge" on the right side of his groin which is not painful, but is "uncomfortable." Upon examination the FNP is unable to reduce the inguinal hernia found in the right groin area. The best next step for the FNP to do for management of this problem is:

Instruct the patient to avoid any heavy lifting, and to go to the emergency department with any severe pain. Also let the patient know you are calling in a referral for consultation with a general surgeon today.

44. D. A 78-year-old male patient walks in to the office complaining of feeling light-headed for a few hours. He appears pale and anxious. Past medical history includes controlled atrial fibrillation, hypertension, and hyperlipidemia. The patient's vital signs are: Temp-98.2 f, B/P 100/58, heart rate-92, resp. rate=16, O2 sat-94%

Which one of the following findings on physical exam are most concerning? Cullen's sign. Bluish discoloration in the periumbilical area strongly indicates retroperitoneal bleeding which can occur in patients on warfarin.

45. A. A recently divorced 59-year-old female patient comes to the clinic with complaints of new onset diarrhea and alternating constipation over the past 3 months, occasional blood in stool, and unintentional 5 pound weight loss over the past 6 weeks. This patient's BMI is 30, vital signs are all within normal limits. Her social history includes smoking ½ ppd for 20 years, as well as one glass of wine per day, and she works as a receptionist. The physical examination is unremarkable. What are the best choices for the top 3 differential diagnoses? Diverticulitis, colon cancer, intestinal parasites. Of these three, colon cancer is the most likely diagnosis and needs immediate diagnostic testing and follow up.

46. D. For the above 59-year-old female patient, which of the following genetic disorders increases her risk for colon cancer: Lynch syndrome. Lynch syndrome testing is for HNPCC or hereditary nonpolyposis colon cancer which is usually seen in persons under the age of 50.

47. A. What is the best initial diagnostic test to find out if a patient actually has colon cancer? Colonoscopy and biopsy. While there are other diagnostic tests that may be a part of evaluating any spread of cancer, a biopsy is required for definitive diagnosis.

48. D. Pain related to acute appendicitis can cause tenderness at: McBurney's point. This is over the right side of the abdomen that is one-third of the distance from the anterior superior iliac spine to the umbilicus.

49. D. A 72-year-old male presents to the office with severe abdominal pain that radiates to the back and genital area. The FNP knows that this may indicate which of the following conditions requiring immediate intervention? Dissection or rupture of abdominal aortic aneurysm. This is an emergency and requires immediate transfer to the emergency department.

50. A. A 19-year-old male football player has suffered an injury during the game. The patient is pale, anxious, and complains of left upper quadrant abdominal pain radiating to the left shoulder. The FNP recognizes that this most likely indicates possible: Ruptured spleen. This is a true emergency and requires immediate transfer to the emergency department.

• • • References

Ahnen, D., Macrae, F., and Bendell, J. (2015). Uptodate. *Clinical presentation, diagnosis and staging of colorectal cancer.* Retrieved from www.uptodate.com/contents/clinical-presentation-diagnosis-and-staging-of-colorectal-cancer?source=preview&language=en-US&anchor=H1&selectedTitle=1~150#H1

Alexandraki, I., & Smetana, G. (2015). Uptodate. *Acute viral gastroenteritis in adults.* Retrieved from: www.uptodate.com/contents/acute-viral-gastroenteritis-in-adults?source=preview&language=en-US&anchor=H17733722&selectedTitle=1~150#H17733722

American Cancer Society. (2015). *Colorectal cancer detection and early prevention.* Retrieved from http://www.cancer.org/cancer/colonandrectumcancer/moreinformation/colonandrectumcancerearlydetection/colorectal-cancer-early-detection-acs-recommendations

American Family Physician. (2015). *Evaluation of acute abdominal pain in adults.* Retrieved from http://www.aafp.org/afp/2008/0401/p971.html

Bleday, R., & Breen, E. (2015a). Uptodate. *Hemorrhoids: Clinical manifestations and diagnosis.* Retrieved from www.uptodate.com/contents/hemorrhoids-clinical-manifestations-and-diagnosis?source=search_result&search=hemorrhoids&selectedTitle=2~150

Bleday, R., & Breen, E. (2015b). Uptodate. *Treatment of hemorrhoids.* Retrieved from www.uptodate.com/contents/treatment-of-hemorrhoids?source=see_link

Breen, E., & Bleday, R. (2015). Uptodate. *Anal fissure: Medical management.* Retrieved from www.uptodate.com/contents/anal-fissure-medical-management?source=see_link

Farrell, R., & Peppercorn, M. (2015). Uptodate. *Overview of the medical management of mild to moderate Crohn's disease in adults.* Retrieved from www.uptodate.com/contents/overview-of-the-medical-management-of-mild-to-moderate-crohn-disease-in-adults?source=machineLearning&search=inflammatory+bowel+disease+treatment&selectedTitle=1~150&sectionRank=1&anchor=H11241188#H11241188

Gilbert, D., Chambers, H., Eliopoulos, G., Saag, M., Black, D., Freedman, D., Pavia, A., & Schwartz, B. (2015). *Sanfort antimicrobial guide 2015* (45th ed.). Antimicrobial Therapy, Inc, Sperryville, VA.

GlobalRPh. (2015). *Infectious disease database.* Retrieved from http://www.globalrph.com/antibiotic/diverticulitis.htm

Goolsby, M. J., & Grubbs, L. (2011). *Advanced assessment: Interpreting findings and formulating differential diagnoses* (2nd ed.). Pennsylvania, PA: F. A. Davis Company,

Kahrilas, P. (2015). Uptodate. *Medical management of gastroesophageal reflux disease in adults.* Retrieved from: www.uptodate.com/contents/medical-management-of-gastroesophageal-reflux-disease-in-adults?source=search_result&search=gerd+adult&selectedTitle=2~150

MacDermott, R. (2015). Uptodate. *Management of mild to moderate ulcerative colitis.* Retrieved from www.uptodate.com/contents/management-of-mild-to-moderate-ulcerative-colitis?source=machineLearning&search=ulcerative+colitis+treatment&selectedTitle=1~150&sectionRank=2&anchor=H27#H27

Martin, R. (2015). *Acute appendicitis in adults: Clinical manifestations and differential diagnosis.* Retrieved from http://eresources.library.mssm.edu:2226/contents/acute-appendicitis-in-adults-clinical-manifestations-and-differential-diagnosis?source=search_result&search=appendicitis+adult&selectedTitle=1~150

Mayo Clinic. (2015). *Diseases and conditions: Viral gastroenteritis.* Retrieved from: http://www.mayoclinic.org/diseases-conditions/viral-gastroenteritis/basics/definition/con-20019350

Peppercorn, M., & Kane, S. (2015). Uptodate. *Clinical manifestations, diagnosis, and prognosis of ulcerative colitis in adults.* Retrieve from www.uptodate.com/contents/clinical-manifestations-diagnosis-and-prognosis-of-ulcerative-colitis-in-adults?source=machineLearning&search=inflammatory+bowel+disease&selectedTitle=1~150&sectionRank=1&anchor=H1844647392#H1844647392

U.S. National Library of Medicine. (2015). *Medline Plus.* Retrieved from https://www.nlm.nih.gov/medlineplus/ency/article/003458.htm

Vakil, N. (2015). Uptodate. *Peptic ulcer disease: Clinical manifestation and diagnosis.* Retrieved from: www.uptodate.com/contents/peptic-ulcer-disease-clinical-manifestations-and-diagnosis?source=machineLearning&search=peptic+ulcer+disease&selectedTitle=2~150&anchor=H3&sectionRank=1#H3

Wald, A. (2015a). Uptodate. *Management of chronic constipation in adults.* Retrieved from www.uptodate.com/contents/management-of-chronic-constipation-in-adults?source=machineLearning&search=constipation+adult&selectedTitle=1~150&sectionRank=1&anchor=H30890974#H30890974

Wald, A. (2015b). Uptodate. *Treatment of irritable bowel syndrome in adults.* Retrieved from www.uptodate.com/contents/treatment-of-irritable-bowel-syndrome-in-adults?source=machineLearning&search=irritable+bowel+syndrome&selectedTitle=1~150&sectionRank=3&anchor=H26#H26

Young-Fadok, T., & Pemberton, J. (2015). Uptodate. *Nonopeartive management of acute uncomplicated diverticulitis.* Retrieved from www.uptodate.com/contents/nonoperative-management-of-acute-uncomplicated-diverticulitis?source=machineLearning&search=diverticulitis&selectedTitle=1~19&sectionRank=1&anchor=H432554965#H432554965

Zakko, S., & Afdhal, M. (2015). Uptodate. *Acute cholecystitis: Pathogenesis, clinical features and diagnosis.* Retrieved from: www.uptotade.com/contents/acute-cholecystitis-pathogenesis-clinical-features-and-diagnosis?source=machineLearning&search=cholecystitis&selectedTitle=1~150&sectionRank=1&anchor=H15#H15

9

Musculoskeletal Review

Frank Tudini, PT, DSc, OCS, COMT, FAAOMPT

Kevin Chui, PT, DPT, PhD, GCS, OCS, CEEAA, FAAOMPT

In the primary care setting, 10–20% of outpatient primary care visits are for musculoskeletal injuries. These injuries may be traumatic (injury related) or atraumatic (i.e., overuse or degenerative syndromes) as well as acute or chronic.

1. Sprains and strains are the most common.

2. Injury to ligaments occur secondary to sudden stress on an affected joint.

3. Ankle (inversion) sprains are the most common and may be sports related, or occur with normal daily activities such as stepping off a curb or stepping into a hole.

Assessment of the injury in the primary care setting:

1. Chief complaint

2. HPI: Onset history & location—typically pain, instability, or dysfunction—ask patient to "point to pain" Remember the seven attributes of a symptom OLDCART: Onset, Location, Duration, Characteristic, Aggravating or Alleviating factors, and Timing.

3. ROS: Assess the MS system, the patient's injury and include safety and mobility considerations.

4. Physical Exam: Inspection (swelling, erythema, atrophy, deformity, surgical scars), palpation, range of motion (ROM), and neurovascular status

5. Tests that can be done in the primary care setting by the practitioner:

   i. Provocative: Recreate mechanism of injury to reproduce pain

   ii. Stress: apply load to ligament of concern

   iii. Functional: Simple tasks performed with activities of daily living

Imaging Considerations:

1. Standard (2 planes/views—AP & lateral or both obliques—mortise) radiographs for bony pathology assessment

2. CT visualize bony pathology & morphology of fractures

3. Nuclear bone scans identify stress fractures, infection, malignancy, or multisite pathology.

4. MRI visualizes ligaments, cartilage, and soft tissues

5. Ultrasound identifies superficial tissue problems, including tendinopathies and synovial problems

Foot and Ankle

Morton (Interdigital) Neuroma

- A non-neoplastic perineural fibrous proliferation involving the plantar digital nerve usually between the 3 and 4 toes or less commonly the 2 and 3 toes and affecting women more than men

- Symptoms include pain in the involved web space that often radiates to the toes. Numbness, burning, and tingling may also be present.
- Diagnosis includes clinical exam, Mulder click sign, and MRI or US. Rule out metatarsal fracture.
- Treatment includes shoe wear modification, orthotics with possible metatarsal pad, rocker bottom shoes.

Plantar Fasciitis

- The most common cause of plantar heel pain
- Characterized by heel pain with the first steps in the morning or when standing up after prolonged sitting, and tenderness at the calcaneal tuberosity that is increased with passive dorsiflexion of the toes. There is often a history of prolonged WB (weight bearing) activity either recreationally or occupationally resulting in repetitive microtrauma to the heel. Can occur in isolation or be a manifestation of systemic disease such as RA (Rheumatoid arthritis) or other spondyloarthropathy.
- Diagnosis includes clinical exam and possibly MRI, US (ultrasound), or bone scintigraphy.
- Treatment includes analgesics, stretching, exercise, orthotics, night splints, taping, physical therapy, and corticosteroid injections. In severe cases, a plantar fasciotomy can be performed.

Bilateral Heel Pain

- Bilateral heel pain has several causes including: plantar fasciitis, Achilles tendonopathy (pain is usually more posterior heel), Achilles bursitis, calcaneal stress fractures, tarsal tunnel syndrome (consider if pain is accompanied by tingling, burning, or numbness in the heel which may radiate into the sole of the foot and is worse with ankle dorsiflexion and eversion), heel pad atrophy especially in older and obese patients, osteomyelitis (signs of infection especially in those with vascular compromise), peripheral nerve entrapment (especially if there are sensory changes), and as a result of rheumatologic disorders or malignancy

Achilles Tendinopathy

- Pain in the posterior ankle and heel, which is worse with running, jumping, and quick motions. Risk factors include abnormal ankle dorsiflexion motion, increased foot pronation, obesity, HTN (hypertension), hyperlipidemia, DM (diabetes mellitus), and training errors.

- Diagnosis consists of subjective pain reports with local pain, swelling, and stiffness in the Achilles tendon region especially following a period of inactivity. Initially, these symptoms may lessen with activity and then increase again after activity. Clinical tests include tenderness to palpation over the tendon or posterior calcaneus, a positive arc sign and positive Royal London Hospital Test, as well as pain with resisted plantar flexion. Diagnosis can be aided by US and MRI.
- Interventions include modalities (laser, iontophoresis), stretching, foot orthoses, manual therapy, physical therapy, taping, heel lifts, and night splints.

Pes Planus

- A foot deformity that occurs when the head of the talus is displaced in a medial and plantar direction, stretching the spring ligament and tibialis posterior muscle and resulting in a loss of the medial longitudinal arch. May be asymptomatic.
- Present clinically with a pronated foot, tenderness over the plantar fascia, with laxity of the medial foot ligaments and tibialis posterior muscle. Callus formation may develop where the talus presses against the medial counter of the shoe.
- Treatment includes shoe modification, orthotics such as arch supports, as well as pain-relieving modalities.

Pes Cavus

- Abnormal foot position characterized by a high arch which causes WB to be asymmetric and uneven along the metatarsal heads and lateral border of the foot.
- May be susceptible to metatarsal head and calcaneal contusions and osteophyte formation, as well as heel pain and stress fractures.
- Interventions include shoe modification and orthoses, as well as stretching of tight musculature, and physical therapy to address lower extremity muscle imbalances.

Charcot Neuropathic Osteoarthropathy

- Foot pathology that occurs in the presence of a peripheral neuropathy (usually diabetic) where inflammation leads to osteolysis, subluxation, dislocation, and deformity of the foot. Due to a loss of pain sensation, WB activities may continue to cause further repetitive trauma.

- Diagnosis: The hallmark sign is mid-foot collapse, described as a "rocker-bottom foot" (see picture below). There is neuropathy present with reduced sensation of pain, swelling, warmth, erythematous foot with mild to moderate pain. Clinical diagnosis is aided by radiographs for fracture and subluxation, as well as MRI. Cellulitis, DVT (deep vein thrombosis), and gout should be ruled out.

- Treatment includes offloading the foot to arrest progression of the deformity. Immobilization with cast and assistive devices such as crutches or wheelchair may be used initially until swelling has resolved. Transition to a walking boot and maybe eventually custom footwear. Surgery may be required to resect any infection or bony prominences that cannot be accommodated for. Achilles tendon lengthening and arthrodesis may be last-resort surgeries. Pharmacologically, anti-resorption bone therapy such as calcitonin may be initiated.

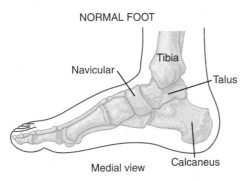

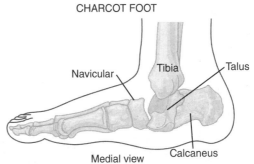

Ankle Sprain Lateral/Medial

- Trauma involving inversion for a lateral ankle sprain or eversion for a medial ankle sprain. Clinical presentation includes tenderness over the involved ligaments, swelling, limited motion, pain, possible bruising or discoloration, decreased strength, and (depending on the severity) altered gait and balance.

- Risk factors include previous ankle sprain, improper warm up and decreased ankle dorsiflexion motion.

- Interventions include initial external support and assistive gait device, physical therapy consisting of manual therapy, physical agents, therapeutic exercise, and eventual return to sports training.

Compartment Syndrome

- Severe uncontrolled pain, swelling, and pain resulting as a complication of a foot crush injury, fracture, surgery, vascular injury, and rarely ankle sprain. Compartment syndrome can be acute or chronic.

- Presentation also includes pain with motion of the foot and toes which increases with exertion. Compartment pressure may be measured by using an intra-compartment pressure monitor. Long-term sequelae may include contracture, deformity, weakness, paralysis, and sensory neuropathy.

- Intervention: Acute compartment syndrome is a medical emergency, while chronic compartment syndrome typically is not. In severe cases, surgery may be necessary to decompress the limb. Also: activity modification, anti-inflammatory modalities, pain medication, physical therapy to improve mobility and strength and reduce pain.

Ottawa Ankle Rules

- X-rays are indicated if there is trauma to the foot or ankle, bony pain in the malleolar zone, and any one of the following:

  1. Tenderness at the distal 6 cm of the posterior edge of the tibia or tip of medial malleolus

  2. Tenderness at the distal 6 cm of posterior edge of the fibula or tip of the lateral malleolus

  3. Inability to bear weight both immediately after the injury and in the ED (Emergency Department) for four steps

Ottawa Foot Rules

- X-rays are indicated if there is trauma to the foot or ankle, bony pain in the mid-foot zone, and any one of the following:

  1. Tenderness at the base of the 5th metatarsal

  2. Tenderness at the navicular bone

  3. Inability to bear weight both immediately after the injury and in the ED for four steps

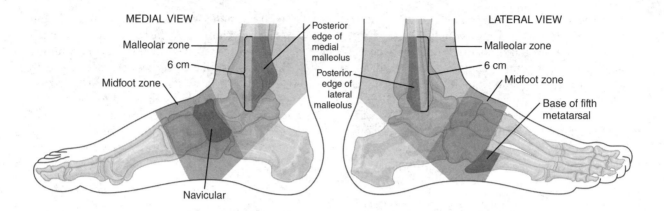

Knee

Osgood Schlatter Disease

- A traction injury of the tibial tuberosity by the quadriceps, affecting children involved in sports (boys > girls) between 11–15 years of age. Usually occurs unilateral but may be bilateral and often during a growth spurt.
- Clinical presentation includes pain, swelling, and enlargement of the proximal tibia where the patellar tendon inserts.
- Treatment includes over-the-counter pain relievers, physical therapy for stretching, strengthening, and modalities, activity modification, and patellar tendon straps. The condition is usually self-limiting with good long-term outcomes.

Bursitis—Patellar, Pes Anserine, Baker Cyst
Prepatellar Bursitis

- Inflammation of the bursa between the patella and the overlying subcutaneous tissue
- Caused by acute trauma to the patella or chronic trauma in the form of prolonged or repeated kneeling
- Presents with pain, swelling, and tenderness over the patella. MRI or, US can be used to confirm diagnosis or rule out other potential diagnoses.
- Intervention includes ice, compression, rest, anti-inflammatory and pain medications. Physical therapy is prescribed for modalities, stretching, and progressive strengthening and return-to-play activities. Occasionally, aspiration or surgical removal of the bursa is necessary.

Pes Anserine Bursitis

- Inflammation of the bursa on the medial proximal tibia where the sartorius, gracilis, and semitendinosus muscles insert.

- Caused by acute trauma, infection, or complications from OA, RA, or gout in the knee, as well as overuse and a lower extremity biomechanical fault. Diagnosis can be confirmed with MRI.
- Treatment same as earlier listing.

Popliteal Cyst (Baker Cyst)

- Inflammation of the gastrocnemius-semimembranosus bursa which is located on the posterior aspect of the knee. May be correlated with meniscus tears.
- Diagnosis can be confirmed with MRI.
- Treatment same as earlier listings.

Patellar Subluxation

- Occurs when the patella slides out of the trochlea laterally and temporarily.
- The patient may be asymptomatic, or if the condition progresses, could lead to patellar dislocation. Usually, there is discomfort with activity, pain around the sides of the patella, sensations of the knee buckling, the patella slipping or catching, and pain with sitting, stiffness, crepitus, swelling.
- Cause is usually multifactorial but often includes anatomic abnormality in the trochlea which can be observed with X-rays.
- Intervention includes physical therapy for strengthening, bracing, neuromuscular reeducation, and in severe cases, surgery consisting of medial patellofemoral ligament reconstruction.
- Reconstruction of the medial patellofemoral ligament for painful patellar subluxation in distal torsional malalignment: A case report

Meniscus Tear

- Traumatic or degenerative condition of the medial and/or lateral meniscus of the knee.

Traumatic injuries usually include a WB and rotation mechanism. Depending on the location and shape of the tear, they can be classified as bucket handle, flap, and radial.

- Clinical presentation includes a history of mechanical catching or locking in the knee, joint line tenderness, pain with knee hyperextension, and maximum passive knee flexion. Pain or clicking. There may be stiffness, swelling, and a sensation of the knee giving way as well. X-ray and MRI can assist diagnosis.

- Interventions include physical therapy and possible arthroscopic surgery.

MCL

- Trauma caused to the medial knee ligament by external force to the leg or rotational trauma.

- The patient presents with pain and laxity with valgus stress test at 30 degrees of knee flexion. There is medial knee swelling with possible locking or catching and tenderness over the ligament. Diagnosis can be aided with MRI.

- Treatment includes physical therapy, ice, anti-inflammatory modalities, compression, NSAID, and possibly bracing depending on severity. Surgery is usually not necessary.

LCL

- Usually traumatic injury resulting from pressure pushing the knee medial to lateral into varus

- Knee swelling lateral with possible locking or catching of the knee and pain and tenderness over the ligament, knee may give way and positive varus stress test at 30 degrees of knee flexion

- Treatment includes physical therapy, ice, anti-inflammatory modalities, compression, NSAIDs, and possibly bracing depending on severity. Surgery is usually not necessary.

ACL

- An acute contact or non-contact injury to the knee, usually involving hyper-extension or rotation with rapid effusion occurring in less than 2 hours, an inability to continue to play sports, knee instability, and a positive lachman and lateral shift test. The reporting of an audible pop increases the likelihood of an ACL injury.

- A-P radiographs are used to rule out fracture and dislocation, and an MRI to provide confirmation.

- Interventions vary depending on the activity level of the patient from conservative to surgical. After surgical intervention, there is usually a 6–9-month rehabilitation process.

PCL

- An injury affecting men more than women, resulting from a direct blow to the front of the knee, such as a bent knee hitting the dashboard in a car crash.

- Patient presentation includes pain with swelling that occurs relatively quickly after injury and may cause a limp, difficulty walking, and an unstable knee that gives way. X-ray and MRI can aid in diagnosis.

- Intervention depends on the activity level of the patient and may range from conservative to surgical. Conservative care begins with immobilization and RICE principles followed by physical therapy for motion and strengthening. Surgical recovery normally includes a 6–9 month rehabilitation process.

Patellar Fracture

- An injury to the patella caused by a direct blow such as a fall or MVA (motor vehicle accident). It is an uncommon fracture comprising only 1% of all fractures. The fracture can be classified as stable, displaced, comminuted (three or more pieces) or open.

- Patient presents with pain and swelling in the anterior knee with bruising and an inability to straighten the knee fully or walk. X-ray used to confirm diagnosis.

- Intervention: If the fracture is non-displaced, surgery may be unnecessary, with treatment including casting and splinting and a time period of NWB (non-weight bearing) with crutch use followed by physical therapy. If displaced, the usual intervention is surgery followed by physical therapy.

Knee OA

- Degenerative condition of the knee joint that is characterized by progressive loss of motion and strength as well as pain. Plain radiographs can aid diagnosis. Altman Criteria for knee DJD (degenerative joint disease) includes three or more of the following positives:
  - Age > 50 years
  - Morning stiffness < 30 minutes
  - Crepitus with active knee motion
  - Bony tenderness
  - Bony enlargement
  - No palpable warmth

- Treatment includes acetaminophen, capsaicin, and corticosteroids for pain relief. Physical therapy provides therapeutic exercise, manual therapy, weight management for overweight or obese patients (BMI > 25 kg/m^2) with a goal of losing 5% of their body weight, as well as aquatic therapy and assistive devices to aid ambulation. In severe cases, joint replacement surgery may be indicated, followed by physical therapy and rehabilitation.

Medial Tibial Stress Syndrome (MTSS) (Shin Splints)

- Overuse injury caused by repetitive stress and injury to the anterior shin area. It is multifactorial and may involve tendinopathy, periostitis, stress reaction of the tibia, dysfunction of the tibialis posterior, tibialis anterior and/or soleus muscles. Stress fractures may need to be ruled out if symptoms persist using X-ray, bone scan, or MRI.

- Patient presents with vague and diffuse pain and tenderness to palpation along the middle and distal tibia, which is associated with exertion and activity. Seen commonly in runners who log > 20 miles per week.

- Treatment involves activity modification and assessment of possible training errors, as well as muscle imbalances, inflexibility, foot pronation, and weakness. RICE (rest, ice, compression, elevation), physical therapy for strengthening and education on footwear, possible orthotics and balance training. In severe cases, a posterior fasciotomy may be performed.

Ottawa Knee Rules

- With a history of recent trauma, the presence of one positive finding indicates the need to order radiographs
  - Age is 55 years and more
  - Isolated tenderness of the patella
  - Tenderness of the fibular head
  - Inability to flex the knee to 90 degrees
  - Inability to WB both immediately after injury and in the ED for 4 steps

Hip

Legg-Calve-Perthes Disease

- Osteonecrosis of the femoral head epiphysis in children less than 15 years of age with boys being affected four times more than girls. Etiology is not completely understood but there is an association with passive smoking, small stature, skeletal retardation, and low birth weight.

- Patient presents with limping, pain, and stiffness in the hip, groin, thigh, or knee, with limited hip ROM. Diagnosis is confirmed with X-ray, MRI, and bone scan.

- Interventions include physical therapy, especially in children under 6 years of age, for stretching, activity limitation, and gait training with emphasis on avoiding WB. If pain is severe, bed rest and traction may be indicated, as well as leg casting. In individuals greater than 6–8 years of age, surgery may be recommended and include contracture release, joint realignment, and removal of excess bone or loose bodies. Pain medication is provided and physical therapy when cleared by the physician.

Intertrochanteric Fracture

- A fracture occurring between the greater and lesser trochanters of the femur. There are 252,000 hip fractures in the United States each year. Affects women twice as often as men, especially in those older than 60 years. Typical mechanism is a fall with a history of osteoporosis. There is a 20–30% mortality rate in the first year after a fracture in the elderly. Can also occur in younger male patients in high-force injuries. Patient presents with pain and decreased ability to bear weight and move the involved limb. AP radiographs of the pelvis and hip, frog lateral views, traction AP, or CT will confirm diagnosis.

- Intervention includes ORIF, followed by rehabilitation unless severe arthritis is present, in which case a THA may be recommended. In the younger population, surgery will be followed by a course of physical therapy.

Hip Dislocation

- Traumatic injury to the hip such as an MVA or fall. Posterior dislocations occur 90% of the time with the patient presenting with the knee and foot medially rotated.

- Patient presents in extreme pain with an inability to move the leg. If a nerve has been injured, there may be a loss of sensation as well.

- Intervention: In the ED, the MD will administer anesthetic and manipulate or reduce the hip. This will be followed by another set of X-rays or CT to rule out fracture. Osteonecrosis is also a complication.

- Normally a 2–3 month recovery with physical therapy focusing on assisted walking, hip motion, and strengthening.

Hip Impingement

- Pain in the hip or groin stemming from multiple causes including intra-articular loose bodies, labral injuries, or bony anomalies (cam or pincer deformity). Usually seen in younger to middle ages individuals and athletes.

- Patient presents with groin and/or hip pain, which is worse with hip flexion and medial rotation and may be worse with walking. Complaints are of a sharp pinching pain with twisting and squatting and sometimes a dull ache. X-rays, CT, and MRI can identify lesions in the hip contributing to the impingement.

- Intervention includes activity changes, NSAID, and physical therapy to address muscle imbalances and provide modalities. If conservative treatment fails, arthroscopic debridement may be performed followed by physical therapy.

Groin Strain

- An injury to the hip adductors that is usually traumatic, involving excessive hip abduction. The adductor longus is the most commonly strained hip adductor muscle.

- The patient presents with pain and tenderness in the groin and inner thigh, pain with active hip adduction, as well as possible popping or snapping. X-rays and MRI can confirm the diagnosis and rule out other potential diagnoses.

- Interventions include ice, compression, anti-inflammatory medications and pain medication, stretching, soft tissue mobilization, and physical therapy for stretching and strengthening

Sports Hernia (Athletic Pubalgia, Sportsman's Hernia)

- Overuse syndrome affecting the muscles that attach to the pubic bones, such as the abdominal obliques, hip adductors, and rectus abdominis.

- Commonly caused by planting and twisting motions in sports such as ice hockey, soccer and football, and wrestling. The symptoms typically get better with rest but then return.

- Patient presents with severe pain in the groin, which is increased during sit-up maneuvers and active use of the hip adductors. Tissue damage can be confirmed by an MRI.

- Interventions include rest for 7–10 days and physical therapy to improve strength and flexibility. Anti-inflammatory medication is usually prescribed. In severe and persistent cases, open or endoscopic surgery may be performed, followed by approximately 3 months of rehabilitation.

Shoulder

Labrum Tear

- Damage to the fibrocartilagenous ring around the glenoid. Typically injured by either acute trauma (fall, direct blow, sudden pull, or a violent overhead reach) or by repetitive micro-trauma to the joint. Tears can be superior (SLAP +/− involvement of the biceps tendon) or inferior (Bankart lesion).

- The patient presents with shoulder pain, and often catching, locking, popping, grinding, occasional night pain, a sense of instability, and limited ROM and strength. CT or MRI with contrast can be used to aid diagnosis, with the gold standard being arthroscopic surgery.

- Interventions include anti-inflammatory medication, rest, activity modification, and physical therapy for mobility and strengthening. With a lack of improvement, arthroscopic surgery may be recommended, followed by a period of immobilization and physical therapy.

AC Joint Injury/Dislocation

- An injury sustained by direct force to the acromioclavicular joint, usually caused by a fall directly onto the point of the shoulder or a fall onto an outstretched hand. Five times more common in men than women.

- The patient presents with pain at the superior-anterior aspect of the shoulder with swelling and point tenderness. There may be a loss of motion and pain with resisted testing of the muscles around the shoulder. Depending on the severity of the injury, there may be a displacement between the clavicle and acromion. Diagnosis is aided with standard GH radiographs, which also rule out corocoid fracture.

- Intervention is usually non-operative for 3 months, except in severe cases, with brief immobilization, ice, and oral analgesics, followed by physical therapy for mobility exercise and strengthening over the next 6–12 weeks.

If symptoms persist, surgery may be indicated, including instrumentation, distal clavicle excision, reconstruction, or suture fixation.

Subacromial Pain (Subacromial Impingement)

- Refers to compression of subacromial structures between the coracoacromial arch and the humerus. The most common cause of shoulder pain. May be related to a bony anomaly, rotator cuff weakness, impaired scapular motion and stability, and poor posture.

- The patient presents with shoulder pain during elevation of the arm.

- Intervention includes physical therapy to reduce pain and improve function as well as provide exercise to the rotator cuff and patient education. Oral analgesics and corticosteroid injections may also be provided by the MD.

Rotator Cuff (RTC) Injury

- The RTC is the primary stabilizer of the glenohumeral joint. When injured, there is little potential for spontaneous healing. The RTC can be injured through trauma or from repetitive overuse and gradual degradation. Injuries are classified as small to massive with large tears being > 3 cm, and as partial thickness or full thickness (complete) tears.

- The patient presents with shoulder pain that may radiate down the lateral aspect of the arm, usually not past the elbow. There is limited and painful ROM. Pain may be particularly intense at night when lying on the affected shoulder. There is weakness, +/− crepitus, and snapping. Plain radiographs, US, MRI, and MRI-arthrography aid in diagnosis.

- Interventions include physical therapy, activity modification, strengthening, steroid injections. Acute or chronic partial thickness tears often improve with conservative management. If symptoms persist, surgery may be indicated, followed by a lengthy rehabilitation course. There is a high failure rate for RTC repairs at 5 years.

Adhesive Capsulitis (Frozen Shoulder)

- A disease process of the shoulder that causes glenohumeral capsular thickening. It is classified as either primary, which has an unknown cause, or secondary, which is often caused by immobilization after an injury or mastectomy. More likely in women over 40 years of age who have been immobilized, have DM, cardiovascular disease, a thyroid condition, TB, or Parkinson's disease.

- Patient presentation varies depending on which of three stages they are within. Stage 1 lasts 1–3 months and is characterized by progressive pain with little to no motion loss and is often misdiagnosed. Stage 2 lasts 3–9 months and is characterized by less pain but diminishing shoulder motion and increased stiffness. Stage 3 occurs from 9–14 months and ROM begins to improve. It is primarily a clinical diagnosis, but X-rays and MRI may help to rule out other diagnoses.

- Interventions include over-the-counter pain medications, anti-inflammatory medications, steroid injections, joint distension, physical therapy, shoulder manipulation under anesthesia, TENs, and rarely surgery to remove scar tissue.

Glenohumeral Osteoarthritis (GH OA)

- A progressive degenerative condition of the glenohumeral joint affecting mainly older adults.

- The patient presents with progressive pain and stiffness which may interfere with sleep. Pain is over the joint line, as well as anterior and/or posterior. There is restricted shoulder motion with pain, +/− crepitus. Differential diagnosis includes RTC tear and RA. Plain radiographs help to confirm the diagnosis and can visualize joint space, osteophytes, and sclerosis, as well as bone cysts.

- Interventions include medications such as NSAIDs and tramadol and physical therapy to maintain and improve ROM and strength. If conservative treatment fails, surgery may include a TSA, hemiarthroplasty, humeral head resurfacing, or a reverse TSA. In less severe cases, arthroscopic debridement may be performed. After surgery, there is a period of immobilization, followed by rehabilitation.

Wrist and Hand

Distal Radius Fracture

- The radius is the most commonly fractured bone in the body. Fractures are usually caused by a fall onto an outstretched hand. Fractures can be intra-articular, extra-articular, open, comminuted, or Colles. Risk factors include osteoporosis and age > 60, but fractures can occur in healthy bones with enough force.

- Patient presents with immediate pain, tenderness, bruising, swelling, and possible deformity. X-ray is diagnostic.

- Intervention includes casting up to 6 weeks if boney alignment is preserved. If the fracture is displaced, it must be reduced and then casted. If the damage is severe enough, surgery is recommended with instrumentation or an external fixator. After immobilization, physical therapy is prescribed for restoration of motion, strength, and function. Full recovery may take more than 1 year.

Avascular Necrosis/Scaphoid Fracture/ Hamate Fracture

- **Avascular Necrosis (Osteonecrosis)**

  1. Death of bone from an interruption in blood supply. Variable history of trauma and tenderness at the scaphoid or lunate (Keinbock's disease). Diagnosed with radiography or MRI.

  2. Patient presents with pain and swelling at the base of the thumb, usually after a fracture or dislocation.

  3. Intervention may be conservative but is usually surgical with immobilization for as long as 6 months. Physical or occupational therapy assist in return of motion, strength, and function.

- **Scaphoid Fracture**

  1. Usually a history of trauma from a fall on an outstretched hand. Represents 71% of all carpal bone fractures and 2–9% suffer avascular necrosis. Occurs usually in younger adults.

  2. The patient presents with tenderness at the anatomic snuffbox and limited motion and strength in the hand and wrist. Radiograph with a scaphoid view is diagnostic.

  3. Intervention includes immobilization or, depending on severity, surgery followed by immobilization. Therapy is prescribed for restoration of ROM, strength, and function.

- **Hamate Fracture**

  1. Stress fracture from repetitive trauma or blunt trauma from swinging a bat, club, or racquet.

2. Patient presents with pain and tenderness 1 cm distal to the flexion crease of the wrist and swelling. Grip is weak and there is occasionally an ulnar or median neuropathy. There is often pain with resisted flexion of the fourth and fifth digit. X-ray is initially performed, but if negative, an MRI may be performed. Differential diagnosis includes TFCC tears and ligamentous injuries.

3. Intervention: If diagnosed quickly, conservative treatment, including casting, can be successful. If diagnosis is delayed or the fracture is displaced, surgery may be necessary, including removal of the hook of the hamate, followed by immobilization and rehabilitation.

Ligament Strain

- Usually occurs as a result of a fall onto an outstretched hand. Up to 2% of patients diagnosed as having a sprained wrist have a more significant injury.

- Patient presents with swelling, pain with movement, possible bruising or discoloration, tenderness, popping, and warmth over the injured ligament. X-rays and CT may be used to rule out fracture.

- Intervention for grade I sprains may include rest, or rest and splinting, for approximately 1 week, followed by a gradual return to activity. For moderate to severe strains, treatment includes immobilization, followed by a course of rehabilitation. In very severe cases, surgery may be required to repair the torn ligament, followed by rehabilitation, which may take several months.

De Quervain's Tenosynovitis

- Painful inflammation of the extensor pollicis brevis and/or abductor pollicis longus, usually related to repetitive overuse. Risk factors include being female with a history of inflammatory arthritis or RA (rheumatoid arthritis), being 30–50 years of age, and pregnancy.

- The patient presents with swelling and pain near the base of the thumb, which can spread up the forearm. Clinical diagnosis is aided by the Finkelstein test.

- Interventions attempt to reduce inflammation and pain and include pain relievers, corticosteroid injections, immobilization, activity modification, ice, PT or OT, and surgery in very serious cases.

Carpal Tunnel Syndrome

- Increased pressure in the carpal tunnel resulting in mechanical compression and ischemia to the median nerve. More common in women and in those with DM, inflammatory conditions such as RA, pregnancy, thyroid disorders, kidney failure, obesity, menopause, and workplace factors such as repetitive wrist and hand movements. There is eventual hand weakness. Diagnosis is aided by NCV (Nerve conduction velocity) and EMG (Electromyography).

- Patient presents with pain, numbness, and tingling in the median nerve distribution of the hand. Symptoms are often increased with upper limb tension testing, as well as the Phalen's test and the reverse Phalen's test. There is often a positive flick sign.

- Interventions include splinting and therapy for exercise, modalities, corticosteroids, therapeutic US, corticosteroid injections, nocturnal hand braces, and ergonomic workstation modifications. In severe cases, surgery may be necessary, followed by PT or OT.

Deformities: Boutonniere Deformity, Mallet Finger, & Swan Neck Deformity

- Boutonniere deformity: Caused by damage to the central slip of extensor tendon and is characterized by disfigurement and impaired function due to hyperextension of the DIP and flexion of the PIP. Treat with splinting initially (within 6 weeks) and then surgery to reconstruct the proximal and distal joints. Therapy is beneficial both before and after surgery.

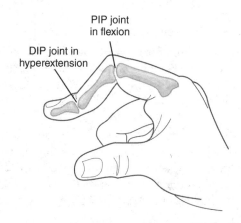

- Mallet finger: Disruption of the terminal extensor tendon, usually from a forceful blow to the tip of the finger. Often seen in athletes. Fracture must be ruled out in the DIP. Patient presents with an extensor lag of the distal IP joint. Treated with splinting in hypertextension approximately 6 weeks. Surgery is controversial but may be the only option with open injuries and with large avulsion fragments.

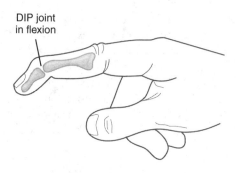

- Swan neck: Deformity consists of hyperextension of the PIP and flexion of the DIP joints. It is the result of excessive extension force, posttraumatic wrist or MP joint flexion contractures, tightness of intrinsic muscles, chronic volar subluxation, or degeneration of the volar structures of PIP joint. There is usually a history of prior injury. If inflammatory arthritis or autoimmune synovitis or RA is suspected, the patient is referred to a rheumatologist. Radiography is performed to rule out fracture. If only a mild deformity is present, a splint can be used. Otherwise, surgery is indicated, ranging from soft tissue procedures to FDS tenodesis, after which therapy is prescribed.

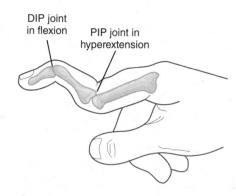

Trigger Finger (Stenosing Tenosynovitis)

- Etiology is unclear, but the condition is more common in women and in those with DM, and those whose work requires repetitive gripping.

- The patient presents with stiffness which is worse in the morning, painful snapping of the affected finger with movement, and tenderness.

There may be an inability to straighten the finger or locking.

- Interventions include splinting, NSAIDs, corticosteroids, injections, rest, ice or heat, and stretching. In severe cases, percutaneous or open surgery is indicated, followed by rehabilitation.

Dupuytren's Contracture

- Fibroproliferative condition of the hand that affects older patients, causing a digital flexion contracture. The prevalence varies but typically affects elderly men of northern European descent.

- The patient presents with a thickening of the palmar skin and a nodule in the early stages. As the condition progresses, a cord develops that gradually contracts and pulls the MCP and PIP joint into flexion. Commonly affects the ring and little fingers and can be bilateral.

- Intervention is almost always surgical when function is impeded or the deformity is disabling. Fasciotomy is usually performed in an outpatient setting; rarely is a digital amputation performed if an irreversible joint contracture is present. Prognosis is good and many patients never develop contracture.

Degenerative Joint Disease (DJD)

- Inflammation and degradation of the distal and proximal IP joints. Predominantly affects postmenopausal women and the elderly.

- Patient presents with pain, stiffness, heat, redness and swelling, a loss of motion, and eventual loss of function in the involved fingers and hand. There is decreased grip strength, and Heberden (DIP) or Bouchard nodes (PIP) may be present. X-ray is the gold standard, but MRI and US can be used as well as lab values.

- Intervention includes controlling pain and inflammation, activity modification, splinting, ice, heat, joint injection. If symptoms are persistent, referral to a hand surgeon is indicated. Surgery is usually reconstructive, followed by rest and splinting for 4–6 weeks, followed by therapy for 4–8 weeks.

Osteomyelitis

- Pyogenic bone infection (frequently *Staphylococcus aureus*) that can occur in any bone usually after penetrating trauma. Risk factors include DM, sickle cell disease, HIV, RA, intravenous drug use, alcoholism, long-term steroid use, hemodialysis, poor circulation, and recent injury.

- Patient presents with redness, warmth, inflammation, stiffness, pus drainage, loss of ROM, +/− fever or chills. The gold standard for diagnosis is bone biopsy, but X-ray, MRI, and CT may be used.

- Interventions include antibiotic therapy and possibly the need to drain the infection or debride the dead bone or other surrounding tissue. Therapy may be beneficial once cleared by the MD.

Ganglion Cyst

- 1–2 cm cystic structures that are more commonly seen on the dorsal aspect of the wrist, particularly over the scapholunate ligament. The origin is unknown but may theoretically be related to acute or chronic stress, allowing leakage of synovial fluid.

- Patient presents with a firm cystic structure in the wrist with no warmth or erythema. Often accompanied by aching that may radiate up the arm. There is tenderness with activity or palpation and decreased ROM and grip strength. If the ulnar or median nerve is compressed, paresthesia may be present. X-rays are usually not indicated.

- Interventions with variable success include repeated pressure on the cyst or cyst removal with an incision or aspiration.

Raynaud's Phenomenon

- Recurrent, long-lasting, and episodic vasospasm of the fingers and toes, often associated with exposure to cold. Risk factors include associated diseases such as scleroderma, lupus, occupations with vibration, exposure to smoking, and medications that affect blood vessels. Prevalence is increased in women, cold climates, and in those with a family history. Age, thin body type, and underlying cardiovascular disease may also be associated with this disease.

- Patient presents with typical episodes of pallor in the digits followed by rubor (cyanosis may be present in severe disease). They may complain of cold or throbbing in the digits. Diagnosis is aided by capillaroscopy. If a secondary disease process is suspected, an antinuclear antibody or ESR test may be performed.

- Intervention includes pharmacological medications that promote vasodilation (calcium channel antagonists), smoking cessation, avoidance and coping of emotional stress, decreasing cold exposure, and improved clothing and measures to protect the skin.

Pelvis and Sacrum

Ankylosing Spondylitis

- Inflammatory arthritis primarily affecting the spine and SI joints. Affects men > women and usually begins in early adulthood. Hereditary and genetic factors such as HLA-B27 may be risk factors. Complications may include uveitis and compression fractures, as well as spinal vertebrae fusing.
- The patient presents with progressive stiffening of spine and thorax, and pain in the lower back and hips, especially in the morning and after activity. As the disease progresses, a rigid thoracolumbar kyphosis and stooped posture may be noticed. X-rays may aid diagnosis, showing a "bamboo spine," as well as lab tests.
- Interventions include medications such as tumor necrosis factor, and physical therapy for stretching and strengthening.

Lumbar Spine

Degenerative Lumbar Disc Disease

- Discogenic low back pain (LBP) is the most common type of chronic LBP.
- Patient presents with deep and dull low-grade midline back ache that may radiate into the gluteal area and rarely to the knees and lower legs. The pain worsens with prolonged sitting and axial loading and sometimes with prolonged standing. Symptoms increase with bending, twisting, and lifting. There is usually no sensory or motor loss, but in severe cases or during acute exacerbations there may be numbness and tingling. MRI is the most commonly used method of diagnosis, but discography is the gold standard.
- Interventions include activity modification, heat and ice, patient education, physical therapy for flexibility, and lumbar stabilization exercises. Medications include NSAIDs and epidural steroid injections. If symptoms fail to improve, lumbar fusion is the most common surgical intervention, but lumbar disc replacements are beginning to become more popular. Rehabilitation follows the surgical interventions.

Radiculopathy

- Pain secondary to compression or inflammation of a spinal nerve(s). May be referred to as sciatic type pain. May be caused by herniated lumbar disc, stenosis, or trauma.
- The patient presents with pain that often radiates from the back into the lower limb and may include numbness, electric type symptoms, paresthesia, and myotomal muscle weakness. Pain may increase with coughing, sneezing, or straining. Clinical examination may reveal a positive straight leg raise test (SLR), altered reflexes and sensory deficits. Diagnostic tests include radiographs, EMG, MRI, and CT Scan.
- Interventions include physical therapy, pain and anti-inflammatory medication, as well as spinal injections. If there is a lack of improvement after 6–8 weeks, surgical intervention such as a laminectomy, discectomy, or microdiscectomy may be considered. These procedures have high success rates and are generally followed by a period of healing and then progressive rehabilitation.

Abdominal Aortic Aneurysm (AAA)

- Dilation of the abdominal aorta. Classified by size. Small is 4 cm or less and is usually observed by MD. Medium aneurysm is 4–5.3 cm, and if so, the physician may continue to observe the aneurysm or perform surgery. Large is 5.6 or growing more than 0.5 cm every 6 months. This is treated surgically. A ruptured abdominal aorta carries an 80% mortality rate. Risk factors include men > 60 years of age, smoking, and family history of AAA and atherosclerosis.
- This is a rare finding in the orthopedic setting and most of these patients do not have symptoms. However, some people present with a pulsating feeling near their navel, deep and constant pain in the abdomen or side of the abdomen, with back pain. Clinically, there may be an alteration of pulse that can be detected with a stethoscope. Diagnosis is confirmed with abdominal US, CT scan, or MRI.
- Intervention is a medical referral to a cardiologist.

Spinal Stenosis

- Narrowing of the spinal canal or nerve root foramen. The narrowing can be congenital or part of a degenerative condition of the joint surrounding the spine and transverse foramen. The symptoms may intensify if there is a concomitant disc herniation, further narrowing the foramen for the nerves. Can mimic vascular insufficiency. This is the most common cause for lumbar surgery in the United States.

- The patient presents with pain in the lower back, buttock, thigh which may be unilateral or bilateral. The pain may be claudicating in nature and is usually worse with extension activities such as standing and walking, and is relieved with sitting or laying down in a hook-lying position. Paresthesia may accompany the pain and there may be LE weakness.

- Intervention includes pain and anti-inflammatory medication (NSAIDs) and referral for physical therapy for education, flexibility, and lumbar stabilization training. If conservative measures fail, lumbar surgery may be indicated, with the most popular being a decompressive laminectomy.

Spondylolisthesis

- Occurs when a superior vertebra slides forward over the vertebra below it. It may be caused by disc degeneration, which results in a loss of intervertebral disc height, from traumatic fracture or stress fracture to the pars interarticularis, an anatomic anomaly, or from joint damage as a result of infection or arthritis. In the aging adult, the overall incidence is 8.7% with the L4–5 level being most affected. In the older adult, the symptoms are similar to spinal stenosis.

- In degenerative conditions, the patient is older but the typical presentation is a child or teenager who is active in sports. They complain of lower back pain with sharp pain, +/− paresthesia, and neurogenic claudication into one or both LEs. The pain is worse with walking, standing, and when they bend over or twist and play sports. In rare cases, bowel and bladder function may become impaired. X-ray, MRI, and CT scan are common diagnostically.

- Interventions include pain medication, NSAIDs, steroid injections, and physical therapy which include hamstring stretching and lumbar flexibility, and strengthening exercises, as well as a bracing/lumbar corset. Conservative measures are usually successful, but if they fail, surgical options include laminectomy and spinal fusion, followed by rehabilitation.

Cauda Equina Syndrome

- The most frequent cause of a neurologic disability syndrome. It involves urinary, defecation, and sexual function. Caused by the compression of the sacral nerve roots inside the lumbosacral vertebral canal from tumor, infection, fracture, or stenosis. Overall incidence is 1 in 33,000 to 1 in 100,000. Occurs in 2% of all lumbar disc herniations.

- Patient presents with low back pain with bilateral sciatica, saddle anesthesia, and bilateral LE motor weakness, and often gait abnormalities. There are variable rectal and urinary tract complaints.

- Interventions include medical referral and usually surgery (laminectomy) to decompress the nerve roots, followed by rehabilitation when cleared by the physician.

Clinical Lumbar Instability

- Benign joint hypermobility syndrome, characterized by an inability to control the lumbar spine at a segmental level.

- Patient presents as a younger individual (up to 4th decade) with complaints of clicking, crunching, or clunking in the low back. The pain usually remains in the lumbar region and is intermittent and at a mild to moderate level. Exam is clinically based and includes joint mobility testing and ROM testing (Gower's sign), as well as a positive score on the Beighton scale. A Gower's sign is observed when the patient flexes forward and then pushes him/herself upright using their hands on their thighs. X-rays are usually negative but may be used in conjunction with MRI to rule out other diagnoses.

- Intervention includes physical therapy, with emphasis on education, ergonomics, and lumbar stabilization. Anti-inflammatory and pain medication may be used during exacerbations. Depending on the degree of instability, outcomes of conservative treatment are generally good.

Thoracic Spine

Rib Dysfunction: Costochondritis

- Refers to inflammation of the cartilage connecting the ribs to the sternum, most often the second to fifth ribs. The condition usually affects people older than 40 years, and in the majority of cases more than one site is affected. Women have a higher incidence than men. Due to the chest wall pain, heart conditions are a differential diagnosis.

- Patient usually complains of chest wall pain with an insidious onset, but may have a history of an injury to the chest, physical strain using the pectoralis muscles, arthritis, or infection including tuberculosis. The pain may be sharp, aching, or give a feeling of pressure that worsens with deep breathing or coughing. There is tenderness to palpation over the sternocostal junction, and swelling may be present. The diagnosis is clinical, but imaging may be performed to rule out other conditions.

- Interventions include NSAIDs, corticosteroid injections, narcotics, antidepressants such as amitriptyline, and anti-seizure drugs such as gabapentin. Physical therapy provides stretching and modalities such as TENS, heat, and ice. The condition often improves over several weeks.

Thoracic Disc Herniation

- Bulging or extrusion of the thoracic disc, which incites an inflammatory reaction and may provide compression on thoracic nerve roots and inflame the dura.

- The patient's main complaint is of sharp pain in the thoracic spine, which is exacerbated with coughing or sneezing. Pain may radiate around the chest or into the belly. If the disc herniation is central and encroaches on the spinal canal, there may be signs and symptoms of myelopathy with sensory disturbances at the level of compression, difficulty walking/ataxic gait, abnormal reflexes, decreased proprioception, multi-segmental LE weakness, or bowel and bladder dysfunction. Usually, X-ray is the first imaging performed; however, with the severity of myelopathy an MRI, CT, or myelogram may be performed.

- Interventions include rest, narcotic and non-narcotic analgesic medications, epidural injections, ice packs and physical therapy for gentle exercise, manual therapy, and back strengthening. If conservative treatment fails, surgery is indicated and includes doral laminectomy. In the case of thoracic myelopathy, surgery is the preferred and immediate treatment, and a thoracotomy or costotransversectomy may be performed.

Stress Fracture Ribs

- Common pathology in rowers and in other sports with repetitive and vigorous shoulder motion, such as baseball. Low bone mineral density, as well as poor diet, amenorrhea, poor mechanics during athletics, and changes in training are risk factors. Occurs most frequently with the first rib. Can also occur traumatically.

- The patient presents with a gradual onset of pain in the side of the neck and upper back or back of the shoulder. The pain is worse with activity and better with rest. Pain worsens with deep breaths and coughing, as well as overhead activity. They may feel a popping, snapping, or grinding sensation in the area of the involved rib, as well as tenderness. Diagnosis is confirmed with X-ray, bone scan, MRI, or CT scan.

Shingles

- Varicella zoster virus (VZV) is a neurotropic herpes virus that infects nearly all humans. The primary infection causes chickenpox, after which the virus becomes dormant in the cranial nerve ganglia, dorsal root ganglia, and autonomic ganglia. Risk factors include individuals older than 50 years, those with diseases that weaken the immune system (HIV, cancer), those undergoing radiation or chemotherapy, and those taking medications that weaken the immune system, such as after an organ transplant.

- The patient presents with pain, burning, numbness, tingling and sensitivity to touch, followed by a red rash that begins a few days after the pain and may follow a single dermatome around the right or left torso. Fluid filled blisters break open and crust over, causing itching. Some patients will also experience fever, headache, fatigue, and sensitivity to light. Skin lesions may resolve in a week, but the pain can last up to 6 weeks. Complications include post-herpetic neuralgia, vision loss, neurologic issues, and skin infections.

- Preventative interventions include vaccines. This disease is particularly dangerous for anyone with a weak immune system, newborns, and pregnant women. Treatment includes anti-viral medication and for pain: Capsaicin cream, lidocaine gel, gabapentin, tricyclic antidepressants, codeine, corticosteroids, and local anesthetics. Modalities such as TENS and MH may provide temporary relief.

Scoliosis

- Three-dimensional deformation of the spine. The cause is multifactorial, including genetic predisposition, abnormal spinal growth, connective tissue disease, CP, MD, and birth defects. Scoliosis can also be acquired by habitually maintaining poor posture. Affects 3% of the population, and the girl:boy ratio is 8:1. Symptoms usually occur in the 9–15 age bracket. The curvature can be in the shape of a "C," or if a compensatory curve is present, in the shape of an "S." In severe scoliosis, the rib cage may press on the lungs and heart.

- The patient presents with back pain, which may be intermittent or constant and is usually dull and achy in nature. There is asymmetry in the height of the shoulders and waist, usually with a leg length discrepancy. A rib hump is present, with forward flexion of the trunk.

- Conservative treatment is generally successful and includes outpatient physical therapy, exercise, electrical stimulation, traction, postural training, manual therapy, and bracing (Milwaukee brace). In severe cases, a spinal fusion with instrumentation may be performed, followed by a course of physical therapy. For the altered appearance of the spine and asymmetry in shoulders and hip, support groups may be beneficial.

Cervical Spine

Torticollis

- Shortening of the sternocleidomastoid muscle (SM) on one side, leading to an ipsilateral side flexion and contralateral rotation of the head. Non-muscular causes contribute to over 18% of torticollis cases. These causes include tumor, syringomyelia, Klippel-Feil syndrome, ocular deficiency, and infection. Affects 1:250 live births.

- The patient presents with an abnormal head posture, with pain, stiffness, and tightness in the SCM muscle. Myofascial pain may radiate into the cranium, producing a headache. There is limited ROM in contralateral side flexion and ipsilateral rotation and decreased flexibility in the SCM muscle. Medical referral is indicated to assure that the cause is muscular in nature.

- If the cause is muscular in nature, pain medication, muscle relaxers, and/or anti-inflammatory medications are prescribed with physical therapy for postural education, possible bracing, modalities, stretching, manual therapy, and exercise. If a non-muscular cause of torticollis is found, the underlying condition is treated medically. Physical therapy and bracing may occur simultaneously.

Acute Disc Herniation/Radiculopathy

- Bulging or extrusion of the cervical disc, which incites an inflammatory reaction and may provide compression on cervical nerve roots and inflame the dura. Can occur over time from cervical degeneration or habitually poor posture, or more acutely from an injury such as whiplash.

- The patient presents with neck pain that is sharp initially but may become dull over time. There is often tingling and paresthesia in the fingers or hand, with UE weakness and a loss of sensation. The pain is worse with certain neck motions, especially quick motions, but is better at rest. Radiographs are typically performed, but MRIs and CT scans are more diagnostic, and an EMG is used if neural involvement in the UE is suspected.

- Interventions include NSAIDs, corticosteroids, steroid injections, soft cervical collars, and physical therapy for modalities, including traction, stretching, and neck strengthening. Conservative treatment is often successful, but surgery may be indicated in severe cases (laminectomy and fusion).

Spinal Stenosis

- Narrowing of the spinal canal or nerve root foramen. The narrowing can be congenital or part of a degenerative condition (OA) of the joint surrounding the spine and transverse foramen. Occasionally caused by herniated discs, thickened ligaments, tumors, and vertebral fractures as well. Usually occurs in patients older than 50 years of age.

- Patient presents with neck pain and stiffness, +/− paresthesia, and numbness. There is often weakness in the neck and bilateral UEs. If the stenosis is central, cervical myelopathy may occur and cause issues in the LEs with weakness, decreased balance, coordination, and incontinence. Radiographs, MRIs, and CTs are diagnostic.

- Interventions include NSAIDs, muscle relaxants, anti-depressants for chronic pain, anti-seizure drugs, opioids, and steroid injections. Physical therapy is used for education, as well as modalities, including traction, MH, TENS, manual techniques, and exercise for strength and flexibility. If conservative treatment fails, surgery is indicated usually in the form of laminectomy.

Rheumatoid Arthritis (RA)

- A chronic progressive inflammatory condition affecting the synovium and joints. Although mainly seen in the hand, wrist, and extremities, it can affect the cervical spine. Of particular concern is that it can lead to upper cervical instability and atlanto-axial subluxation, which can be a life-threatening condition and cause symptoms of cervical myelopathy, including spastic gait, balance, and bowel and bladder dysfunction.

- Patient presents with neck pain and limited motion. The pain is generally dull and achy but can become sharp during a period of exacerbation. X-rays can be diagnostic and are used during cervical flexion to assess the integrity of the AA joint. MRI is also commonly used.

- Interventions include cervical fusion if myelopathy is present. Otherwise, cervical collars can provide relief, along with pain and anti-inflammatory medication/injections. Physical therapy can assist with education, pain-relieving modalities, gentle ROM, and strengthening. After the period of exacerbation passes, therapy can become more aggressive.

Concussion

1. Falls under the category of a traumatic brain injury. The effects are usually temporary but complications such as post-concussion syndrome occur and last for weeks to months after the initial injury.

2. Patient presents after a blow to the head, +/− LOC. Complaints often include headaches, problems with concentration, memory, balance, and coordination. Feelings of "being foggy," ringing in the ears, fatigue, nausea, vomiting, slurred speech, sleep disturbance, and sensitivity to light and noise are common. Neurologic exam and cognitive testing should be performed, as well as possible MRI or CT of the brain in severe cases.

3. Interventions include medications for pain, vestibular therapy if balance is affected, optical exam if vision is impaired, including prism glasses, physical therapy for pain, and to address any cervical spine issues that may have occurred simultaneously with the concussion. Once the concussion has resolved, athletes may receive additional therapy and conditioning for return to play.

Elbow

Lateral Epicondylalgia (Tennis Elbow)

- Pain in the region of the lateral epicondyle caused by mechanical overloading and abnormal microvascular response in the extensor carpi radialis longus or brevis muscles, affecting 1–3% of the population.

- Patient presents with pain and tenderness over the lateral epicondyle, which is increased with wrist motion, gripping, and resisted finger extension of the second or third digits. Grip strength is decreased. Often an overuse injury, training error for athletes, or work-related cause (manual labor or prolonged computer use and keyboarding), but some onsets are insidious.

- Interventions include: rest, NSAIDs, extracorporeal shock wave therapy, ultrasound therapy, Botox injections, and corticosteroid injections. Physical therapy provides modalities, stretching, manual techniques including joint mobilization and soft tissue work, strengthening (emphasis on eccentric), ergonomic recommendations and counter-force bracing. Recalcitrant cases may undergo surgical release. More recently, platelet-rich plasma injections have shown promise in the treatment of lateral epicondylalgia. Cervical spine should be ruled out as contributing to symptoms.

Medial Epicondylalgia (Golfer's Elbow)

- An overuse syndrome characterized by pain at the flexor/pronator tendinous origin (most commonly the flexor carpi radialis and pronator teres muscles) on the medial epicondyle. Ulnar neuropathy is the most common cause of medial elbow pain. Ulnar neuropathy may be present in up to 50% of cases.

- Patient presents as an athlete participating in sports with repetitive valgus stress, flexion, and pronation (e.g., golf), or in occupations that require frequent elbow, wrist, and hand motion. There is pain and tenderness over the medial epicondyle, which often radiates into the forearm. There is decreased grip strength, pain with resisted wrist flexion, limited elbow motion, and in chronic cases, decreased flexibility in the forearm.

- Interventions include prevention and patient education on training errors if athletic, ergonomics if work-related, activity modification, counterforce bracing, massage, stretching, strengthening (eccentric emphasis), rest, ice, ultrasound, NSAIDs, and corticosteroid injection.

Review Questions

1. For which of the following diagnoses are patients most likely to complain of pain on the plantar surface of the foot?
   A. Metatarsal stress fracture
   B. Pes cavus
   C. Pes planus
   D. Morton's neuroma

2. What is the most common cause of heel pain?
   A. Plantar fasciitis
   B. Achilles tendonopathy
   C. Ankle sprain
   D. Compartment syndrome

3. Pain with a standing (weight bearing) heel raise will occur with which of the following diagnoses?
   A. Achilles tendonopathy
   B. Lateral ankle sprain
   C. Compartment syndrome
   D. Medial ankle sprain

4. The following picture shows a foot deformity that is characteristic of which of the following diagnoses?
   A. Compartment syndrome
   B. Diabetes mellitus
   C. Charcot foot
   D. Pes cavus

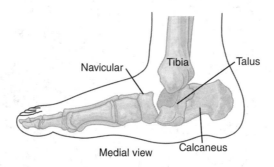

5. Which of the following is true of the Ottawa foot and ankle rules?
   A. Has a high specificity for foot and ankle fractures
   B. Has high sensitivity for foot and ankle fractures
   C. Is specific for fractures of the cuboid bone
   D. Is correlated with decreased foot and ankle ROM

6. Severe uncontrolled pain, swelling, and pain with a history of foot trauma is consistent with which of the following diagnoses?
   A. Pes cavus
   B. Pes planus
   C. Achilles tendonopathy
   D. Compartment syndrome

7. Which of the following is true of a lateral ankle sprain?
   A. Trauma involving an eversion force
   B. Decreased ankle plantar flexion ROM
   C. Treatment may involve an external support initially
   D. Tenderness over the deltoid ligament

8. A traction injury to the tibial tuberosity in adolescents is termed what?
   A. Osgood–Schlatter disease
   B. Prepatellar bursitis
   C. Infrapatellar bursitis
   D. Quadriceps tendonopathy

9. Which of the following knee conditions may require surgery?
   A. Osgood Schlatter disease
   B. Medial tibial stress syndrome
   C. Pes anserine bursitis
   D. Patellar subluxation

10. Pes anserine bursitis:
    A. Describes inflammation of the gastrocnemius-semimembranosus bursa.
    B. Is also known as a Baker's cyst.
    C. Includes the semimembranosus tendon.
    D. Can be caused by an LE biomechanical fault.

11. Swelling on the posterior aspect of the knee:
    A. May be repatellar bursitis.
    B. May be pes anserine bursitis.
    C. May be associated with meniscus tears.
    D. Usually indicates popliteal artery compromise.

12. A patient with a meniscus tear may present with which of the following?
    A. A history of patellar subluxation
    B. Mechanical catching and joint line tenderness
    C. Trauma involving valgus stress to the knee
    D. Trauma involving varus stress to the knee

13. A football player is hit on the lateral side of the right knee while twisting to the left. Which ligament is most likely to be injured?
    A. LCL
    B. MCL
    C. ACL
    D. PCL

14. Which of the following injuries results in rapid and moderate to severe effusion?
    A. LCL
    B. MCL
    C. ACL
    D. Meniscus tear

15. Medial tibial stress syndrome may involve which of the following muscles?
    A. Quadriceps femoris
    B. Gastrocnemius
    C. Soleus
    D. Peroneal brevis

16. Limping and pain in a child's leg of insidious onset may be indicative of what?
    A. Intertrochanteric fracture
    B. Hip dislocation
    C. Legg-Calve-Perthes disease
    D. Hip impingement
17. Which of the following is true of intertrochanteric fractures?
    A. Affects men more than women
    B. Has a 50–60% mortality rate in the first year after the fracture
    C. Primary intervention is ORIF
    D. Carries a 30% chance of re-fracture
18. A patient is involved in an MVA where his knee hits the dashboard of the car. Which of the following are possible injuries?
    A. Anterior hip dislocation
    B. PCL ligament tear
    C. Patellar dislocation
    D. ACL tear
19. Which of the following is true of hip dislocations?
    A. 75% of dislocations are anterior.
    B. With a posterior dislocation, the femoral nerve may be injured.
    C. After a posterior dislocation, the limb is held in full external rotation.
    D. Osteonecrosis is a potential complication.
20. What is the most commonly injured hip adductor muscle?
    A. Adductor magnus
    B. Adductor brevis
    C. Pectineus
    D. Adductor longus
21. A tear to the inferior portion of the shoulder labrum is termed:
    A. A Bankart lesion.
    B. A SLAP tear.
    C. An inferior AC joint strain.
    D. An inverse biceps tear.
22. A patient falling directly on the shoulder with tenderness over the superior-anterior shoulder is present in what?
    A. Subacromial pain syndrome
    B. Rotator cuff strain
    C. AC joint injury
    D. First rib stress fracture
23. Shoulder pain radiating down the lateral side of the humerus to the elbow after a fall on to an out-stretched arm could be caused by what?
    A. Adhesive capsulitis
    B. AC joint strain
    C. RTC tear
    D. Biceps tear

24. Which of the following is true of adhesive capsulitis (frozen shoulder)?

    A. It is correlated with RTC tears.

    B. It is more likely to occur in patients under 30 years of age.

    C. It may take upward of 14 months to resolve.

    D. It is treated with immobilization in the freezing stage.

25. Of the following, which is the most commonly fractured bone in the body?

    A. The scaphoid

    B. The humerus

    C. The ulna

    D. The radius

26. Kienbock's disease refers to what?

    A. Avascular necrosis of the scaphoid bone

    B. Osteonecrosis of the lunate

    C. Partial subluxation of the TFCC

    D. Non-union fracture of the distal radius

27. A patient is being evaluated for a complaint of pain at the base of the thumb. The provider performs a Finkelstein test and the results are positive. This is indicative of which of the following disease processes?

    A. DeQuervain's tenosynovitis

    B. Carpal tunnel syndrome

    C. Ligamentous strain

    D. Trigger finger

28. The picture below depicts which deformity?

    A. Boutonniere deformity

    B. Mallet finger

    C. Swan neck deformity

    D. Subluxed DIP

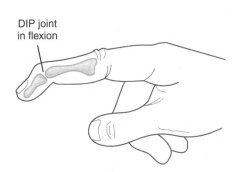

DIP joint in flexion

29. Thickening of the palmar skin of the hand in older adults is termed what?

    A. DeQuervain's tenosynovitis

    B. Trigger finger

    C. Dupuytren's contracture

    D. Swan neck deformity

30. Trigger finger is the layperson's term for:
    A. Dupuytren's contracture.
    B. DeQuervain's tenosynovitis.
    C. Ligamentous strain of the DIP joint.
    D. Stenosing tenosynovitis.

31. Raynaud's phenomenon is associated with which of the following?
    A. Men, cold climates, and a history of hypothyroid
    B. Women, scleroderma, and cold climates
    C. Men, stroke, and DM
    D. Women, sedentary occupation, smoking

32. What is ankylosing spondylitis?
    A. An inflammatory arthritis affecting adolescent girls
    B. An inflammatory arthritis more commonly seen in men
    C. A genetic disease affecting older men
    D. An infective arthritis affecting teenage boys

33. What is the most common type of chronic LBP?
    A. Degenerative lumbar disc disease
    B. Spinal stenosis
    C. Rheumatoid arthritis
    D. Osteoarthritis of the sacroiliac joint

34. Which of the following is associated with lumbar radiculopathy?
    A. Negative SLR
    B. Muscle weakness in particular distribution
    C. Dull achy pain in the back
    D. Usually occurs bilateral

35. Which of the following is true of AAA?
    A. Common cause of LBP in older men
    B. Can cause bilateral LE radicular symptoms in feet and ankles
    C. Surgery recommended even with small aneurysms
    D. Usually asymptomatic

36. The most common cause for lumbar surgery in the United States is:
    A. Spinal tumor.
    B. Ankylosing spondylitis.
    C. Spondylolisthesis.
    D. Spinal stenosis.

37. Which of the following is true of a patient with lumbar spinal stenosis?
    A. Symptoms are improved with standing.
    B. Symptoms are relieved by walking for 15–30 minutes.
    C. Symptoms are worsened by laying on their stomach and pressing upward.
    D. Symptoms are improved when walking bent over a shopping cart.

38. Which of the following lumbar conditions are most likely to occur in adolescents?
    A. Spondylolisthesis
    B. Spinal stenosis
    C. Lumbar disc herniation
    D. Degenerative lumbar disc disease

39. An abnormal gait pattern is associated with which of the following lumbar conditions?
    A. Lumbar instability
    B. Cauda equina syndrome
    C. Spondylolisthesis
    D. AAA

40. A positive Gowers' sign is often found in which of the following conditions?
    A. Lumbar disc herniation
    B. AAA
    C. Lumbar radiculopathy
    D. Clinical lumbar instability

41. Insidious chest wall pain can occur with which of the following?
    A. AAA
    B. C5-6 radiculopathy
    C. Costochondritis
    D. Lumbar facet syndrome

42. Which of the following can cause thoracic pain that may radiate around to the front of the chest?
    A. Thoracic disc herniation
    B. Rib stress fracture
    C. Shingles
    D. All of the above

43. Which of the following is true of scoliosis?
    A. Associated with uneven shoulders, a leg length discrepancy, and rib hump
    B. Usually affects teenage boys and those with birth defects
    C. Onset occurs in women in their third to fourth decade of life
    D. Affects approximately 20% of the population

44. A Milwaukee brace is a conservative treatment for which condition?
    A. Torticollis
    B. Lumbar stenosis
    C. Scoliosis
    D. Thoracic disc herniation

45. Torticollis is a shortening or spasm of which of the following muscles?
    A. Anterior scalene
    B. Subclavius
    C. Latissimus dorsi
    D. Sternocleidomastoid

46. Which of the following can cause sensory changes in the hand?
    A. Thoracic disc herniation
    B. Cervical stenosis
    C. Lumbar stenosis
    D. Torticollis

47. Bowel and bladder dysfunction can occur with which of the following?
    A. Cervical myelopathy
    B. Thoracic myelopathy
    C. Lumbar myelopathy
    D. All of the above

48. Concentration and visual disturbances are common in which of the following conditions?

    A. Cervical disc herniation

    B. RA affecting the cervical spine

    C. Cervical radiculopathy

    D. Concussion

49. A patient presents with pain, swelling and tenderness over the patellar area. The patient states that she has been doing a lot of kneeling in her garden lately. The PCP recognizes that the patient has symptoms consistent with:

    A. Pes anserine bursitis.

    B. Baker cyst.

    C. Prepatellar bursitis.

    D. LCL grade II sprain.

50. If the person in the preceding question added that they felt a "pop" in the knee before the swelling occurred, this would change the potential diagnosis from bursitis or sprain to which of the following?

    A. LCL tea

    B. MCL tear

    C. Quadriceps tear

    D. ACL tear

Answers and Rationales

1. D. Morton's neuroma is a painful condition that affects the ball of the foot, most commonly between the area of the third and fourth toe.

2. A. Plantar fasciitis is one of the most common causes of heel pain. It involves pain and inflammation of a thick band of tissue, called the plantar fascia that runs across the bottom of the foot and connects the calcaneus bone to the toes. Plantar fasciitis commonly causes stabbing pain that usually occurs with the very first steps in the morning.

3. A. When performing a physical exam, most people with Achilles tendinopathy will complain of pain when they stand on the affected leg and raise their heel off the ground. This movement reproduces their pain.

4. C. Diabetes damages blood vessels, decreasing the blood flow to the feet. Poor circulation weakens bone, and can cause disintegration of the bones and joints in the foot and ankle. As a result, people with diabetes are at a high risk for developing Charcot foot. The combination of bone disintegration and trauma can warp and deform the shape of the foot.

5. B. Evidence supports the Ottawa ankle rules as an accurate instrument for excluding fractures of the ankle and mid-foot. The instrument has a sensitivity of almost 100% and a modest specificity, and its use should reduce the number of unnecessary radiographs by 30–40%.

6. D. Compartment syndrome causes severe pain that does not go away with analgesic medications and is not relieved when the foot is raised. In more severe cases, it may include paresthesia, pallor, and pulselessness.

7. C. Early management of a lateral ankle sprain includes RICE (rest, ice, compression, and elevation). External support may allow the structures around the ankle to rest, provide compression and support, and prevent recurrence.

8. A. Osgood–Schlatter disease is a common cause of knee pain in growing adolescents. It is an inflammation of the area just below the knee where the patellar tendon attaches to the tibia.

9. D. Some patients with patellar subluxation are not cured by conservative treatment and may need surgery. The surgeon may initially perform an arthroscopy to assess the mechanics of the knee joint and ascertain if there is an issue that can be corrected.

10. D. Pes anserine bursitis can be caused by repetitive activities, incorrect sports training techniques (e.g., a lack of stretching), obesity, osteoarthritis of the knee, incorrect positioning of the knee, turning the leg sharply with the foot planted on the ground, injury such as a direct hit to the leg, a tear in the cartilage of the knee, or flat feet.

11. C. Symptoms of a torn knee meniscus include pain, swelling posteriorly, popping, and the feeling that the knee is "locking."

12. B. Symptoms of a torn meniscus commonly include the patient stating that there is a feeling of mechanical "catching" and joint line tenderness.

13. B. The MCL (medial collateral ligament) can be injured during activities that involve bending, twisting, or a quick change of direction. The MCL can be injured in football when the outside of the knee is hit (i.e., a valgus force). This type of injury can also occur during skiing and in other sports with lots of stop-and-go movements, jumping, or weaving.

14. C. A gross effusion will most commonly be present within a few hours after an ACL injury; however, absence of an effusion does not mean an ACL injury has not occurred.

15. C. Medial tibial stress syndrome (MTSS), commonly known as "shin splints," is a frequent injury of the lower extremity and one of the most common causes of exertional leg pain. It is related to inflammation of the soleus muscle that is located in the posterior part of the calf.

16. C. Legg–Calvé–Perthes disease occurs when the blood supply is temporarily interrupted to the femoral head of the hip joint. Without sufficient blood flow, the bone begins to die and can break easily, and subsequently may heal poorly.

17. C. Open reduction and internal fixation (ORIF) is indicated for all intertrochanteric fractures, unless the patient's medical condition is such that any anesthesia, general or spinal, is contraindicated.

18. B. PCL tears make up less than 20% of injuries to the knee ligaments. Injuries that tear the PCL often damage some of the other ligaments or cartilage in the knee as well. PCL injuries are often due to a blow to the knee while it's bent. Common causes include: striking the knee against the dashboard during an auto accident or falling on the knee while it's bent.

19. D. Osteonecrosis of the hip may occur with any hip dislocation. It occurs when the blood supply to the bone is disrupted. Osteonecrosis is also called avascular necrosis or aseptic necrosis. Although it can occur in any bone, osteonecrosis most often affects the hip.

20. D. The adductor muscles of the thigh are responsible for moving the leg across the body and are susceptible to muscle strains. Strains of the adductor muscles occur where the muscle tendons attach to the pelvic bone.

21. A. A Bankart lesion is an injury of the anterior (inferior) glenoid labrum of the shoulder due to anterior shoulder dislocation. When this happens, a pocket at the front of the glenoid forms that allows the humeral head to dislocate into it.

22. C. Acromioclavicular joint injuries are often seen with contact sports injuries and car accidents. The acromioclavicular joint is located at the top of the shoulder where the acromion process and the clavicle meet to form a joint.

23. C. A rotator cuff tear may result from an acute injury such as a fall or may be caused by chronic wear and tear with degeneration of the tendon. Typically, there is pain in the front of the shoulder that radiates down the side of the arm. It may be present with overhead activities such as lifting or reaching.

24. C. Shoulder pain associated with adhesive capsulitis is progressive and initially felt mostly at night, or when the shoulder is moved close to the end of its range of motion. The pain usually progresses to constant pain at rest that is aggravated by all movements of the shoulder. In approximately 90% of patients with adhesive capsulitis, the pain may last 1–2 years.

25. D. Arm fractures account for almost 50% of all broken bones. The radius is commonly fractured when a person tries to break their "fall on an outstretched hand" (FOOSH).

26. B. Kienbock's disease is a condition where the blood supply to one of the small bones in the wrist, the lunate, is interrupted. Without adequate blood supply, the bone can die. This is called osteonecrosis. Damage to the lunate causes a painful, stiff wrist and, over time, can lead to arthritis.

27. A. The test known as the Finkelstein test can help the clinician confirm De Quervain's tenosynovitis. To perform the test, the thumb is bent down across the palm of your hand, and then covered with the fingers. The patient then bends the wrist toward their little finger. If this causes pain, it is likely due to De Quervain's tenosynovitis.

28. B. Commonly associated with a sports or baseball injury. A flexion force on the tip of the extended finger jolts the DIP joint into flexion. Active extension power of the DIP joint is lost, and the joint rests in an abnormally flexed position.

29. C. Dupuytren's contracture is a hand deformity that usually develops over years. Knots of tissue form under the skin, eventually creating a thick cord that can pull one or more fingers into a bent position.

30. D. Stenosing tenosynovitis is a condition commonly known as "trigger finger." It is sometimes also called "trigger thumb." Trigger fingers are more common with certain medical conditions such as rheumatoid arthritis, gout, and diabetes. Repeated and strong gripping may lead to the condition. In most cases, the cause of the trigger finger is not known.

31. B. People of all ages can have Raynaud's phenomenon. Raynaud's phenomenon may run in families, especially in families that typically have autoimmune disorders. The primary form is the most common. It most often starts between age 15 and 25, and is most common in women and people living in cold places.

32. B. Ankylosing spondylitis is an inflammatory disease that can cause some of the vertebrae in the spine to fuse together. This fusing makes the spine less flexible and can result in a hunched-forward posture. Ankylosing spondylitis affects men more often than women. Signs and symptoms of ankylosing spondylitis typically begin in early adulthood.

33. A. Degenerative joint disease is the most common type of low back pain. The lumbar facet joints are susceptible to wear and tear, degeneration, inflammation, and arthritic changes. This may result in pain or limited range of motion.

34. B. Radicular pain radiates into the lower extremity (thigh, calf, and occasionally the foot) directly along the course of a specific spinal nerve root. The most common symptom of radicular pain is sciatica caused by compression of a spinal nerve in the low back. It often will be caused by compression of the lower spinal nerve roots (L5 and S1). With this condition, leg pain and weakness may occur and will depend on which nerve in the low back is affected.

35. D. Abdominal aortic aneurysms often grow slowly and usually without symptoms, making them difficult to detect. Some aneurysms will never rupture. Many start small and stay small, others may enlarge over time. As an abdominal aortic aneurysm enlarges, some people may notice a pulsating feeling near the navel, deep constant pain in the abdomen, or back pain.

36. D. A lumbar laminectomy is typically performed to alleviate pain from lumbar spinal stenosis. Spinal stenosis is caused by degenerative changes that lead to enlargement of the facet joints in the back of the vertebrae.

37. D. Standing upright and bending backward (extension) can make the symptoms of spinal stenosis worse. This is because lumbar flexion (bending forward) increases the diameter of the transverse foramen. It is therefore more comfortable for patients to sit or lean forward. Patients are frequently unable to walk for long distances and often state that their symptoms are improved when bending forward while walking with the support of a walker or shopping cart.

38. A. The most common cause of low back pain in adolescent athletes is a stress fracture in one of the vertebrae. This condition is called spondylolysis and usually affects the fifth lumbar vertebra in the lower back. If the stress fracture weakens the bone so much that it is unable to maintain its proper position, the vertebra can start to shift out of place. This condition is called spondylolisthesis.

39. B. Although early treatment is required to prevent permanent problems, cauda equina syndrome may be difficult to diagnose. Symptoms vary in intensity and may evolve slowly over time. The patient may exhibit an unusual gait pattern, bladder and/or bowel dysfunction, urinary retention, severe or progressive problems in the lower extremities, including loss of or altered sensation between the legs, over the buttocks, along the inner thighs, and the back of the legs and feet.

40. D. Generally, Gowers' sign is identified by the way people with proximal muscle weakness stand up from the floor. A patient with lumbar instability or weakness may bend the top half of his or her body forward, place weight on the knees using the hands, transfer the body weight supported by the hands up the legs and then raise to a standing position.

41. C. Costochondritis is inflammation of the junctions of the ribs with the cartilage where it attaches at the sternum. Costochondritis causes localized chest wall pain and tenderness that can be reproduced by pushing on the involved cartilage in the front of the rib cage. Costochondritis is a relatively harmless musculoskeletal chest pain and usually resolves without treatment.

42. D. When considering the differential diagnoses for a patient complaining of thoracic pain, the possibility of disc herniation, rib fracture, and shingles should all be considered as potential diagnoses.

43. A. Scoliosis most typically occurs in those 10 to 18 years old, females more than males, and is often detected by school screenings or regular physician visits. A medical professional will look for: curvature of the spine, uneven shoulders and/or protrusion of one shoulder blade, asymmetry of the waistline, or one hip higher than the other.

44. C. The Milwaukee brace is also known as a cervico-thoraco-lumbo-sacral orthosis. It is a back brace used in the treatment of spinal curvatures such as scoliosis. It is a full-torso brace that extends from the pelvis to the base of the skull. This brace is normally used with growing adolescents to hold a 25° to 40° advancing curve. The brace is intended to minimize the progression to an acceptable level, not to correct the curvature.

45. D. Torticollis results in a fixed or dynamic posturing of the head and neck in tilt, rotation, and flexion. Spasms of the sternocleidomastoid, trapezius, and other neck muscles, usually more prominent on one side than the other, may cause turning or tipping of the head.

46. B. Cervical stenosis can cause numbness, weakness, or tingling in the arm hand, leg or foot. Tingling in the hand is the most common symptom.

47. D. Myelopathy is a collective name for many different types of problems involving the spinal cord. When myelopathy occurs because of an accident or trauma, it is called a spinal cord injury. In other cases,

myelopathy occurs as a result of a disease process. Symptoms of bowel or bladder dysfunction may be caused by myelopathy along any area of the spinal cord.

48. D. A concussion is a traumatic brain injury that alters the way your brain functions. Effects are usually temporary but can include headaches, visual disturbances, and problems with concentration, memory, balance, and coordination.

49. C. Prepatellar bursitis is an inflammation of the bursa in the front of the patella. It occurs when the bursa becomes irritated and produces too much fluid, which causes it to swell and put pressure on the adjacent parts of the knee. Prepatellar bursitis is often caused by pressure from constant kneeling. Plumbers, roofers, and gardeners are at greater risk for developing this condition.

50. D. When the anterior cruciate ligament (ACL) is injured, the patient may state that they had heard a "popping" noise and then felt the knee "give out." Other symptoms may include pain with swelling of the knee, loss of full range of motion, and discomfort with walking.

● ● ● **References**

Aldridge, T. (2004). Diagnosing heel pain in adults. *American Family Physician, 70,* 332–342.

Almond, L. M., Hamid, N. A., & Wasserberg, J. (2007). Thoracic intradural disc herniation. *British Journal of Neurosurgery, 21*(1), 32–34.

American Academy of Orthopaedic Surgeons (AAOS). (2014). American Academy of Orthopaedic Surgeons clinical practice guideline on management of anterior cruciate ligament injuries. Rosemont (IL): *American Academy of Orthopaedic Surgeons,* Sep 5, 619.

Bare, A. A., & Guanche, C. A. (2005). Hip impingement: The role of arthroscopy. *Orthopedics, 28*(3), 266–273.

Block, J. A., & Sequeira, W. (2001). Raynaud's phenomenon. *The Lancet, 357*(9273), 2042–2048.

Bontempo, N. A., & Mazzocca, A. D. (2010). Biomechanics and treatment of acromioclavicular and sternoclavicular joint injuries. *British Journal of Sports Medicine, 44*(5), 361–369.

Bozkurt, M., Unlu, S., Cay, N., Apaydin, N., & Dogan, M. (2014). The potential effect of anatomic relationship between the femur and the tibia on medial meniscus tears. *Surgical and Radiologic Anatomy, 36*(8), 741–746.

Çakmak, S., Tekin, L., & Akarsu, S. (2014). Long-term outcome of Osgood-Schlatter disease: Not always favorable. *Rheumatology International, 34*(1), 135–136.

Carcia, C. R., Martin, R. L., Houck, J., & Wukich, D. K. (2010). Orthopaedic Section of the American Physical Therapy Association. Achilles pain, stiffness, and muscle power deficits: Achilles tendinitis. *Journal of Orthopaedic & Sports Physical Therapy, 40*(9), A1–26.

Cheung, J. P. Y., Fung, B., & Ip, W. Y. (2012). Review on mallet finger treatment. *Hand Surgery, 17*(03), 439–447.

Cortina, J., Amat, C., Selga, J., & Corona, P. S. (2014). Isolated medial foot compartment syndrome after ankle sprain. *Foot and Ankle Surgery, 20*(1), e1–e2.

Debarge, R., Demey, G., & Roussouly, P. (2011). Sagittal balance analysis after pedicle subtraction osteotomy in ankylosing spondylitis. *European Spine Journal, 20*(5), 619–625.

de Souza, M. C., de Ávila Fernandes, E., Jones, A., Lombardi Jr., I., & Natour, J. (2011). Assessment of cervical pain and function in patients with rheumatoid arthritis. *Clinical rheumatology, 30*(6), 831–836.

Do, T. T. (2006). Congenital muscular torticollis: Current concepts and review of treatment. *Current Opinion in Pediatrics, 18*(1), 26–29.

El-Sallakh, S., Aly, T., Amin, O., & Hegazi, M. (2012). Surgical management of chronic boutonniere deformity. *Hand Surgery, 17*(03), 359–364.

Forman, T., Forman, S., & Rose N. A. (2005). A clinical approach to diagnosing wrist pain. *American Family Physician, 72*(9), 1753–1758.

Franco, A. H. (1987). Pes cavus and pes planus analyses and treatment. *Physical Therapy, 67*(5), 688–694.

Fritz, J. M., Piva, S. R., & Childs, J. D. (2005). Accuracy of the clinical examination to predict radiographic instability of the lumbar spine. *European Spine Journal, 14*(8), 743–750.

Gautam, V. K., Verma, S., Batra, S., Bhatnagar, N., & Arora, S. (2015). Platelet-rich plasma versus corticosteroid injection for recalcitrant lateral epicondylitis: Clinical and ultrasonographic evaluation. *Journal of Orthopaedic Surgery, 23*(1), 1–5.

Gervais, J., Périé, D., Parent, S., Labelle, H., & Aubin, C. E. (2012). MRI signal distribution within the intervertebral disc as a biomarker of adolescent idiopathic scoliosis and spondylolisthesis. *BMC Musculoskeletal Disorders, 13*(1), 239.

Gilden, D., Mahalingam, R., Nagel, M. A., Pugazhenthi, S., & Cohrs, R. J. (2011). Review: The neurobiology of varicella zoster virus infection. *Neuropathology and Applied Neurobiology, 37*(5), 441–463.

Gude, W., & Morelli, V. (2008). Ganglion cysts of the wrist: Pathophysiology, clinical picture, and management. *Current Reviews in Musculoskeletal Medicine, 1*(3–4), 205–211.

Guly H. R. (2002). Injuries initially misdiagnosed as sprained wrist (Beware the sprained wrist). *Emergency Medicine Journal, 19*, 41–42.

Hailer, Y. D., Montgomery, S., Ekbom, A., Nilsson, O., & Bahmanyar, S. (2012). Legg-Calve-Perthes disease and the risk of injuries requiring hospitalization: A register study involving 2579 patients. *Acta Orthopaedica, 83*(6), 572–576.

Hardy, P., & Sanghavi, S. (2009). Rotator cuff injury: still a clinical controversy? *Knee Surgery, Sports Traumatology, Arthroscopy, 17*(4), 325–327.

Herman, A. M., & Marzo, J. M. (2014). Popliteal cysts: A current review. *Orthopedics (Online), 37*(8), e678.

Honda, H., & McDonald, J. R. (2009). Current recommendations in the management of osteomyelitis of the hand and wrist. *The Journal of Hand Surgery, 34*(6), 1135–1136.

Huisstede, B. M., Fridén, J., Coert, J. H., Hoogvliet, P., & European HANDGUIDE Group. (2014). Carpal tunnel syndrome: Hand surgeons, hand therapists, and physical medicine and rehabilitation physicians agree on a multidisciplinary treatment guideline—results from the European HANDGUIDE Study. *Archives of Physical Medicine and Rehabilitation, 95*(12), 2253–2263.

Huisstede, B. M., Hoogvliet, P., Coert, J. H., & Fridén, J. (2014). Multidisciplinary consensus guideline for managing trigger finger: Results from the European HANDGUIDE Study. *Physical Therapy, 94*(10), 1421–1433.

Ilahi, O. A., Cosculluela, P. E., & Ho, D. M. (2008). Classification of anterosuperior glenoid labrum variants and their association with shoulder pathology. *Orthopedics, 31*(3), 226.

Iversen, T., Solberg, T. K., Romner, B., Wilsgaard, T., Nygaard, Ø., Waterloo, K., . . . & Ingebrigtsen, T. (2013). Accuracy of physical examination for chronic lumbar radiculopathy. *BMC Musculoskeletal Disorders, 14*(1), 206.

Kasai, Y., Akeda, K., & Uchida, A. (2007). Physical characteristics of patients with developmental cervical spinal canal stenosis. *European Spine Journal, 16*(7), 901–903.

Kontopodis, N., Metaxa, E., Papaharilaou, Y., Tavlas, E., Tsetis, D., & Ioannou, C. (2014). Advancements in identifying biomechanical determinants for abdominal aortic aneurysm rupture. *Vascular, 23*(1), 65–77.

Kosashvili, Y., Drexler, M., Backstein, D., Safir, O., Lakstein, D., Safir, A., . . . & Gross, A. (2014). Dislocation after the first and multiple revision total hip arthroplasty: Comparison between acetabulum-only, femur-only and both component revision hip arthroplasty. *Canadian Journal of Surgery, 57*(2), E15.

Lamba, D., Pant, V. S., Joshi, M., Sah, H., & Mahara, M. (2011). A comparison study of the effects of massage therapy with and without ultrasonic therapy in medial epicondylitis. *Journal of Physiotherapy & Occupational Therapy, 5*(2), 54–57.

Lau, L. H., Kerr, D., Law, I., & Ritchie, P. (2013). Nurse practitioners treating ankle and foot injuries using the Ottawa Ankle Rules: A comparative study in the emergency department. *Australasian Emergency Nursing Journal, 16*(3), 110–115.

Liporace, F. A., Adams, M. R., Capo, J. T., & Koval, K. J. (2009). Distal radius fractures. *Journal of Orthopaedic Trauma, 23*(10), 739–748.

Maffey, L., & Emery, C. (2007). What are the risk factors for groin strain injury in sport? *Sports Medicine, 37*(10), 881–894.

Martin, R. L., Davenport, T. E., Paulseth, S., Wukich, D. K., & Godges, J. J. (2013). Orthopaedic Section American Physical Therapy Association. Ankle stability and movement coordination impairments: ankle ligament sprains. *Journal of Orthopaedic & Sports Physical Therapy, 43*(9), A1–40.

Melvin, J. S., & Mehta, S. (2011). Patellar fractures in adults. *Journal of the American Academy of Orthopaedic Surgeons, 19*(4), 198–207.

McKeon, K. E., & Lee, D. H. (2015). Posttraumatic boutonnière and swan neck deformities. *Journal of the American Academy of Orthopaedic Surgeons, 23*(10), 623–632.

Miao, J., Wang, S., Wan, Z., Park, W. M., Xia, Q., Wood, K., & Li, G. (2013). Motion characteristics of the vertebral segments with lumbar degenerative spondylolisthesis in elderly patients. *European Spine Journal, 22*(2), 425–431.

Moore, J. S. (1997). De Quervain's tenosynovitis: Stenosing tenosynovitis of the first dorsal compartment. *Journal of Occupational and Environmental Medicine, 39*(10), 990–1002.

Moen, M. H., Bongers, T., Bakker, E. W., Zimmermann, W. O., Weir, A., Tol, J. L., & Backx, F. J. G. (2012). Risk factors and prognostic indicators for medial tibial stress syndrome. *Scandinavian Journal of Medicine & Science in Sports, 22*(1), 34–39.

Mulligan, J., & Amblum, J. (2014). Diagnosis and Treatment of Scaphoid Fracture. *Emergency Nurse, 22*(3), 18–23.

Non-Surgical Management of Hip and Knee Osteoarthritis Working Group. (2014). VA/DoD clinical practice guideline for the non-surgical management of hip and knee osteoarthritis. Washington (DC): Department of Veterans Affairs, Department of Defense; 126 p.

Pearce, J. M. S. (2008). Observations on concussion. *European Neurology, 59*(3–4), 113–119.

Proulx, A. M., & Zryd, T. W. (2009). Costochondritis: Diagnosis and treatment. *Am Fam Physician, 80*(6), 617–620.

Rambani, R. & Hackney, R. (2015). Loss of range of motion of the hip joint: A hypothesis for etiology of sports hernia. *Muscles, Ligaments and Tendons Journal*, 5(1), 29.

Ramonda, R., Frallonardo, P., Musacchio, E., Vio, S., & Punzi, L. (2014). Joint and bone assessment in hand osteoarthritis. *Clinical Rheumatology*, 33(1), 11–19.

Roddy, E., Zwierska, I., Hay, E. M., Jowett, S., Lewis, M., Stevenson, K., . . . & Foster, N. E. (2014). Subacromial impingement syndrome and pain: Protocol for a randomised controlled trial of exercise and corticosteroid injection (the SUPPORT trial). *BMC Musculoskeletal Disorders*, 15(1), 81.

Rogers, L. C., Frykberg, R. G., Armstrong, D. G., Boulton, A. J., Edmonds, M., Van, G. H., . . . & Uccioli, L. (2011). The Charcot foot. *Diabetes Care*, 34(9), 2123–2129.

Rosenthal, M. D., Rainey, C. E., Tognoni, A., & Worms, R. (2012). Evaluation and management of posterior cruciate ligament injuries. *Physical Therapy in Sport*, 13, 196–208.

Schwartz, E. N., & Su, J. (2014). Plantar fasciitis: A concise review. *The Permanente Journal*, 18(1), e105.

Shakil, H., Iqbal, Z. A., & Al-Ghadir, A. H. (2013). Scoliosis: Review of types of curves, etiological theories and conservative treatment. *Journal of Back and Musculoskeletal Rehabilitation*, 27(2), 111–115.

Sinha, I., Lee, M., & Cobiella, C. (2008). Management of osteoarthritis of the glenohumeral joint. *British Journal of Hospital Medicine (London, England: 2005)*, 69(5), 264–268.

Stein, G., Koebke, J., Faymonville, C., Dargel, J., Müller, L. P., & Schiffer, G. (2011). The relationship between the medial collateral ligament and the medial meniscus: A topographical and biomechanical study. *Surgical and Radiologic Anatomy*, 33(9), 763–766.

Szucs, P. A., Richman, P. B., & Mandell, M. (2001). Triage nurse application of the Ottawa knee rule. *Academic Emergency Medicine*, 8(2), 112–116.

Takao, T., Morishita, Y., Okada, S., Maeda, T., Katoh, F., Ueta, T., . . . & Shiba, K. (2013). Clinical relationship between cervical spinal canal stenosis and traumatic cervical spinal cord injury without major fracture or dislocation. *European Spine Journal*, 22(10), 2228–2231.

Tamburrelli, F. C., Genitiempo, M., Bochicchio, M., Donisi, L., & Ratto, C. (2014). Cauda equina syndrome: Evaluation of the clinical outcome. *Eur Rev Med Pharmacol Sci*, 18(7), 1098–1105.

Townley, W. A., Baker, R., Sheppard, N., & Grobbelaar, A. O. (2006). Dupuytren's contracture unfolded. *BMJ: British Medical Journal*, 332(7538), 397.

Urrutia, J., & Fadic, R. (2012). Cervical disc herniation producing acute Brown–Sequard syndrome: Dynamic changes documented by intraoperative neuromonitoring. *European Spine Journal*, 21, 418–421.

Van Demark, Jr., R., Van Demark, III, R., & Helsper, E. (2015). Stress fracture of the hook of the hamate: A case report. *South Dakota Medicine*, 68(4), 157–9, 161.

Vinther, A., Kanstrup, I. L., Christiansen, E., Alkjær, T., Larsson, B., Magnusson, S. P., & Aagaard, P. (2005). Exercise-induced rib stress fractures: Influence of reduced bone mineral density. *Scandinavian Journal of Medicine & Science in Sports*, 15(2), 95–99.

Walmsley, S., Osmotherly, P. G., & Rivett, D. A. (2014). Clinical identifiers for early-stage primary/idiopathic adhesive capsulitis: Are we seeing the real picture? *Physical Therapy*, 94(7), 968–976.

Weinstein, J. N., Tosteson, T. D., Lurie, J. D., Tosteson, A. N., Blood, E., Hanscom, B., . . . & An, H. (2008). Surgical versus nonsurgical therapy for lumbar spinal stenosis. *New England Journal of Medicine*, 358(8), 794–810.

Werner, B. C., Fashandi, A. H., Gwathmey, F. W., & Yarboro, S. R. (2015). Trends in the management of intertrochanteric femur fractures in the United States 2005–2011. *Hip International*, 25(3), 270–276.

Wise, J. N., Weissman, B. N., Appel, M., Arnold, E., Bancroft, L., Bruno, M. A., et al. (2013). Expert Panel on Musculoskeletal Imaging. ACR Appropriateness Criteria® chronic foot pain. [online publication]. Reston (VA): American College of Radiology (ACR); 10 p.

Yan, J., Sasaki, W., & Hitomi, J. (2010). Anatomical study of the lateral collateral ligament and its circumference structures in the human knee joint. *Surgical and Radiologic Anatomy*, 32(2), 99–106.

CHAPTER

10

Nervous System

Rebecca Smart, MPH, MSN, APRN, NNP-BC, FNP-BC

Review

- Exam findings can be deduced from a careful history
- Initial MINIMAL screening exams should include the following:
  - Mental status—Oriented to person, place, and time; follow commands and respond appropriately
  - Cranial nerves—Visual fields, pupillary light reflex (PERRLA), EOMs, facial strength, and hearing to whisper test or finger rub
  - Motor system—Strength in upper and lower extremities, pronator drift, tandem gait walking on heels; coordination: RAMs, finger-to nose, heel-knee-shin
  - Reflexes—DTRs; plantar, biceps, triceps, patellar, and ankle bilaterally (Graded 0 = absent, 1 = hypoactive, 2 = normal, 3 = hyperactive, 4 = clonus)
  - Sensation—Light touch, two-point discrimination, all four distal extremities, vibration on great toe bilaterally

Deficits in any area, or neurologic complaints or findings, require an expanded exam. Figure 10-1 illustrates the functional areas of the cerebral cortex.

Cranial Nerves

To remember the cranial nerves (see Figure 10-2), use a mnemonic "On Old Olympus's Towering Top, A Finn and German Viewed Some Hops":

- **CN I:** Olfactory
- **CN II:** Optic
- **CN III:** Oculomotor
- **CN IV:** Trochlear
- **CN V:** Trigeminal
- **CN VI:** Abducens
- **CN VII:** Facial
- **CN VIII:** Acoustic
- **CN IX:** Glossopharyngeal
- **CN X:** Vagus
- **CN XI:** Spinal Accessory
- **CN XII:** Hypoglossal

Red Flags for Referral for Adults

- No response to treatment or improvement from standard therapy
- Focal findings suggestive of space occupying lesion of brain or spinal cord (unequal pupil size, papilledema with headache)

215

- Peripheral nerve compression
- Acute or sudden onset of symptoms—headache, change in level of consciousness (LOC), aphasia, visual change = IMMEDIATE consult/hospital
- Headaches requiring emergency care:
  - "Worse headache of my life"
  - Thunderclap headache (abrupt onset of severe pain)
  - Sudden onset of exertional headache (after sex, coughing, straining)

Brain Tumors

May be associated with signs of increased intracranial pressure (ICP): Vomiting without nausea and neuro deficits; headache may be in morning, usually dull aching and increasing over time. New onset seizures consider mass lesion.

- Tumors can be benign or malignant symptoms; deficits depend upon location.

* Triad: papilledema, morning headache, vomiting

Stroke and Transient Ischemic Attack

Leading cause of adult long-term disability in the United States.

Higher incidence in men, elderly (> 60), Asian, Hispanic, African American + family history and lower socioeconomic status (non-modifiable risk factors).

- Modifiable risk factors: Hypertension, hyperlipidemia, carotid stenosis or dissection, cardiac disease, atherosclerosis, previous stroke or TIA, diabetes, obesity and sedentary lifestyle, poor nutrition, cigarette smoking, alcohol consumption, Obstructive Sleep Apnea (OSA), stress
- Women: Oral contraceptive use is linked to small increase in risk of thrombosis. Risk increased significantly with women who smoke. Estrogen should also not be used with vascular disease (pre-eclampsia).
- Pregnant and postpartum have higher association (coagulopathy and pre-eclampsia).
- Migraine with aura is associated with 2-fold risk of stroke.
- Illicit drug use of cocaine, heroin, and amphetamine abuse is linked to stroke.

"Time is brain"—onset of symptoms is important to assess (thrombolytic therapy window of 4.5 hours).

Sensitive Test for Stroke

- Pronator drift—Observe: Facial droop, arm weakness, and speech abnormalities—probability of stroke = 72%
  - Pt stands with arms outstretched fully extended, palms up, eyes closed. Watch 5–10 seconds for pronation and downward drift. (+ test)

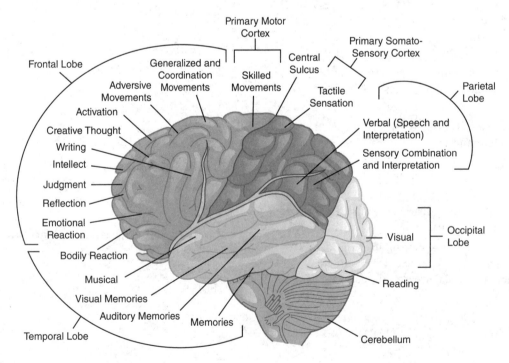

Figure 10-1 Functional Areas of Cerebral Cortex.

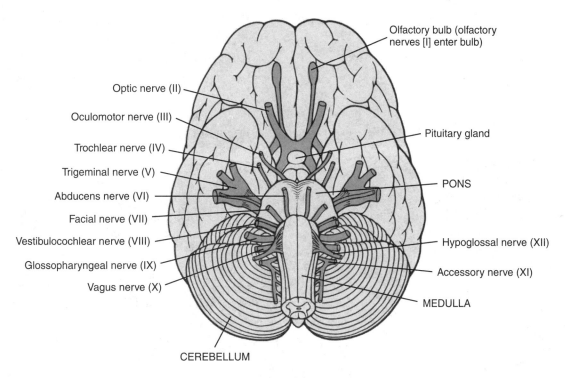

Figure 10-2 Cranial nerves

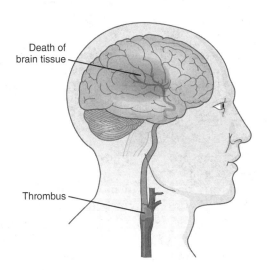

Figure 10-3 Ischemic Stroke

TIA

A transient episode of neurological dysfunction caused by focal brain, spinal cord, or retinal ischemia, without acute infarction.

- Episode lasts less than 10 minutes and not greater than 24 hours.
- Increased risk of stroke (5%) within 48 hours.

Stroke

Reduction in cerebral blood flow to a region of the brain resulting in vascular injury.

Types:
- Ischemic—(most common—85%) occlusion or stenosis caused by the following:

  atherosclerosis of large vessels extra- or intracranial (ICA, MCA); small vessel disease-lacunar stroke; cardioembolic (atrial fibrillation), hypercoaguable states, vasculitis or dissection, infarcts of unknown origin. (cryptogenic); Figure 10-3 illustrates an Ischemic stroke.

- Hemorrhagic—(15%) subarachnoid, intracerebral

Neurologic deficits represent the decreased blood flow in the affected region of the brain

**Sickle cell disease is the most common cause of ischemic stroke in AA children.

Treatment: IMMEDIATE REFERRAL TO ER for suspected stroke. Image within 24 hours of symptom onset for TIA.

*Look for red flags—arm drift (pronator drift), weakness, facial droop, or abnormal speech

Red Flags for Stroke

- Sudden severe headache/nausea/vomiting
- Sudden dizziness or inability to walk
- Sudden confusion
- Sudden difficulty seeing in one/both eyes
- Sudden difficulty speaking or understanding

- Sudden numbness/weakness of one side of the body or face
- Sudden altered level of consciousness

Management

- Pulse oximetry and BP

Testing

- Immediate non-contrast CT to exclude intracerebral hemorrhage (ICH) (stroke)
- Anticoagulation studies—PT < INR, APTT, chemistry panel, CBC with platelet count, cardiac troponins, creatine kinase
- ECG
- Non-urgent labs to consider—Lipid panel, Hgb A1C, ESR, LFTs, CRP
- MRI with DWI (TIA)
- MRA
- Echocardiography—transthoracic and or transesophageal
- CT angiography
- Consider hypercoagulation panel—(if history warrants) APA, Factor V Leiden, B2 glycoprotein IgM, IgG, Protein C, Protein S, Antithrombin III

Antiplatelet Drugs: recommended for reduction of vascular events

- Aspirin (50–325 mg)
- Combination aspirin/dipyridamole (25 and 200 mg BID ER dipyridamole)
- Ticlopidine
- Clopidogrel 7 mg
- CHADS2 VAS score is used for risk of stroke in non-valvular atrial fibrillation patients to determine the level of anticoagulation needed. The variables include congestive heart failure or LVEF < 35, hypertension, age > 75 years, diabetes, stroke/TIA/systemic thromboembolism, vascular disease (MI/PAD/aortic atheroma), age 65–74, sex (http://www.mdcalc.com/cha2ds2-vasc-score-for-atrial-fibrillation-stroke-risk/)

Anticoagulants

- Warfarin—Prevent stroke in aFib, coagulopathies, cardiomyopathy. INR 2–3 diet/vitamin K issues
- New Oral Anticoagulants—All have bleeding risk, no reversibility—though currently working on it, short half life, NO INR; check renal clearance/creatinine
- Dabigatran—Direct thrombin inhibitor: 150 mg po (by mouth) twice daily
- Rivaroxaban factor Xa inhibitor—20 mg po daily
- Apixaban factor Xa inhibitor—5 mg po twice daily

Concussion

Direct impulsive force is delivered to head, face, or body resulting in rapid acceleration, deceleration, or rotation of the brain.

- Mild TBI or concussion used interchangeably—accounts for 75% of TBI @ 3 million cases annually
- Sports related concussion—< 10% have LOC
- Sports with greatest risk—Males: football and rugby, hockey and soccer; Females: soccer and basketball
- Loss of consciousness is not a reliable indicator for dysfunction or recovery.

Symptoms may present in a delayed fashion.
  Three categories of signs and symptoms:

- Somatic—Headaches, sleep disturbance, tinnitus, nausea/vomiting, visual disturbance, imbalance
- Cognitive—Poor concentration, memory impairment, complaints of mental fog, confusion about recent events, repeating or answering questions slowly
- Neuropsychiatric—Anxiety, increased fatigue, depressed mood, irritability

Additional tools used to identify athletes with concussion besides direct physical exam: Post-concussive symptom scale, Sensory Organization test, Balance Error Scoring System. Neuropsychological testing.

- CT imaging is used for LOC with more serious TBI, rule out subarachnoid hemorrhage, post-traumatic amnesia, focal neurologic deficits, skull fracture, or an alteration in mental status that persists
- Encourage "cocooning" after injury—Physical and cognitive rest, no video, schoolwork, TV, texting
- For athletes: No return to play until complete resolution of symptoms during exercise and rest
- Athletes who return to play too soon are at risk for additional concussions, cognitive issues, and vestibular disturbance
- Risk factors for prolonged recovery: younger age, previous concussions, headaches, and "fogginess"

- Post-concussive syndrome can develop (headache, dizziness, concentration/processing disturbance)
- Patients who experience repetitive concussions are at risk for permanent impairment which may lead to psychiatric illnesses, dementia, and chronic traumatic encephalopathy (CTE)

Treatment

Medications may mask recovery.

- Melatonin 1–5 mg at bedtime OR
- Trazadone 25–50 mg as first-line therapy for sleep disturbance
- Amitryptylline is very effective in treating post concussive headache and sleep—10–25 mg at bedtime (age > 12). Increase weekly—50 mg is typical dosing. *Consider baseline ECG due to conduction disturbances.

Meningitis

Inflammation of the meninges due to bacterial infection. Extremes of age (newborns, elderly) most at risk.

Etiology

- Bacterial—*Steptococcus pneumoniae. Haemophilus influenzae* type B, and *Neisseria meningitidis*. Hib vaccine now given and has decreased incidence of H. flu), Listeria monocytogenes
- Viral—coxsackie, echo, herpes, West Nile, EBV, CMV
- Other—Lyme, syphilis, fungal, protozoal
- Bacterial is fatal in 5–40% of cases

Risk

HIV, alcoholism, malignancy, head trauma, asplenia, complement deficiency, college students living in dormitories, TB, infective endocarditis

Presentation: Rapid development of fever and chills (85%), headache, photophobia, nuchal rigidity, seizures, somnolence, (rashes or petechiae), nausea, vomiting

*May see findings consistent with viral presentation (e.g., tonsillar exudates, vesicular rashes, cervical adenopathy)

Signs of meningeal irritation:

- Kernig's sign—In supine position with hip flexed at 90 degrees, resistance or discomfort is felt in back and posterior thigh with passive knee extension
- Brudzinski's sign—Passive flexion of neck causes knee or hip flexion

Prevention: **Hib vaccine, conjugate meningitis, and pneumococcal vaccine

Management

This is a medical emergency.
***Lumbar puncture—CSF culture and gram stain—only way to differentiate between viral and bacterial

- Elevated WBC count is seen > 1000 cells/ul—predomination of neutrophils (neutrophilic pleocytosis) bacterial
- WBC < 1000 in aseptic or viral meningitis, negative gram stain, no bacteria
- PCR for rapid identification
- Labs: CBC, blood cultures, serum electrolytes, glucose, LFTs, HIV—specific tests per history

Treatment

Empiric therapy with antibiotics based on susceptibilities in specific populations and guidelines, THEN targeted therapy dictated by organism and patient population

- Age > 50 years: Vancomycin + ampicillin plus third-generation cephalosporin
- Age 18–50 years: Vancomycin + third-generation cephalosporin
- Age 1–18: Vancomycin + third-generation cephalosporin
- Age < 1 month—Ampicillin, + gentamicin or cephalosporin
- Treatment of close contacts: meningococcal meningitis (roommates, crowded environments: prisons, military)
- Ciprofloxacin, Rifampin
- Risk of neurologic sequelae, follow-up for hearing and neuropsych required

PROGRESSIVE DEGENERATIVE DISORDERS

Dementia

Chronic deterioration in cognitive function with impairment in activities of daily living (ADLs), behavior, and deficits in intellectual functioning.

- Different variations (Table 10-1 describes the global deterioration scale)

Alzheimer's Disease (AD)

Most common form in ages 65 and over. Prevalence doubles every 5 years after age 65 with genetic and environmental influence. ApoE e4 gene, Down syndrome and family history increase risk. More common in women. Early onset is rare (10%)—age 30–60 (familial, inherited 50%). Other:

- Hypertension, diabetes, hyperlipidemia increase risk
- Lower education level and depression association

    ****Advancing age is the greatest risk

Due to neuritic amyloid plaques and neurofibrillary tangles in brain

- Insidious onset and gradual progression (continuing cognitive decline)
- Impairment in memory plus aphasia, apraxia, or agnosia (impairment in two cognitive domains): attention, executive function, language, social cognition
- Deficits are a significant decline in previous level of functioning. Patient often unaware of deficits. Forgetfulness and losing items common, disorientation, poor short-term memory
- Deficits do not occur exclusively during a course of delirium
- Experience behavioral problems with sleep disturbance, wandering, agitation, "sundowning," may have hallucinations and delusions
- Exam: May appear normal; abnormal coordination and motor exam in advanced disease
- MMSE/Neuropsych testing; clock draw test
- Labs: Metabolic panel, CBC, ESR, serum TSH, serum Vit B12 and folic acid, LFTs, RPR. Urine drug screen (genetic testing for familial type)
- CT/MRI—hippocampal volume loss, temporal lobe, or posterior cortical atrophy
- PET/SPECT scanning
- EEG (If seizures suspected)
- Elevations in tau protein on CSF (not done routinely)

Stages

Progression varies by patient—Mild/Mod/Severe by MMSE

Frontotemporal Dementia

Picks disease atrophy of frontal lobe. *Think Behavior and Language—Apathy and language

Table 10-1	Global Deterioration Scale

- Used with primary degenerative dementia. (Reisberg Stages) 7 different stages. Stages 1–3 are the pre-dementia stages. Stages 4–7 are the dementia stages. Beginning in stage 5, an individual can no longer survive without assistance—Each Stage lasts 3–4 years and progression is very different among patients.
1. No impairment
2. Very mild symptoms with indistinguishable changes (mild cognitive impairment MCI). Age-associated memory impairment
3. Mild cognitive decline
4. Moderate cognitive decline (clear but early AD) moderate dementia
5. Moderately severe decline (clear functional impairment)
6. Severe decline (can no longer care for self)
7. Very severe decline (around-the-clock care or institutional care)

Data from Reisberg, B., Ferris, S. H., de Leon, M. J., and Crook, T. (1982). Global Deterioration Scale. *American Journal of Psychiatry,* 139:1136–1139.

disturbance, difficulty understanding or making speech, disinhibition

Dementia with Lewy Body

Fluctuating cognition and visual hallucinations common. Presence of Lewy bodies in subcortical and cortical structures (absence of neurofibrillary tangles).

Vascular

Second most common form

- Due to multiple infarcts, often comorbid with AD
- **STEPWISE** progression of decrease in cognition with memory loss occurring later than AD
- History of hypertension, stroke, TIA, hyperlipidemia, vascular disease, and diabetes
- May see abnormal neuro exam (weakness, gait disturbance, exaggerated DTR)
- Lesions on CT/MRI appear in white and gray matter

Other

- Treatable types
  - Neoplasm
  - Metabolic encephalopathy
  - Normal pressure hydrocephalus
  - Psychiatric

Treatment of AD

Cholinesterase inhibitors—mild–moderate
Side effects: GI, caution with cardiac conduction abnormalities; syncopal/bradycardic episodes, caution with asthma, COPD, seizure, GI history

- Donepizil
- Rivastigmine
- Glantamine

Moderate AD

- N-methl1-D-aspartate receptor antagonist: Memantine and or cholinesterase inhibitor

No efficacy demonstrated for antioxidants or hormones.

- Antipsychotics used to treat agitation/hallucinations, delusions *Black Box Warning—increase morbidity, cardiovascular events (have not been determined to be more effective than placebo)
  - Haloperidol—risk of tardive dyskinesia
  - Risperidone—extrapyramidal symptoms
  - Olanzapine—metabolic effects, diabetes
  - Quetiapine—orthostasis, sedating
    - Other—Antidepressants: Sertaline; Anticonvulsants: valproic acid

Non-pharmacologic: psychosocial intervention, physical exercise, cognitive exercise, ADL training, reality orientation, socialization in familiar surroundings with routine.
There is no cure.

ACUTE NEUROLOGICAL DISORDERS

Delirium

Acute disturbance in mental functioning characterized by confusion, impaired thinking, cognition and attention deficit with a fluctuating course

- Patient may be hypo or hyperalert and demonstrate incoherent or illogical speech
- Risk—age, elderly, hospitalized patients

Causes

- Metabolic—Electrolyte imbalance, dehydration, hypoxia, vitamin deficiency
- Medications—Anticholinergics, antihistamines, lithium, sedatives, narcotics
- Withdrawal—Alcohol, benzodiazepines, narcotic
- Infections—UTI, pneumonia, sepsis, influenza
- Neurologic—Intracranial hemorrhage, stroke, subdural hematoma, seizure
- Endocrine—Hypo/hyperthyroid
- Cardiovascular—CHF, MI, arrhythmia

Diagnostics

MMSE, CBC, chemistry profile, thyroid panel, LFTs, urinalysis, toxicology screen, CXR. Additional tests as indicated (CT, MRI, LP EEG)
Treatment: Treat underlying illness (restore electrolyte imbalance or discontinue medication)
Haldol for agitation—.25 mg q 4 hour/max 2 mg/d

Headache

Diagnosis is established based on clinical findings—History is most important tools in evaluation and PE.

- Special attention to gait, motor, sensory, and fundoscopic exam

Primary

- Migraine (with and without aura)—Aura 20%
- Tension type—most common
- Cluster

Secondary

- Result of abnormal anatomical pathology
- Abnormal neurologic exam, change in pattern of headache, systemic disease
- Increased intracranial pressure
- Intracerebral hemorrhage
- Concussion
- Tumor
- Infection
- Psychiatric

Immediate referral/treatment needed for: Subarachnoid hemorrhage, giant cell arteritis, brain tumor, meningitis, ischemic stroke, Chiari I malformation AND RED FLAGS

- **HEADACHE DON'T MISS DIAGNOSIS**
  - **SA hemorrhage**
  - **Meningitis/encephalitis**
  - **Temporal arteritis**
  - **Acute strokes**
  - **Trigeminal neuralgia**

- Hypertensive emergencies
- Mass lesions

IDENTIFY RED FLAGS (These headaches should prompt a CT.)

- Change in basic headache pattern
- Sudden onset, worst headache ever
- Headache accompanied by neurological signs and symptoms.
- Sudden onset, especially after age 50.
- Physical illness (i.e., fever, chills, nuchal rigidity, rash)
- Headache followed by physical exertion: trauma, exercise, sexual activity
- Or use mnemonic from American Headache Society—**SNOOP**:

  Systemic symptoms (fever, weight loss) or secondary headache risk factors (HIV, systemic cancer)

  Neurologic symptoms or abnormal signs (confusion, impaired alertness, or consciousness)

  Onset: Sudden, abrupt, or split-second

  Older: New onset and progressive headache, especially in middle age > 50 (giant cell arteritis)

  Previous headache history or headache progression: first headache or different (change in attack frequency, severity, or clinical features)

Migraine

- Usually unilateral with or without aura associated with nausea, with or without vomiting, photophobia; phonophobia; osmophobia, persisting 4–72 hours
- Aura may precede 20 min—1 hour before; Visual: scotoma: (blindspots), zigzag, flashing lights, paresthesia/weakness, hemianopsia
- More common in women, strong familial pattern, menstrual pattern is a trigger in 50% of cases; > white and lower socioeconomic class
- Triggers include fatigue, environment, weather, food, alcohol, caffeine, change in meal, menstruation, change in sleep
- Diagnostics: NONE required except for neurologic findings, history or secondary headache LABORATORY TESTING: metabolic profile, thyroid function, ESR, RA, Lyme, coagulation workup.

Treatment

Decrease the number/severity and duration of attacks and reduce impairment

Episodic Migraines:

- Non-Specific: Acetaminophen, aspirin, and caffeine can be effective for mild, or infrequent headache. NSAIDs, combination analgesics, narcotics, steroids, anti-nausea medications.
- Triptans—GOLD STANDARD
  - Sumatriptan, eletriptan, rizatriptan, naratriptan, almotriptan: First-line for treatment chosen by type of headache, administration (injection, intranasal, po), half-life and side effects
  - Contraindication: Cardiovascular disease, cerebrovascular disease, breastfeeding
  - Side effects: flushing, tingling, chest/neck/sinus/jaw discomfort. Risk of serotonin syndrome with SSRI
- Ergots—acute treatment—usually migraines lasting > 72 hours

  CI: Cadiovascular disease, cerebrovascular disease

  Side effects: powerful vasoconstrictor; nausea; don't mix with triptan/decongestant
- NSAIDs—naproxen, ketoprofen

  Contraindications: CABG, renal impairment, gastric or peptic ulcer
- Antiemetics: metoclopramide, proclorperazine, diphenhydramine for acute nausea and vomiting

Prophylaxis

- When migraine attacks are severe and frequent enough to interfere with patient's daily activities despite appropriate medical management
- Two or more headaches each week
- Medication overuse during attacks
- Severe adverse effects from medications to treat migraines or unresponsive to abortive treatment
- Contraindications to acute treatment

Treatment

Beta-blockers—propranolol, timolol

- Preferred for patients with hypertension, angina
- Side effects: fatigue, drowsiness, contraindicated in asthma, COPD, CHF, type 1 diabetes

- Anticonvulsants—topiramate, gabapentin, divalproex sodium, sodium valproate
  - Topiramate-SE-paresthesia, hyperthermia, cognitive impairment, CI: kidney stones
  - Vaproate: teratogenic, SE—weight gain, tremor, monitor LFTs
  - Gabapentin-SE—drowsiness, excreted renally
- Antidepressant—amitryptyline—preferred for anxiety, mood disorder, insomnia
  - Anticholinergic—CI: elderly, urinary retention or heartblock
  - Side effects: increased appetite and weight gain, watch for rashes, dry mouth
  - Antidepressant—fluoxetine-SSRI—dose every other day (off label)
  - Acetaminophen—Used in pediatric population and pregnancy CI: liver disease/cirrhosis

Other Therapies

- Magnesium, Butterbur, feverfew, Riboflavin, Co-enzyme Q-10
- Biofeedback, behavioral changes, acupuncture,
- Lifestyle changes, trigger management

Cluster

- M: F 4:1 > 30—lancinating, severe, boring to eye. Lasts 20–30 minutes, often several times/night, every other day up to 8/day. "Ice pick" or suicide headaches
- May demonstrate ipsilateral Horner's syndrome with conjunctival injection, lacrimation, nasal congestion, rhinorrhea, miosis, ptosis, eyelid edema, facial sweating
- Cluster periods may last 2–16 weeks than remit for 1 year or more (chronic patients have no remission period)
- No specific testing, rule out secondary causes; can be confused with trigeminal neuralgia or giant cell arteritis.

Treatment

Acute therapy—Severity of the pain requires acute abortive therapy that responds quickly

- Oxygen: via FM at 7–12 liters/min for 10–20 minutes per attack
- Triptans: Sumatriptan shot, nasal spray 1 shot or spray with headache, repeat in 2 hours as needed. Zomig can also be used for relief of cluster headaches.
- Lidocaine intranasally
- Ergots: DHE shot or spray—1 shot every 8 hours, 1–2 sprays in each nostril can repeat in 8 hours, up to 6 sprays per day.
- Prophylaxis: Usual Verapamil. Can use Depakote, Lithium, Topamax all titrated up.
- Steroid tapers and Medrol dose pac until preventative is effective

Tension

Bilateral band like with steady pain, pain is mild to moderate, lasting 30 minutes—2 days

Does not interfere with activities and not aggravated by physical activity

Episodic tension-type headache: the most common headache disorder—aggravated by stress

Seen in adolescents and adults

Treat with simple analgesia, ASA, NSAIDs, Tylenol, combine analgesics with caution, biofeedback, physical therapy, stress reduction, relaxation.

Red Flags for Headache—Pedi

- Unequal pupils
- Cannot awaken
- Worsening HA
- Repeated vomiting
- Seizure
- Slurred speech
- Increased confusion LOC
- Don't forget to check for hyphemas (pooling of blood in anterior chamber between cornea and iris)

Temporal Arteritis

(Giant cell arteritis) vasculitis involving ophthalmic, temporal, and carotid system

- Medical emergency in the elderly
- Age of onset 50–70 F > M
- Concerns of vision loss—visual disturbances in 50% of patients
- Headache localized over eye and scalp tenderness
- Associated with polymyalgia rheumatic (PMR) with joints and muscle aches

- ESR elevation 100, elevated CRP
- Associated symptoms: fever, jaw or tongue claudication, weight loss, fatigue
- Labs: ESR, CBC, LFTs, CRP
- Surgical referral: For unclear diagnosis—temporal artery biopsy
- Imaging: Duplex ultrasonography of temporal and axillary arteries

Prompt Treatment

Oral corticosteroids—40–60 mg/d for 4 weeks until symptom resolution/ESR normal. Then slow taper over 1–2 year.

Follow-up/Referral: rheumatologist, ophthalmologist, risk of recurrence followed every 4–6 weeks.

Trigeminal Neuralgia

Onset > 50, mostly idiopathic

- Lasts seconds to minutes, shock-like severe lancinating unilateral pain in sensory distribution of trigeminal nerve (CN V)
- Increase in frequency, arises spontaneously, triggered by sensory stimulus; chewing, talking, touching.

  *No neurologic deficit noted

- Exclude temporal arteritis; post-herpetic neuropathy (PHN), and multiple sclerosis if bilateral

Treatment

- First-line—Carbamazepine initially 100 mg/d, gradually titrated up. 400–800 mg/d
- Monitor CBC, platelets for bone marrow suppression
- Other—Oxcarbamazapine, lamotrigene

Bell's Palsy

Unilateral paralysis of CN VII, acute onset, idiopathic etiology

Cause: HSV 1 or 2, EBV, Lyme, MS, neoplasm, aneurysm of basilar artery

Risk—pregnancy (3-fold increase), diabetes, trauma, syphilis

Recovery in 65% at 3 months, 85% at 9 months
– Steroids and Valtrex in 72 hrs

Bilateral Excludes Bell's

- Forehead sparing of motor function indicates upper motor lesion (stroke, infarction)
- Symptoms: Pain near ear, hyperacusis, may have distortion of taste, weakness on one side of face, weakness of eye closure
- No sensory loss on affected side
- Asymmetry of mouth
- Increased tear flow, dry eye, corneal reflex intact
- Rash or vesicles around ear—herpes zoster; **Think Ramsay Hunt *Don't Miss
- Diagnostics/Evaluation—none required; testing dependent on history
- Tests: CBC, ESR, Lyme, HIV, glucose, CT dependent on history
- Treatment: Antivirals: Valtrex 1000 mg TID × days—not given routinely
- Prednisone 1 mg/kg/d 6 mg/kg × 7 days without taper
- Eye protection: patch at night, artificial tears

MOTOR NEURON DISORDERS

Multiple Sclerosis

Autoimmune progressive neurodegenerative disease characterized by demyelination and inflammation with axonal loss in the spinal cord and brain.

- Deficits vary in time and location (CNS location and episodes)
- More common in northern latitudes, 15% have family history
- Clinical features: CN dysfunction—VI, palsy, nystagmus, vision loss, optic neuritis
- Impaired motor—weakness, increased tone, + Babinski, action tremor
- Sensory—changes in sensation, proprioception, vibration, numbness, tingling, paresthesias, c/o itching
- Cerebellar—+ Romberg, gait imbalance, gait ataxia
- Bowel or bladder—urgency or incontinence
  - Fatigue
  - Lhermitte's sign: Electrical sensation down back of legs produced with flexion of neck

Three types:

- Relapsing Remitting—Acute onset, self-limiting, recovery, some residual deficit
- Secondary Progressive—Develops after relapsing, remitting with slow deterioration in function, may still have some acute attacks
- Primary Progressive—Steady functional decline without acute onset

Diagnosis

- MRI—90% multifocal T2 abnormalities brain and spinal cord
- LP—CSF—Oligoclonal bands (neurologist)
- Bloodwork: Screening—CBC, chem panel, HIV, ANA, B12, ESR

Treatment

- Acute Exacerbations: IV methylprednisone × 5 days
- Interferon B, glatiramir acetate, natalizumab, fingolimod. Reduce frequency of relapse and long-term disability
- Treat depression and symptoms (spasticity, bladder dysfunction) with disease progression

Parkinson's Disease

- Clinical symptom of tremor at rest (usually 1 hand) due to loss of dopaminergic cells in substantia nigra
- Gradual onset asymmetric is most common presentation. (insidious)
- Decreased arm swing, bradykinesia and rigidity detected on symptomatic side (cogwheel)
- Clinical diagnosis, routine labs are not helpful
- Balance and gait affected with progression—risk of falls
- Rigidity and freezing

- Autonomic disturbance: constipation, urinary urgency, sweating, orthostatic hypotension
- Decreased blink rate, masked facies, anosmia
- Seborrhea

Neuroimaging is used to exclude other conditions.

Treatment with dopamine agonists, levo dopa-cabidopa, and MAO-B inhibitor, anticholinergics Physical and Occupational Therapy

(Benign) Essential Tremor

Rhythmic oscillation of body part—present on movement, absent at rest

- Most common movement disorder
- M > W, median age of onset 15
- 2/3 family history, 1st-degree relatives

Clinical Diagnosis

- Action tremor of upper distal arms and hands, partial tremor of head
- Symmetrical presentation
- Voice may be affected
- Does not appear in sleep
- Alcohol often suppresses the symptoms
- Nicotine, caffeine, stress, anxiety, hypoglycemia, fatigue, some medications worsen symptoms
- Handwriting demonstrates problem

Exclude hyperthyroidism, neurologic causes and deficits

Treatment

- Beta adrenergic blocker
- Primidone
- Patients self-treat with pre-meal cocktails
- Evaluate treatment and progression with drawing of pinwheel

PD patients may have both types of tremor.

Review Questions

1. A 76-year-old patient arrives at the office with his wife with complaints of episodes of slurred speech, word-finding difficulties, and numbness in his arm. The first priority in management is:

    A. Tell him to take an aspirin right away.

    B. Order a CT scan.

    C. Send him to the ER.

    D. Perform an EKG.

2. Which one of these patients are most at risk for ischemic stroke?

    A. A patient with atrial fibrillation on Coumadin with INR of 1.2

    B. A patient with 2ppd tobacco history $\times$ 40 years who quit 5 years ago

    C. A patient on anticoagulation therapy with INR of 4.0

    D. A hypertensive patient currently being treated with Losartan

3. Initial urgent treatment for dizziness is associated with which of the following?

    A. Tinnitus

    B. Diabetes

    C. Nausea and vomiting

    D. Dysphasia

4. Which of the following situations is NOT considered a "Red Flag" for referral for a patient the FNP is seeing in his/her practice?

    A. A patient who presents with an abnormal perception of movement (sensation of spinning)

    B. A patient with peripheral nerve compression

    C. A patient with no response to treatment or improvement from standard therapy

    D. Acute or sudden onset of symptoms—change in LOC, visual change

5. What is the first symptom seen in the majority of Parkinson's patients?

    A. Intention tremor

    B. Bradykinesia

    C. Rest tremor

    D. Rigidity

6. A 73-year-old female patient presents with limb paralysis nystagmus, vertigo, nausea, slurred speech, and cerebellar ataxia. An occlusion of which part of the brain is suspected?

    A. Occipital and temporal lobes, dorsal surface of thalamus, upper part of cerebellum, midbrain

    B. Anterior cerebral surfaces

    C. Posterior cerebral surfaces

    D. Parts of the medulla

7. Dysarthria, dysphagia, and diplophia are signs of which of the following?

    A. Peripheral vertigo

    B. Central vertigo

    C. Presyncopal causes of vertigo

    D. Psychogenic causes of vertigo

8. What diagnostic maneuver reproduces the characteristics of vertigo?

    A. Epley maneuver

    B. Dix–Hallpike maneuver

    C. Lying prone on the exam table

    D. VNG (video nystagnography)

9. A patient presents with dizziness, delayed clockwise rotational clockwise nystagmus, and spinning for less than a minute after position change and denial of hearing loss and headache. The appropriate diagnostic evaluation to use would be what?

    A. MRI

    B. CT with contrast

    C. No studies are necessary.

    D. EKG

10. An 82-year-old patient presents with a history of TIA and confusion. A sensitive neurologic test for stroke would be what?

    A. The pronator drift

    B. Epley maneuver

    C. Visual field exam

    D. Get-up-and-go test

11. The CHA2DS2–VASc Index is used for categorizing patients according to risk. These risk factors include all of the following EXCEPT:

    A. Diabetes.

    B. Stroke/TIA.

    C. Age 65–74.

    D. Drugs.

12. A patient with multiple sclerosis presents with concerns of exacerbation. The nurse practitioner knows the examination will likely present with the following:

    A. Tremor at rest

    B. Hyperreflexia + Babiniski, upper motor neuron signs, ataxic gait

    C. Hyporeflexia, decreased reflexes, hypotonia, sensory disturbance

    D. Sensory deficit that follows a single dermatomal distribution

13. A child presents with febrile seizures. Which statement offers the BEST information for the education of the family by the NP?

    A. These types usually present as absence or simple partial seizures.

    B. The child will usually need anticonvulsant therapy for 6 months.

    C. There is a higher risk of developing epilepsy later in life (greater than the general population).

    D. Most occur on the first day of fever; > 75% > 102 degrees.

14. Ménière's disease is an idiopathic disorder that is characterized by which of the following?

    A. Episodic attacks of vertigo lasting less than a minute and hearing loss

    B. Dizziness, double vision, hearing loss, tinnitus, vertigo

    C. Episodic attacks of vertigo, tinnitus, aural fullness, and hearing loss

    D. Disabling attacks of vertigo, diplopia, hearing loss, tinnitus, and aural fullness

15. A primary headache differs from a secondary headache in what way?

    A. A primary headache is the first headache of someone's life.

    B. A secondary headache presents with an aura.

    C. A secondary headache is a result of abnormal anatomic pathology.

    D. A primary headache is due to systemic disease.

16. First-line treatment for essential tremor is which of the following?

    A. Propranolol (Inderal)

    B. Alprazalam (Xanax)

    C. Amitryptylline (Elavil)

    D. Alcohol

17. A 62-year-old woman complains of severe lancinating pain in her right cheek that worsens with cold drinks or teeth brushing. She is afraid to chew or eat because it seems to initiate the attack. The most likely diagnosis is which of the following?

    A. Sinus infection

    B. Abscessed tooth

    C. Trigeminal neuralgia

    D. Bell's palsy

18. What test for carpal tunnel syndrome reports a positive finding for tingling after passive flexion of the wrist for 1 minute?

    A. Tinel's sign

    B. C-T-S test

    C. Radial test

    D. Phalen's Sign

19. A 35-year-old male c/o (complaints of) the abrupt onset of recurrent "ice pick" headaches behind one eye. He presents to the NP's office with an acute episode. On physical exam, the patient is noted to have tearing in one eye, ptosis, and nasal discharge/congestion. The NP's plan for therapeutic management would be which of the following?

    A. High-dose NSAIDs

    B. High-dose oxygen 7–10 L

    C. Send to the ER for CT scan

    D. Verapamil

20. A 72-year-old patient presents with c/o headache with unilateral marked scalp tenderness. You note induration of the temporal artery. Upon checking his labs, the FNP expect to find which of the following?

    A. Normal CRP

    B. ESR 100 mm or >

    C. WBC >15,000

    D. Positive western blot

21. When the FNP administers the Mini-mental status exam (MMSE) and asks what is the difference between a river and a lake? He/she is actually measuring which of the following?

    A. Education level

    B. Memory

    C. Abstract thinking

    D. Plasticity

22. A 22-year-old patient with no cardiovascular history presents with a history of a unilateral headache accompanied by nausea, vomiting, photophobia, or phonobia. What further diagnostics are required to establish the diagnosis?

    A. CT

    B. MRI

    C. No further laboratory investigation is needed

    D. CBC with differential

23. Which of the following medications is the best choice for acute treatment of the patient who presents with unilateral headache accompanied by nausea, vomiting, photophobia or phonophobia?

    A. Triptans

    B. Beta-blockers

    C. NSAIDs

    D. Narcotics

24. Which CN is responsible for shoulder shrugging?
    A. CN X
    B. CN XI
    C. CN IX
    D. CN XII

25. Which CNs are being tested with EOM?
    A. A CN III, IV, VI
    B. CN III, IV, V
    C. CN II, III, IV
    D. CN II, IV, V

26. The next patient to be seen by the FNP is a 16-year-old old high school soccer player who suffered a Gr 1 concussion. The best advice at this time would be which of the following?
    A. Pupillary checks every hour, monitor vital signs
    B. You may return to play as soon as your symptoms have resolved
    C. Physical rest × 2 weeks, no contact sports with medical follow-up
    D. Physical and cognitive rest monitored by medical personnel. Monitor for emotional symptoms, headaches difficulty remembering, feeling foggy, trouble concentrating

27. The classic presentation of carpal tunnel syndrome includes repetitive use and gradual onset of tingling (paresthesias) in which fingers?
    A. Thumb, index, and middle finger
    B. Index, middle, and fifth finger
    C. All the fingers of the hand
    D. Thumb

28. During the neurologic exam, a patient has had a positive Romberg test. This highlights an issue in what part of the neurologic system?
    A. The sensory system and balance
    B. Mental status
    C. The motor system
    D. The reflex system

29. Which statement below best describes a positive Romberg test?
    A. The patient is unable to walk in a straight line with one foot in front of the other.
    B. The patient holds arms straight forward with eyes closed.
    C. The patient stands with feet together, eyes closed, arms at side with excessive swaying—begins to fall down and keeps feet far apart to maintain balance.
    D. Patient places outstretched arms with palms facing up and closed eyes. One arm goes downward after 5–10 seconds.

30. Serious causes of headache that require immediate urgent referral include which of the following?
    A. Migraine
    B. Hypertension
    C. Cervical spondylosis
    D. TIA

31. An 18-year-old male college student is being evaluated by the FNP at the student health center. He has had a fever > 102 F for approximately 24 hours and c/o severe headache. During the examination, the patient is directed to lay in a supine position and passively bend his neck toward his chest; he flexes his knees and hips. What is the name of this maneuver?
    A. Brudzinksi
    B. Kernig
    C. Cullens
    D. Lachman

32. Which of the following factors is NOT contributory toward the development of Bell's palsy?
    A. Pregnancy
    B. Diabetes
    C. Lyme disease
    D. Heart disease

33. Bell's palsy presents as acute weakness or paralysis of the muscles supplied by which cranial nerve(s)?
    A. VI
    B. V
    C. VII
    D. VII and VIII

34. A 32-year-old patient with migraines and a history of asthma is complaining of two migraine headaches per week despite treatment with triptans. The next consideration for treatment is which of the following?
    A. Discontinue triptans and offer NSAIDs.
    B. Start topiramate as preventative therapy.
    C. Start propranolol or timolol as preventative therapy.
    D. Order an MRI.

35. A new patient explains that she has a history of migraines with aura. Counseling should include which of the following?
    A. Headaches that occur as a result of aura may last much longer and be more serious than those without.
    B. There is controversy over the use of oral contraceptives and she may want to consider another form of contraception.
    C. A visual scotoma (circumscribed vision loss) is caused by cerebral ischemia in the middle or posterior cerebral artery.
    D. The aura can be a jabbing "ice pick" feeling in the head or over one eye that lasts seconds.

36. An 80-year-old patient was admitted to the hospital with confusion this week. Her daughter tells the hospitalist her memory may be slipping a bit, but she was oriented and independent last week, driving herself to the market. Upon admission to the hospital, she is found to have pneumonia. Currently, she is difficult to arouse and has incoherent speech. Last night, she was up all night and seemed to know her daughter but was confused regarding place and time. Her CT was normal. The most appropriate diagnosis of consideration at this time is which of the following?
    A. Dementia
    B. Parkinson's Disease
    C. Stroke
    D. Delirium

37. A 70-year-old patient has c/o of gradual memory loss without neurologic deficits. The best method of evaluation at this time would be which of the following?
    A. Administering a MMSE
    B. CT of the brain
    C. Neuropsychological testing
    D. Meeting with the family to obtain a history

38. A family member of an 85-year-old Alzheimer's patient wants to know what the risk factors are for getting the disease? Which of the following statements would be the best response?
    A. "If we can scan your brain and offer you treatment, we can prevent the disease from progressing."
    B. "They have not found an association with vascular disease, diabetes, or hypertension."
    C. "There is some genetic risk, but advancing age is the biggest risk factor."
    D. "More men than women get the disease; there is a protective effect with estrogen."

39. Which of the following medications should be considered as first-line therapy for patients with mild to moderate Alzheimer's disease?

    A. Anticholinergics

    B. Ace inhibitors

    C. Cholinesterase inhibitors

    D. Antidepressants

40. A patient presents with decreased arm swing and cogwheel rigidity. What conditions are these a manifestation of?

    A. Multiple sclerosis

    B. Vascular dementia

    C. Parkinson's disease

    D. Rheumatoid arthritis

41. A 28-year-old female presents with weakness, complaints of fatigue, recent problems with diplopia, numbness of her left arm, and some bladder changes. She remembers something similar happening last year. What would be in the differential?

    A. Migraine with aura

    B. Multiple sclerosis

    C. Meningitis

    D. Pituitary tumor

42. A 22-year-old college student presents with an acute onset of high fever, chills, nausea, slight confusion, and is noted to have a headache and petechiae. The exam reveals a + Kernig's sign. The most appropriate next step in management would be which of the following?

    A. Tell him this looks viral, offer NSAIDs around the clock, check a throat culture to verify, and have the patient come back in 24–48 hours if he's not feeling better.

    B. Perform throat culture; treat empirically since he lives in a college dorm.

    C. Check for mono—Send off EBV/Mono spot, throat culture, treat empirically.

    D. Send him to the ER for an LP and further evaluation.

43. What recommendation should the NP offer to a high school soccer player who has suffered a mild concussion?

    A. "You may return to play in 1 week."

    B. "You may not return to play until resolution of all of your symptoms during both exercise and rest."

    C. "You may return to play after resolution of your symptoms and a follow-up CT scan."

    D. "Since you did not suffer loss of consciousness (LOC), you may return to play."

44. Patients who have experienced concussive events are at risk for developing which of the following?

    A. Headache

    B. Dizziness

    C. Processing disturbance

    D. All of the above

45. Which type of dementia has a step-wise progression in memory loss, may present with an abnormal neuro exam or gait, and is often seen with multiple infarcted areas of the brain?

    A. Metabolic encephalopathy

    B. Alzheimer's dementia

    C. Lewy body dementia

    D. Vascular dementia

46. A patient presents with complaints of moderate headache pain that is bilateral, does not increase with activity level, but is aggravated by stress. It seems to come and go at times, but can last from one hour to sometimes all day. This is likely which of the following?

    A. Migraine headache

    B. Potential brain tumor

    C. Tension headache

    D. Cluster headache

47. A 60-year-old man with TIA and atrial fibrillation is currently being treated with Apixaban, one of the new oral anticoagulants. What is an important teaching point for this patient today?

    A. He must watch the vitamin K in his diet because it can interfere with the medication.

    B. He must continue to have his INR monitored, although it is less frequent than with warfarin.

    C. There is a bleeding risk; discuss sign and symptoms of bleeding, bruising (GI, etc.).

    D. This drug has a very long half-life, so you can take it any time you want during the day.

48. Modifiable risk factors for stroke include which of the following?

    A. Male

    B. Age > 60

    C. Socioeconomic status

    D. Obstructive sleep apnea, alcohol consumption, obesity

49. A patient presents with morning headaches that has been increasing over time, papilledema, and vomiting. What is the prioritized diagnosis?

    A. Meningitis

    B. Migraine

    C. Brain tumor

    D. Stroke

50. First-line therapy for a patient with trigeminal neuralgia is which of the following?

    A. Prednisone 1/kg/d × 7 days without taper

    B. Carbamazepine

    C. Valtrex and prednisone

    D. Amitryptilline

Answers and Rationales

1. C. An aspirin is incorrect if you are concerned of stroke and you are not sure if it is hemorrhagic or ischemic in origin. A CT is reasonable, but should be done emergently upon admission to the ER. An EKG would be applicable for chest pain or hospital admission.

2. A. The patient who is out of his therapeutic window and at risk for a thromboembolic event (INR range 2–3). Smokers who quit are at greater risk than non-smokers, but at 5 years their risk drops to half that of smokers.

3. D. is the only correct answer because it could be associated with stroke or TIA. The others are all non-urgent symptoms or associations.

4. A. All of the answers are red flags for referral except vertigo.

5. C. Asymmetric tremor at rest is usually seen in one hand as a presenting symptom for PD. Intention tremor is also known as essential tremor and presents symmetrically in a different population. The other symptoms are seen later in the disease.

6. A. The most common areas of occlusion are the ICA or MCA. The midbrain, upper part of the cerebellum and dorsal surface of the thalamus receive blood from the basilar artery, which also supplies the temporal and occipital lobes. Thus, the patient exhibits symptoms in the regions of the brain that have been affected with slurred speech, cerebellar ataxia, nausea and vertigo, and limb paralysis, nystagmus. The posterior cerebral surface would result in bilateral motor sensory, visual complaints, and contra-lateral hemiplegia. Answer D would result in pain, temperature, and sensation impairment, as well as vertigo and dysphagia—in a contralateral fashion.

7. B. These are all signs of stroke, therefore they are not consistent with A, C, or D.

8. B. The Epley maneuver is the repositioning maneuver used to treat BPPV, while the Dix–Hallpike will elicit nystagmus and vertigo.

9. C. Vertigo without neurologic deficits requires no imaging. It is a clinical diagnosis.

10. A. The pronator drift will show upper motor neuron weakness if the patients arm drifts, as well as confusion if they are unable to follow instructions. The Epley maneuver is done for vertigo. Visual fields should be assessed as part of a neuro exam, and the get-up-and-go test is a timed mobility test for the elderly.

11. D. All of the answers are variables used to assess the risk to start anticoagulation except for drugs. Additional variables include sex, vascular disease, LVEF, thromboembolism, PAD, CHF.

12. B. Would be a Parkinson's patient, C is incorrect. D: In MS, it does not follow single dermatomal distributions.

13. D. Febrile seizures occur with fever $> 100, 75\% > 102$, and in the absence of an identifiable cause. They do not require treatment and usually occur on the first day the fever does. They are typically generalized, less than 15 minutes in duration, and may have tonic clinic activity. The risk for developing epilepsy later in life is slightly increased from that of the general population (1%).

14. C. By definition, Ménière's has the classic symptoms of vertigo tinnitus and hearing loss accompanied by aural fullness. The condition can be chronic or can resolve. There is an extensive differential for dizziness and double vision, including stroke; MS is not associated with Ménière's.

15. C. It is also due to systemic disease. A migraine presents with an aura 20% of the time.

16. A. Though many patients will self-medicate with alcohol, and it will suppress the symptoms, beta-blockers are the first-line treatment.

17. C. Classic symptoms of trigeminal neuralgia is shock-like severe lancinating unilateral pain in the sensory distribution of the trigeminal nerve (CN V), often initiated by cold, chewing, or a sensory stimulus. The etiology is often unknown. Bell's palsy does not present this way or with the same distribution.

18. D. Phalen's sign—numbness and tingling in the median nerve distribution of the fingers.

19. B. This patient meets the classic presentation for cluster headache. He does not need to go to the ER, especially with a "recurrent" history. The presentation of a Horner's-like syndrome is normal. He will respond to high-dose oxygen for acute treatment. Verapamil should also be titrated or adjusted for prevention.

20. B. The ESR would be elevated with a diagnosis of temporal arteritis, which is what this patient most likely has. The CRP should be elevated. The other findings are not consistent with the condition.

21. C. Asking about similarities and differences is abstract thinking. Memory testing would be day, date, month, season etc. The test does not take into account the educational level or measure plasticity.

22. C. The diagnosis is established on the basis of clinical findings. If there are clinical features that may suggest an alternative diagnosis, then additional laboratory investigations are necessary. If appropriate therapy is initiated and there is a lack of response, than an alternate diagnosis would also be considered.

23. A. Beta-blockers are preventative therapy. NSAIDs may be used for tension headache or episodic headache. Narcotics are not first-line. Triptans are first-line therapy for a patient without cardiovascular history.

24. B. The vagus nerve is 10, the hypopharyngeal nerve is 9, and hypoglossal is 12; the nerve responsible for the shoulder shrug is CN 11.

25. A. CN 3—oculomotor medial deviation and all other directions, 4-trochlear (innervates superior oblique and downward gaze), 6 abducens (innervates lateral rectrus and lateral gaze). Extraocular range of motion. CN V is the trigeminal nerve.

26. B. It needs to be monitored by medical personnel; some athletes will be inappropriately anxious to return to sport.

27. A. Median nerve compression results in thumb, index finger, and middle finger symptoms.

28. A. The Romberg test helps assess proprioception—sensory and balance.

29. C. Tandem gait test. B is a negative test. D is a motor exam for pronator drift.

30. D. A careful history and physical would delineate the cause. Migraine can be diagnosed clinically and does not need further workup. Hypertension can be serious if not controlled, but is not usually the reason for immediate urgent referral. Patients with hypertensive crisis would require an urgent referral. Answer C is a primary cause that can contribute to headaches, but if you have excluded life-threatening reasons, there is no urgency. D is correct. It is necessary to exclude S/A hemorrhage, ICH, and stroke that may be presenting as TIA.

31. A. The Lachman test is a test for integrity of the ACL. Kernig's sign is also a test for meningeal irritation: In the supine position, with the hip flexed at 90 degrees, resistance or discomfort is felt in the back and posterior thigh with passive knee extension. Cullen's sign is superficial edema and bruising in the subcutaneous fatty tissue around the umbilicus, following rupture of ectopic or intraperitoneal hemorrhage.

32. D. All but heart disease are contributory. Between 7–9% of patients have recurrence.

33. C. The facial nerve is CN VII. It is the only one affected.

34. B. The patient is a candidate for prophylaxis because she is having two or more migraines per week, and may be heading toward medication overuse. She should not use a beta-blocker with asthma; topiramate or another option should be considered. An MRI is not necessary because there is no acute change, neurologic deficits, or red flags.

35. B. Migraine with aura may be an independent risk factor for stroke in women < 45. Headaches following an aura do not have to last longer or be worse than those without, and the aura is not due to ischemia. The last answer describes cluster symptoms.

36. D. This meets the criteria of the acute mental disturbance characterized by confusion, impaired thinking, and cognition and attention deficit with a fluctuating course.

37. A. The Mini-Mental Status Exam is a screening tool that would give you a baseline. Neuropsychological testing would be beneficial depending on the findings. Meeting with the family is always important to obtain a thorough history and for verification. The FNP would not want to do that first; only after issues were identified.

38. C. There is no preventive treatment at this time. The medications are only for once the disease is diagnosed. There is an association with vascular disease, diabetes, and hypertension. Advancing age is the biggest risk factor, with prevalence doubling every 5 years after 65. More women than men have AD.

39. C. The only drugs approved for use for mild–moderate AD are the anticholinesterase inhibitors.

40. C. Patients with Parkinson's disease may demonstrate decreased arm swing, and cogwheel rigidity in upper limbs as a result of increased tone. Upon exam, there is resistance and a ratchetlike rhythmic contraction of the muscle as the practitioner moves the limb through the range of motion (elbow, wrist).

41. B. Multiple sclerosis presents with varying deficits at different times due to the multifocal demyelination and inflammation. Common symptoms include gait ataxia, visual loss, diplopia, paresthesias, weakness, and fatigue.

42. D. This patient matches all the features of meningitis; sudden onset fever chills, systemic illness, neck stiffness in a previously healthy young adult in group living puts him at high risk. Concerning features are the change in mental status and meningeal irritation.

43. B. Loss of consciousness is not a reliable indicator for dysfunction or recovery. CT imaging is only used LOC with more serious TBI, rule out subarachnoid hemorrhage, post-traumatic amnesia, focal neurologic deficits, skull fracture, or an alteration in mental status that persists. For athletes, there is no set time period: There should be no return to play until there is complete resolution of all symptoms at exercise and rest.

44. D. Post-concussive syndrome can develop (headache, dizziness, concentration/processing disturbance) after concussion, as well as other long-term permanent impairment for repetitive concussions.

45. D. Vascular Dementia is a **STEPWISE** progression of decrease in cognition with memory loss occurring later than AD. It often presents with an abnormal neuro exam, exaggerated DTR, weakness. AD is a gradual decline with a normal exam. There can be mixed dementia. A is treatable, and C is in same category with AD: degenerative type with fluctuating cognition.

46. C. Episodic tension headache is the most common, bilateral type headache and can last anywhere from 30 min to 2 days. The pain can be mild to moderate.

47. C. The new anticoagulant (Eliquis) apixaban blocks the blood-clotting factor Xa. It has a lower bleeding risk than warfarin, but it does remain. It does not require frequent bloodwork. It is taken twice daily and has a 12-hour half-life.

48. D. The others are non-modifiable risk factors.

49. C. The classic triad of dull morning headache, papilledema, and vomiting are signs of increased intra-cranial pressure. Stroke would likely present with other neurologic deficits, but would also be ruled out with further evaluation. The other two do not fit the presentation.

50. B. Carbamazepine initially 100 mg/d, gradually titrated up to 400–800 mg/d.

References

Bushnell, C., McCullough, L. D., Issam, A. Awad, M. V., Chireau, W. N., Fedder, K. L., . . . Walterson, M. R. on behalf of American Heart Association Stroke Council, Council on Cardiovascular and Stroke Nursing, Council on Clinical Cardiology, Council on Epidemiology and Prevention, and Council for High Blood Pressure Research. (2014). Guidelines for the prevention of stroke in women: A statement for healthcare professionals from the American Heart Association/American Stroke Association. *Stroke, 45*(5), 1545–1588. doi:10.1161/01.str.0000442009.06663.48

Centers for Disease Control and Prevention. (2014). Injury prevention and control: Traumatic brain injury. Retrieved from www.cdc.gov/traumaticbraininjury/.

Dodick, D. W. (2003). Clinical clues and clinical rules primary vs. secondary headache. *Advance Studies in Medicine, 3*(6C), S550–S555.

Kernan, W. N., Oybiagele, B., Black, H. R., Bravata, D. M., Chimowitz, M. I., Ezekowitz, M.D., . . . Wilson, J. A. (2014). Guidelines for the prevention of stroke in patients with stroke and transient ischemic attack: A guideline for healthcare professionals from the American Heart Association/American Stroke Association. *Stroke, 45*(7), 2160–2236. doi:10.1161/STR.0000000000000046

Halstead, M. E., McAvoy, K., Devore, C. D., Carl, R., & Lee, M. (2013). Returning to learning following a concussion. *Pediatrics, 132*(5), 948–957. doi:10.1542/peds.2013-2867

Harmon, K. G., Drezner, J. A., Gammons, M., et al. (2013). American Medical Society for Sports Medicine position statement: Concussion in sport. *British Journal of Sports Medicine, 47*(1), 15–26.

Reisberg, B., Ferris, S. H., de Leon, M. J., and Crook, T. (1982). The global deterioration scale for assessment of primary degenerative dementia. *American Journal of Psychiatry, 139*, 1136–1139.

Rowland, L., & Pedley, T. (Eds.). (2009). *Merritt's neurology* (12 ed.). Philadelphia, PA: Lippincott Williams & Wilkins.

Siberstein, S. D., Holland, S., Freitag, F., Dodick, D. W., Argoff, C., & Ashman, E. (April, 2012). Evidence-based guideline update: Pharmacologic treatment for episodic migraine prevention in adults. Report of the Quality Standards Subcommittee of the American Academy of Neurology and the American Headache Society. *Neurology*, *78*(17), 1337–1345. doi: http://dx.doi.org/10.1212/WNL .0b013e3182535d20

Silberstein, S. D., Lipton, R. B., & Dalessio, D. J. (2001). Overview, diagnosis, and classification. In S. D. Silberstein, R. B. Lipton, & D. J. Dalessio (Eds.), *Wolff's Headache and Other Head Pain* (7th ed.). Oxford, England: Oxford University Press.

Suchowersky, O., Reich, S., Perlmutter, J., et al. (2006). Practice parameter: Diagnosis and prognosis of new onset Parkinson's disease (an evidence-based review): Report of the Quality Standards Subcommittee of the American Academy of Neurology. *Neurology*, *66*, 968–975.

Tunkel, A., Hartman, B. J., Kaplan, S. L., Kaufman, B. A., Roos, K. L., Scheld, W. M., & Whitley, R. J. (2004). IDSA guideline: Practice guidelines for the management of bacterial meningitis. *Clinical Infectious Diseases*. *39*(9), 1267–1284. doi:10.1086/425368

Zesiewicz, T. A., Elble, R., Louis, E. D., et al. (2005). Practice parameter: Therapies for essential tremor: Report of the Quality Standards Subcommittee of the American Academy of Neurology. *Neurology*, *64*, 2008–2020.

Endocrine System

Nancy L. Dennert, MS, MSN, FNP-BC, CDE, BC-ADM

Diabetes mellitus is a chronic illness requiring continuous medical care. The nurse practitioner must work with the patient and the patient's health care team to identify a therapeutic treatment plan that optimizes risk-reduction strategies. The plan should be patient-centered, tailored to the individual, and supportive of the concept of diabetes self-management.

Diabetes Facts

- 29.1 million Americans or 9.3% of the entire population has diabetes.
- 8.1 million have undiagnosed diabetes.
- 37% of U.S. adults > 20 years have pre-diabetes.
- 1 in 5 health care dollars is spent caring for people with diabetes.
- Racial disparities in diagnosed diabetes in the U.S.:
  - 12.6% of African Americans
  - 11.8% of Hispanics
  - 8.4% of Asian Americans
  - 7.1% of non-Hispanic whites
  - 24.1% of Native Americans in southern Arizona

Diagnosis of Pre-Diabetes

- Pre-diabetes is the term used for an individual who has one or more of the following characteristics (should have at least one confirmatory test)

- FPG 100–125 mg/dL (impaired fasting glucose)

  Or

- 2-hour post 75 gm. OGTT 140–199 mg/dL (impaired glucose tolerance)

  Or

- A_{1C} 5.7–6.4% (those with A_{1C} of > 6% should be considered very high risk for development of DM)

The majority of individuals with pre-diabetes will develop type 2 diabetes within 10 years.

Diagnosis of Diabetes Mellitus

Diagnosis of diabetes mellitus occurs if the individual has one the following characteristics. (The individual should have at least one confirmatory test if there is only one positive test result.) If the individual presents with a positive result for more than one of these tests, confirmatory testing is not necessary.

- AIC ≥ 6.5%

  Or

- FPG ≥ 126 mg/dL (No caloric intake × 8 hours)

  Or

- 2-hour post 75 gm OGTT of ≥ 200 mg/dL

  Or

- Patients with symptoms, a random glucose of ≥ 200

Screening Recommendations for Both Pre-Diabetes and Diabetes
Adults

- Asymptomatic adults of any age who have a BMI ≥ 25 (or if Asian American, a BMI ≥ 23), with one or more additional risk factors for diabetes, which may include: high-risk ethnicity, family history, central obesity, dyslipidemia (particularly those with high triglycerides and low HDLs), hypertension.
- All individuals over the age of 45 who are overweight or obese.
- Screening can be done with the A_{1C}, FPG, or a 2-hour 75 gram OGTT. Diagnosis of asymptomatic individuals should only occur with repeat confirmatory testing.
- Normal tests of individuals meeting the criteria should be repeated at a minimum of every three years.

Children

Screen asymptomatic children who are overweight (>85th percentile) and who have two or more of the following risk factors:

- Family history of type 2 DM in 1st- or 2nd-degree relative
- High-risk ethnicity
- Have a condition associated with insulin resistance: HTN, dyslipidemia, PCOS, acanthosis nigricans, or were SGA.
- Maternal history of gestational diabetes during the child's gestation
- Frequency: every 3 years

There are four recognized types of diabetes mellitus.

1. Type 1 diabetes (formerly known as juvenile diabetes): Type I diabetes is now called "Immune-mediated diabetes" to more closely identify the pathology of the disease. There are approximately 1 million immune mediated type I diabetics in the United States Etiology: Immune-mediated pancreatic beta cell destruction usually leading to absolute insulin deficiency.

2. Type 2 diabetes: Results from a progressive loss of insulin secretion on the background of insulin resistance. A strong association with both a genetic predisposition (inherited), as well as obesity. This is the fastest-growing population of all types of diabetes mellitus. There are approximately 30 million type 2 diabetics in the United States.

3. Gestational diabetes (GDM). Diabetes that develops in the second or third trimester of pregnancy.

   * Clinical pearl: Diabetes that occurs in the first trimester is considered to be overt diabetes and is not considered gestational diabetes.

4. Diabetes that is due to other causes—e.g., diseases or disorders that affect the pancreas, such as cystic fibrosis, partial pancreatectomy, or pancreatic cancer. Additionally, diabetes that develops as a result of exposure to certain medications or chemical agents such as glucocorticoids, medications that are used to treat HIV/AIDS or some immunosuppressive medications.

Goals for the Diabetic Individual: The ABC's of Diabetes

A = A_{1C}
B = Blood Pressure
C = Cholesterol

The Hemoglobin A_{1C}

The hemoglobin A_{1C} is a reflection of the approximate average of blood glucose levels over the most recent 3 months.

The ADA goal for *most** diabetics is an A_{1C} < 7% (equates to an average blood glucose of 154). (AACE: American Association of Clinical Endocrinologists set this goal at ≤ 6.5%.)

In theory, an individual can achieve an A_{1C} of < 7% if they meet the following criteria:

1. Fasting (8-hour minimum fasting period) blood glucose level of between 80–130 mg/dL.

2. A two-hour post-meal (post-prandial) blood glucose of less than 180. Additionally, the patient should maintain a blood glucose throughout the day of less than 180 mg/dL.

   * Both the ADA and the AACE recognize that there are times when a less stringent A_{1C} goal is appropriate. Although an A_{1C} of < 7% is ideal, other factors to consider are: disease duration, life expectancy, significant comorbidities, patient attitude, available resources, and support systems.

Blood Pressure/Renal Function Assessment

Clinical trials have demonstrated that keeping the blood pressure less than 140/90 for most diabetic individuals can help reduce the risk of developing kidney damage.

- Most diabetics with hypertension or the presence of microalbumin in the urine will be placed on an ACE inhibitor (angiotensin converting enzyme inhibitor) or an ARB (angiotensin receptor blocker) to maintain blood pressure at a goal of less than 140/90 and to prevent or reduce the presence of microalbuminuria.

- The clinician should measure for microalbuminuria annually. If positive, a confirmatory test measurement should be repeated within 3 months. If the patient continues to have a positive result with a micoralbumin level > than 30 mcg/ml, the patient and clinician should institute measures to reduce microalbuminuria and improve renal function.

- The microalbumin test can be performed as a random spot collection of urine, and when positive with confirmatory testing, should be checked by the clinician every three months to assess for progression or improvement in renal function.

- Diabetic individuals should be referred to a nephrologist in the presence of persistent microalbuminuria, a glomerular filtration rate of less than 30, and/or hematologic evidence of a decline in renal function.

Cholesterol

The 2015 ADA Standards of Medical Care have been revised to recommend when to initiate and intensify statin therapy.

- < age 40 with no CVD factors: No statin therapy

  With CVD factors: Moderate-high dose statin therapy

  With overt CVD: High-dose statin therapy

- Age 40–75 with no CVD risk factors: Moderate statin therapy.

  Age 40–75 with CVD risk factors: High-dose statin therapy.

- Age > 75, same recommendation as for age 40–75, except consider risk/benefit profile and titrate downward as needed.

  * Clinical pearl: All patients over the age of 40 with diabetes are recommended to be on statin therapy.

DKA and HHS

Both DKA (diabetic ketoacidosis) and HHS (hyperglycemic hyperosmolar states) are severe and potentially life-threatening diabetic complications. DKA is more commonly seen in Type I DM but can occur with Type II DM especially in the case of illness.

DKA and HHS are 40% more likely to occur when patients have times of physiologic stress such as infections (UTIs pneumonia), myocardial ischemia, or other medical or surgical-related illnesses. Hyperglycemia is noted in both conditions, but frequently > 600 mg/dL for the patient with HHS and sometimes as high as 1000 mg/dL. HHS develops more slowly and more subtly than DKA. It may take days to weeks to develop, and the hyperosmolar state results in severe fluid loss and dehydration. DKA will usually develop faster than HHS. Sometimes, DKA will develop in < 24 hours. Clinical features of DKA may include Kussmaul's respirations (hyperventilation that occurs as a compensatory mechanism to counteract the metabolic acidosis), as well as nausea, vomiting, abdominal pain, anorexia, dehydration, and fatigue. Generally speaking, only patients with advanced DKA become comatose. Most patients with HHS will have some degree of neurologic disturbance, which may manifest as irritability, stupor, spasticity, hyperreflexia, seizures, and coma. Both DKA and HHS require hospitalization to provide fluid and electrolyte repletion, along with insulin administration. Regular insulin is given via IV after approximately one hour of the initiation of fluid replacement.

DKA: Laboratory Findings

- PH < 7.3
- Bicarbonate < 18
- Anion gap > 10
- Osmolality < 320
- Hyperglycemia > 250 mg/dL
- Ketones: present

HHS: Laboratory Findings

- PH > 7.3
- Bicarbonate > 18
- Anion gap: Variable
- Osmolality > 320
- Hyperglycemia > 600 mg/dL
- Ketones: Rare

Therapeutic Agents for Type 2 Diabetes Mellitus

Biguanides

Typically, the first agent used for the Type 2 DM individual is a biguanide (metformin).

Metformin will:

- Reduce hepatic glucose production
- Enhance insulin sensitivity in muscle and fat cells

- Lower blood glucose by 1–1.5%
- Usual dose is 1000 mg BID; needs to be titrated to that dose
- Adverse effects: GI distress in up to 50% of pts (patients).
- May promote weight loss
- No hypoglycemia
- Risk of lactic acidosis
- Caution in patients with: renal disease (creatinine > 1.4 women; > 1.5 men)
- ETOH abuse
- Elderly (> age 80)
- With radiological studies: d/c metformin 24 hours before procedure until 48 hours afterward, (until hydration is reestablished).
- Can improve ovulatory function (think pregnancy)
- Approved for use in children over the age of 10

DPP-4 Inhibitors (dipeptidyl peptidase)

- Inhibits the enzyme that breaks down GLP-1 and GIP
- 2006: Januvia (sitagliptin) 100 mg daily (adjust dosage downward for renal impairment)
- 2009: Onglyza (saxagliptin) 5 mg daily (adjust dosage downward for renal impairment)
- 2011: Tradjenta (linagliptin) 5 mg daily (no adjustment needed for renal impairment)
- 2013: Nesina (alogliptin) 6.25, 12.5, 25 mg (adjust dosage downward for renal impairment)
- Can be monotherapy. Often used in combination with metformin
- No hypoglycemia and weight neutral
- Can be expensive
- Additional $\downarrow A_{1C}$ by 0.5–1.0

GLP-1 RAs (glucagon-like peptide receptor agonists)

Daily: Byetta (exenatide), Victoza (liraglutide)

Weekly: Bydureon (long-acting exenatide), Tanzeum (albiglutide), Trulicity (dulaglutide)

Increases insulin secretion in response to carbohydrates

Prevents excessive hepatic glucose production by suppressing glucagon release

Slows gastric emptying and signals the brain to recognize increased satiety. This results in reduced food intake and increased satiety.

Promotes weight loss

Decreases A_{1C} by 0.5–1.5% when used as monotherapy

GI adverse events: Nausea and diarrhea are usually self-limiting (approx. 8–10 weeks for most)

Post marketing reports of an increased risk of pancreatitis

If patient is on a DPP4 inhibitor, stop the DPP4 inhibitor when initiating a GLP-1 (both together will increase the risk of pancreatitis)

In clinical trials in rats, development of medullary thyroid carcinoma. (Do not use in patients with personal or family history of medullary thyroid cancer.) Do not use in patients with history of MEN 2 (multiple endocrine neoplasia type 2).

SGLT-2 Inhibitors (sodium-glucose co-transporter 2 inhibitors)

Examples of the SGLT-2 co-transport inhibitors are:

- Invokana (canagliflozin) (FDA approval—March, 2013) 100 mg or 300 mg QD
- Farxiga (dapagliflozin) (FDA approval—January, 2014) 5 mg or 10 mg QD
- Jardiance (empagliflozin) (FDA approval—August, 2014) 10 mg or 25 mg QD
- Blocks glucose reabsorption by the kidney. Increasing glucosuria.
- No hypoglycemia
- Decrease in blood pressure
- Weight loss occurs as a result of the loss of glucose (calories) in the urine.
- Approx. A_{1C} reduction of 1% as monotherapy

SGLT-2 disadvantages:

- May cause genitourinary infections
- May cause volume depletion/hypotension/dizziness
- Transient increase in K+ or creatinine
- May cause increase in LDL

Thiazolinediones (TZDs)

- Actos (pioglitazone) 15–45 mg/daily. Avandia (rosiglitazone)
- Decrease insulin resistance in peripheral tissue/decrease hepatic glucose production
- May also decrease TG and increase HDL.
- SE: weight gain, edema (contraindicated for patients with CHF)
- Need to monitor LFTs.
- $\downarrow A_{1C}$ by 1–1.5%

Takes 6–12 weeks for maximum effectiveness.

New warning regarding increased risk of bladder cancer.

Alpha-Glucosidase Inhibitors

- Precose (acarbose) and Glyset (miglitol)
- Delays CHO digestion and decreases post-prandial glucose
- Useful in patients with mild glucose intolerance associated with post prandial hyperglycemia
- Can cause bloating and flatulence due to the increased transit time of food through the digestive system
- $\downarrow A_{1C}$ by 0.5%

Sulfonylureas

Glyburide, Glipizide, Glimepiride

Stimulates insulin secretion

Risk of hypoglycemia

Weight gain

Caution in patients with sulfa allergies, and renal or liver impairments

Cost-effective

Improve A_{1C} by 1–2%

Meglitinides

- Repaglinide (Prandin) and Nateglinide (Starlix)
- Similar to sulfonylureas in that they stimulate the pancreas to produce more insulin. More rapid onset/shorter duration
- SE: hypoglycemia and weight gain
- Frequent dose scheduling (with each meal)
- Useful for those with sulfa allergy
- Monotherapy or use with metformin
- $\downarrow A_{1C}$ by 1–1.5%

Insulin

Start insulin when the following conditions are present:

- Any newly diagnosed type 1
- Severe hyperglycemia (> 400 mg/dL)
- Signs of dehydration
- Signs of acidosis or ketosis

Clinical Pearl

If the diabetic has an A_{1C} >10% or if blood sugar is commonly > 300, the patient is considered to be glucose toxic and should have insulin therapy. Insulin can be removed from the regimen of the type 2

diabetic once the glucose toxicity resolves and the patient's condition improves.

It is important to remember that insulin can be added to the regimen at any time. It can be added to oral therapy whenever necessary. Usually, initiation for a type 2 diabetic is done with basal insulin (glargine, detemir). They are typically taken before bed and provide background insulin (no peak) for an approximately 24-hour duration.

When initiating prandial insulin (short-acting insulins given prior to meals), consider discontinuing the sulfonylurea.

Short-acting insulins are lispro (HumaLOG), aspart (NovoLOG), and glulisine (Apidra).

* The greatest risk of insulin therapy is hypoglycemia.

Hypoglycemia

The rule of "15"

If the individual has symptoms of low blood sugar, they should check their blood sugar. If low (below 70), follow the rule of "15."

Eat or drink 15 grams of fast-acting sugar (4 glucose tablets, 4 ounces of fruit juice, ½ can of regular soda).

Check blood sugar again after 15 minutes. If it is still low, repeat with 15 grams of fast-acting sugar.

Once blood sugar is over 100, the individual should have a small snack with protein and carbohydrate such as a ½ sandwich and milk to sustain the blood glucose level.

* Sometimes a patient will feel symptomatic even when their blood sugar is not low (below 70). This commonly occurs in individuals who have chronically high blood sugars. In that case, the diabetic individual can initiate the same treatment as is done for "true" hypoglycemia. However, the clinician should reinforce with the diabetic individual that this is not a normal physiologic response and they should work together to bring the patient to a more normal state of hypoglycemic awareness.

Thyroid Disorders

- Bi-lobar structure located in the neck.
- 2 lobes connected by isthmus at the level of the cricoid cartilage.
- Thyroid gland produces and stores thyroid hormone.
- Production of thyroid hormone is dependent on ingestion of iodine.
- T3 and T4 are bound to plasma proteins.
- Thyroxine (T4): Majority of T4 is bound to plasma proteins; small amount of free T4 that is circulating in serum reflects thyroid activity.
- Triiodothyronine (T3): 80% is formed in liver, kidney, and muscle as breakdown of

T4; the remaining 20% is secreted directly by thyroid.

- TSH (thyroid stimulating hormone) is released by anterior pituitary in response to TRH (thyrotropin releasing hormone).
- TSH is inhibited by circulation of T3 and T4 (negative feedback system).
- TSH level is a good indicator of thyroid function; sensitive and specific.
- TSH normal range 0.40–4.5u/ml (normal levels may vary slightly depending on assay used by laboratory).
- Hyperthyroid (TSH < 0.40)
- Hypothyroid (TSH > 4.5)
- Euthyroid (TSH = 0.40–4.5)
- American Thyroid Association: Screen men and women every 5 years beginning at 35 y.o. Screen women over 50 years of age or with any symptoms.
- USPTF does not recommend routine screening.

Interpretation of Diagnostic Tests

1. Free T4 and TSH
   - Free T4 (thyroxine) normal range is 4.5–12.0.
   - Low T4 with elevated TSH confirms hypothyroidism.
   - High T4 with low TSH confirms hyperthyroidism.
   - TSH may rise before drop in T4 is observed (subclinical hypothyroidism).
2. RAI Uptake Test (Radioactive Iodine Uptake Test)
   - Useful for diagnosing hyperthyroidism
   - Measures amount of iodine taken up by thyroid gland
   - Increased uptake of iodine in hyperthyroid, goiter
   - Decreased uptake of iodine in subacute thyroiditis, hypothyroidism
   - Check for allergy to shellfish
   - Not useful if patients are already on thyroid replacement
3. Thyroid Ultrasound
   - Measures size and shape of gland, homogenous, solid, or cystic nodule
   - If suspicious for cancer, can obtain sample of cells with ultrasound guided FNA (fine needle aspiration)
4. Radionucleotide Thyroid Scan
   - (if suspecting nodule, cancer)
   - "Hot area" hyper-functioning nodule is present – 90% benign
   - "Cold area" hypo-functioning nodule is present – 5–10% malignant

Hypothyroidism

- Most common form of thyroid disorders
- Symptoms can mimic normal aging.
- 10 × more common in women
- 1 out of every 50 people, age 60 and older
- Low levels of circulating thyroid hormone causes clinical manifestations
- High TSH and low free T4
- 95% of all cases are primary hypothyroidism caused by underfunctioning of the thyroid gland.
- Autoimmune (Hashimoto's Thyroiditis) is the most common cause.
- Goiter may or may not be present.
- Check antithyroid antibody titer (TPO: thyroid peroxidase autoantibody). A positive result means it is Hashimoto's disease.

Other less common causes of primary hypothyroidism are:

- Ablative therapy
- Thyroidectomy (for goiter or cancer)
- Iodine deficiency
- Pharmacologic agents such as lithium or amiodarone
- Transient postpartum thyroiditis. May occur in 5–10% of postpartum women.

Secondary Hypothyroidism

- Rare 5% of all cases
- Neoplasm of the pituitary gland or hypothalamus
- Hypopituitarism (pituitary adenoma)
- Congenital (cretinism)

Symptoms of Hypothyroidism

- Cold intolerance
- Hair loss
- Constipation
- Arthralgias
- Weight gain

- Goiter
- Dry skin
- Depression, irritability, poor concentration
- Fatigue
- Menstrual disturbance

Physical exam and laboratory findings may include:

- Pale/cool/coarse/dry skin
- Dry coarse hair
- Eyelid and facial edema (lid lag or ptsosis)
- Slow speech
- Neurologic signs such as delayed reflexes (patellar "hang-up" reflex)
- Bradycardia
- Cardiomyopathy
- Anemia
- Dyslipidemia
- Hyponatremia (if edema present)

Hyperthyroidism

- Excess secretion of Thyroid Hormone (T4 and T3)
- a.k.a., thyrotoxicosis
- Common causes:

   Graves' disease 60–80% of all cases (autoimmune)

   15% of cases > 60-year-old

   May be related to a hyperfunctioning thyroid nodule.

   Toxic nodular goiters account for 5% of cases.

   More common in patients > 40 y.o. with long-standing history of multinodular goiter

   Thyroid Inflammatory Diseases: Leakage of thyroid hormone from damaged or inflamed gland (post-viral illness, postpartum thyroiditis)

Symptoms of Hyperthyroidism

- Weight loss despite good appetite
- Nervousness, emotionally labile, tremors
- Sweating, heat intolerance
- Insomnia
- Increased BMs
- Amenorrhea
- Elderly symptoms: weak, depressed, palpitations

*Clinical pearl: Both endogenous and exogenous hyperthyroidism (caused by over-replacement of thyroid hormone) can cause tachyarrhythmia and/or atrial fibrillation. Include a cardiac assessment when performing the workup of a patient who has hyperthyroidism.

Physical exam findings:

- Skin smooth, soft, palmar erythema, diaphoresis
- Nails clubbing, onycholysis
- Eye exam may show exophthalmos, lid lag, palpebral fissures
- Neck: thyroid enlargement – goiter
- Respiratory: dyspnea
- Cardiac: tachycardia, arrhythmias
- MS: proximal weakness, tremors, hyperreflexia
- Neuro/MS: restless, labile, irritable, decreased concentration, memory loss

Treatment options for hyperthyroidism:

- There is no treatment to reverse the underlying autoimmune cause of Graves' disease
- Treatment options to control production of thyroid hormone and/or symptom control include:
   - Beta-blockers to control sympathomimetic symptoms (usually propranolol unless contraindicated); may also use CCBs
   - Antithyroid drugs (thioamides)
   - Ablative therapy with radioactive iodine (RAI-131).
   - Surgical thyroidectomy (may be partial or total)

Ablative Therapy with RAI 131

- Now the first-line treatment option
- Concentrates in the thyroid gland, causing atrophy of thyroid tissue
- Adverse side effect development of permanent hypothyroidism
- Not to be used in pregnancy or nursing. Patients should wait at least 6 months post-RAI ablative therapy.

Thioamides: Inhibit formation of T3 and T4. Examples of thioamides include:

- MMI (methimazole) 10–20 mg q 8 hrs (daily, every 8 hrs)
- PTU (propylthiouracil) 50–100mg q 6–8 hrs (daily, every 6 to 8 hrs)
- The patient typically will obtain a euthyroid state in 4–6 weeks

- Generally, thioamides are not the first-line choice of treatment, due to the risk of agranulocytosis and hepatitis.

Thryoidectomy (partial or total)

- Occasionally used in patients with large goiters and thyroid nodules that are resistant to radio-iodine therapy.
- Pregnant women, children
- Complications:
  - laryngeal nerve damage
  - hypoparathyroidism (hypocalcemia)

Adrenal Disorders

Chronic Adrenal Insufficiency: Addison's disease

A deficiency of the adrenal hormones: cortisol and aldosterone. Addison's disease usually develops slowly, most commonly during a person's middle age, and is often undiagnosed until it has progressed beyond the early stages. However, during a stressful period, the symptoms can worsen very quickly and cause an Addisonian crisis which may be life threatening.

Primary adrenal insufficiency—Caused by damage to the adrenal gland from autoimmune disease, infection, TB, or cancer

Secondary adrenal insufficiency—Caused by failure of the pituitary gland to produce ACTH, or due to a reduction of CRH (corticotropin releasing hormone) from the hypothalamus.

Symptoms of Addison's disease are:

- Fatigue
- Muscle weakness
- Hypotension
- Hypoglycemia
- Nausea/vomiting
- Salt cravings
- Weight loss
- Hyperpigmentation
- Diagnosis

Diagnosis of Addison's Disease (H & P)

- The most unique symptom is hyperpigmentation – Often in non-sun-exposed areas.
- ACTH stimulation test. A patient is given ACTH, and subsequent cortisol levels are measured in both the serum and the urine. (People with Addison's disease do not respond to the ACTH hormone.)
- If ACTH is positive, may have a CRH stimulation test. The patient is given IV CRH, and serial measurements are taken of both cortisol and ACTH. Patients with Addison's disease have low cortisol levels and high ACTH levels if the secondary cause is related to the hypothalamus.
- Additional tests for primary adrenal insufficiency are:
  - Ultrasound of the abdomen, kidneys, and adrenal glands
  - TB skin testing
  - Antibody testing to assess for autoimmune origin
  - MRIs and CT scans can help assess for secondary causes such as abnormalities within the pituitary gland or the hypothalamus.

Treatment of Addison's Disease

- Patients are typically referred to an endocrinologist for care, treatment, and follow-up.
- Patients are treated with cortisol replacement, such as hydrocortisone, prednisone, or dexamethasone.
- With primary adrenal insufficiency, there is a greater chance of aldosterone deficiency, and the patient is maintained with fludrocortisone (Florinef) daily.
- Dosages are adjusted during times of increase stress, illness, surgery, or trauma. Patients should carry injectable hydrocortisone to inject in case of emergency.

Cushing's Syndrome (CS)

Caused by an excessive production of cortisol, the excessive production may be ACTH independent or ACTH dependent.

ACTH: Pituitary adenomas account for 70% of all ACTH-dependent Cushing's syndrome. They are almost always benign microadenomas.

ACTH independent: Exogenous—Occurs when excess steroids are taken into the body. Drug induced Cushing's syndrome is the most common reason for ACTH-independent CS.

ACTH independent: Endogenous—Caused by adrenal adenomas or carcinomas. Excess cortisol is rarely due to excess production by the adrenal gland itself.

Diagnostic Tests

First-line tests: Establish diagnosis

- 24-hour urinary test for free cortisol (UFC: Three samples are taken. Normal levels are < 100 mcg/24 hours.
- Dexamethasone suppression test (DST). Patient is given 1 mg of dexamethasone between 11:00 and 12:00 midnight. In the a.m., serum cortisol measurements above 5 mcg/dL indicate CS.

Second-line tests: Differentiate the cause

- ACTH measurements
- High-dose DST testing
- CRH stimulation test
- Pituitary MRI

Treatment:

- Discontinue the causative medication
- Inhibit steroid synthesis with pharmacologic treatments such as ketoconazole, mitotane (Lysodren), metyrapone (Metopirone), and etomidate (Amidate).
- Transphenoidal surgery for pituitary tumors or radiation therapy.

Review Questions

1. The nurse practitioner is reviewing the laboratory values of a 28-year-old male patient who presents to the office to establish care with a primary care provider. The lab results from the previous week indicate an A_{1C} of 7.2. The nurse practitioner obtains a fasting blood sugar in the office of 142. The patient denies any significant past medical history and states that he "feels fine." The nurse practitioner recognizes that:

   A. The patient has developed type 1 diabetes.

   B. The patient has developed type 2 diabetes.

   C. The patient has diabetes and further testing is required.

   D. The patient has pre-diabetes.

2. The nurse practitioner has been working with a 40-year-old diabetic, single mother of two teenage children. The patient has an A_{1C} of 8.0%. The patient and provider agree upon a plan that is designed to achieve glycemic control and set a target date of 6 months. When the patient returns six months later, her A_{1C} is 7.8%. The NP would then:

   A. Encourage the patient to take a greater responsibility for her health, reinforcing the concept that she is a role model for her children.

   B. Reassess the plan and consider barriers such as income, health literacy, and family dynamics.

   C. Encourage the patient to design a plan that will meet the needs of both herself and her family.

   D. Explain to the patient that as long as there was improvement in her A_{1C}, the plan is a success.

3. The nurse practitioner is reviewing the laboratory values of a patient during a follow-up office visit. The NP observes the following results in the chart:

   September: A_{1C} = 6.6 Fasting glucose = 118

   December: A_{1C} = 6.8 Fasting glucose = 122

   The nurse practitioner is correct in noting:

   A. The patient does not meet the criteria to establish a diagnosis of diabetes mellitus.

   B. The patient partially meets the criteria to establish a diagnosis of diabetes mellitus, but further confirmatory testing is required.

   C. The patient has diabetes mellitus.

   D. The A_{1C} and fasting tests should be repeated in 3 months to confirm a diagnosis of diabetes mellitus.

4. The American Diabetes Association (ADA) recommends the use of laboratory testing to screen for pre-diabetes in asymptomatic people. The recommendation is to perform this screening on:

   A. All children who are overweight or obese.

   B. All adults with a BMI > 25 with one or more risk factors for diabetes mellitus.

   C. All adults and children as part of their complete routine physical exams.

   D. All children who were born to mothers that have had gestational diabetes.

5. Impaired fasting glucose (IFG) and impaired glucose tolerance (IGT) are both markers for pre-diabetes. Both IFG and IGT are closely associated with:

   A. Autoimmune disorders such as hypothyroidism, rheumatoid arthritis, and Sjögren's syndrome.

   B. Elevations in liver enzymes and inflammatory markers such as C-reactive protein.

   C. Obesity, coronary artery disease, and peripheral vascular disease.

   D. Central obesity, high triglycerides, low HDLs, and hypertension.

6. Which of the following laboratory results would be a strong indicator that the patient has pre-diabetes?

   A. An A_{1C} between 5.5 and 5.7

   B. A 2-hour post-prandial glucose between 110 and 140, after a 75 gm oral glucose tolerance test.

   C. A fasting glucose between 100 and 125 after an 8-hour fasting interval.

   D. An A_{1C} of greater than or equal to 6.5%.

7. Immune mediated diabetes accounts for 5–10% of all diabetes mellitus and is caused by autoimmune destruction of the pancreatic beta cells. Which of the following statements is true regarding immune-mediated diabetes?

   A. It will develop during early childhood or adolescence.

   B. Patients with immune-mediated diabetes have a BMI less than 25.

   C. The rate of beta cell destruction is more rapid in some individuals and slower in others.

   D. Initial treatment with oral hypoglycemic agents is appropriate until there is a complete loss of beta cell function.

8. Type 2 diabetes mellitus is associated with insulin resistance. Which of the following statements about insulin resistance is true?

   A. Patients with insulin resistance have decreased insulin production.

   B. Insulin resistance may improve with weight loss.

   C. Insulin resistance and type 2 diabetes mellitus are progressive diseases that will eventually lead to absolute insulin deficiency.

   D. Insulin resistance is a genetic trait and thus cannot be altered or improved.

9. Treatment plans for the diabetic patient should be individualized. In developing the plan, consideration should be given to: (check all that apply)

   A. Age.

   B. Culture.

   C. Medical condition.

   D. Social situation.

   E. School or work schedule.

   F. Hereditary factors.

   G. Gender.

10. The most common comorbidities that occur with type 2 diabetes mellitus are:

    A. Depression, cancer, obstructive sleep apnea.

    B. Obesity, coronary artery disease, sedentary lifestyle.

    C. Hypertension, hyperlipidemia, obesity.

    D. Hypothyroidism, hyperlipidemia, chronic kidney disease.

11. DSME (diabetes self-management education) encourages the patient to make informed decisions. This approach is most successful when:

    A. The diabetic is provided with enough education and information that he or she can make an informed decision.

    B. It is patient-centered and responsive to individual preferences, needs, and values.

    C. The patient is given written directions that outlines a specific medication regimen and goal.

    D. A consensus model is used which considers multiple disciplines involved in the care of the diabetic individual.

12. Medical nutritional therapy (MNT) is an integral part of diabetes self-management education. Which of the following aspects of MNT would be most supportive to the patient?

    A. All patients with type 2 diabetes should be encouraged to lose between 2 and 8 kilograms of their body weight.

    B. All members of the health care team involved with the diabetic individual should be knowledgeable about MNT and support its implementation.

    C. All patients with diabetes mellitus need to know how to count carbohydrates and limit the amount of carbohydrates in each meal.

    D. Provide the patient with menus and recipes that will be easy for the patient to create at home.

13. Patients that are diagnosed as pre-diabetic may begin pharmacologic therapy. The strongest evidence-based pharmacologic therapy to prevent the patient's progression to diabetes is to initiate therapy with:

    A. A DPP4 such as saxagliptin.

    B. A basal insulin such as glargine.

    C. A GLP-1 receptor agonist such as liraglutide.

    D. A biguanide such as metformin.

14. Patients who are on intensive insulin regimens should monitor their blood glucose multiple times throughout the day. The patient should be instructed that monitoring of blood glucose is essential:

    A. Before every meal.

    B. Before engaging in exercise.

    C. Upon awakening in the morning.

    D. Before driving a car.

15. The "Rule of 15" is used when the diabetic experiences hypoglycemia. The "Rule of 15" instructs the patient to:

    A. Take 15 units of insulin for every 15 grams of carbohydrate ingested.

    B. The patient should try to have 15 grams of protein, 15 grams of fat, and 15 grams of carbohydrate in equal portions for each meal.

    C. The patient should ingest 15 grams of carbohydrate, wait 15 minutes, and re-check their blood glucose level. Repeat as necessary until symptoms abate or blood glucose is > 100.

    D. Immediately inject 15 milligrams of a glucagon hypoglycemic emergency kit into their mid-thigh muscle.

16. The patient is started on metformin therapy. The nurse practitioner should explain to the patient that a potentially fatal side effect of metformin is:

    A. Nausea and diarrhea.

    B. Lactic acidosis.

    C. Ketoacidosis.

    D. Pancreatitis.

17. An overweight diabetic patient verbalizes that he is interested in beginning therapy with a GLP-1 RA to improve his diabetic control and assist with weight loss. The nurse practitioner must first assess the patient for:

    A. A personal or family history of medullary thyroid cancer.

    B. A personal or family history of papillary thyroid cancer.

    C. A personal or family history of familial hereditary polyposis.

    D. A personal or family history of polycystic kidney disease.

18. A patient presents to the primary care office for an initial evaluation. The patient is complaining of polyuria and polydipsia and exhibits symptoms of dehydration. An A_{1C} is obtained that reveals an A_{1C} of 12.7%. The nurse practitioner should initiate therapy with:

    A. Metformin.

    B. A GLP-1 RA.

    C. Insulin.

    D. A sulfonylurea.

19. The patient is reviewing her labs with the nurse practitioner. She inquires about the significance of the hemoglobin A_{1C} test. The nurse practitioner explains:

    A. "It represents the serum glucose level."

    B. "It reflects the post-prandial (after-meal) increase of the serum glucose."

    C. "It represents the percentage of red blood cells that contain hemoglobin."

    D. "It correlates with the average serum glucose level of the previous 90 days."

20. A type 2 diabetic patient is started on pharmacologic therapy that is expected to assist with weight loss. Which pharmacologic therapy may assist with weight loss?

    A. A dipeptidyl peptidase inhibitor (DPP-4 inhibitor)

    B. A thiazolinedione (TZD)

    C. A sodium-glucose co-transporter 2 inhibitor (SGLT-2 inhibitor)

    D. A sulfonylurea

21. What is the most common side effect of metformin therapy?

    A. Hypoglycemia

    B. Gastrointestinal upset

    C. Weight gain

    D. Fungal infections

22. A type 2 diabetic patient presents for a diabetic follow-up visit. The patient has a history of hypertension and persistent microalbuminuria. The patient verbalizes that he regularly takes lisinopril (20 milligrams daily). The nurse practitioner observes that the patient's most recent GFR (glomerular filtration rate) is 29 and knows that the recommended management for this patient is to:

    A. Refer them to a nephrologist.

    B. Repeat the GFR in 3 months and monitor electrolytes, bicarbonate, and calcium.

    C. Obtain a 24-hour urine sample for creatinine clearance.

    D. Obtain a renal ultrasound to assess for renal artery stenosis.

23. Diabetic retinopathy is the most common cause of new cases of blindness among adults age 20–74 years. It is associated with the duration of the disease, as well as microvascular damage. Which of the following conditions, when present, would alert the nurse practitioner to recommend an immediate ophthalmic evaluation?

    A. Orthostatic hypotension

    B. Nephropathy

    C. Coronary artery disease

    D. Gastroparesis

24. A 38-year-old female patient with type 1 diabetes has developed persistent microalbuminuria, as evidenced by two specimens collected over a 6-month period. The patient is normotensive. The nurse practitioner would be correct in recommending that the patient:

    A. Continue with watchful waiting and repeat urine microalbumin annually.

    B. Restrict the protein in their diet to no more than 60 kilograms of protein per day.

    C. Obtain a serum pregnancy test, and if negative, initiate ACE-inhibitor therapy.

    D. Repeat the test using a first morning urine sample obtained with a clean-catch, midstream collection method.

25. A 75-year-old patient with a 20-year history of type 2 diabetes presents to the office for a follow-up evaluation. She brings her most recent 3 months of blood glucose logs, which reveal a morning fasting glucose of 58–75. Her A_{1C} is 6.0%. The nurse practitioner reviews her medication regimen, which is:

    Metformin 1000 mg po BID

    Sitagliptin 100 mg po once daily

    Glargine insulin 10 units SQ at HS

    The nurse practitioner discusses with the patient her concerns regarding persistent hypoglycemia and recommends that the patient:

    A. Discontinue the metformin.

    B. Discontinue the sitagliptin.

    C. Discontinue the glargine insulin.

    D. Reduce the metformin dose to 1000 mg daily in the a.m.

26. A 10-year-old male patient is seen in his PCP's office. The patient has a negative PMH and a glucose reading of 626. The patient has been complaining of abdominal pain and nausea. The NP notes that the patient is breathing with deep, labored, and rapid respirations, and is lethargic. What is the most likely cause of the patient's condition?

    A. HHS caused by type II DM

    B. DKA caused by type I DM

    C. Uncontrolled hyperglycemia with dehydration

    D. Diabetes exacerbation related to pneumonia

27. The NP is working in the ED when a patient with known DM 1 is brought in by ambulance. The patient states that she has been sick with the flu and has not been able to control her blood sugar despite taking her usual doses of short-acting insulin. The patient's BS is 522 upon admission to the ED. Serum and urine Ketones are +. Blood gas reveals a PH of 7.25. The NP is aware that the first step in treatment is:

    A. Initiate hydration with IV NS.

    B. Initiate a regular insulin IV.

    C. Initiate IV bicarbonate therapy.

    D. Initiate treatment of the underlying causes of elevated BS.

28. A female patient with type II DM on oral hypoglycemic therapy is seen in the office for a follow-up evaluation. The patient states that she was recently diagnosed with a UTI over the weekend and went to a walk-in treatment center. She started on antibiotic therapy 24 hours ago. She continues to complain of UTI symptoms. Additionally, her BS has been consistently elevated in the 250–300 range. The NP would be correct in considering:

    A. Sending the patient to the ED for evaluation of HHS.

    B. Initiating treatment with insulin in the office and adding an insulin regimen at home to cover the patient's "sick days."

    C. Intensifying the oral hypoglycemic therapy.

    D. Obtaining stat ABGs to assess for acidosis.

29. Both DKA and HHS can be seen in the diabetic patient. The NP should be aware that the most common reason for development of these two conditions are:

    A. Non-adherence to the diabetic medication regimen.

    B. Non-adherence to the diet and exercise regimen.

    C. An underlying medical condition causing physiologic stress.

    D. A lack of understanding by the patient about these two conditions.

30. A patient with type 2 DM is being evaluated in the NP's office. The patient states that she has lost a lot of weight lately "without even trying" and expects that the NP will be pleased. The patient's BS in the office is 524. She has lost 20 pounds since her last visit one month ago. The patient verbalizes profound fatigue. The NP is aware that the patient is most likely experiencing:

    A. Fatigue related to her rapid weight loss and malnutrition.

    B. Fatigue related to severe dehydration, which is likely caused by HHS.

    C. Fatigue related to an underlying infection.

    D. Fatigue related to severe hyperglycemia.

31. The most sensitive laboratory indicator of overall thyroid function is to evaluate the level of circulating:

    A. Free T4.

    B. Free T3.

    C. TSH.

    D. TPO (thyroid peroxidase antibody).

32. An individual is being evaluated by the NP for a thyroid disorder. The NP notes that the TSH is 0.01 mcg U/L. What should the NP do next?

    A. Repeat the TSH.

    B. Obtain total T3 and free T4 levels.

    C. Perform an ultrasound-guided FNA (fine needle aspiration) of the thyroid gland.

    D. Order a test of TBGs (thyroid binding immunoglobulins).

33. A 38 y.o. female with a negative past medical history is being evaluated by the NP. The patient complains of weight loss, hand tremors, and "feeling like my heart is pounding." Her apical pulse is regular at 104 BPM. The NP orders TFTs (thyroid function tests) which reveal a TSH of < .01 mcg U/L. What should the NP do next?

    A. Obtain a stat pregnancy test. If negative, order ablative therapy with radioactive iodine 131.

    B. Obtain a stat pregnancy test. If negative, order a benzodiazepine to reduce tremors and anxiety.

    C. Obtain a stat pregnancy test. If negative, initiate therapy with a thioamide.

    D. Obtain a stat pregnancy test. If negative, initiate beta-blocker therapy with propranolol.

34. Thioamides may cause severe side effects. Before initiating treatment with a thioamide, the NP should obtain a baseline:

    A. Coagulation study.

    B. Renal function test.

    C. CBC with differential.

    D. Dexa scan.

35. Appropriate thyroid hormone biosynthesis is dependent on the dietary intake of:

    A. Calcium.

    B. Iron.

    C. Magnesium.

    D. Iodine.

36. The NP is evaluating the lab results of a 52-year-old female patient with a history of Hashimotos hypothyroidism. The NP observes that the patient's TSH indicates overtreatment with her thyroid replacement medication. She instructs the patient to reduce her dosage by taking her levothyroxine 6 days per week instead of 7. The patient responds "I don't want to do that since it will make me gain weight. Why can't I just stay at this dose?" What is an appropriate response from the NP?

    A. "Thyroid replacement medication is not to be used for weight loss."

    B. "Decreasing the medication dosage one day a week will not have any effect on your weight."

    C. "You may continue at the same dosage for now. If you should start to feel jittery or have symptoms consistent with hyperthyroidism, we will need to reduce your dosage at that time."

    D. "Over-replacement with thyroid hormone puts you at risk for developing cardiac arrhythmias."

37. A patient is at risk for secondary hypothyroidism if they have which of the following conditions?

    A. Adrenal insufficiency

    B. Cushing's disease

    C. Pituitary adenoma

    D. Systemic lupus erythematous

38. The most common clinical presentation of a patient with hypothyroidism is:

    A. The presence of a goiter.

    B. Hair loss.

    C. Fatigue.

    D. Parasthesias.

39. A patient is diagnosed with subclinical hypothyroidism. The NP would expect the laboratory findings to include:

    A. An elevated TSH with a normal free T4 level.

    B. A suppressed TSH level with a normal free T4 level.

    C. A suppressed TSH level with a low free T4 level.

    D. An elevated TSH with a low free T4 level.

40. A patient with a known history of hypothyroidism and bipolar disorder informs the NP that lately she has been feeling very sluggish. Her TSH is 12.4 mcg U/L. Upon review of the patient's medication, the NP observes that the patient is on levothyroxine 112 mcg daily and lithium 300 mg TID. The NP instructs the patient to:

    A. Increase the levothyroxine to 125 mcg daily and repeat TSH in 6 weeks.

    B. Reduce the lithium dose to 300 mg bid and repeat the TSH in 6 weeks.

    C. Reduce the dose of levothyroxine to 100 mcg daily since the TSH level is too high. Repeat TSH in 6 weeks.

    D. Stop the lithium and use an alternative treatment for the patient's bipolar disorder.

41. A patient with primary adrenal insufficiency will often have which of the following classic presenting symptoms?

    A. Hypertension

    B. Weight gain

    C. Hyperpigmentation

    D. Increased appetite

42. A patient with primary adrenal insufficiency might be expected to have which of the following lab results?

    A. Hypokalemia

    B. Hyponatremia

    C. Hyperglycemia

    D. Hypocalcemia

43. A patient is suspected to have *primary* adrenal insufficiency. The nurse practitioner notes that the 8:00 a.m. cortisol is low. What would the NP expect to find with regard to other lab values?

    A. An elevated plasma ACTH

    B. A decreased plasma ACTH

    C. Positive adrenal antibodies

    D. Elevated aldosterone levels

44. A patient is diagnosed with primary adrenal insufficiency. What is an important educational point that the patient needs to understand?

    A. The patient will need to take a glucocorticoid replacement during times of physiologic stress.

    B. The patient will need glucocorticoid replacement daily and lifelong.

    C. Patients should have their glucocorticoid levels checked prior to any surgical or invasive procedure.

    D. The patient should always take the glucocorticoid replacement at bedtime.

45. Clinical features that can be expected of a patient with Cushing's syndrome are:

    A. Multiple small striae over the hips and breast areas.

    B. Hyperpigmentation of skin areas that have not been exposed to the sun.

    C. Dizziness and syncopal episodes.

    D. Easy bruising and skin atrophy.

46. Which of the following is a test that is most helpful in diagnosing Cushing's syndrome?

    A. An MRI of the pituitary gland with and without a contrast medium

    B. A random serum cortisol level

    C. A 1 mg overnight dexamethasone suppression test

    D. A random ACTH level

47. Of the following, which is associated with Cushing's syndrome?

    A. Hypothalmic-pituitary axis tumors

    B. Pituitary tumors

    C. Disorders involving the thymus gland

    D. Adrenal tumors

48. Which of the following is the most common cause of Cushing's syndrome?

    A. Autoimmune disorders

    B. Exogenous replacement with corticosteroids

    C. Pituitary microadenomas

    D. Adrenal insufficiency

49. A patient that has hypercortisolemia and an elevated ACTH level would be interpreted as having which of the following?

    A. Cushing's syndrome

    B. Cushing's disease

    C. Addison's disease

    D. Primary adrenal insufficiency

50. A patient with an elevated 24-hour urine for cortisol can be diagnosed as having which of the following?

    A. Cushing's disease

    B. Cushing's syndrome

    C. Hypercortisolemia of undetermined origin

    D. Primary adrenal hyperplasia

Answers and Rationales

1. C. The patient meets the criteria to be diagnosed with diabetes. The clinician would be unable to determine what type of diabetes the patient has without further testing.

2. B. The clinician needs to reassess the plan and work with the patient to identify barriers that are preventing the patient from achieving the goal.

3. C. The patient has diabetes mellitus and meets the criteria to establish diagnosis with an $A_{1C} \geq 6.5\%$ and confirmatory testing.

4. B. The ADA recommends screening for pre-diabetes and diabetes in all adults with a BMI > than 25 and at least one other risk factor.

5. D. Central obesity, high triglycerides, and low HDLs are consistent with metabolic syndrome and are closely associated with pre-diabetes and diabetes.

6. C. An individual may be diagnosed with pre-diabetes if the fasting glucose (8-hour fast) is 100–125. If the fasting glucose is > 125 on two or more occasions, the patient would be diagnosed with diabetes mellitus.

7. D. The rate of beta cell destruction with immune-mediated diabetes mellitus is highly individualized.

8. B. Weight loss is one of the only non-pharmacologic interventions that may reduce insulin resistance.

9. A, B, C, D, E, and F are all correct. All answers are correct except G "gender." Rationale: The sex of the patient is not a determinant of therapeutic recommendations.

10. C. The most common comorbid conditions associated with type 2 diabetes are hyperlipidemia, hypertension, and obesity. There is a strong correlation between metabolic syndrome and the development of type 2 diabetes.

11. B. DSME must be patient-centered and responsive to the individual's needs, otherwise it is unlikely to be successful.

12. B. All members of the health care team involved in the care of a diabetic individual should be familiar with MNT (medical nutrition therapy) and be consistent with the recommendations of these life-long behavioral modifications.

13. D. Metformin has the strongest evidence-base as a pharmacologic therapy for diabetes prevention.

14. D. Although all answers are acceptable, the patient treated with an intensive insulin therapy poses the greatest risk to self and others when driving.

15. C. The "Rule of 15" was created to simplify treatment for the hypoglycemic patient while that person remains capable of assisting themselves to correct their hypoglycemia. When patients are hypoglycemic, they often have impaired judgment. Teaching the patient this simple rule can help prevent a further decline in blood glucose and prevent overcorrection of their low blood sugar.

16. B. All patients that are on metformin therapy must be aware of the potential for lactic acidosis, which can be fatal.

17. A. A black box warning exists for all GLP-1 RAs if there is a family or personal history of medullary thyroid cancer or a history of MEN2 (multiple endocrine neoplasia syndrome). During clinical trials conducted on rats, there was an increase in the development of medullary thyroid cancer when given high-dose concentrations of GLP-1 RA.

18. C. A patient with an A_{1C} of 12.7% is considered to be "glucose toxic," and insulin is the recommended therapy. Later, when the A_{1C} improves to < 9%, the patient may consider alternative therapies.

19. D. The A_{1C} reflects the average percentage of glucose within the red blood cells. RBCs have a life expectancy of approximately 90 days.

20. C. Of the pharmacologic therapies listed, only the SGLT-2 inhibitor contributes to weight loss through the loss of glucose (and therefore calories) by increasing glucose filtrate in the urine.

21. C. Metformin commonly causes gastrointestinal side effects.

22. A. A diabetic patient that has either persistent microalbuminuria or a GFR < 30 should be referred to a nephrologist.

23. B. Nephropathy, retinopathy, and DPN (diabetic peripheral neuropathy) are all manifestations of long-term microvascular damage. The presence of one of these is a strong indicator for the presence of another.

24. C. ACE inhibitors have been shown to decrease and sometimes reverse the progression of microalbuminuria and so should be initiated on all non-pregnant females with persistent microalbuminuria. ACE inhibitors are not necessarily recommended for normotensive patients that do not have microalbuminuria present.

25. C. The patient is demonstrating significant hypoglycemia, which is particularly dangerous in the elderly diabetic patient. Metformin and sitagliptin are unlikely to cause any hypoglycemia. The insulin should be discontinued.

26. B. The patient is exhibiting Kussmaul's respirations and clinically presents as diabetic ketoacidosis.

27. A. Initial treatment for DKA is hydration with an IV of normal saline until euvolemia is established.

28. B. All patients with diabetes mellitus should have a "sick days" plan in place in order to prevent more severe consequences of hyperglycemia. It is reasonable to have this patient use short-term insulin therapy while recovering from her UTI. The patient does not exhibit any signs or symptoms of HHS or DKA.

29. C. Both DKA and HHS are often associated with underlying physiologic stress. 40% of the time it is associated with an illness that is either medical or surgical in origin.

30. B. The 20-pound weight loss in a 30-day period is most likely caused by severe dehydration. This is consistent with the very high blood sugar and profound fatigue. The patient is exhibiting signs of HHS and should be hospitalized for treatment.

31. C. TSH is both sensitive and specific for determining circulating T4 and T3 and is used for evaluating both hyperthyroidism and hypothyroidism.

32. B. Total T3 and free T4 levels can help the NP evaluate whether the patient has overt or subclinical hyperthyroidism. There is no need to repeat the TSH at this time.

33. D. The patient's lab values reveal hyperthyroid state. The patient is symptomatic. Therapy with a beta-blocking agent should be initiated to alleviate symptomology. Treatment with radioactive iodine or thioamides will be necessary, but will not provide immediate relief of the symptoms.

34. C. Thioamides have been implicated in causing agranulocytosis in a small number of individuals. A baseline CBC with differential should be obtained.

35. D. The presence of iodine in the body is essential for the production of thyroid hormone.

36. D. This response by the NP will answer the patient's question, as well as explain the rationale for avoiding over-replacement with thyroid hormone.

37. C. Most secondary thyroid disorders can be traced to a problem with the pituitary gland or the pituitary-hypothalmic axis.

38. B. The most common presenting complaint of untreated hypothyroidism is fatigue. A goiter may be present in both hypothyroidism and hyperthyroidism, and therefore is not useful in determining the disease state.

39. A. By definition, subclinical hypothyroidism is an elevated TSH (thyroid stimulating hormone) level with a normal thyroxine level (T4).

40. A. Lithium interferes with the synthesis of thyroid hormone. The patient's thyroid dose will need to be increased to accommodate for this. It would not be appropriate to adjust the lithium dose.

41. C. Hyperpigmentation of the skin is a classic hallmark sign for adrenal insufficiency.

42. B. A patient with Addison's disease will often have low aldosterone levels. Aldosterone increases the retention of sodium and causes the excretion of potassium. Therefore, low aldosterone levels may result in hyponatremia.

43. A. Primary adrenal insufficiency means that the adrenal glands are the source of the deficiency in adrenal hormone. ACTH (from the pituitary gland) should be elevated in an effort to try to increase the cortisol levels through a negative feedback system.

44. B. A patient with primary adrenal insufficiency will need glucocorticoid replacement every day for life.

45. D. The patient often presents with bruising and thin, friable skin. Although the patient will also have striae, the striae seen in Cushing's disease are characteristically wide and purplish in color and widely distributed over all areas of the trunk.

46. C. The 1 mg overnight dexamethasone suppression test is the "gold standard" for determining if the patient has Cushing's syndrome or Cushing's disease. Further differentiation is then needed to determine if it is primary (Cushing's syndrome—adrenal origin) or secondary (Cushing's disease—pituitary origin)

47. D. Adrenal tumors are a common cause of Cushing's syndrome (second only to exogenous replacement).

48. B. The most common cause of Cushing's syndrome is exogenous replacement with glucocorticoids.

49. B. The patient has Cushing's disease because the problem is originating in the pituitary gland, which is demonstrated by an inappropriately elevated ACTH level in the presence of high cortisol levels.

50. C. The patient has elevated cortisol levels; however, the source of the high levels cannot be determined without further testing.

• • • References

Bancos, I., Hahner, S., Tomlinson, J., & Arlt, W. (2015). Diagnosis and management of adrenal insufficiency. *The Lancet Diabetes & Endocrinology, 3*(3), 216–226. doi: 10.1016/S2213-8587(14)70142-1

Black, C., Donnelly, P., McIntyre, L., Royle, P., Shepherd, J. J., & Thomas, S. (2007). Meglitinide analogues for type 2 diabetes mellitus. *Cochrane Database of Systematic Reviews*, Issue 2. Art. No.: CD004654. doi: 10.1002/14651858.CD004654.pub2

DeFronzo, R. A. (2011). Bromocriptine: A sympatholytic, D2-dopamine agonist for the treatment of type 2 diabetes. *Diabetes Care, 34*(4):789–794. doi:10.2337/dc11-0064

Standards of medical care in diabetes. (2015). *Diabetes Care, 38*(S1):S1–S93.

Dicker, D. (2011). DPP-4 Inhibitors: Impact on glycemic control and cardiovascular risk factors. *Diabetes Care*, vol. 34 (supplement 2). http://doi.org/10.2337/dc11-s229

FDA approves once-daily basal insulin toujeo. (n.d.). Retrieved March 28, 2015, from http://www.endocrinologyadvisor.com/toujeo-insulin-approved-by-fda-for-diabetes/article/400320/

Frank, M. L. & Gerhardt, A. M. (2015). Treating dyslipidemia in patients with type 2 diabetes mellitus. *The Nurse Practitioner*, August, vol. 40, no. 8.

Garber, J. F., Cobin, R. H., Gharib, H., Hennessey, V., Klein, I., Mechanick, J. I., . . . Woeber, K. A. (2012). *Clinical practice guidelines for hypothyroidism in adults: Cosponsored by the American Association of Clinical Endocrinologists and The American Thyroid Association.* Retrieved from https://www.aace.com/files/final-file-hypo-guidelines.pdf

Heidelbaugh, Joel. J. (2014). *Type II diabetes mellitus, a multidisciplinary approach.* Philadelphia: Elsevier.

Henske, J. A., Griffith, M. L., & Fowler, M. J. (2009). Initiating and titrating insulin in patients with type 2 diabetes. *Clinical Diabetes, 27*(2), 72–76 doi: 10.2337/diaclin.27.2.72

Inzucchi, S. E., Berganstat, R. M., Buse. J. B., Diamant, M., Ferranini, E., Nauck, M., . . . Matthews, D. (2015). Management of hyperglycemia in type 2 diabetes: A patient-centered approach. *Diabetes Care, 38*(140), 140–149. doi: 10.2337/dc14-2441

Korytkowski. M. T. (2004). Sulfonylurea treatment of type 2 diabetes mellitus: Focus on glimeperide. *Pharmacotherapy, 24*(5), 606–620.

Norman, J. (2014). Diseases of the adrenal cortex: Cushing's syndrome. Retrieved from http://www.endocrineweb.com/conditions/cushings-syndrome/diseases-adrenal-cortex-Cushing's-syndrome

Reid, T. S. (2013). Practical use of glucagon-like peptide-1 receptor agonist therapy in primary care. *Clinical Diabetes, 31*(4), 148–157.

Toft, D. J., & Spinasanta, S. (2014) Addison's disease and adrenal insufficiency. Retrieved from http://www.endocrineweb.com/conditions/addisons-disease/addison-disease-adrenal-insufficiency-overview

Van de Laar, F. (2005). Alpha glucosidase inhibitors for patient with type 2 diabetes. *Diabetes Care, 28*(1):154–163. doi: 10.2337/diacare.28.1.154

12

Hematology

Julie A. Koch, DNP, RN, FNP-BC
Lindsay A. Munden, DNP, RN, FNP-BC

The FNP is often called upon to review lab analyses prior to, during, or following patient visits. These clinical tools provide essential information that can be used to confirm a suspected diagnosis and rule out multiple differential diagnoses. Although the development of the presumed diagnosis depends upon obtaining a detailed history and physical examination, the FNP must rely on knowledge of the underlying etiology, and the development of an asystematic approach to evaluating the complete blood count (CBC) is beneficial.

Anemia

One of the most common hematological conditions encountered in primary care is anemia. Anemia is defined as a quantitative deficiency of hemoglobin (Hgb), often accompanied by a reduced number of red blood cells (RBCs) that results in a decreased oxygen-carrying capacity of the blood. Although anemia is associated with a number of diagnostic codes, the condition is not a disease. Rather, it is a manifestation of an underlying pathology that disturbs hematological homeostatic mechanisms.

Hemoglobin, Hematocrit, and RBCs

A decrease in Hgb, hematocrit (Hct), and/or the RBC count is indicative of anemia. Normally, the Hgb to Hct ratio is 1 to 3 (i.e., 14 grams of Hgb correlates with an Hct of 42%). This ratio is relatively

constant, even in most anemic states, but may be altered in cases of severe dehydration or overhydration. When evaluating Hgb, Hct, and RBCs in the individual with anemia, it is important to remember that anemias are commonly classified according to cell size (microcytic, macrocytic, or normocytic) and cell color (hypochromic or normochromic). This knowledge leads to a systematic approach in the evaluation of anemia, and consistency is key.

MCV

The first RBC index that should be evaluated in the individual with anemia is the mean corpuscular volume (MCV). MCV measurement, reported in femtoliters, is a measure of the average volume (or size) of an RBC. The MCV allows the anemia to be classified normocytic [800–100fL], microcytic [< 80fL], or macrocytic [>100fL]) and can be used to further determine the etiology.

MCHC

The MCHC (mean corpuscular Hgb concentration), the average concentration of Hgb in RBCs, is commonly evaluated next. The MCHC provides the practitioner with information regarding the color of the cells (32–37 g/dl = normochromic; < 32 g/dl = hypochromic). The MCHC is diminished in microcytic anemias and is normal in macrocytic anemias. Table 12-1 identifies the common indices that are used to evaluate patients with anemia.

Table 12-1	Hematological Indices Evaluated in Patients with Anemia
Index	**Normal Value**
RBC	4.5–6.0 million/mm3
Hgb	Male 14–18 gm/100 mL; Females 12–16 gm/100 mL
Hct	Male 40–54%; Females 37–48%
Platelets	150,000–450,000
MCV	80–100 fL
MCHC	32–37 g/dL
Reticulocyte Count	1–2%

Peripheral Smear

A peripheral blood smear is often triggered to be performed on an automated CBC if abnormal cells are detected, but should be ordered when the FNP has a particular concern for a specific diagnosis. The peripheral smear allows the practitioner an opportunity to evaluate the health of the bone marrow since it provides an evaluation of the shape of RBCs and the presence of abnormal circulating cells (see Table 12-2).

RDW

Red cell distribution width (RDW) is a component of an electronic CBC that indicates the degree of variation in size (homogeneity or heterogeneity) among the circulating RBCs. Cells developed in a

Table 12-2	Clues to Causes of Anemia Found within the Peripheral Smear
RBC Morphology	**Common Causes or Associated Conditions**
Spherocytes	Hereditary Spherocytosis Autoimmune Hemolytic Anemia
Schistocytes	Hemolysis Microangiopathic Hemolytic Anemias
Elliptocyte/Ovalocyte	Iron Deficiency Anemia
Teardrop Cells	Iron Deficiency Anemia
Sickle Cells	Sickle Cell Disease
Target Cells	Thalassemia
Bite Cells	G6PD Deficiency
Basophilic Stippling	Thalassemia Lead Toxicity

healthy environment should be similar in size; thus, a variation of < 15% is considered normal. In *acute* states, RDW is often increased (reported as anisocytosis; RDW > 15%), but in *chronic* states of anemia, RDW may normalize as more circulating RBCs are produced of abnormal size.

Reticulocyte Count

A reticulocyte count (normal = 1–2%) measures the proportion of immature RBCs in the blood. The reticulocyte count helps to determine if the bone marrow is functioning properly and responding adequately to the need for additional RBCs. The reticulocyte count is also helpful in monitoring the response to therapy for iron deficiency anemia and the return to bone marrow function following chemotherapeutic assault. In anemic states, it is best to evaluate the absolute reticulocyte count (a corrected allocation that uses the patient's Hct to calculate results and compensates for the anemia).

Microcytic Anemia

Microcytic anemias are characterized by the presence of smaller-sized RBCs (microcytes) that are represented on the hemogram as a decreased MCV. The most common cause of microcytic anemia in children and adults, and the number one cause of anemia worldwide, is iron deficiency anemia. Anemia of chronic disease is most often a normocytic anemia, but can be microcytic in 20% of cases. Thalassemia is a less likely cause of microcytic anemia.

Iron Deficiency Anemia

Although iron deficiency anemia (IDA) affects only 7–10% of Americans, it impacts 1–20% of infants and toddlers, and 15–45% of pregnant women. Blood loss is the number one cause of IDA in Americans over the age of 4; other causes include increased need during pregnancy, impaired absorption, and inadequate dietary intake. IDA results in the production of cells that are microcytic and hypochromic. Other abnormal laboratory findings in IDA include decreased serum iron (the amount of iron in circulation), decreased serum ferritin (the amount of iron in storage), and increased total iron binding capacity (the capacity to bind iron) as more sites are available to bind iron, which is lacking in the circulation. A serum ferritin level of < 16 micrograms/liter is considered diagnostic of IDA. Treatment of IDA commonly includes oral replacement with up to 300 mg of elemental iron daily in divided doses for adolescents and adults. Ferrous sulfate, which contains

65 mg of elemental iron in each 325 mg tablet, is better absorbed than other preparations. With supplementation, iron stores (serum ferritin) may take 4–6 months to return to normal levels. Serum iron levels rise earlier in the treatment process and reflect recent intake. A noticeable increase in Hgb may not occur until after 2–4 weeks of supplementation, but reticulocytosis should be noted within 3–10 days.

Thalassemias

Thalassemias are a group of autosomal recessive hematologic disorders caused by defects in the synthesis of one or more of the hemoglobin alpha or beta chains, which results in the malformation of RBCs, increasing hemolysis. In most people, thalassemia is found incidentally on a CBC that shows mild microcytic, hypochromic anemia. However, the gold standard test for diagnosis is hemoglobin electrophoresis. *Alpha thalassemia* occurs more commonly in people originating from Southeast Asia, China, and occasionally Africa. The alpha thalassemia trait is a mild form of anemia, not requiring therapy. Alpha thalassemia major, however, requires frequent RBC transfusions, and in some instances, iron chelation therapy. *Beta thalassemia* occurs in those originating from Mediterranean countries. Those with the beta thalassemia trait are asymptomatic and usually do not require treatment. Thalassemia major, also known as Cooley's anemia, is detected during infancy and is treated lifelong with frequent RBC transfusions. Beta thalassemia major causes hemolytic anemia, poor growth, and skeletal abnormalities during development. Transfusion dependent patients are at risk for iron overload, and chelation therapy with SQ or IV Desferal is often needed to remove the excess iron. Persons with the thalassemia trait have a normal life expectancy, but those with beta thalassemia major often die from cardiac complications of iron overload by 30 years of age. Parents with any combination of alpha or beta thalassemia syndromes place a child at risk for the disorder. Each child of two carrier parents is at a 25% risk of the disease. Preconception genetic counseling and screening of parents is recommended. If a parent is positive for the trait, a prenatal diagnosis can be made with fetal blood sampling or chorionic villi sampling.

Macrocytic Anemia

Macrocytic anemia represents a group of pathological conditions associated with RBCs of insufficient numbers in which the cells are larger than normal. Although many specific etiologies are known to cause macrocytic anemias, the two most common are vitamin B12 and folic acid deficiency.

Vitamin B12 Deficiency Anemia

The most common cause of macrocytic anemia is vitamin B12 deficiency, and pernicious anemia (lack of intrinsic factor to absorb B12) is the most prevalent underlying etiology, especially in those between the ages of 50 and 60 years. Symptoms of vitamin B12 deficiency include a smooth, beefy red tongue, which is frequently very sore, and the presence of an insidious onset of neurological symptoms: e.g., paresthesia (pins and needles in a stocking and glove distribution), extremity weakness, incoordination, and/or decreased position and vibratory sense. When macrocytic anemia is detected, the next step is to obtain a vitamin B12 level. To determine if the vitamin deficiency is caused by a deficiency in the intrinsic factor, rather than other malabsorptive conditions, increased needs, impaired metabolism, or deficits in dietary intake, a Schilling test should be ordered. When the FNP is unable to determine if macrocytic anemia is related to vitamin B12 or folic acid deficiency, homocysteine (Hcy) and methylmalonic acid (MMA) levels should be drawn. Both MMA and Hcy will be elevated in vitamin B12 deficiency, while only the Hcy will be elevated in folate deficiency. When treating the patient with vitamin B12 deficiency, consideration of (a) the patient's condition and (b) convenience of therapy should heavily influence the method and dosage selected for replacement. The traditional approach is to give 1000 mcg weekly for eight weeks and then monthly for life. More severe anemic states often require daily IM injections, initially followed by tapered therapy. More recent research has demonstrated that 1000 micrograms of oral replacement daily may be an acceptable alternative for those who have sufficient absorption in the small intestine. The response time to appropriate vitamin B12 replacement is usually rapid, with reticulocytosis occurring within 2 to 5 days and peaking within 5 to 7 days. Hct normalization occurs within weeks, but full hematological recovery may take up to 2 months.

Folate Deficiency Anemia

Awareness of folic acid deficiency has become paramount due to its association with an increased risk of embryonic neural tube defects. Despite the focus on supplementation for pregnant women, the FNP needs to be aware that folic acid deficiency anemia is most common between the ages of 60 and 70 years; it is also prevalent among alcoholics, those living in poverty, those undergoing hemodialysis, and those with malabsorptive conditions. Individuals are often asymptomatic, but may develop glossitis resembling pernicious anemia when the folate deficiency is severe. It is important to remember that folic acid deficiency is not characterized by neurological changes, even in its most severe state. Serum folate levels reflect the short-term balance of folate and are very sensitive to dietary changes, thus serum levels should be obtained fasting. A serum folic acid > 4 ng/mL essentially rules out folate deficiency. But, intermediate results (2–4 ng/mL) warrant further testing, such as the RBC folate level (a time-averaged value that is less affected by recent dietary intake) and MMA and Hcy levels to rule out a coexisting vitamin B12 deficiency. The most commonly recommended folic acid replacement for adults is 1 mg/day. To minimize the risk of neural tube defects, the CDC recommends that all women between the ages of 15 and 45 years consume 0.4 mg of folic acid daily. Women with a previous history of birthing a child with a neural tube defect should increase their folic acid intake to 4 mg daily beginning one month prior to planned conception and continue this dose through the first three months of pregnancy. In response to supplementation, reticulocytosis occurs rapidly and peaks within 7 to 10 days. Hct levels usually return to normal within one month. If levels are not rising as expected, and coexisting vitamin B12 anemia has been ruled out, the FNP should keep in mind that IDA coexists in 1/3 of patients with vitamin B12 or folate deficiency.

Normocytic Anemias

Normocytic anemias can be divided into two major etiologies: (1) decreased RBC production and (2) increased RBC loss or destruction. Anemia of chronic disease (ACD), the most common form of normocytic anemia and the second most common cause of anemia worldwide, is associated with decreased RBC production.

Anemia of Chronic Disease

The underlying pathophysiology of ACD is multifactorial; there is decreased activity of the bone marrow, inadequate production of erythropoietin or decreased response to erythropoietin, and decreased RBC lifespan. ACD is associated with a variety of chronic disorders: infection, inflammation, malignancy, and other systemic diseases (i.e., renal disease, liver disease, rheumatic arthritis, and/or endocrine disorders). Common lab findings include low circulating serum iron and transferrin levels. But, unlike IDA, the TIBC in ACD is also low, and serum ferritin will be normal or increased. In ACD,

it is also rare for the Hct to drop below 25%, and the Hgb usually is maintained at 8–12 g/dL. The treatment of ACD is dependent on the timely identification and management of the underlying etiology. Since anemia of chronic disease is often relative to underproduction of erythropoietin, recombinant human erythropoietin (EPO) supplementation is common: 50–150 IU/kg three times a week. FNPs should be aware that the target goal for correction of Hgb with EPO is 11–12 g/dL; Hgb levels greater than this have demonstrated no additional health benefits, but are associated with an increased risk of cardiovascular events. Because IDA frequently coexists with ACD and iron is necessary for proper erythropoiesis, many patients with ACD will benefit from iron supplementation. As with other anemias, blood transfusions are reserved for patients with severe or life-threatening anemia.

Normocytic Hemolytic Anemias

Hemolytic anemia represents approximately 5% of all anemias and can be categorized as congenital/inherited (e.g., sickle cell disease, hereditary spherocytosis or elliptocytosis, thalassemia, or G6PD deficiency) or acquired (e.g., microangiopathic hemolytic anemias [DIC, HUS, or TTP], transfusion of ABO-incompatible blood, use of toxic chemicals or drugs, presence of prosthetic heart valves, or hemodialysis). The practitioner should consider hemolysis if there is a precipitous fall in Hgb, if there is significant reticulocytosis, and/or there is the presence of spherocytes (small, dense RBCs with a loss of biconcave shape) or RBC fragments on the peripheral smear. In addition to a precipitous decline in indices within the hemogram, the most sensitive measure of hemolysis is LDH (lactate dehydrogenase). When RBCs are destroyed, their LDH is released into circulation and Hgb is released from damaged erythrocytes, leading to an increase in indirect bilirubin (typically not exceeding 3 mg/dl) and urobilinogen levels. Serum haptoglobin (which binds to free Hgb) is also sensitive for hemolytic anemia; with intravascular hemolysis, Hgb is released from cells and is bound by haptoglobin. Thus, circulating free haptoglobin levels decline. If checking for autoimmune hemolytic anemia, the FNP should order a direct Coombs' test; the test evaluates for IgG alloantibodies or autoantibodies and their complement proteins, which bind to and destroy erythrocytes. Persistent hemolysis may result in the development of jaundice, bilirubin gallstones, or staining of the skin from hematosiderosis. Iron overload may occur in patients who have received multiple transfusions. Others may have an increased need for folic acid during erythropoietic recovery.

G6PD Deficiency Anemia

Glucose-6-phosphate dehydrogenase (G6PD) deficiency is the most common enzyme deficiency worldwide, impacting 400 million people. The X-linked inherited disorder has multiple variants, with different gene mutations resulting in varying levels of enzyme deficiency and symptom manifestation, including neonatal hyperbilirubinemia and acute or chronic hemolysis. G6PD most commonly affects persons of African, Mediterranean, Asian, or Middle-Eastern descent. The conversion of nicotinamide adenine dinucleotide phosphate to its reduced form in erythrocytes is the basis of diagnostic testing for the deficiency, which is confirmed by fluorescent spot test. Because acute hemolysis, which is typically self-limiting but can be severe enough to warrant transfusion, is caused by exposure to an oxidative stressor (i.e., infection, oxidative drugs, and/or fava beans), treatment is geared toward avoidance of these and other stressors. Medications to avoid include quinolones, sulfonamides, nitrofurans, antimalarials, and antihelminitics.

Sickle Cell Anemia

The term sickle cell disease (SCD) is used to describe a group of blood cell disorders in which individuals inherit abnormal Hgb, Hgb S. Approximately 100,000 Americans have SCD, and while the majority of these are African American, a number of individuals are of Hispanic, southern European, Middle Eastern, and Asian Indian descent. The most severe form of the disease occurs when individuals inherit Hgb SS, one Hgb S gene from each parent. Individuals who have inherited normal Hgb (Hgb A) from one parent and Hgb S from the other are known to have sickle cell trait and may transmit the defective gene to offspring. Approximately 1 in 13 African American babies is born with sickle cell trait, while 1 in every 365 is born with SCD. All 50 states and the District of Columbia require newborn screening for SCD.

Because sickle cells lack the flexibility of normal RBCs, they adhere to vessels walls, impeding flow and limiting oxygenation to tissues, which results in the symptomatology associated with SCD: dactylitis, acute pain/vaso-occlusive crises, acute chest syndrome, stroke (up to 24% of those with Hgb SS will suffer a stroke by age 45), retinal detachment, heart failure, pulmonary hypertension, leg ulcers, and kidney or liver damage. SCD patients are also prone to hemolytic anemia. While normal RBCs live 90–120 days, sickle cells last only 10–20 days. Individuals with SCD live with mild to moderate anemia, but severe, life-threatening anemia in children can occur with splenic sequestration crisis (trapping of RBCs in the spleen) or an aplastic crisis (acute bone marrow suppression usually caused by parvovirus B19 infection). Hematopoetic stem cell transplant is the only cure for SCD. Individuals require frequent visits for health care maintenance because infections are the number one cause of mortality. Influenza, meningococcal, and pneumococcal vaccinations are imperative. Children are often prophylactically treated with penicillin until age 5. Transcranial Doppler stroke screening is initiated annually between the ages of 2 and 16 years. Annual opthamology referral is appropriate for those $\geqq$ age 10 years. Increasing fluids and administering ibuprofen or acetaminophen may be helpful for acute pain syndrome, but hospitalization is often required. Hydroxyurea can decrease the number and severity of pain episodes and acute chest events and is commonly prescribed as long-term prophylactic therapy.

Aplastic Anemia

Aplastic anemia is a rare but serious hematologic disorder that is characterized by pancytopenia and bone marrow hypoplasia. Aplastic anemia can occur at any age, but is most common in those 10–25 years old and those older than 60 years. Aplastic anemia is more common in Asia than other countries, and occurs with equal frequency among males and females. Aplastic anemia can progress insidiously over weeks or months or may come on suddenly. The majority of cases are acquired and idiopathic. Infections, environmental factors (e.g., exposure to toxic chemicals, radiation, and/or chemotherapy), autoimmune disorders, pregnancy, and medications may precipitate the bone marrow failure. The timeframe from exposure to symptom presentation is typically between 6 and 12 months. Patients often present with symptoms of anemia and thrombocytopenia, but may also report fatigue, dyspnea, tachycardia, pallor, easy bruising/bleeding, overt and/or recurrent infections, and oropharyngeal ulcerations. To be diagnosed with aplastic anemia, at least two of the following must be present: (1) Hgb < 10g/dL, (2) platelet count < 50×10^9/L, and/or (3) absolute neutrophil count < 1.5×10^9/L. The corrected reticulocyte percentage will be < 1%. Bone marrow biopsy typically demonstrates hypocellular marrow without abnormal cells. Severe aplastic anemia is a hematologic emergency and care should be instituted immediately. Non-pharmacologic management includes support with RBC and platelet transfusions, hematopoietic cell transplantation (HCT), and supportive care. Pharmacologic measures include immunosuppressive agents, hematopoietic growth factors, antimetabolites, and chelating agents. The major causes of morbidity and mortality from aplastic anemia are infection and bleeding.

Abnormalities of the White Blood Cells (WBCs)

In addition to evaluating the RBCs and their indices, the FNP should have foundational knowledge of conditions that are associated with abnormalities of WBCs. WBCs can be categorized into two groups: granulocytes (basophils, eosinophils, and neutrophils) and agranulocytes (lymphocytes and monocytes). WBC counts in adults range from 4,500–10,500/mm^3, and differential components are helpful in determining the body's response to acute and chronic infections, inflammatory conditions, allergic reactions, immunodeficiencies, and hematologic malignancies (see Table 12-3).

Leukocytosis is usually indicative of benign conditions including infections and inflammatory processes, but can be a manifestation of a more serious etiology such as leukemia or a myeloproliferative disorder. An elevated WBC count can also be caused by stress, anemia, immune system disorders, severe allergic reactions, trauma, bronchogenic carcinomas, uremia, medications (quinine, corticosteroids, and epinephrine), acute hemolysis, hemorrhage, splenectomy, polycythemia vera, and pregnancy. Leukocytosis is most commonly associated with an increase in the absolute number of mature neutrophils, but can also reflect an increase in lymphocytes, eosinophils, monocytes, or basophils.

Leukopenia, often used interchangeably with neutropenia, is observed when the WBC supply is depleted by infection or treatments, such as chemotherapy or radiation, or when stem cell abnormalities disrupt bone marrow function. Leukopenia may also be caused by viral infections, congenital disorders characterized by diminished bone marrow function, cancer or other diseases that damage bone marrow, or autoimmune disorders. Symptoms may include anemia, fatigue, fever, headache, stomatitis, pneumonia, menorrhagia, and thrombocytopenia. Treatment is aimed at managing the underlying condition and minimizing the risks for infection.

Neutrophils

Neutrophils (polys or segs) are the most numerous and important leukocytes in the body. Through phagocytosis, they constitute the body's preliminary defense against infection. In a healthy adult, most neutrophils circulating in the bloodstream are mature (segmented); however, the term "left shift" refers to an increase in the proportion (>10%) of bands (stabs), immature neutrophils with a banded-appearing nucleus. The left shift typically indicates bacterial infection, but may also occur when there is inflammation or necrosis. *Neutrophilia* is typically caused by bacterial infections and is the most

Table 12-3	Common Conditions Resulting in Elevations of Circulating WBCs		
WBC Component	**Function**	**Normal Range**	**Conditions Resulting in Elevated Levels**
Neutrophils (Polys or Segs)	First responders to bacterial infections	30–70%	Acute bacterial infections
Lymphocytes	Immune responses against antigens	15–40%	Viral infections Leukemia
Monocytes	Assist with phagocytosis; regulate immunity	2–8%	Autoimmune disorders Severe bacterial infections Chronic infections
Eosinophils	Target antigen antibodies for destruction; regulate inflammation	0–5%	Allergic disorders Parasitic infections
Basophils	Hypersensitivity reactions; allergic responses	0–3%	Parasitic infections Some allergic disorders Inflammation
Bands	Triggered to target bacterial infections with neutrophils	0–4%	Severe bacterial infections

common form of leukocytosis. The condition may also be caused by trauma, inflammatory disorders, burns, acute hemorrhage, sepsis, cigarette smoking, malignancy, uremia, and metabolic processes. *Neutropenia* can be caused by insufficient or injured bone marrow stem cells, increased destruction of neutrophils in circulation, shifts in neutrophils from circulating blood to the tissues, infections (e.g., tuberculosis and viral infections), or nutritional deficiencies.

Eosinophils

Eosinophils play two major roles in the body: destroying foreign substances and regulating inflammation. Eosinophils are (a) phagocytic, (b) target antigen-antibodies for destruction, and (c) become increasingly active during allergic reactions and parasitic infections. *Eosinophilia* can occur in the blood or body tissues and may be due to asthma, autoimmune disorders, infections, dermatologic conditions, allergic events, eczema, hay fever, or leukemia. *Eosinopenia* can occur with Cushing's syndrome, stress, or corticosteroid therapy. Treatment is generally not necessary because the immune system is able to compensate adequately with other WBC components.

Basophils

Basophils are the least numerous of the WBCs and are responsible for hypersensitivity reactions and allergic responses with receptors for IgE. Basophils contain a multi-lobed nucleus and granules comprised of histamine, heparin, and serotonin. The cells can be stained with a base dye (methylene blue), hence the name basophil, meaning "baseloving." *Basophilia* may be indicative of asthma, allergic reactions to food, drugs or parasites, anaphylaxis, infections, inflammatory conditions (e.g., IBD dermatitis), or myeloproliferative disorders. *Basopenia* may stem from thyroid disorders, urticaria, ovulation, pregnancy, radiation, chemotherapy, or infections.

Lymphocytes

Lymphocytes are the primary components of the body's immune system and are the second most common WBCs. Lymphocytes circulate in blood, lymph fluid, and in body tissues such as the spleen, thymus, bone marrow, lymph nodes, tonsils, and liver. The three main types are T cells, B cells, and natural killer cells which are critical for immune responses against antigens. *Lymphocytosis* may indicate acute or chronic infections (viral or bacterial) including

mononucleosis or tuberculosis, cancer of the blood (leukemias) or lymphatic system, or an autoimmune disorder causing chronic inflammation. A common reason for lymphocytosis is lymphocytic leukemia. *Lymphocytopenia* may be caused by acquired diseases such as infectious diseases, autoimmune disorders, steroid therapy, aplastic anemia, Hodgkin's disease, radiation, and chemotherapy. Inherited disorders causing lymphocytosis are rare.

Monocytes

Monocytes are structurally the largest of the WBCs. Monocytes migrate from blood to tissue within a few hours after bone marrow production and develop into macrophages and dendritic cells. Once converted, monocytes assist other WBCs to remove dead or damaged tissues, destroy cancer cells, and regulate immunity against foreign substances. *Monocytosis* occurs in response to chronic infections, autoimmune disorders, blood disorders, and cancers. *Monocytopenia* can occur in response to toxins released by bacteria into the bloodstream and those receiving chemotherapy.

Abnormalities of Platelets

The final factor of the CBC that FNPs are commonly required to evaluate is the platelet count. Platelets are components of blood cells developed from megakaryocytes in the bone marrow that are essential for coagulation. The majority of platelets circulate in the blood; however, approximately one-third are stored in the spleen. The typical life cycle of a platelet is 7–10 days. The normal range of platelets, also referred to as thrombocytes, is 150,000–450,000/μL.

Thrombocytosis

Thrombocytosis is defined as a platelet count of more than 450,000/μL. *Primary thrombocytosis* is caused by an overproduction of platelets in the bone marrow. Most patients with primary thrombocytosis are asymptomatic and treatment entails the use of hydroxyurea lifelong to suppress platelet production. Low-dose aspirin is occasionally needed to reduce the risk of thrombus formation. Complications of primary thrombocytosis include thrombosis, bleeding (GI), and in rare instances, progression to acute myeloid leukemia. *Secondary thrombocytosis*, is caused by an underlying disease such as anemia, cancer, inflammation, infection, surgery (splenectomy), or certain medications. Symptoms of secondary thrombocytosis may include headaches, weakness, dizziness, bruising, bleeding, chest pain, and loss of consciousness. A diagnosis is made during the interpretation of a routine CBC; however, bone marrow aspiration may be needed. Treatment is aimed at resolving the underlying cause.

Thrombocytopenia

Thrombocytopenia is defined as a platelet count of less than 150,000/µL and is often found incidentally when obtaining a CBC. Symptoms, if present, may include easy bruising (ecchymosis and petechiae), bleeding from mucous membranes, spontaneous epistaxis, excessive bleeding from wounds, and hematuria. Causes of thrombocytopenia stem from the impaired production of platelets (i.e., viral infections, aplastic anemia, chemotherapeutic drugs, cancers, alcohol, myelodysplastic syndrome), increased destruction of platelets (i.e., transfusion reactions, medications such as digoxin, quinine, quinidine, acetaminophen, rheumatologic conditions, autoimmune conditions, TTP, ITP, HIT, severe infections, HELLP), or splenic sequestration (i.e., chronic alcohol abuse, liver disease, gestational thrombocytopenia). Treatment depends on the severity and underlying cause. Most patients do not require regular transfusions of platelets. In severe thrombocytopenia, steroids are used to suppress the autoimmune attack on platelets. IV antibodies or IVIG can be used in patients who are not responsive to steroids.

Thrombotic Thrombocytopenic Purpura (TTP) is a syndrome of decreased platelets causing a pentad of clinical features: microangiopathic hemolytic anemia, thrombocytopenic purpura, neurologic abnormalities, fever, and renal disease. Peripheral blood smears reveal moderate-to-severe schistocytosis. Most cases are associated with a deficiency in a metalloproteinase enzyme ADAMTS13 contributing to autoantibody development. Patients with TTP are found to have large multimers of von Willebrand factor (vWF) in their plasma, and the deficiency of ADAMTS13 results in a reduced ability to break down these multimers. Diagnosis is confirmed by ADAMTS13 activity and antibody levels; additional diagnostics may focus on organ involvement (comprehensive metabolic profiles) and contributing factors (HIV, Hepatitis B and C, ANA, and pregnancy test). The treatment of choice is the prompt initiation of plasma exchange. Evidence also supports the use of corticosteroids. Untreated, TTP has a high mortality rate near 90%, but with initiation

of prompt plasma exchange this rate is reduced to 10–20%. Once stable, recommendations for follow-up include weekly CBC and LDH for 2 weeks, then biweekly lab analyses for a month. Relapse and reoccurrence is not uncommon.

Idiopathic Thrombocytopenic Purpura (ITP) is characterized by a decreased number of platelets and a reduced ability for primary clotting. Signs and symptoms include prolonged purpura, bruising tendency, gingival bleeding, menorrhagia, epistaxis, and petechiae, without hepatosplenomegaly. In children (ages 2–6 years), most cases are acute and tend to follow a viral illness. Adult cases are more commonly chronic in nature, sometimes persisting for 6 months or longer. The condition is diagnosed with a CBC; isolated thrombocytopenia is the hallmark finding. Treatment is rarely indicated when platelet counts are greater than 50,000/µL unless there is evidence of active bleeding. For those requiring treatment, a single dose of IVIG (0.8–1g/kg) or a short course of corticosteroids should be used first-line. Rituximab or high-dose dexamethasone should be considered for those who do not respond to initial therapy. Splenectomy may be helpful for those with refractory or recurrent thrombocytopenia.

Heparin Induced Thrombocytopenia (HIT) is a complication of heparin therapy that is caused by antibodies that bind to heparin and platelet factor 4 (PF4), causing a prothombotic state. In *nonimmune HIT*, which occurs most frequently, there is a mild decrease in the platelet count within the first 2 days after initiating heparin, which normalizes with continued therapy. In *immune-mediated HIT*, platelets are affected 4–10 days following exposure to heparin. Unlike other forms of thrombocytopenia, HIT presents without bleeding; rather, venous thromboembolism, pulmonary embolism, MI, and CVA are the causes for concern. HIT is typically diagnosed by evaluating a platelet count and PF4 antibody level. Erythematous or necrotizing skin reactions at the site of heparin injections should prompt the health care provider to consider HIT in the differential. Treatment entails the immediate discontinuation of heparin and treatment with an alternate anticoagulant (e.g., direct thrombin inhibitors) until the INR is therapeutic. Patients with HIT should be anticoagulated for 3 months (if there is a history of thrombotic complication) or 4 weeks (in patients without a history of thrombotic complication).

Review Questions

1. Iron deficiency typically manifests as:

   A. Macrocytic, normochromic anemia.

   B. Microcytic, hypochromic anemia.

   C. Microcytic, normochromic anemia.

   D. Normochromic, normocytic anemia.

2. A 20-year-old college student presents with complaints of excessive fatigue, fever, and exudative pharyngitis, which is accompanied by anterior and posterior cervical lymphadenopathy. What WBC findings would support the suspected diagnosis?

   A. Increased neutrophils with more than 10% bands

   B. Increased lymphocytes with more than 10% atypical lymphocytes

   C. Increased total leukocytes, with an increased proportion of basophils

   D. Increased total leukocytes, with an increased proportion of eosinophils

3. Which of the following laboratory findings are most consistent with anemia related to folic acid deficiency?

   A. Decreased MCV and decreased MCHC

   B. Decreased MCV and normal MCHC

   C. Increased MCV and normal MCHC

   D. Normal MCV and normal MCHC

4. The FNP is evaluating a CBC that reveals an abnormally low Hgb, Hct, and RBC count. Which of the following lab values would assist the FNP in determining if the anemia was microcytic or macrocytic?

   A. Ferritin level

   B. MCV

   C. MCHC

   D. TIBC

5. Which of the following conditions is associated with normocytic anemia?

   A. A deficiency in vitamin B12 intake or absorption

   B. Chronic blood loss

   C. Concurrent chronic illness (i.e., chronic kidney disease)

   D. Inadequate globin synthesis

6. The FNP is following up with a patient previously diagnosed with anemia who complains of a sore tongue and numbness and tingling of the hands and feet. The FNP recognizes that she needs to address that you need to address the patient's response to:

   A. Administration of erythropoietin.

   B. Ferrous sulfate supplementation.

   C. Folic acid supplementation.

   D. Vitamin B12 supplementation.

7. The FNP is following up with a young adult woman previously diagnosed with microcytic, hypochromic anemia. The FNP recognizes that it is important to rule out:

   A. Abnormal uterine bleeding.

   B. Gastrointestinal bleeding.

   C. Inadequate intake of folic acid.

   D. Low carbohydrate diet fads.

8. What laboratory finding on the white blood cell count would lead the nurse practitioner to suspect acute appendicitis as the cause of a client's right lower quadrant abdominal pain?

   A. Increased lymphocytes with more than 10% atypical lymphs

   B. Increased neutrophils with more than 10% bands

   C. Increased total leukocytes, with an increased proportion of basophils

   D. Increased total leukocytes, with an increased proportion of eosinophils

9. When interpreting findings in an individual with leukocytosis, the FNP recognizes that a "left shift" is represented by an increase in the proportion of:

   A. Eosoniphils.

   B. Lymphocytes.

   C. Monocytes.

   D. Neutrophils.

10. What organ system is responsible for the majority of the body's production of erythropoietin?

    A. Bone Marrow

    B. Kidneys

    C. Liver

    D. Spleen

11. An elevated red cell distribution width (RDW) correlates with which of the following findings on the peripheral smear?

    A. Anisocytosis

    B. Microcytosis

    C. Poikilocytosis

    D. Reticulocytosis

12. Women of childbearing age should have an adequate intake of what micronutrient to decrease the risk of fetal neural tube defects?

    A. Folic acid

    B. Iron

    C. Vitamin B6

    D. Vitamin B12

13. The most appropriate additional diagnostic test for the patient with decreased WBCs, RBCs, and platelets is a:

    A. Bone marrow biopsy.

    B. Direct Coombs' test.

    C. Hemoglobin electrophoresis.

    D. Serum haptoglobin.

14. The presence of schistocytes on the peripheral smear of a patient with decreased platelets should raise the suspicion of:

    A. Autoimmune hemolytic anemia.

    B. Erythroblastisfetalis.

    C. Thalassemia major.

    D. Thrombotic thrombocytopenic purpura.

15. The FNP is educating an anemic patient about the procedure(s) for a Schilling test. The practitioner recognizes that a Schilling test involves:

    A. An early morning, fasting lab draw.

    B. Collecting urine for 24 hours.

    C. Endoscopic sampling of the gastric mucosa.

    D. Serial collections of serum vitamin B12 levels.

16. What is the most likely diagnosis for a patient with the following CBC findings?

    WBC: $7.1 \times 10^3/\mu l$

    RBC: $3.32 \times 10^3/\mu l$

    Hgb: 11.3 g/dL

    Hct: 34.4%

    MCV: 91 fL

    MCHC: 32 g/dL

    Plt: $364 \times 10^3/\mu l$

    RDW: 13.4%

    Reticulocytes: 0.9%

    A. Anemia of chronic disease

    B. Folate deficiency anemia

    C. Iron deficiency anemia

    D. Vitamin B12 deficiency anemia

17. What is the most likely diagnosis for a patient with the following CBC findings?

    WBC: $8.8 \times 10^3/\mu l$

    RBC: $3.01 \times 10^3/\mu l$

    Hgb: 10.3 g/dL

    Hct: 32.2%

    MCV: 74 fL

    MCHC: 28.3 g/dL

    Plt: $400 \times 10^3/\mu l$

    RDW: 18.4%

    Reticulocytes: 2.1%

    A. Anemia of chronic disease

    B. Folate deficiency anemia

    C. Iron deficiency anemia

    D. Vitamin B12 deficiency anemia

18. Which diagnostic test could help identify whether the cause of anemia is hemolytic in nature?

    A. Bone marrow aspiration

    B. Direct antiglobulin test

    C. Hemoglobin electrophoresis

    D. Serum haptoglobin

19. The lab index that has demonstrated reliability as an *early* marker of microcytic and macrocytic anemias is the:
    A. MCH.
    B. MCHC.
    C. MCV.
    D. RDW.

20. The FNP is seeing a patient who has been taking ferrous sulfate. Which statement by the patient demonstrates a need for additional education?
    A. "I should take my medication with orange juice to increase absorption."
    B. "I should take one tablet twice a day."
    C. "It is best to take the iron on an empty stomach."
    D. "It is recommended that I take enteric coated iron with meals."

21. An older adult with ESRD who is undergoing hemodialysis is in the office for follow-up. The patient is on erythropoietin therapy, but has not been able to attain a hemoglobin level greater than 9.2 g/dL despite negative assessment for blood loss and other common etiologies known to contribute to hyporesponsiveness to erythropoietin. The patient's haptoglobin and LDH are elevated. Which of the following causes of hemolysis is most likely contributing to the patient's anemia?
    A. Autoimmune
    B. Drug-induced
    C. Hereditary
    D. Mechanical

22. Which of the following is the leading cause of death in individuals with sickle cell anemia?
    A. Bacterial infection
    B. Heart failure
    C. Kidney failure
    D. Stroke

23. When evaluating the patient with megaloblastic anemia who does not have neurological symptoms, the FNP recognizes that the most likely diagnosis is:
    A. An underlying hemolytic process.
    B. Folic acid deficiency.
    C. Iron deficiency.
    D. Suppression of the bone marrow.

24. An older adult who has been hospitalized with macrocytic anemia with an Hgb of 8 g/dl is being seen for follow-up. Because of the degree of anemia, daily vitamin B12 injections for one week have been ordered. What additional labs will be drawn during this follow-up visit?
    A. Calcium level
    B. Creatinine and BUN
    C. Fasting glucose
    D. Potassium level

25. The gold standard for diagnosing sickle cell disease is a(n):
    A. Bone marrow aspiration.
    B. Direct antiglobin test.
    C. Hemoglobin electrophoresis.
    D. Indirect Coombs' test.

26. What therapy is commonly used to prevent acute pain syndrome in children and adults with SCD?

    A. Hydroxyurea

    B. Ibuprofen

    C. Intravenous iron infusions

    D. Monthly blood transfusions

27. A seven-year-old boy, recently diagnosed with acute lymphocytic leukemia (ALL), has been receiving induction chemotherapy treatments. Current lab values indicate a WBC count of 4,300/mm^3, neutrophils 50%, lymphocytes 15%, monocytes 2%, eosinophils 3%, and basophils 1%. What is his absolute neutrophil count (ANC)?

    A. 86/mm^3

    B. 645/mm^3

    C. 2,150/mm^3

    D. 3,440/mm^3

28. A 19-year-old male has beta thalassemia major, which was detected during infancy. He receives frequent RBC transfusions for severe anemia. Which of the following supplements should the patient avoid?

    A. Folic acid

    B. Multi-vitamins with iron

    C. Vitamin B12

    D. Vitamin C

29. A mother of an exclusively breast fed 4-month-old infant presents to the nurse practitioner for a well-child examination. Which of the following recommendations is appropriate at this time to reduce the risk for iron deficiency anemia in the infant?

    A. Begin supplementation with an iron-rich formula.

    B. Have the mother take an iron supplement.

    C. Initiate an oral multivitamin with iron for the baby.

    D. Introduce iron-rich foods for the baby.

30. A 20-year-old African American male was recently treated for a minor skin infection with sulfamethoxazole/trimethoprim DS twice daily for 10 days. He returns to the clinic complaining of fatigue, yellowing of his skin and eyes, and dark urine. These symptoms lead the nurse practitioner to suspect which of the following?

    A. G6PD deficiency

    B. Pernicious anemia

    C. Sickle cell disease

    D. Thalassemia

31. The nurse practitioner is caring for the mother of three children under the age of 5 years who recently began supplementation with ferrous sulfate over-the-counter. What is the most important educational focus for her at this follow-up visit?

    A. Addressing the importance of taking the medication at the same time every day.

    B. Determining where she keeps her medication bottles.

    C. Ensuring that she understands the rationale for her current therapy.

    D. Identifying the underlying pathophysiology leading to anemia.

32. A 16-year-old female is experiencing an asthma exacerbation following exposure to cats at her neighbor's home. Which leukocyte will likely be elevated?

    A. Basophils

    B. Eosinophils

    C. Monocytes

    D. Neutrophils

33. Which of the following conditions is a common reason for lymphocytosis?
    A. Acute rhinosinusitis
    B. Leukemia
    C. Malaria
    D. Streptococcal pharyngitis

34. A 33-year-old pregnant female with a history of beta thalassemia trait consults with the nurse practitioner about her child's risk for inheriting the disorder. The father of the child is uninvolved in the prenatal planning, and it is unknown whether he is a carrier. The most appropriate action by the nurse practitioner is to:
    A. Counsel the mother about pregnancy termination options.
    B. Discuss that a prenatal diagnosis cannot be made.
    C. Discuss that the chances of the child inheriting the disease are 50%.
    D. Refer the patient for genetic counseling.

35. Which of the following lab tests confirms a diagnosis of iron deficiency when evaluating microcytic anemia?
    A. Hgb electrophoresis
    B. Platelet count
    C. Serum ferritin
    D. Vitamin B12 level

36. A 30-year-old female recently began treatment with ferrous sulfate 325 mg PO TID between meals. She presents to the nurse practitioner for a repeat CBC after one month of iron therapy. Lab values are as follows: Hgb 12.0 g/dL, Hct 36%, MCV 82, and MCHC 32 g/dL. What is the most appropriate follow-up course of action by the nurse practitioner?
    A. Continue current treatment regimen.
    B. Decrease oral iron supplementation.
    C. Increase oral iron supplementation.
    D. Switch to IV iron therapy.

37. A 60-year-old female is following up with the nurse practitioner for a recent diagnosis of pernicious anemia, and she would like to know how long she will need to continue treatment with Vitamin B12. The most appropriate response by the nurse practitioner is:
    A. 1–3 months.
    B. 3–6 months.
    C. 6–12 months.
    D. Lifelong.

38. An 80-year-old Caucasian alcoholic male complains of fatigue, glossitis, and occasional palpitations. He denies neurological complaints. His CBC reveals the following: Hgb 8.0 g/dL, Hct 24%, and MCV 110. Which would be the most likely diagnosis?
    A. Anemia of chronic disease
    B. Folic acid deficiency anemia
    C. Iron deficiency anemia
    D. Vitamin B12 deficiency anemia

39. The nurse practitioner is following up with a patient who was recently diagnosed with vitamin B12 deficiency. To assess the effectiveness of dietary education, the FNP should focus on the patient's intake of which food source?

    A. Broccoli

    B. Chicken

    C. Legumes

    D. Lettuce

40. A monocyte count comprising 20% of leukocytes within the CBC is likely a result of which of the following?

    A. An allergic response

    B. An autoimmune disorder

    C. An acute bacterial infection

    D. A parasitic disease

41. Microangiopathic hemolytic anemia, thrombocytopenic purpura, neurologic abnormalities, fever, and renal disease are associated with which hematologic syndrome?

    A. Idiopathic thrombocytopenic purpura

    B. Immune heparin induced thrombocytopenic purpura

    C. Nonimmune heparin induced thrombocytopenic purpura

    D. Thrombotic thrombocytopenic purpura

42. The nurse practitioner is following up with a patient who was recently diagnosed with beta thalassemia major. The nurse practitioner recognizes that the life expectancy of someone with this disorder is:

    A. 15 years.

    B. 30 years.

    C. 45 years.

    D. 60 years.

43. Following an upper respiratory infection, a 5-year-old boy presents to the clinic with his mother for complaints of unexplained purple discolorations to his upper and lower extremities, frequent nose-bleeds, and petechiae. The CBC reveals a decreased platelet count. Which diagnosis is most likely?

    A. Aplastic anemia

    B. Idiopathic thrombocytopenia purpura

    C. Sickle cell disease

    D. Thrombotic thrombocytopenia purpura

44. Which of the following is a potential complication for a patient diagnosed with heparin-induced thrombocytopenia?

    A. Bleeding

    B. Epistaxis

    C. Pulmonary embolism

    D. Purpura

45. The nurse practitioner recognizes that the first-line treatment of choice for ITP in children includes which of the following therapies?

    A. RBC transfusion

    B. Rituximab

    C. Single dose of IVIG

    D. Splenectomy

46. A 12-year-old boy with fatigue, dyspnea, pallor, and easy bruising presents for evaluation by the nurse practitioner. Hemogram evaluation reveals pancytopenia. Which test should be utilized to confirm the suspected diagnosis?

    A. ANA screen

    B. Bone marrow biopsy

    C. Folate level

    D. Hgb electrophoresis

47. Bleeding and bruising are most likely to occur as a result of which condition?

    A. Leukopenia

    B. Lymphocytopenia

    C. Thrombocytopenia

    D. Thrombocytosis

48. Within which timeframe should the nurse practitioner reevaluate the hemogram of an anemic patient who has started folic acid supplementation?

    A. 2 weeks

    B. 4 weeks

    C. 6 weeks

    D. 8 weeks

49. A 40-year-old female with iron deficiency anemia returns to the clinic for an early morning appointment after 3 months of iron supplementation to have her CBC and serum iron level drawn. Which statement by the patient may cause the nurse practitioner to reschedule the lab draw?

    A. "I had a large cup of coffee this morning with breakfast."

    B. "I have been exercising for 45 minutes every evening."

    C. "I think the iron pills are causing my stomach to be upset."

    D. "I took my iron pill while I was in the waiting room."

50. A 20-year-old Asian man presents to your clinic for follow-up. He has a history of aplastic anemia and has recently received a hematopoietic cell transplantation. Upon his examination, a generalized maculopapular pruritic rash, with sparing of the scalp, is noted. Which of the following is most imperative for the nurse practitioner to rule out?

    A. An allergic reaction to a newly initiated medication

    B. Graft versus host disease

    C. Recent exposure to school-age children

    D. Worsening symptomatology of aplastic anemia

Answers and Rationales

1. B. Iron deficiency results in the development of cells that are smaller in size (microcytic) and more pale in color (hypochromic) due to the lack of Hgb during cell synthesis. In the early phases of iron deficiency, cells may actually remain normocytic and normochromic because the bone marrow draws upon stored iron reserves during erythropoiesis. Once the stores have been depleted, the production the erythrocytes formed become microcytic and hypochromic.

2. B. The case scenario is consistent with the classic triad seen with infectious mononucleosis: fever, exudative pharyngitis, and adenopathy. Within mono, the characteristic CBC findings include absolute lymphocytosis in which more than 10% of the cells are atypical.

3. C. Folic acid deficiency results in impaired RNA and DNA synthesis within the developing erythrocyte and the development of immature and dysfunctional enlarged RBCs (megaloblasts). Because hemoglobin synthesis is not impaired, RBCs formed in the presence of folic acid deficiency retain their normal concentration of hemoglobin (MCHC) and normal color.

4. B. The mean cell volume is the lab value that reflects RBC size or average volume. Based on MCV, cells are classified as normocytic (80–100 femtoliters [fL]), microcytic (< 80 fL), or macrocytic (> 100 fL).

5. C. Normocytic anemia, with an MCV of 80–100fL, correlates with anemia of chronic disease. Chronic blood loss is associated with iron deficiency anemia, a microcytic anemia. Deficiency in vitamin B12 results in the development of macrocytic anemia. Inadequate globin synthesis occurs in beta thalassemia, a microcytic anemia.

6. D. The case presentation is that of vitamin B12 deficiency. Although glossitis may occur with folic acid deficiency, parasthesias of the hands and feet in a stocking/glove distribution are characteristic of pernicious anemia; thus, it is important to evaluate the patient's response to vitamin B12 supplementation.

7. A. In young adult women, abnormal uterine bleeding is a common cause of iron deficiency anemia, a microcytic, hypochromic anemia. Bleeding from the GI tract is a more common cause of IDA in older adults. Inadequate intake of folic acid would result in macrocytic anemia. Low carbohydrate diets still allow for adequate intake of iron from meats and green leafy vegetables.

8. A. Acute infectious processes stimulate an increase in the production and release of mature neutrophils and mobilization of less mature neutrophils or bands. Normally, the vast majority of neutrophils circulating in the bloodstream are in the mature form, but with acute infectious processes, mobilization of bands can increase the proportion of immature neutrophils to greater than 10%.

9. D. The term "left shift" is almost always associated with neutrophils. The left shift means that the population of cells is shifted toward most immature cells, with an increased percentage of immature neutrophils (i.e., bands, metamyeloctyes, and myelocytes) being present to fight infection.

10. B. 90% of the body's erythropoietin is produced by the kidneys; only about 10% is produced in the liver.

11. A. Anisocytosis describes variance in RBC sizes that is common in anemia as new cells formed are larger (macrocytic) or smaller (microcytic) than the healthy cells which were formed prior to the underlying processes that resulted in anemia. This variance in sizes of circulating red blood sizes correlates with an increased RDW.

12. A. Folic acid deficiency in early pregnancy has been linked to the teratogenic effect of neural tube defects.

13. A. Pancytopenia (a deficiency in all three cellular components of the blood) is indicative of aplastic anemia. A bone marrow aspiration biopsy is needed to rule out myelodysplastic syndrome and metastatic tumor deposits. The hypoplastic bone marrow of aplastic anemia will have fatty replacement which is often accompanied by a relative increase in nonhematopoietic elements (i.e., mast cells).

14. D. Thrombotic thrombocytopenic purpua is a microangiopathic hemolytic anemia that is accompanied by systemic microvascular thrombosis that can impact any organ(s) within the body. Within this potentially fatal condition, RBCs within the circulation become severed as they come in contact with thrombi within the vessels. The remaining fragmented cell is known as schistocyte. An initial schistocyte count of greater than 1% strongly suggests a diagnosis of TTP in the absence of other known causes of thrombotic microangiopathy.

15. B. The Schilling test is used to determine whether the body absorbs vitamin B12 normally. Patients undergoing testing receive two doses of vitamin B12: The first is an oral radioactive form; an intramuscular injection of non-radioactive vitamin B12 is administered one hour later. The patient then collects urine over the next 24 hours, and the specimen is evaluated to determine how much vitamin B12 is excreted in the urine.

16. A. The MCV of this patient with anemia reveals a normocytic anemia. Iron deficiency anemia is a microcytic anemia, while folic acid and vitamin B12 deficiencies result in the production of RBCs that are larger in size than normal cells, macrocytic anemia.

17. C. The MCV of this patient with anemia reveals a microcytic anemia. Anemia of chronic disease is most commonly a normocytic anemia, while folic acid and vitamin B12 deficiencies result in the production of RBCs that are larger in size than normal cells, which is called macrocytic anemia.

18. D. Standard blood tests for the workup of suspected hemolytic anemia include a CBC with peripheral smear, serum LDH, serum haptoglobin, and indirect bilirubin. Changes in the LDH and serum haptoglobin are the most sensitive of these tests. Within intravascular hemolysis, free hemoglobin is released into the circulation and quickly bound by haptoglobin; thus, circulating haptoglobin levels decline.

19. D. An increase in RDW beyond the normal range of 15% is seen in early attempts to maintain hematologic homeostasis. Marked reticulocytosis results in transient changes to the RDW because the reticulocytes differ in size from the cells produced under healthy conditions.

20. D. Iron is best absorbed when taken on an empty stomach, but does have GI effects that limit tolerability (i.e., nausea and epigastric discomfort); taking iron supplementation with food can decreased absorption by two-thirds and the use of enteric-coated preparations limits the absorption in the duodenum. Ascorbic acid does enhance iron absorption in the GI tract.

21. D. Patients undergoing hemodialysis are at risk for physical damage to the RBC membranes because it causes them to break down faster than normal. Autoimmune hemolytic anemia is linked to specific diseases (lupus, hepatitis, leukemia, and lymphoma) and infections (EBV, CMV, and HIV). Drug-induced hemolytic anemia is linked to chemotherapy, quinine and antimalarial medications, levodopa, and anti-inflammatories, among others. Hereditary or inherited hemolytic anemias (including sickle cell anemia, thalassemia, G6PD deficiency, and hereditary spherocytosis and elliptocytosis) most commonly have manifestations that begin earlier in the lifespan.

22. A. Although the risk of bacterial infections does decrease in the individual with sickle cell anemia after the age of three years, bacterial infections are still the most common cause of death at any age.

23. B. Megaloblastic anemia correlates with macrocytic anemia. Of the macrocytic anemias, vitamin B12 commonly produces a variety of neurological symptoms because of its relationship with methylmalonic acid and methionine, while folic acid deficiency does not manifest with neurological symptoms.

24. D. Vitamin B12 replacement is accompanied by a shift of potassium from the serum to within the cells during reticulocytosis; the risk for hypokalemia is more common in the individual with severe anemia and can be compounded by coexisting conditions or medications that place the individual at risk for hypokalemia or the negative consequences associated with this electrolyte imbalance (e.g., those on diuretics or digoxin).

25. C. Hemoglobin electrophoresis identifies variant and abnormal hemoglobins, including hemoglobin S (HbS) or sickle hemoglobin. It can be used to differentiate those who have sickle cell disease (in which at least one of the two abnormal inherited genes will result in the production of hemoglobin S) and sickle cell anemia (in which the individual has inherited two hemoglobin S genes, hemoglobin SS [HbSS], the most common and severe type of the disease).

26. A. Several studies in children and adults have revealed that hydroxyurea reduces the number of episodes of vaso-occlusive or pain crises and hospitalizations. Therapy with hydroxyurea has also been shown to decrease the need for transfusions. Experts recommend that children and adults with hemoglobin SS who have frequent, painful episodes, recurrent chest crises, or severe anemia requiring transfusions take hydroxyurea daily. Some experts initiate this therapy to all hemoglobin SS children over the age of 9 months to prevent or reduce the chance of complications; safety and effectiveness in children under the age of 9 months has not been established. Ibuprofen is helpful when mild pain crises occur.

27. C. The absolute neutrophil count (ANC) refers to the number of neutrophil granulocytes in the blood and is utilized as a measure of risk for infection in patients undergoing chemotherapy. The ANC is calculated by multiplying the WBC count by the percent of neutrophils (segs and bands) present in the blood. The ANC can be interpreted as follows:

    ANC greater than 1500/mm^3: No increased risk of infection

    ANC 1000–1500/mm^3: Slight increase in risk of infection

    ANC 500–1000/mm^3: Moderate increase in risk of infection

    ANC 100–500/mm^3: High risk of infection

    ANC less than 100/mm^3: Extremely high risk of infection

28. B. Iron overload is a major concern for transfusion-dependent patients with thalassemia major, contributing to morbidity and mortality. Each unit of transfused blood has approximately 250 mg of iron, which accumulates in the tissues, especially the liver and heart. Thalassemia major patients commonly undergo iron chelation therapy to minimize their risk of transfusion-induced iron overload complications. Supplementation with iron should be avoided unless there is substantial evidence of an iron deficiency.

29. C. The American Academy of Pediatrics (2010) identifies that iron deficiency anemia is a common yet undetected problem among children. Current recommendations include universal iron supplementation for all children, with dosing dependent on the child's age and the anticipated amount of iron consumed. Term, healthy infants have sufficient iron for the first 4 months of life. Human breast milk contains very little iron, and therefore, breastfed infants should be supplemented with 1 mg/kg per day of oral iron from 4 months of age until iron-rich foods are introduced. Formula-fed infants receive adequate iron from formula and complementary foods, and supplementation is not required.

30. A. Glucose-6-Phosphate Dehydrogenase deficiency is a genetic disorder in which the body doesn't have enough of the G6PD enzyme to help protect the RBCs from oxidative insult. The most common presentation is hemolytic anemia, leading to symptoms of jaundice, pallor, fatigue, dark urine, tachycardia, and dyspnea. G6PD is on the X chromosome and tends to affect more men than women. The hemolytic anemia is most often triggered by an oxidative stressor such as bacterial or viral infections and certain medications (sulfonamides, analgesics, antimalarials, antihelminths). Hemolytic anemia can also occur after eating fava beans or inhaling pollen from fava plants (a reaction called favism), or exposure to mothballs.

31. B. Iron poisoning is a common toxicologic emergency in young children. Education is essential in the prevention of such events. More than 15,000 cases of iron exposure are reported to poison control centers across the nation annually. Approximately 1/5 of cases result in unintentional ingestion in children under the age of 6. The medication is available in many forms, including tablets, capsules, drops, syrups, and elixirs contained in bottles both with and without child-proof closures. The availability of the medication within reach of children in the home and the candy-like appearance contributes to these avoidable occurrences.

32. B. The leukocytes that increase during an allergic reaction are the eosinophils. Eosinophils regulate inflammation and destroy foreign substances. The normal percentage of eosinophils on a CBC differential is 0–5%. Eosinophilia occurs when a large amount of eosinophils are recruited to a particular site in the body and are most commonly triggered by allergic disorders and parasitic infections.

33. B. The majorities of both acute and chronic forms of leukemia affect lymphocytes and are a common reason for leukocytosis. Lymphocytes are the primary components of the body's immune system and are the second most common WBCs, second to neutrophils. Lymphocytosis may also indicate acute or chronic infections, cancer of the blood or lymphatic system, or autoimmune disorders causing chronic inflammation.

34. D. Parents with any combination of alpha or beta thalassemia syndromes place a child at risk for the disorder. Each child of two carrier parents is at a 25% risk of the disease. If a parent is positive for the trait, a prenatal diagnosis can be made with fetal blood sampling or chorionic villi sampling. Genetic counseling is an integral and necessary component of comprehensive care for patients and parents affected by all forms of thalassemia disease and trait. Genetic counseling is the process of providing

information and support to individuals and families with a diagnosis and/or risk of occurrence of an inherited disorder. Services should be provided by a licensed genetic counselor.

35. C. Ferritin is a protein found within cells that stores iron for later use. Serum ferritin reflects the iron storage capacity of the body and is the most useful test to diagnose iron deficiency anemia. Serum ferritin levels are often ordered in conjunction with other iron tests such as the total iron binding capacity (TIBC). Ferritin levels are low in iron deficiency anemia and elevated in iron overload, inflammation, or infection. A normal ferritin level is 12–300 ng/mL in males and 12–150 ng/mL in females.

36. A. An increase in hemoglobin by 1g/dL within one month of iron supplementation demonstrates an adequate response to treatment and confirms the diagnosis of IDA. In adults, therapy should be continued for 3 months after hemoglobin is corrected to restore ferritin stores.

37. D. Pernicious anemia is an autoimmune disorder caused by the destruction of parietal cells in the gastric fundus, resulting in the cessation of intrinsic factor production. The intrinsic factor is important for the absorption of vitamin B12 from the small intestine. Since pernicious anemia is irreversible, lifetime supplementation of B12 (injections, nasal, or high-dose oral route) is necessary.

38. B. A deficiency in folate typically causes macrocytosis without neurological manifestations. The most common causes are inadequate dietary intake, malnutrition, and excessive alcohol intake. Folate food sources include green leafy vegetables, grains, beans, and liver. The classic presentation is an elderly patient and/or alcoholic older male with signs and symptoms of anemia such as weakness, fatigue, difficulty concentrating, irritability, headache, palpitations, or shortness of breath.

39. B. Vitamin B12 is naturally found in animal products, including fish, meat, poultry, eggs, milk, and milk products. Vitamin B12 is generally not present in plant-based foods, but fortified breakfast cereals are an option for strict vegetarians.

40. B. Monocytes are the largest of the WBCs and comprise 2–8% of the leukocyte count. Monocytes are produced in the bone marrow and migrate from blood to tissue within a few hours, where they develop into macrophages and dendritic cells. Monocytes assist other leukocytes to remove dead or damaged tissues, destroy cancer cells, and regulate immunity against foreign substances. Monocytosis may occur in response to chronic infections, autoimmune disorders, blood disorders, or cancers.

41. D. Thrombotic thrombocytopenic purpura is a syndrome of decreased platelets causing microangiopathic hemolytic anemia, thrombocytopenic purpura, neurologic abnormalities, fever, and renal disease. Although not all patients present with the classic pentad of symptoms, the presence of microangiopathic hemolytic anemia and thrombocytopenia alone should prompt suspicion of TTP.

42. B. Although persons with thalassemia trait have a normal life expectancy, patients with beta thalassemia major often die from cardiac complications from iron overload related to regular blood transfusions by 30 years of age.

43. B. Idiopathic thrombocytopenia purpura (ITP) is a syndrome characterized by a decreased number of platelets causing a reduced ability for primary clotting leading to purpura and petechiae. The cause is unknown, but in children, most cases are acute and tend to follow a viral illness. The condition is diagnosed with a CBC and isolated thrombocytopenia is the hallmark finding.

44. C. Heparin-induced thrombocytopenia (HIT) is a complication of heparin therapy and is caused by antibodies that bind to heparin and platelet factor 4 (PF4), causing a prothombotic state. Unlike other forms of thrombocytopenia, HIT presents without bleeding; rather, venous thromboembolism, pulmonary embolism, MI, and CVA are the causes for concern.

45. C. Acute cases of ITP in children generally do not require treatment and resolve spontaneously within 2 months. For children requiring treatment (platelets less than 50,000/µL), a single dose of IVIG dosed at 0.8–1g/kg or a short course of corticosteroids should be used as first-line therapy. Rituximab is used for those with refractory disease.

46. B. Aplastic anemia is a serious blood disorder caused by bone marrow failure characterized by pancytopenia and marrow hypoplasia. Therefore, the first tests to order when evaluating a patient for suspected aplastic anemia include a CBC with differential reticulocyte count, peripheral blood smear, and a bone marrow biopsy with cytogenic evaluation. A bone marrow biopsy typically demonstrates hypocellular marrow without abnormal cells.

47. C. Thrombocytopenia is defined as a platelet count of less than 150,000/µL and is often found incidentally when obtaining a CBC. Most patients with thrombocytopenia are asymptomatic. However, when platelet counts decrease to less than 50,000/µL, symptoms may include easy bruising (ecchymosis, petechiae), bleeding from mucous membranes, spontaneous epistaxis, excessive bleeding from wounds, and hematuria.

48. B. The most common recommended dose of folic acid replacement for adults with folic acid deficiency is 1 mg/day. In response to supplementation, reticulocytosis occurs rapidly and peaks within 7 to 10 days. Hematocrit levels usually return to normal within one month and evaluating the hemogram within this timeframe is considered standard. If levels are not rising as expected, and coexisting B12 anemia has been ruled out, the practitioner should keep in mind that iron deficiency anemia coexists in 1/3 of patients with B12 or folate deficiency.

49. D. Serum iron levels are highest in the morning and this is an ideal time to evaluate these lab values; however, for the most accurate results, patients should be advised to fast for 8–12 hours prior to the blood draw. Serum iron levels rise earlier in the treatment process and reflect recent intake. Therefore, iron levels are impacted if the patient ingests oral iron supplements within 24–48 hours of a lab evaluation.

50. C. Patients who undergo hematopoietic cell transplantation have a risk for developing graft versus host disease (GVHD), and possibly graft failure, and should therefore be monitored frequently. The clinical manifestations of acute GVHD occur in the skin, GI tract, and liver, with the skin the most commonly affected organ. The characteristic rash of GVHD is pruritic, maculopapular, and scalp-sparing.

• • • References

Baker, R., Greer, F., & The Committee on Nutrition American Academy of Pediatrics. (2010). Diagnosis and prevention of iron deficiency and iron-deficiency anemia in infants and young children (0–3 years of age). *Pediatrics, 126*(5), 1040–1050.

Bakhshi, S. (2014). *Aplastic anemia: Practice essentials, background, etiology.* Retrieved from http://emedicine.medscape.com/artcile/198759-overview

Braden, C. (2015). *Neutropenia: Practice essentials, background, pathophysiology.* Retrieved from http://emedicine.medscape.com/article/204821-overview

Camaschella, C. (2015). Iron-deficiency anemia. *New England Journal of Medicine, 372,* 1832–1843.

Carson, S., & Martin, M. (2014). Effective iron chelation practice for patients with β-thalassemia major. *Clinical Journal of Oncology Nursing, 18*(1), 102–111.

Chabot-Richards, D. S., & George, T. I. (2014). Leukocytosis. *International Journal of Laboratory Hematology, 36,* 279–288.

Copelan, E., & Avalos, B. (2014). *Evaluation of neutropenia.* Retrieved from https://online.epocrates.com/u/2911893/Evaluation+of+neutropenia

Gauer, R. L., & Braun, M. M. (2012). Thrombocytopenia. *American Family Physician, 85*(6), 612–622.

Janus, J., & Moerschel, S. K. (2010). Evaluation of anemia in children. *American Family Physician, 81,* 1462–1471.

Kaferle, J., & Strzoda, C. E. (2009). Evaluation of macrocytosis. *American Family Physician, 79,* 203–208.

Krzych, L. J., Nowacka, E., & Knapik, P. (2015). Heparin-induced thrombocytopenia. *Anaesthesiology Intensive Therapy, 47*(1), 63–76.

Marsh, J., Ball, S., Cavenagh, J., Darbyshire, P., Dokal, I., Gordon-Smith, E., . . . Yin, J. (2009). Guidelines for the diagnosis and management of aplastic anaemia. *British Journal of Haematology, 147,* 43–70.

Muncie, H., & Campbell, J. (2009). Alpha and beta thalassemia. *American Family Physician, 80*(4), 339–344.

Neunert, C., Lim, W., Crowther, M., Cohen, A., Solberg, L, Crowther, M., & The American Society of Hematology. (2011). The American Society of Hematology 2011 evidence-based practice guideline for immune thrombocytopenia. *Blood, 117*(16), 4190–4207.

Pagana, K. (2009). What does the absolute neutrophil count tell you? *American Nurse Today, 4*(2), 12–13.

Powers, J. M., & Buchanan, G. R. (2014). Diagnosis and management of iron deficiency anemia. *Hematology/Oncology Clinics, 28,* 729–745.

Rees, D. C., Williams, T. N., & Gladwin, M. T. (2010). Sickle-cell disease. *The Lancet, 376,* 2018–2031.

Scully, M., Hunt, B., Benjamin, S., Liesner, R., Rose, P., Peyvandi, F., . . . Machin, S. (2012). Guidelines on the diagnosis and management of thrombotic thrombocytopenic purpura and other thrombotic microangiopathies. *British Journal of Haematology, 120*(4), 556–573.

Thomas, D., Hinchliffe, R., Briggs, C., Macdougall, I., Littlewood, T., Cavill, I., & The British Committee for Standards in Haematology. (2013). Guideline for the laboratory diagnosis of functional iron deficiency. *British Journal of Haematology, 161*(5), 639–648.

Urrechaga, E., Hoffmann, J. J., Izquierdo, S., & Escaneor, J. F. (2014). Differential diagnosis of microcytic anemia: The role of microcytic and hypochromic erythrocytes.

International Journal of Laboratory Hematology, 37(3), 334–340.

Vieth, J. T., & Lane, D. R. (2014). Anemia. *Emergency Medicine Clinics of North America, 32,* 613–628.

Watson, H., Davidson, S., & Keeling, D. (2012). Guidelines on the diagnosis and management of heparin-induced thrombocytopenia: Second edition. *British Journal of Haematology, 159*(5), 528–540.

13

Renal/Urinary System

Sylvie Rosenbloom, DNP, APRN, FNP-BC, CDE

Normal Findings

- The kidneys are found in the retroperitoneal space.
- The right kidney is slightly displaced by the liver and is located somewhat lower than the left one.
- Nephrons, containing the glomeruli, are the kidney's functional units.
- The kidneys produce approximately 1,500 mL of urine daily.

Function

The kidneys are involved in the regulation of fluids and electrolytes. The antidiuretic hormone and aldosterone produced by the kidneys help promote water reabsorption in the body and excrete waste products. Kidneys are also involved in the production of red blood cells through the production of erythropoietin, which stimulates the production of bone marrow. In addition, the kidneys secrete the following hormones: renin and bradykinin, which play a role in blood pressure; prostaglandins, calcitrol, and vitamin D3 production.

Laboratory Findings

- Serum creatinine: male 0.7–1.3 mg/dL; female 0.6–1.1 mg/dL
- Normal: eGFR > 90 mL/min; Renal failure: < 15 mL/min

Urinary Tract Infections

A urinary tract infection (UTI) can also be referred to as acute cystitis. It is an inflammation of the urinary tract epithelium, most often originating from the fecal flora. Bacteria usually ascend via the urethra into the bladder. The most common pathogen responsible for outpatient or hospital-acquired UTI is *Escherichia coli*. Most common signs and symptoms are dysuria, frequency, urgency, suprapubic tenderness, and hematuria.

When bacteria migrate to the kidneys, pyelonephritis can ensue. Pyelonephritis results when one or both upper urinary tracts are involved. Signs and symptoms include those involved in acute cystitis, as well as fever, chills, and flank or groin pain. Causes of pyelonephritis include nephrolithiasis/urolithiasis, pregnancy, neurogenic bladder, and vesicoureteral reflux.

Epidemiology

- There are an estimated 7 million office UTI visits yearly with an estimated cost of over $1 billion.
- Approximately 4–6% of women will have asymptomatic bacteriuria at any given time. This number increases to 26% in women with diabetes mellitus.
- The incidence of resistant UTI continues to increase.

Diagnosis

- Made primarily by history (dysuria and frequency); physical exam is often not necessary.

- Urinalysis (microscopic or dipstick): Positive nitrites. Sensitivity 80–90%; specificity 94–98%.
- Urine culture often unnecessary in acute cystitis but should be obtained if pyelonephritis is suspected or if complicating factors are present, as well as for recurrent UTI. Sensitivity > 90%.
- Imaging studies should be obtained in infants or children with an initial febrile UTI or recurrent cystitis.
- No imaging studies needed for patients with uncomplicated UTI. However, in healthy adults with febrile UTI, persistent bacteriuria, or a suspicion of foreign bodies or obstructions, imaging studies (sonography) should be obtained.

Differential Diagnosis

- Vaginitis
- Urethritis
- Structural urethral abnormalities
- Painful bladder syndrome
- Pelvic inflammatory disease
- Nephrolithiasis/urolithiasis
- Prostatitis

Treatment

Resolution of symptoms should occur approximately 48 hours after initiation of therapy. A urinary analgesic (pyridium) can be given, in addition to the antibiotic regimen, to help alleviate symptoms.

Uncomplicated

First line:
- 3-day course of Bactrim (trimethoprim/sulfa)
- 5–7 day course of Macrobid (nitrofurantoin)

Second line:
- 3-day course of quinolone (contraindicated in pregnancy)
- 7-day course of amoxicillin or first-generation cephalosporin

Complicated

Initial empiric treatment should be initiated, and then guided/changed as per urine culture and sensitivity results.

Follow-up

- No test of cure necessary for uncomplicated UTI.
- Urine culture and sensitivity should be obtained for persistent symptoms.
- Rule out bacterial prostatitis in men.
- Refer to urologist if persistent bacteriuria or recurrent UTI.

- May consider antibiotic prophylaxis for recurrent UTI (>3/year).
- In pregnancy, refer to obstetrician if pyelonephritis is suspected or develops.

Prevention

- Encourage patients to remain well hydrated. The recommended daily allowance (RDA) for fluids in healthy adults is 30 mL/kg/day.
- Instruct female patients on proper hygiene.
- Avoid constipation.
- Use of spermicide/diaphragm increases the risk of UTI.
- Encourage micturition after intercourse.
- Currently, there is no sufficient evidence to promote the use of cranberry products.
- Educate patient that using pyridium may cause an orange-red discoloration to bodily fluids (urine, sweat, tears).

Glomerulonephritis

Glomerulonephritis is an inflammation of the glomeruli leading to a decrease in the kidney's filtration ability. It can be caused by infection such as streptococcus, bacterial endocarditis, viral infections such as HIV and hepatitis, autoimmune disorders such as lupus, and other conditions such as diabetes and hypertension or those that are idiopathic (Berger disease). Signs and symptoms include hematuria, proteinuria, hypertension, edema (hands and feet), fatigue from anemia, and kidney failure (acute and chronic) can ensue.

Treatment

The treatment of glomerulonephritis involves treating and managing the underlying cause to prevent further kidney damage. Prompt referral to a nephrologist is key. A biopsy is often done in idiopathic cases. Corticosteroids and immunosuppressive agents are utilized. Hypertension and diabetes control are key to prevent further kidney damage.

Follow-up

- Restrict sodium intake to minimize and prevent fluid retention and control hypertension.
- Reduce protein and potassium intake to prevent proteinuria and hyperkalemia.
- Maintain a healthy body mass index.
- Improve diabetes and hypertension control.
- Smoking cessation.

Nephrotic Syndrome

Nephrotic syndrome often occurs as a result of glomerular injury. It is characterized by the presence of heavy proteinuria (3–3.5 g/24 hr), hypoalbuminemia (<3 g/dL) and peripheral edema. Patients with nephrotic syndrome are at increased risk of infection and thromboembolic events. If untreated, the condition can lead to acute kidney injury and/or renal failure. Diagnosis is made with a 24-hr urine collection measuring protein excretion. A renal biopsy is often done to determine the cause of proteinuria.

Epidemiology

About 30% of adults with diabetes mellitus, systemic lupus erythematosus, or amyloidosis will develop nephrotic syndrome.

Clinical Manifestations

- Proteinuria
- Hypoalbuminemia
- Edema
- Hyperlipidemia/hypertriglyceridemia
- Vitamin D deficiency
- Hypothyroidism

Signs/Symptoms

- Weight gain (edema)
- Fatigue
- Foamy urine
- Loss of appetite
- Signs/symptoms of hypothyroidism

Treatment

- Proteinuria—The administration of angiotensin converting enzymes (ACE) or angiotensin-receptor blockers (ARB) with the close monitoring of serum potassium and creatinine levels. Normal protein diet.
- Edema—Diuretics and low-sodium diet (2 g/day) and loop diuretics (Lasix/furosemide) as needed.
- Hyperlipidemia/hypertriglyceridemia—This will subside with the treatment of nephrotic syndrome. Initiation of HMG CoA reductase inhibitor (statins) may be required.
- Hypercoagulability state—If thrombosis occurs, heparin followed by the administration of Coumadin (warfarin) is given.

Follow-up

- Monitor kidney functions/electrolytes.
- Advise your patient to perform daily weights to assess for improvement of edema.

- Educate patient on signs/symptom of deep vein thrombosis/pulmonary embolism and teach them to seek prompt medical attention should they arise.
- Encourage a low-sodium, low-fat diet.
- Fluid restrictions may be advised.

Nephrolithiasis/Urolithiasis

Urinary lithiasis (kidney stones) are the result of an accumulation of protein, crystals, or other substances resulting in an obstruction of the urinary flow. These can be located in the kidney, bladder, ureters, or urethra. The most common type of stone is calcium oxalate (70–80%), struvite (magnesium, ammonium, or phosphate) (15%), uric acid (7%), or cysteine (<1%). The most common manifestation of kidney stones is renal colic. This presents as moderate to severe pain at the costovertebral angle junction or flank area, often radiating to the groin area. Dysuria, frequency, urgency, pink-tinged urine, nausea, and vomiting can also be present. Fever and chills may indicate infection. Complications of untreated nephrolithiasis can lead to kidney damage and/or renal failure.

Epidemiology

- The U.S. prevalence of kidney stones is approximately 15% in men and 6% in women.
- Kidney stones are more prevalent in Caucasians.
- Recurrence rate is 30–50% over a 5-year period.
- The majority of kidney stones occur in persons under the age of 50.
- A family history of nephrolithiasis increases one's risk.

Evaluation

Often made with a good history and focused physical examination. Testing of choice is renal ultrasonography (sensitivity 54%) or computed tomography scan (sensitivity 70%). A complete blood count may be ordered to rule out infection; a metabolic panel to assess levels of calcium and a uric acid level can also be ordered. A urinalysis and 24-hour urine collection will be obtained to assess for pH and calcium citrate, oxalate, or other sedimentation, respectively.

Differential Diagnosis

- Hydronephrosis
- Glomerular nephritis
- UTI
- Pyelonephritis

- Ectopic pregnancy in females
- Dysmenorrhea
- Acute intestinal obstruction
- Acute mesenteric ischemia
- Herpes zoster

Treatment

- Initial treatment usually focuses on pain management. Both opioids and non-steroidal anti-inflammatory (NSAIDs) are utilized.
- Urine straining to identify stone type.
- Urology referral for urosepsis, acute renal failure, anuria, unremitting pain, nausea, or vomiting.
- Stone removal via lithotripsy, ureteroscopy, percutaneous nephrolithotomy.
- Calcium stones – A thiazide diuretic or potassium citrate may be ordered.
- Uric acid stones – Allopurinol may be prescribed to decrease uric acid levels.
- Cystine stones – Increase fluid intake and urinary alkalinization.

Follow-up/Prevention

- Encourage adequate fluid intake.
- Calcium oxalate stone formation can be minimized by decreasing the intake of oxalate-rich foods such as rhubarb, beets, okra, spinach, and chocolate.
- Increase intake of calcium-rich foods but caution patients about calcium supplements.
- A low-sodium and low-animal-protein diet has been shown to decrease the incidence of nephrolithiasis.
- Referral to a urologist.

Acute Kidney Injury

Classification

- Renal Insufficiency—Defined as a GFR of 25 to 30 mL/minute or a reduction in renal function of 25%. There is a mild elevation of urea and serum creatinine.
- Acute Kidney Injury—Diagnosed with sudden onset of increased BUN, serum creatinine and elevation of other kidney waste products. It can potentially progress to complications such as fluid overload, hyperkalemia, metabolic acidosis, hypocalcemia, hyperphosphatemia, and uremia.

- Chronic Kidney Injury—Occurs when the GFR if less than 60 mL/min for 3 or more months.
- Renal Failure—also known as end-stage kidney disease; occurs with significant loss of kidney function (<10% functioning).
- Uremia—Consequence of renal failure manifested by elevations of blood urea and serum creatinine levels, as well as symptoms of fatigue, anorexia, nausea, vomiting, pruritus, and neurological changes.
- Azotemia—described as elevations in blood urea levels with/without elevated serum creatinine levels.

Acute Kidney Injury (AKI)

Most often occurs in hospitalized patients and is characterized by a sudden decline in renal function, with a decreased GFR and a rise in renal waste products (serum creatinine and blood nitrogen levels). It is associated with a 50–80% mortality rate, and is a result of hypovolemia, decreased kidney perfusion, and/or toxic/inflammation of renal cells, leading to decreased kidney function. Risk factors include hypertension, heart failure, diabetes mellitus, sepsis, hypovolemia, use of nephrotoxic medication and contrast materials, and hospitalization. Can occur in up to 5% of hospitalized patients. Assessment and treatment of the causes of AKI are imperative.

Chronic Kidney Injury (CKI)

As stated earlier, CKI is diagnosed when there is a decrease in kidney function present for three or more months. It is most often seen in individuals with a history of hypertension, diabetes mellitus, systemic lupus erythematosus, or other kidney diseases such as renal lithiasis, chronic pyelonephritis, and chronic glomerulonephritis.

Signs/Symptoms of AKI/CKI

- Decreased kidney functions can lead to edema, hypertension, and decreases in urinary output (oliguria).
- Symptoms of nephrotic syndrome: proteinuria, hyperlipidemia, hypothyroidism, decreased vitamin D levels.
- Prolonged renal failure leads to fatigue, anemia, electrolyte imbalances, acid-base disturbances, anorexia, vomiting, change in mental status, seizures.
- Assess for other comorbidities such as congestive heart failure, diabetes mellitus, and liver disease that can potentially cause AKI/CKI.
- Assess for use of nephrotoxic drugs.

Table 13-1		Stages of Chronic Kidney Diseases	
Stage	GFR*	Description	Treatment
1	90+	Normal kidney function but urine findings or structural abnormalities or genetic trait point to kidney disease	Observation, control of blood pressure. More on management of Stages 1 and 2 CKD.
2	60–89	Mildly reduced kidney function, and other findings (as for stage 1) point to kidney disease	Observation, control of blood pressure and risk factors. More on management of Stages 1 and 2 CKD.
3A	45–59	Moderately reduced kidney function	Observation, control of blood pressure and risk factors. More on management of Stages 3 CKD.
3B	30–44		
4	15–29	Severely reduced kidney function	Planning for endstage renal failure. More on management of Stages 4 and 5 CKD.
5	<15 or on dialysis	Very severe, or endstage kidney failure (sometimes call established renal failure)	Treatment choices. More on management of Stages 4 and 5 CKD.

*All GFR values are normalized to an average surface area (size) of $1.73m^2$

Reproduced from The Renal Association. (2013). CKD Stages. Retrieved from http://www.renal.org/information-resources/the-uk-eckd-guide/ckd-stages#sthash.0McZtzkn.dpbs.

Stages of CKI

The five stages of chronic kidney diseases are described in Table 13-1.

Evaluation

Upon diagnosing kidney disease, renal function must be assessed and etiology determined. In both AKI and CKI, a thorough history is conducted, including a review of medications and physical examination. Initial testing will include serum urea and creatinine levels, urine dipstick/urinalysis for evaluation of sedimentation, hemoglobin, and leukocytes. Imaging studies such as ultrasonography may be performed to rule out obstructions, cysts, or masses. If nephritic or nephrotic glomerular disease is present, serologic testing may ensue to identify the etiology of kidney disease.

Treatment

Recognition and prompt treatment of AKI is key. The purpose of treatment is to preserve kidney function and prevent future deterioration (CKI/renal failure):

1. Manage hypertension
2. Correct fluid/electrolyte abnormalities
3. Treat/prevent infections
4. Ensure adequate nutrition
5. Drug regimen review and discontinuation of nephrotoxic medications

Follow-up/Prevention

- Educate your patient regarding the importance of controlling their hypertension and diabetes.
- Maintain dietary changes (low-sodium, low-potassium, low-protein as prescribed).
- Avoid nephrotoxic drugs such as non-steroidal anti-inflammatory drugs (NSAIDs) and contrast imaging drugs.
- Maintain proper hydration.
- Promptly report any decreases in urination, hematuria, edema, nausea, vomiting, feeling fatigued, changes in mental status, or seizures as these can indicate worsening of kidney injury.

Urinary Incontinence

Urinary incontinence (UI) is defined as a lack of bladder control resulting in involuntary urine leakage. It can majorly impact one's quality of life, leading to depression, anxiety, and social isolation. Classified as follows:

1. Urge incontinence – Involuntary urine leakage occurring with strong symptoms of urgency; also known as overactive bladder.
2. Stress incontinence – Involuntary urine loss with the increase of intra-abdominal pressure occurring with coughing, sneezing, and laughing in the absence of bladder contraction.
3. Overflow incontinence – Urine leakage occurring with an overdistended bladder, often seen with incomplete emptying of the bladder. It is caused by detrusor underactivity of bladder outlet obstruction.

4. Mixed incontinence – Stress and urge incontinence.

5. Functional incontinence – Involves a fully functional urinary system but occurs with the inability to toilet one's self in a timely manner.

Epidemiology

The prevalence of UI increases with advanced age and in long-term care residents. Stress incontinence is most commonly seen in younger females; the highest incidence is seen between the ages of 45 to 49, while urgency incontinence is more prevalent in older females. Risk factors include:

1. Obesity
2. Parity, including mode of delivery: Higher rates in vaginal delivery
3. Age
4. Ethnicity/Race – More prevalent in Caucasians than African Americans
5. Tobacco use and caffeine intake
6. Vaginal atrophy
7. Medical history of hypertension, diabetes, stroke, depression, hormone replacement therapy, neurologic disorders, cognitive impairment, cancer, genitourinary radiation, or surgery such as hysterectomy
8. Medications (reversible)

Evaluation

Initial evaluation will attempt to distinguish the type of UI and identify potential reversible causes. This may necessitate tact and discretion because many patients are reluctant to discuss this issue. Often diagnosed with a thorough history and physical examination, including a pelvic exam to rule out vaginal atrophy. A urinalysis is obtained to rule out infection. Kidney function testing is not routinely done except in cases of urinary retention to rule out hydronephrosis. Further testing such as bladder stress test, postvoid residual, urodynamic testing and urethral mobility evaluation may be undertaken. Refer to urology in cases of hematuria, abdominal/pelvic pain associated with incontinence, abnormal physical exams such as prolapsed bladder, and incontinence associated with new neurologic symptomatology.

Treatment

- Anticholinergic medications such as oxybutynin (Ditropan, Oxytrol), tolterodine (Detrol), darifenacin (Enablex), solifenacin (Vesicare), trospium (Sanctura), fesoterodine (Toviaz) are utilized.
- Exercises such as pelvic floor muscle training with or without biofeedback and bladder training.
- Medical devices such as electric or magnetic electrostimulation.
- Treatment of underlying reversible causes, such as infection, or obstructions such as those caused by prostate enlargement or pelvic organ prolapse

Follow-up/Prevention

- Discuss weight loss if patient is obese.
- Discuss the importance of glycemic control in patients with diabetes.
- Keep a bladder diary.
- Avoid intake of potential triggers such as caffeine, alcohol, and spicy or acidic foods that can irritate the bladder.
- Decrease fluid intake before bed.
- Seek medical care if symptoms such as dysuria, hematuria, pelvic/abdominal pain, fever, and chills develop.

Review Questions

1. The most common bacteria involved in urinary tract infections is:
   A. Klebsiella.
   B. Escherichia coli.
   C. Clostridium difficile.
   D. Staphylococcus.

2. A 25-year-old female comes to the outpatient clinic complaining of suprapubic pressure and burning with urination for the past two days. She denies having any chills but states that she may have had a fever yesterday. The next step will be:
   A. Obtain a urine dipstick.
   B. Get a urine culture and sensitivity.
   C. Ask about previous infections.
   D. Refer the patient to a urologist.

3. Referring to the above case, the patient states that she has not had any prior urinary tract infections. The next step will be to:
   A. Obtain a urine dipstick.
   B. Get a urine culture and sensitivity.
   C. Ascertain any drug allergies.
   D. Refer the patient to a urologist.

4. A mother brings in her 4-month-old boy and states that the baby has had a low-grade fever, been more irritable than usual, and has had foul-smelling urine. What is the most appropriate next step?
   A. Obtain a urine dipstick.
   B. Get a urine culture and sensitivity.
   C. Immediately start the patient on an antibiotic.
   D. Refer the patient to a urologist.

5. A young female visits your clinic and complains of burning with urination. She states that she had these same symptoms about six months ago and was diagnosed with a urinary tract infection. She reports that a 3-day course of antibiotic was effective. Upon further questioning, it is uncovered that she has just become sexually active. Patient education should include all of the following EXCEPT:
   A. Voiding after intercourse may prevent recurrent UTI.
   B. Using a spermicide may increase your risk of UTI.
   C. Drinking 6 ounces of cranberry juice daily may prevent future UTI.
   D. She could use prophylactic antibiotic if she develops recurrent UTI.

6. A 19-year-old boy comes in for a follow-up of exudative tonsillitis with a streptococcus positive throat culture. He states that his throat feels much better but this morning his urine had a pink tinge and was very foamy. What does the FNP suspect is happening with this patient?
   A. Nephrolithiasis
   B. Hydronephrosis
   C. UTI
   D. Glomerulonephritis

7. What are the four criteria in making a diagnosis of nephrotic syndrome?
   A. Proteinuria, hypoalbuminemia, edema, dyslipidemia
   B. Proteinuria, hyperalbuminemia, edema, dyslipidemia
   C. Proteinuria, hypoalbuminemia, edema, hyperthyroidism
   D. Proteinuria, hyperalbuminemia, edema, hypothyroidism

8. In reviewing a 42-year-old female's bloodwork, the results indicate a diagnosis of nephrotic syndrome. Patient education should include all of the following EXCEPT:

    A. This condition increases your risk of infection.

    B. This condition increases your likelihood of clot formation.

    C. She needs to monitor her sodium intake.

    D. She needs to decrease her protein intake.

9. The most common stone composition of nephrolithiasis is:

    A. Struvite (magnesium, ammonium, and phosphate).

    B. Calcium oxalate.

    C. Cysteine.

    D. Uric acid.

10. A 25-year-old female comes to the office complaining of right-sided abdominal pain that has radiated to the groin area for the last 2 days. She has felt nauseated and has had a decreased appetite. The differential diagnosis will include all of the following EXCEPT:

    A. Ectopic pregnancy.

    B. Pyelonephritis.

    C. Constipation.

    D. Acute intestinal obstruction.

11. In educating a female patient with nephrolithiasis, the FNP reviews with the patient all of the following EXCEPT:

    A. Adequate hydration may decrease her risk of reoccurrence.

    B. How to strain her urine in order to analyze the type of stone.

    C. Advising her to increase her intake of cranberry juice or take cranberry supplements.

    D. Explaining that she has a 50% increased risk of reoccurrence over the next 5 years.

12. The FNP diagnoses a UTI in a 33-year-old female who provides a history of dysuria and frequency × 48 hours, and a urine dipstick that was positive for nitrites. She admits to having had two UTIs in the last 6 months. The FNP initiates antibiotic therapy with ciprofloxacin. The patient calls the FNP two days later to state that she has developed a fever. What is the next step?

    A. Change her antibiotic.

    B. Have her return and obtain a urinalysis and a urine culture and sensitivity.

    C. Refer to urology

    D. Tell her to increase hydration and take Tylenol (acetaminophen) for fever.

13. A 44-year-old male is diagnosed with nephrolithiasis by ultrasonography. He is discharged with a strainer and a follow-up appointment with a urologist two weeks later. Patient education includes all of the following EXCEPT:

    A. Use the strainer when you urinate and bring the stones, if any, to the urologist for analysis.

    B. If fever develops, take Tylenol (acetaminophen) 650 mg q4h (4 hours a day) prn (*pro re nata*).

    C. Tell him to eat foods rich in calcium.

    D. Drink plenty of fluids.

14. While reviewing the laboratory results of a 32-year-old man who came to the office for a complete physical exam two days prior, it is noted that his blood urea nitrogen and creatinine levels are as follows: 19 mg/dL (normal 7–18 mg/dL) and 1.4 mg/dL (normal 0.6–1.2 mg/dL). Previous results from six months prior were within normal limits. What's the next step?

    A. Tell the patient to increase consumption of fluids.

    B. Check a urinalysis.

    C. Repeat the bloodwork and assess medication intake.

    D. Tell the patient "Not to worry." These elevations are minimal and you will recheck them in six months at the next follow-up visit.

15. A patient complains of possible blood in her urine. A urine dipstick is positive for hemoglobin and leukocytes. A urinalysis, urine culture, and sensitivity and renal ultrasound are ordered to rule out all of the following EXCEPT:

    A. Nephrotic syndrome.

    B. Nephrolithiasis.

    C. Glomerulonephritis.

    D. UTI.

16. A 28-year-old woman who is 7 months pregnant comes to the urgent care. She states that she is on the third day of Macrobid (nitrofurantoin) and says she still has some dysuria and had a fever last night. The next step is:

    A. Change her antibiotic and obtain a urine culture.

    B. Start patient on some IV fluids and refer to urology.

    C. Tell her to continue her medication; her symptoms will resolve eventually.

    D. Start her on pyridium.

17. A 44-year-old African American female comes to the office to discuss symptoms of stress incontinence that she has been having for the last three months. The FNP tells her that:

    A. Her symptoms may resolve if she loses some weight.

    B. Her race is associated with a higher prevalence of incontinence.

    C. Stress incontinence is usually seen in older females, while urge incontinence is more prevalent in younger-aged females.

    D. Fluid intake has no impact on her symptoms.

18. The FNP diagnoses a 42-year-old male with glomerulonephritis. Which potential complications will be monitored?

    A. Bradycardia

    B. Hypertension

    C. Decreased cardiac output

    D. Hypotension

19. The FNP sees a 52-year-old man who needs an intravenous pyelogram (IVP). What do you need to assess prior to the procedure?

    A. Ability of patient to pass urine

    B. Ability of patient to tolerate PO fluids

    C. Current medication list.

    D. That the patient is ambulatory.

20. Referring to the preceding case, what is the patient encouraged to do after he returns from his procedure?

    A. Increase fluid intake.

    B. Increase ambulation.

    C. Increase frequent urination.

    D. Continue bed rest.

21. A 26-year-old female is being treated for cystitis. She informs the FNP that this is the third reoccurrence in almost a year. The FNP proceeds to ask her about her fluid intake. Which of the following would the FNP encourage her to stop drinking?

    A. Fruit juice

    B. Tea

    C. Water

    D. Lemonade

22. A 52-year-old male patient presents to the office following a brief hospitalization for pyelonephritis. He is currently on the second day of a 7-day course of antibiotic. Patient education includes which of the following?

    A. If you develop dysuria, increase PO fluids for two days.

    B. Continue your antibiotic until you are asymptomatic.

    C. Return to the office in 7–10 days for a repeat urinalysis, as well as a urine culture and sensitivity.

    D. If you develop urinary frequency, decrease PO fluid intake.

23. Acute renal failure is diagnosed when the estimated glomerular filtration rate is below which of the following?

    A. 5 mL/min

    B. 10 mL/min

    C. 15 mL/min

    D. 25 mL/min

24. What is the leading cause of acute renal failure?

    A. Hypotension

    B. Anemia

    C. Prostate cancer

    D. Diabetes mellitus

25. Kidney disease is associated with which of the most dangerous electrolyte imbalances?

    A. Hypermagnesemia

    B. Hyponatremia

    C. Hyperkalemia

    D. Hypercalcemia

26. A 66-year-old man with a past medical history that includes chronic kidney disease comes to the clinic. When discussing nutrition, he needs to know he should eat which of the following diets?

    A. High carbohydrate, high protein diet

    B. High calcium, high potassium, low protein diet

    C. Low protein, low sodium, low potassium diet

    D. Low protein, high potassium

27. The FNP is seeing a 32-year-old male who states: "I think I'm having kidney stones again." The FNP expects the patient to describe his pain as:

    A. Dull and aching pain in the costovertebral area.

    B. Diffused abdominal aching and cramp-like pain.

    C. Sharp pain radiating to the spine.

    D. Excruciating pain that comes and goes and radiates to the groin.

28. A 44-year-old male with a history of kidney stones is being seen in the primary care clinic. In reviewing his chart, it is noted that the patient's kidney stones are made up of uric acid crystals. He should be told to avoid which of the following?

    A. Milk

    B. Liver

    C. Apples

    D. Carrots

29. A 59-year-old man comes to the office for follow-up of his hypertension. His blood pressure today is 128/82. While reviewing his recent laboratory value, it is noted that his creatinine is 1.9 mg/dL. Which of his following medications should be discontinued at this time?

    A. Beta-blockers
    B. Calcium-channel blockers
    C. Direct-acting vasodilators
    D. Angiotensin-converting enzyme inhibitors

30. Which of the following is NOT a normal kidney change resulting from aging?

    A. Decreased bladder capacity
    B. Nocturnal polyuria
    C. Kidney enlargement
    D. Decreased glomerular filtration rate

Answers and Rationales

1. B. The most common bacteria involved in urinary tract infections is the gut bacteria: *Escherichia coli*. It accounts for 85% of all infections.

2. C. The next step in assessing/treating this patient will depend on whether or not this urinary tract infection is recurrent or a first occurrence.

3. B. In an uncomplicated or non-recurring urinary tract infection, a urinalysis (dipstick or microscopic) can adequately identify urinary tract infections. A urine culture and sensitivity should be performed in the following cases: (1) any patient with a first febrile infection; (2) a recurrent infection with or without fever (more than one per year); (3) a urinary calculi; and (4) a congenital defect.

4. D. Structural defects are the most common cause of urinary tract infections in infant males.

5. C. There is no current evidence supporting the use of cranberry products. Adequate fluid intake (water) is recommended to remain well hydrated.

6. D. Foamy and pink-tinged urine can signify proteinuria and hematuria, respectively. The most common complication of streptococcus is glomerulonephritis.

7. A. The four criteria in diagnosing nephrotic syndrome are: proteinuria (>3g/day), hypoalbuminemia, hypercholesterolemia/hypertriglyceridemia, and edema. Nephrotic syndrome increases one risk of developing hypothyroidism.

8. D. Proteinuria is often treated with the administration of angiotensin converting enzyme (ACE) or angiotensin-receptor blocker (ARB) medications and close monitoring of serum potassium and creatinine levels. A normal protein diet may be consumed.

9. B. Calcium oxalate makes up about 70–80% of kidney stones, followed by struvite (15%), uric acid (7%), and cysteine (1%).

10. C. In the case presentation, the following conditions need to be ruled out: hydronephrosis, glomerular nephritis, UTI/pyelonephritis, dysmenorrhea, acute intestinal obstruction, acute mesenteric ischemia, herpes zoster, and ectopic pregnancy in females.

11. C. The evidence for recommending cranberry juice/supplement is inconclusive. Increased water intake is advised to minimize stone formation.

12. C. Results of a urine culture and sensitivity will take approximately 48 hrs to return. The patient can rapidly deteriorate during this time. It is best to have her seen by a urologist immediately.

13. B. Fever can indicate pyelonephritis. If untreated, pyelonephritis can lead to kidney damage and/or renal failure.

14. C. Repeat the test to ensure that a laboratory error did not occur. Intake of non-steroidal anti-inflammatory medications needs to be ruled out in the acute onset of kidney disease.

15. A. All but nephrotic syndrome may present with hematuria.

16. B. Prompt treatment of UTI is of utmost importance when pregnant. UTI often escalates to pyrlonephritis in pregnancy and complications can ensue.

17. A. Stress incontinence is more prevalent in the obese. Caucasian females have a higher incidence of stress incontinence than African Americans. Adequate hydration is important; however, fluids should be limited at bedtime. Caffeine and alcohol may worsen symptoms. Stress incontinence is more prevalent in younger females, while urge incontinence is more frequently seen in older females.

18. B. Signs and symptoms of glomerulonephritis include: hypertension, tachycardia, edema, decreased urine output (oliguria), lethargy, and other signs of fluid overload. Pre-renal causes of acute renal failure are characterized by signs of hypotension.

19. C. Assessing the patient's current medication list for nephrotoxic medications such as non-steroidal anti-inflammatory drugs and metformin is important to avoid kidney injury. If patient cannot tolerate PO fluids, IV hydration will be maintained.

20. A. The dye utilized to perform the IVP is nephrotoxic. Encouraging an increase in PO fluid intake will aid in clearing the drug from the body.

21. B. Caffeine and alcohol are known bladder irritants, therefore they should be avoided to decrease the risk of cystitis. It is recommended to drink six to eight 8-oz glasses of water daily. Fruit juices are acceptable.

22. C. The patient should complete the entire course of the prescribed antibiotic. If symptoms of cystitis develop, he should contact his health care provider immediately. The patient should return to the office for a repeat urinalysis and urine culture once the antibiotic treatment is completed. Increasing PO fluid intake is also encouraged.

23. C. Acute renal failure, also known as end-stage renal disease, occurs when the eGFR < 15 mL/min.

24. D. Uncontrolled diabetes mellitus and hypertension are the most common causes of kidney disease.

25. C. Kidney disease often causes hyperkalemia, which can lead to dangerous cardiac arrhythmias.

26. C. Patients with chronic kidney disease need to consume a low-protein, low-sodium, and low-potassium diet. The sub-functioning kidney cannot adequately excrete the by-products of protein metabolism. A low-sodium diet will help control hypertension.

27. D. Renal colic pain is often described as excruciating pain that waxes and wanes.

28. B. Uric acid can be decreased by consuming a low purine diet. Cheese, red meats, and wine should be avoided.

29. D. Angiotensin-converting enzyme inhibitors are contraindicated in kidney disease.

30. C. Aging causes the kidneys to shrink resulting in loss of cortical kidney tissue. This is a result of decreased renal blood flow.

● ● ● References

Curan, G., Aronson, M., & Preminger, G. (2015). Uptodate. *Diagnosis and acute management of suspected nephrolithiasis in adults*. Retrieved from resources.library.mssm .edu:2226/contents/diagnosis-and-acute-management-of-suspected-nephrolithiasis-in-adults?source=search_result &search=kidney+stones&selectedTitle=1~150

Herbert, L., & Parikh, L. (2015). *Differential diagnosis and evaluation of glomerular diseases*. Retrieved from http:// eresources.library.mssm.edu:2226/contents/differential -diagnosis-and-evaluation-of-glomerular-disease?source =search_result&search=glomerulonephritis+adult& selectedTitle=1~150#H1

Hooton, T. (2015). Uptodate. *Uncomplicated acute cystitis and pyelonephritis in women*. Retrieved from http://eresources.library.mssm.edu:2226/contents/acute -uncomplicated-cystitis-and-pyelonephritis-in-women? source=search_result&search=urinary+tract+infection& selectedTitle=1~150#PATIENT_INFORMATION

Fatehi, P., & Hsu, C. (2015). Uptodate. *Diagnostic approach to the patient with acute kidney injury (acute kidney failure) or chronic kidney disease*. Retrieved from http://eresources .library.mssm.edu:2226/contents/diagnostic-approach-to -the-patient-with-acute-kidney-injury-acute-renal-failure -or-chronic-kidney-disease?source=machineLearning& search=renal+insufficiency&selectedTitle=1~150&section Rank=1&anchor=H2#PATIENT_INFORMATION

Kelepours, E., & Rovin, B. (2014). Uptodate. *Overview of heavy proteinuria and the nephrotic syndrome*. Retrieved from http://eresources.library.mssm.edu:2226/contents/ overview-of-heavy-proteinuria-and-the-nephrotic-syndrome? source=machineLearning&search=nephrotic+syndrome& selectedTitle=1~150&sectionRank=1&anchor=H20 #H20

Kidney Disease: Improving Global Outcomes (KDIGO) Glomerulonephritis Work Group. (2012). *KDIGO clinical practice guideline for glomerulonephritis*. Retrieved from http://www.guideline.gov/content.aspx?id=38244

Lukacz, E. (2015). Uptodate. *Evaluation of women with urinary incontinence*. Retrieved from http://eresources .library.mssm.edu:2226/contents/evaluation-of-women- with-urinary-incontinence?source=search_result&search =urinary+incontinence&selectedTitle=1~150

Mayo Clinic. (2015a). *Acute kidney diseases*. Retrieved from http://www.mayoclinic.org/diseases-conditions/kidney- failure/basics/complications/con-20024029

Mayo Clinic. (2015b). *Chronic kidney diseases*. Retrieved from http://www.mayoclinic.org/diseases-conditions/ kidney-disease/basics/definition/con-20026778

Mayo Clinic. (2015c). *Glomerulonephritis*. Retrieved from http://www.mayoclinic.org/diseases-conditions/glomerul onephritis/basics/lifestyle-home-remedies/con-20024691

Mayo Clinic. (2015d). *Kidney diseases*. Retrieved from http://www.mayoclinic.org/diseases-conditions/kidney- stones/basics/prevention/con-20024829

Mayo Clinic. (2015e). *Nephrotic syndrome*. Retrieved from http://www.mayoclinic.org/diseases-conditions/nephrotic- syndrome/basics/definition/con-20033385

Mayo Clinic. (2015f). *Urinary incontinence*. Retrieved from http://www.mayoclinic.org/diseases-conditions/urinary- incontinence/basics/definition/con-20037883

National Clinical Guideline Centre. (2013). *Acute kidney injury. Prevention, detection and management of acute kidney injury up to the point of renal replacement therapy.* Retrieved from http://www.guideline.gov/content.aspx?id =47080

Pearle, M. S., Goldfarb, D. S., Assimos, D. G., Curhan, G., Denu-Ciocca, C. J., Matlaga, B. R., . . . White, J. R. (2014). *Medical management of kidney stones.* Retrieved from http://www.guideline.gov/content.aspx?id=48229

University of Michigan Health System. (2012). *Urinary tract infection.* Retrieved from http://www.guideline.gov/ content.aspx?id=34419

U.S. Department of Health and Human Services. (2012). *Effective health care program: Non-surgical treatment for the treatment of incontinence: A review of the research for women.* Retrieved from http://effectivehealthcare.ahrq .gov/index.cfm/search-for-guides-reviews-and-reports/? pageaction=displayproduct&productID=1030

U.S. Department of Health and Human Services. (2014). *Nephrotic syndrome in adults.* Retrieved from http:// www.niddk.nih.gov/health-information/health-topics/ kidney-disease/nephrotic-syndrome-in-adults/Pages/facts .aspx

U.S. National Library of Medicine. (2015). *Medline plus: Urinary incontinence.* Retrieved from http://www.nlm .nih.gov/medlineplus/urinaryincontinence.html#cat78

14

Infectious Diseases

Julie G. Stewart, DNP, MPH, MSN, FNP-BC, APRN

This chapter will review some infectious diseases not covered in system-focused chapters, including human immunodeficiency virus, tick-borne illnesses, agents of bioterrorism, diarrheal diseases, sexually transmitted diseases, and general concepts of antibiotic and antiviral therapy.

Family nurse practitioners are the front line for evaluating patients that may need immediate and/or specialized care as it relates to infectious diseases. Rapid and thorough recognition of signs and symptoms, focused physical examination, and appropriate testing based on a comprehensive evaluation of the patient is essential.

- History of present illness (HPI)—Must include the seven attributes of a complaint/symptom (location, quality, timing, quantity/severity, when does symptom(s) occur, what makes it worse and better, associated symptoms). Include the presence of fever or no fever (temp > 38 °F), the duration and pattern of fever if present, areas of discomfort/pain, recent travel, stool consistency and amount if appropriate, weight loss, etc.

- Allergies—In particular, antibiotics and what allergy manifestations consisted of.

- Past medical and surgical history—Be sure to include immunizations and any history of sexually transmitted diseases (STDs) and/or previous infections.

- Psychosocial—Smoking increases patients' risk for bacterial infections, and alcohol abusers are more susceptible to viral and bacterial infections due to the effect of alcohol on the immune system. Illicit drug users are more likely to

become infected with HIV, hepatitis B and C, as well as tuberculosis, and bacterial endocarditis. Sexual preferences can be a risk for various STDs as well as lack of condom use.

- Family history
- Travel history
- Current medications
- Full review of systems

Clinical Tips

- Any fever (temperature greater than 99.5 °F orally or > 100.4 °F rectally) that has associated neurological symptoms requires immediate attention.

- Infants and children with fever that also are listless need immediate comprehensive evaluation (review Pediatric chapter).

- In general, infants, children, the elderly, and those who are immunocompromised are typically at highest risk for morbidity and mortality associated with infectious diseases.

- Understanding the epidemiological triangle (agent, host, environment), aids the nurse practitioner in rapid evaluation and diagnosis of infectious diseases.

- Culture and sensitivity testing is appropriate to identify the correct medication to use, particularly in illnesses with resistant strains of microbes.

- Special care in choosing appropriate antibiotics, particularly in pregnancy is required.

- The elderly often present with more subdued signs and symptoms and require a thorough evaluation (see Geriatrics chapter).

- Viruses are responsible for approximately 90% of upper respiratory infections.

- Washing hands, and washing and cleaning toys and medical equipment, are vital in preventing the transmission of many infectious diseases.

Human Immunodeficiency Virus (HIV)

- Globally, approximately 35 million people are infected with HIV, with over 70% affected living in sub-Saharan Africa.

- Everyone should be tested for HIV infection as part of routine screening, with CDC guidelines recommending this for those ages 13–64, all prenatal patients, and more frequent screening for those at high risk (every 3–6 months).

- HIV is a retrovirus. Once it enters the host (CD4) cell, it converts its RNA (ribonucleic acid) to DNA (deoxyribonucleic acid) via its enzyme reverse transcriptase. There are two types, HIV-1 and HIV-2. HIV-1 is more common and more easily transmitted.

- HIV is completely dependent upon CD4 cells for replication and survival. HIV gains entry into the CD4 cell by binding onto receptors on the outside of the CD4 cell and fusing with the lipid outer layer of the cell. Once inside the cell, HIV removes its outer coating, exposing its RNA, and releases reverse transcriptase enzyme to convert the HIV RNA to DNA. HIV DNA then enters the nucleus of the CD4 cell and is integrated into the host (CD4) DNA. Once the replicated virus has matured with the assistance of the enzyme protease, new virions are released to infect more CD4 cells to continue the process. Over time, the destruction of CD4 cells leads to severe immune suppression.

- Acute Retroviral Syndrome occurs within the first 2–4 weeks post-infection. Large amounts of the virus are replicating in the body at this time and can cause a rapid depletion of CD4 cells. Symptoms can include flu-like symptoms (fatigue, muscle and joint aches, sore throat, fever, rash, lymphadenopathy, headache). After this primary infection, clinical latency, or asymptomatic HIV infection can last approximately 10 years before signs and symptoms occur.

- Acquired immunodeficiency syndrome (AIDS) defined by the Centers for Disease Control (CDC) as Stage 3 is when the patient's CD4 cell absolute count drops to 200 cells/mm^3 or below, and/or the patient has an opportunistic infection or certain cancers.

- Prevention of opportunistic infections guidelines are found on the CDC website, which gives details for prevention and treatment of various opportunities also based on where the patient lives. The 2015 CDC guidelines for the treatment of sexually transmitted diseases are summarized in Figure 14-1.

  - In general, all patients whose CD4 counts fall **below 200 cells/mm^3** should receive medication to prevent pneumocystis pneumonia (PCP). First-line medication includes TMP-SMX (double strength or single strength) once daily. Alternative options include dapsone or atovaquone.

  - In general, all patients whose CD4 counts fall **below 100 cells/mm^3** should receive medication to prevent toxoplasma gondii encephalitis. First-line medication is TMP-SMX (double strength) once daily.

  - In general, all patients whose CD4 cells **fall to 50 cells/mm^3 or below** need medication to prevent disseminated mycobacterium avium complex (MAC)

  - Disease. First-line treatment includes azithromycin 1200 mg PO once weekly or clarithromycin 500 mg po bid (by mouth, two times a day).

- Patients should receive vaccination for human papilloma virus, pneumonia, hepatitis A, hepatitis B, and influenza as indicated. Vaccination for varicella, Herpes Zoster, and measles/mumps/rubella (MMR) is contraindicated unless the patient's CD4 count is over 200 cells/mm^3.

- Testing for co-infection of syphilis, tuberculosis, and hepatitis A, B, and C should be part of routine surveillance.

- Antiretroviral therapy should be offered to all patients who are willing to start therapy regardless of CD4 cell count. Treatment regimens include three drugs, and guidelines are available on the CDC website to view options. However, consultation with an HIV specialist is strongly recommended prior to initiation of therapy.

- Post-exposure prophylaxis (PEP)—Three-drug regimen should be started as soon as possible (ideally within one hour of exposure)—No later than 72 hours post-exposure. Consultation with an Infectious Disease, HIV, or Emergency Department specialist should be included. Guidelines can be found on the CDC website.

- Pre-exposure prophylaxis (PrEP)—Numerous studies have documented the very low risk of transmission of HIV in a patient who has the undetectable virus, and if the sexual partner is using PrEP, the risk of transmission is extremely low). At this time, Truvada is the drug of choice. Truvada contains two antiretroviral agents (tenofovir and emtricitabine). Close monitoring is required to evaluate for adverse effects.

Vector-Borne Infectious Diseases

- **Malaria**—A parasitic disease found in 97 countries with highest burden is sub-Saharan Africa. *Plasmodium falciparum, P. vivax, P. malariae,* and *P. ovale* which bite between dusk and dawn are the species infecting humans. Children under 5 are the most likely to die from untreated malaria. Clinical signs and symptoms begin 7–15 days after bite. Fever, chills, headache, and vomiting need to be recognized as malaria within first 24 hours to begin treatment and reduce mortality. Anemia, respiratory distress, and multi-organ involvement rapidly occur. Clinical relapse can occur. Antimalarial medications can prevent illness, and are used to treat illness. Treatment is urgent and consult with infectious disease specialist/emergency department is urgent.

- **Chikungunya**—Transmitted by mosquitoes *Aedes aegypti* and *Aedes albopictus*, and can be transmitted by blood-borne routes. Incubation is typically 3–7 days (can be 1–12). Fever and joint pain are most common symptoms, which can last up to 10 days, and persistent rheumatoid type symptoms can last for months. Treatment is supportive.

- **Dengue**—Transmitted by the *aedes aegypti* mosquito. Incubation is 4–10 days after bite. Clinical presentation lasts 2–7 days and includes high fever, severe headache, severe pain behind the eyes, joint, muscle, and bone pain, vomiting, and rash. Treatment for dengue is supportive. When fever declines, severe dengue can occur— the capillaries become permeable/leaky and severe abdominal pain, vomiting, respiratory distress can lead to death if circulatory collapse is not treated appropriately.

- **Lyme Disease**—Transmitted by bite of deer tick *Ixodes scapularis* in the northeast and *Ixodes pacificus* in western United States; intermediate vector is mice and squirrels. Tick needs to feed about 18 hours to transmit the spirochete, *Borrelia burgdorferi*. Transmission of *flavivirus* is primarily through the bite of an infective mosquito. Other routes include exposure to blood of infected person, breast milk from infected mother, perinatal transmission. Incubation period is typically 3 to 14 days after exposure, but can go to 30 days. Clinical presentation varies. Up to 80% of people get a red papule where tick bite was which then enlarges to a concentric circle(s), known as Erythema migrans. As the rash expands, approximately 40% of people will get central clearing which gives a bull's-eye appearance. Some patients get flu-like symptoms with malaise, muscle aches, headache, others have no symptoms. Complications include Bell's palsy, joint effusions, meningitis, Lyme carditis, heart attack, and prolonged arthritic issues. Diagnosis in early disease by clinical picture and history; however, 6–8 weeks post-bite most patients will have developed antibodies which will be detected on Elisa and Western Blot. A positive IgM must have 2 of the following bands (23, 39, 41 kDa), IgG must have 5 out of 10 bands (18, 23, 28, 30, 39, 41, 45, 58, 66, 93 kDa). Treatment with doxycycline (not if female is pregnant) or amoxicillin most commonly used for 14 days minimum. If tick bite is caught within 48 hours, it can be treated with doxycycline 200 mg orally once (adults).

- **Rocky Mountain Spotted Fever**—The most common fatal tick-borne disease in the United States, caused by the bacterium *Rickettsia rickettsia*. Incubation is 5–10 days. Clinical presentation includes fever, headache, rash, vomiting, abdominal pain, and conjunctival injection. When petechial rash occurs (approx. 6 days after onset of symptoms), progression to severe disease is occurring. Treatment with doxycycline should begin as soon as patient presents with any symptoms and there is clinical suspicion based on history and physical.

- **West Nile Virus**—Transmission of this arbovirus is primarily through the bite of an infective mosquito. Other routes include exposure to blood of infected person, breast milk from infected mother, perinatal transmission. Incubation period is typically 3 to 14 days after exposure. Clinical presentation: Most infected people are asymptomatic (80%); however, others may get fever, headache, rash, vomiting, body aches, and weakness. In a small number of cases neurological involvement (meningitis, encephalitis) can occur. Treatment is supportive.

Diarrheal Infectious Diseases

- **Rotavirus and Norovirus**—Transmitted by fecal-oral route. Incubation is 24–72 hours after ingestion. Clinical presentation is fever with nausea, vomiting, abdominal cramps, and watery stools. Treatment is supportive, may treat with ciprofloxacin 500 mg twice a day orally while awaiting stool culture results (other fluoroquinolones, or Bactrim DS may be used).

- *Campylobacter jejuni*—Bacterial infection transmitted by ingesting contaminated foods (ham, chicken, turkey, mayonnaise). Incubation can range from 1–7 days. Clinical presentation includes fever with nausea, vomiting, abdominal pain, fatigue, watery/bloody diarrhea. Treatment is supportive, may treat with ciprofloxacin 500 mg twice a day orally while awaiting stool culture results (other fluoroquinolones, or Bactrim DS may be used). If no fever, adults may use loperamide for diarrhea.

- *Salmonella*—Bacterial infection transmitted by contaminated foods, water, and infected reptiles and turtles. The incubation is fairly short, from 6–72 hours. Clinical presentation includes fever with nausea, vomiting, abdominal pain, fatigue, watery/bloody diarrhea. Treatment is supportive; may treat with ciprofloxacin 500 mg twice a day orally while awaiting stool culture results (other fluoroquinolones, or Bactrim DS may be used). If no fever, adults may use loperamide for diarrhea.

- *Shigella*—Bacterial infection transmitted via water, contaminated food, and fecal-oral route. Incubation can range from 1–7 days after infected. Clinical presentation is fever and abdominal pain with watery stools (occult blood). Treatment is supportive; may treat with ciprofloxacin 500 mg twice a day orally while awaiting stool culture results (other fluoroquinolones, or Bactrim DS may be used). If no fever, adults may use loperamide for diarrhea.

- *Escherichia coli*—Bacterial infection transmitted via contaminated food, water. Known as "traveler's diarrhea." Incubation period ranges from 10 hours to 6 days. Clinical presentation is watery diarrhea with abdominal cramping. Treatment is supportive; may treat with ciprofloxacin 500 mg twice a day orally while awaiting stool culture results (other fluoroquinolones, or Bactrim DS may be used). If no fever, adults may use loperamide for diarrhea.

- *Giardia*—A protozoal organism transmitted via fecal-oral route or contaminated water. Incubation can be from 1–4 weeks. Clinical presentation includes anorexia, abdominal cramping, flatulence, soft-watery stools with a foul smell. Treatment should include Flagyl 250 mg three times a day orally for one week. (Educate patient on no alcohol with Flagyl.)

- *Vibriosis*—A gram-negative rod that is naturally occurring in marine environments. Most commonly *Vibrio parahaemolyticus* and *Vibrio vulnificus* that cause illness when patient is exposed to seawater or inadequately cooked seafood. (This bacteria can also cause cholera.) Clinical presentation is diarrhea, wound infections, or primary septicemia. Treatment for adults includes wound culture and/or blood cultures immediately. Antibiotic treatment can include doxycycline 100 mg twice a day orally for 1–2 weeks and ceftazidime 1–2 g IV/IM every eight hours. (Fluoroquinolones and doxycycline are contraindicated in children, please consult specialist immediately for treatment.)

- **HIV/AIDS (covered earlier)**

- **Chlamydia**—*C. trachomatis* is causative agent for this STD that is the most often reported infectious disease in the U.S. Incubation is 6–14 days. Clinical presentation varies as many infections are asymptomatic, therefore annual screening for those at risk is recommended. Females may complain of mucopurulent vaginal discharge, dysuria, dyspareunia, and lower abdominal discomfort; males may complain of dysuria and/or urethral discharge, inguinal lymphadenopathy may be present in both females and males. Treatment (both partners) is azithromycin 1 gram orally in a single dose or doxycycline 100 mg orally twice a day for 7 days. Patient education includes refraining from sexual intercourse for one week post treatment. Pelvic inflammatory disease (PID) is a risk with this infection and can lead to infertility.

- **Gonorrhea**—*Neisseria gonorrhoeae* is the causative agent. Incubation typically 2–5 days. Clinical presentations include symptoms from localized inflammatory reactions including urethritis, cervicitis, pharyngitis, epididymitis, prostatitis, and PID. In addition, complaints of dysuria, frequency, pelvic or testicular pain, and purulent discharge may be present.

Sexually Transmitted Diseases: Summary of 2015 CDC Treatment Guidelines

These summary guidelines reflect the 2015 CDC Guidelines for the Treatment of Sexually Transmitted Diseases. They are intended as a source of clinical guidance. An important component of STD treatment is partner management. Providers can arrange for the evaluation and treatment of sex partners either directly or with assistance from state and local health departments. Complete guidelines can be ordered online at www.cdc.gov/std/treatment or by calling 1 (800) CDC-INFO (1-800-232-4636).

DISEASE	RECOMMENDED Rx		DOSE/ROUTE	ALTERNATIVES	
Bacterial Vaginosis	metronidazole oral[1]		500 mg orally 2x/day for 7 days	tinidazole 2 g orally 1x/day for 2 days	OR
	metronidazole gel 0.75%[1]	OR	One 5 g applicator intravaginally 1x/day for 5 days	tinidazole 1 g orally 1x/day for 5 days	OR
	clindamycin cream 2%[2]	OR	One 5 g applicator intravaginally at bedtime for 7 days	clindamycin 300 mg orally 2x/day for 7 days	OR
	★ Treatment is recommended for all symptomatic pregnant women.			clindamycin ovules 100 mg intravaginally at bedtime for 3 days	OR
Cervicitis	azithromycin	OR	1 g orally in a single dose	Consider concurrent treatment for gonococcal infection if at risk of gonorrhea or lives in a community where the prevalence of gonorrhea is high. Presumptive treatment with antimicrobials for *C. trachomatis* and *N. gonorrhoeae* should be provided for women at increased risk (e.g., those aged <25 years and those with a new sex partner, a sex partner with concurrent partners, or a sex partner who has a sexually transmitted infection), especially if follow-up cannot be ensured or if NAAT testing is not possible.	
	doxycycline[3]		100 mg orally 2x/day for 7 days		
Chlamydial Infections Adults and adolescents	azithromycin	OR	1 g orally in a single dose	erythromycin base[5] 500 mg orally 4x/day for 7 days	OR
	doxycycline[3]		100 mg orally 2x/day for 7 days	erythromycin ethylsuccinate[5] 800 mg orally 4x/day for 7 days	OR
				levofloxacin[5] 500 mg 1x/day orally for 7 days	OR
				ofloxacin[5] 300 mg orally 2x/day for 7 days	
Pregnancy[5]	azithromycin[7]		1 g orally in a single dose	★ amoxicillin 500 mg orally 3x/day for 7 days	OR
				erythromycin base[5,6] 500 mg orally 4x/day for 7 days	OR
				erythromycin base 250 mg orally 4x/day for 14 days	OR
				erythromycin ethylsuccinate 800 mg orally 4x/day for 7 days	OR
				erythromycin ethylsuccinate 400 mg orally 4x/day for 14 days	
Infants and Children (<45 kg): urogenital, rectal	erythromycin base[8] ethylsuccinate	OR	50 mg/kg/day orally (4 divided doses) daily for 14 days	★ Data are limited on the effectiveness and optimal dose of azithromycin for chlamydial infection in infants and children < 45 kg	
Neonates: ophthalmia neonatorum, pneumonia	erythromycin base[9] ethylsuccinate	OR	50 mg/kg/day orally (4 divided doses) daily for 14 days	★ azithromycin 20 mg/kg/day orally, 1 dose daily for 3 days	
Epididymitis[10,11] For acute epididymitis most likely caused by sexually transmitted CT and GC	ceftriaxone	PLUS	250 mg IM in a single dose		
	doxycycline		100 mg orally 2x/day for 10 days		
★ For acute epididymitis most likely caused by sexually-transmitted chlamydia and gonorrhea and enteric organisms (men who practice insertive anal sex)	ceftriaxone	PLUS	250 mg IM in a single dose		
	levofloxacin	OR	500 mg orally 1x/day for 10 days		
	ofloxacin		300 mg orally 2x/day for 10 days		
For acute epididymitis most likely caused by enteric organisms	levofloxacin	OR	500 mg orally 1x/day for 10 days		
	ofloxacin		300 mg orally 2x/day for 10 days		
Genital Herpes Simplex First clinical episode of genital herpes	acyclovir	OR	400 mg orally 3x/day for 7-10 days[13]		
	acyclovir	OR	200 mg orally 5x/day for 7-10 days[13]		
	valacyclovir[12]	OR	1 g orally 2x/day for 7-10 days[13]		
	famciclovir[12]		250 mg orally 3x/day for 7-10 days[13]		
Episodic therapy for recurrent genital herpes	acyclovir	OR	400 mg orally 3x/day for 5 days		
	acyclovir	OR	800 mg orally 2x/day for 5 days		
	acyclovir	OR	800 mg orally 3x/day for 2 days		
	valacyclovir[12]	OR	500 mg orally 2x/day for 3 days		
	valacyclovir[12]	OR	1 g orally 1x/day for 5 days		
	famciclovir[12]	OR	125 mg orally 2x/day for 5 days		
	famciclovir[12]	OR	1000 mg orally 2x/day for 1 day[13]		
	famciclovir[12]		500 mg orally once, followed by 250 mg 2x/day for 2 days		
Suppressive therapy[14] for recurrent genital herpes	acyclovir	OR	400 mg orally 2x/day		
	valacyclovir[12]	OR	500 mg orally 1x/day		
	valacyclovir[12]	OR	1 g orally once a day		
	famciclovir[12]		250 mg orally 2x/day		
Recommended regimens for episodic infection in persons with HIV infection	acyclovir	OR	400 mg orally 3x/day for 5-10 days		
	valacyclovir[12]	OR	1 g orally 2x/day for 5-10 days		
	famciclovir[12]		500 mg orally 2x/day for 5-10 days		
Recommended regimens for daily suppressive therapy in persons with HIV infection	acyclovir	OR	400-800 mg orally 2-3x/day		
	valacyclovir[12]	OR	500 mg orally 2x/day		
	famciclovir[12]		500 mg orally 2x/day		
Genital Warts[15] (Human Papillomavirus) External genital and perianal warts	**Patient Applied** ★ imiquimod 3.75% or 5%[12] cream	OR	See complete CDC guidelines.		
	podofilox 0.5%[15] solution or gel	OR			
	sinecatechins 15% ointment[2,12]				
	Provider Administered Cryotherapy	OR	Apply small amount, dry, apply weekly if necessary	★ podophyllin resin 10%-25% in compound tincture of benzoin may be considered for provider-administered treatment if strict adherence to the recommendations for application.	OR
	trichloroacetic acid or bichloroacetic acid 80%-90%	OR		intralesional interferon	
	surgical removal			photodynamic therapy	OR
				topical cidofovir	OR

Figure 14-1 Chart of STD Treatments

Reproduced from Centers for Disease Control and Prevention. (2015). Sexually transmitted diseases: Summary of 2015 CDC treatment guidelines. Retrieved from http://www.cdc.gov/std/tg2015/2015-wall-chart.pdf

Sexually Transmitted Diseases: Summary of 2015 CDC Treatment Guidelines

These summary guidelines reflect the 2015 CDC Guidelines for the Treatment of Sexually Transmitted Diseases. They are intended as a source of clinical guidance. An important component of STD treatment is partner management. Providers can arrange for the evaluation and treatment of sex partners either directly or with assistance from state and local health departments. Complete guidelines can be ordered online at www.cdc.gov/std/treatment or by calling 1 (800) CDC-INFO (1-800-232-4636).

DISEASE	RECOMMENDED Rx		DOSE/ROUTE	ALTERNATIVES	
Gonococcal Infections[16]					
Adults, adolescents, and children >45 kg: uncomplicated gonococcal infections of the cervix, urethra, and rectum	ceftriaxone	PLUS	250 mg IM in a single dose	★ If ceftriaxone is not available: cefixime[17] 400 mg orally in a single dose	PLUS
	azithromycin[7]		1 g orally in a single dose	azithromycin[7] 1 g orally in a single dose	
				★ If cephalosporin allergy:	
				gemifloxacin 320 mg orally in a single dose	PLUS
				azithromycin 2 g orally in a single dose	OR
				gentamicin 240 mg IM single dose	PLUS
				azithromycin 2 g orally in a single dose	
Pharyngeal[18]	ceftriaxone	PLUS	250 mg IM in a single dose		
	azithromycin[7]		1 g orally in a single dose		
Pregnancy	See complete CDC guidelines.				
Adults and adolescents: conjunctivitis	ceftriaxone	PLUS	1 g IM in a single dose		
	azithromycin[7]		1 g orally in a single dose		
Children (≤45 kg): urogenital, rectal, pharyngeal	ceftriaxone[19]		25–50 mg/kg IV or IM, not to exceed 125 mg IM in a single dose		
Lymphogranuloma venereum	doxycycline[3]		100 mg orally 2x/day for 21 days	erythromycin base 500 mg orally 4x/day for 21 days	
Nongonococcal Urethritis (NGU)	azithromycin[7]	OR	1 g orally in a single dose	erythromycin base[5] 500 mg orally 4x/day for 7 days	OR
	doxycycline[3]		100 mg orally 2x/day for 7 days	erythromycin ethylsuccinate[5] 800 mg orally 4x/day for 7 days	OR
				levofloxacin 500 mg 1x/day for 7 days	OR
				ofloxacin 300 mg 2x/day for 7 days	
★ Persistent and recurrent NGU[3,20,21]	Men initially treated with doxycycline: azithromycin		1 g orally in a single dose		
	Men who fail a regimen of azithromycin: moxifloxacin		400 mg 1x/day for 7 days		
	Heterosexual men who live in areas where *T. vaginalis* is highly prevalent: metronidazole[22]	OR	2 g orally in a single dose		
	tinidazole		2 g orally in a single dose		
Pediculosis Pubis	permethrin 1% cream rinse	OR	Apply to affected area, wash off after 10 minutes	malathion 0.5% lotion, applied 8-12 hrs then washed off	OR
	pyrethrins with piperonyl butoxide		Apply to affected area, wash off after 10 minutes	ivermectin 250 µg/kg, orally repeated in 2 weeks	
Pelvic Inflammatory Disease[10]	*Parenteral Regimens*			*Parenteral Regimen*	
	Cefotetan	PLUS	2 g IV every 12 hours	Ampicillin/Sulbactam 3 g IV every 6 hours	PLUS
	Doxycycline	OR	100 mg orally or IV every 12 hours	Doxycycline 100 mg orally or IV every 12 hours	
	Cefoxitin	PLUS	2 g IV every 6 hours		
	Doxycycline		100 mg orally or IV every 12 hours		
	Recommended Intramuscular/Oral Regimens				
	Ceftriaxone	PLUS	250 mg IM in a single dose		
	Doxycycline	WITH or WITHOUT	100 mg orally twice a day for 14 days		
	Metronidazole		500 mg orally twice a day for 14 days		
	Cefoxitin	PLUS	2 g IM in a single dose		
	Probenecid,	PLUS	1 g orally administered concurrently in a single dose		
	Doxycycline	WITH or	100 mg orally twice a day for 14 days		
	Metronidazole	WITHOUT	500 mg orally twice a day for 14 days		
Scabies	permethrin 5% cream	OR	Apply to all areas of body from neck down, wash off after 8-14 hours	lindane 1%[23,24] 1 oz. of lotion or 30 g of cream, applied thinly to all areas of the body from the neck down, wash off after 8 hours	OR
	ivermectin		200 µg/kg orally, repeated in 2 weeks		
Syphilis					
Primary, secondary, or early latent <1 year	benzathine penicillin G		2.4 million units IM in a single dose	doxycycline[25] 100 mg 2x/day for 14 days	OR
				tetracycline[25] 500 mg orally 4x/day for 14 days	
Latent >1 year, latent of unknown duration	benzathine penicillin G		2.4 million units IM in 3 doses each at 1 week intervals (7.2 million units total)	doxycycline[25] 100 mg 2x/day for 28 days	OR
				tetracycline[25] 500 mg orally 4x/day for 28 days	
Pregnancy	See complete CDC guidelines.				
Neurosyphilis	aqueous crystalline penicillin G		18–24 million units per day, administered as 3–4 million units IV every 4 hours or continuous infusion, for 10–14 days	procaine penicillin G 2.4 MU IM 1x daily probenecid 500 mg orally 4x/day, both for 10–14 days	PLUS
★ Congenital syphilis	See complete CDC guidelines.			See CDC STD Treatment guidelines for discussion of alternative therapy in patients with penicillin allergy.	
Children: Primary, secondary, or early latent <1 year	benzathine penicillin G		50,000 units/kg IM in a single dose (maximum 2.4 million units)		
Children: Latent >1 year, latent of unknown duration	benzathine penicillin G		50,000 units/kg IM for 3 doses at 1 week intervals (maximum total 7.2 million units)		
Trichomoniasis	metronidazole[22]	OR	2 g orally in a single dose	metronidazole[27] 500 mg 2x/day for 7 days	
	tinidazole[26]		2 g orally in a single dose		
Persistent or recurrent trichomoniasis	metronidazole		500 mg orally 2x/day for 7 days		
	If this regimen fails: metronidazole	OR	2 g orally for 7 days		
	tinidazole		2 g orally for 7 days		
	If this regimen fails, susceptibility testing is recommended.				

Figure 14-1 Chart of STD Treatments (Continued)

Disseminated infection can cause meningitis, endocarditis, and/or arthritis-dermatitis. Many patients may be asymptomatic; therefore, screening patients at risk is indicated. Treatment for uncomplicated infections includes either azithromycin 1 gram orally once or doxycycline 100 mg orally twice a day for 7 days with ceftriaxone 250 mg intramuscularly.

- **Trichomoniasis**—*Trichomonas vaginalis* is the causative agent of this STD. Incubation is typically one week but can be longer. Clinical presentation for females includes profuse malodorous vaginal discharge that is gray or green in color, pruritus, and may include dysuria, dyspareunia, and spotting. Men are often asymptomatic. Treatment is Flagyl 2 grams in one single dose or 500 mg orally twice a day for one week.

- **Herpes Simplex Virus (HSV)**—Type 2 most common genital HSV, although HSV-1 can be transmitted genitally as well. Transmission occurs by direct contact via viral shedding. Many people are aware they are infected with HSV. Lifelong infection with periodic reactivation in neural ganglia occurs. Incubation is 2–14 days after exposure. Primary infection is typically most severe. Clinical presentation includes burning, itching, tenderness, pain, development of vescicles with erythematous base, inguinal lymphadenopathy. Treatment includes Valtrex 1 gram orally twice a day for 10 days (other options on chart), sitz baths, and cotton undergarments. Patient education includes good handwashing, no intercourse with outbreaks, and condoms for any intercourse with the need to know that condoms do not offer 100% reduction in transmission of HSV. Severe, recurrent outbreaks should alert the nurse practitioner to offer HIV testing. Suppressive therapy should be considered.

- **Human Papilloma Virus (HPV)**—Incubation varies from weeks to a year. Often asymptomatic; however, clinical presentation includes visible warts—often type 6 or 11. Types 16, 18, and 31 are associated with cervical dysplasia. Treatment options include Condylox, Aldara, cryotherapy, podohyllin, or TCA (see chart). Vaccination is indicated for females ages 11–26, males ages 11–21, and men who have sex with men through age 26 years.

- **Syphilis**—*Treponema pallidum* is the causative agent of syphilis which can affect many organs. Incubation period is 10–90 days after infected.

Clinical presentation during primary syphilis includes a chancre which is painless but highly infectious, secondary syphilis occurs 6 weeks to 6 months after primary and is very contagious during this time. A macular, popular rash presents often on the palms of the hands and soles of the feet. The rash may also be annular or follicular. Flu-like symptoms may be present. Latent syphilis after the secondary symptoms have disappeared is composed of two states— early latent (< 1 year) and late latent (> 1 year). The patient is not infectious in late latent. Tertiary syphilis includes cardiovascular or neurosyphilis, gumma formations. Congenital infection is asymptomatic under age 2, then children present with rash, jaundice, failure to thrive, and hepatosplenomegaly. See chart for treatment schedule and follow-up. Treatment of pregnant women with syphilis must be penicillin. Those women who are penicillin-allergic require desensitization with a specialist.

Possible Infectious Agents of Bioterrorism

- **Anthrax (*Bacillus anthracis*)**—Transmission occurs by direct contact, inhalation, injection, or ingestion. Incubation period is 2–4 days. Clinical presentation can include cutaneous eschar, fever, chills, and mediastinitis. Treatment options doxycycline or ciprofloxacin for cutaneous, antitoxin, and other medications as required for inhalation, pulmonary edema, and meningitis.

- **Botulism (*Clostridium botulinum*)**—Transmission is by airborne droplet, ingestion, or contaminated wound. Incubation period is 12–36 hours. Clinical presentation consists of descending paralysis starting with diplopia, dysphagia, dysarthria, and dystonia. Treatment is supportive and botulinum antitoxin.

- **Plague (*Yersinia pestis*)**—Transmission most often by flea bite, can also be airborne droplet or direct contact. Incubation is 2–4 days. Clinical presentation can include buboes, fever, pneumonia, acute respiratory distress syndrome, and sepsis. Treatment includes streptomycin or gentamicin.

- **Hemorrhagic Fever Viruses**—Includes Ebola, Marburg, Lassa Fever, Rift Valley Fever, and Yellow Fever. Transmission typically by rodents, mosquitoes, and possibly bats. Clinical presentations vary but typically fever, dizziness, muscle aches, fatigue, and signs of bleeding under the skin or from orifices. Severe cases can involve shock, seizures, coma, and renal failure. Treatment is supportive; ribavirin may be helpful; convalescent phase plasma possibly effective in some cases.

- **Smallpox**—Two clinical forms: variola major (most severe; four types) and variola minor (less common and less severe). Last naturally occurring case was in 1977 in Somalia. Transmission is usually direct, such as prolonged face-to-face contact or coming into contact with infected body fluids or contaminated objects such as bedding/blankets. Incubation period is 7–17 days (not contagious during this time), then prodrome when patient gets high fever, muscle aches, headache, lasts 2–4 days. As soon as rash occurs (typically starting in mouth), patient is very contagious; rash starts on face, then arms and legs, then hands and feet. Within 24 hours, the rash is all over the body. By day 3, the rash turns into raised bumps, which turn into opaque fluid-filled blisters with depression in middle by day 4. The patient is most contagious for 7–10 after rash appears. Fatality is 30%. Vaccination as prevention—no treatment effective.

- **Tularemia (*Francisella tularensis*)**—Transmission occurs if bitten by infected deer tick, deerfly, or by touching infected animal carcasses (usually rabbit, hare, rodents), drinking infected water, or inhaling bacteria. Incubation is 3–14 days after exposure. Clinical signs and symptoms depend on route of transmission; however, fever, chills, headache, muscle aches, joint pain are common. Other symptoms include pharyngitis, ulcers on mouth, lymphadenopathy. Not contagious; however, this disease can be rapidly fatal and treatment urgent, with streptomycin as drug of choice.

Bites—Dog, Cat, Bat, Human

- **Dog**—The most common organisms are from the dog's oral cavity, the patient's skin, and the environment including *Pasteurella* spp. (*Pasteurella multocida* and *Pasteurella canis*), *Staphylococcus* and *Streptococcus* spp., gram-negative rod *Capnocytophaga canimorsus*, and anaerobic pathogens include *Porphyromonas*, *Bacteroides*, and *Fusobacterium* spp. Treatment includes washing the wound for 15 minutes, if dog is unknown to patient, or if not up to date with rabies vaccination, then the dog needs to be reported and monitored per protocol and the patient should undergo rabies vaccination series (human rabies immune globulin day 0, and rabies vaccine day 0, 3, 7, and 14 unless previously vaccinated, then see CDC protocol). Antibiotic options include penicillin, Augmentin, third-generation cephalosporin, for PCN-allergy: doxycycline or fluoroquinolone acceptable. Check if tetanus vaccine needed.

- **Cat Bites**—usually deep puncture wounds that often get infected and can cause abscesses. Typical organisms *Past. Multocida*, *multocida*, and *septica* most common isolates of cat bites. Other common aerobes include *streptococci, staphylococci, moraxella,* and *neisseria*. Common anaerobes included fusobacterium, bacteroides, porphyromonas, and prevotella. *Bartonella henslae* is the causative agent for cat-scratch fever from a cat (kitten usually) bite or scratch. Treatment with Augmentin is first line. Check if tetanus vaccine needed.

- **Bat Bites**—Transmission of rabies is via saliva of an infected host. Typically, humans get rabies via a bite from the infected bat; however, wounds, abrasions, scratches, and mucous membranes that come in contact with infected saliva may also cause transmission and post-exposure prophylaxis should be given. The incubation period ranges from weeks to months. Once the virus reaches the brain, it multiplies rapidly and neurological signs are apparent within 2–5 days. Then the virus migrates to the salivary glands and the saliva and infected host are contagious. Immediate care includes gentle washing of the wound, and if the bat has been captured, it should be sent to the health department for rabies testing. Anyone who may have contact with the bat should begin rabies vaccination series, which can be discontinued if the bat tests negative for rabies. Rabies vaccination series consists of human rabies immune globulin day 0, and rabies vaccine day 0, 3, 7, and 14 (unless previously vaccinated, then see CDC protocol).

Antivirals and Antimicrobials Basics

Antibiotic

The product of a living organism that kills or inhibits the growth of microorganisms.

Antimicrobial

Any naturally occurring or synthetic substance that kills or inhibits the growth of microorganisms.

Bactericidal

The ability to kill bacteria independent of the immune system.

Bacteriostatic

The ability to inhibit the growth and replication of bacteria.

- Inhibit cell wall synthesis
- Direct action on the cell membrane to alter permeability and cause leakage of intracellular compounds
- Affect ribosomal subunits to inhibit protein synthesis
- Bind ribosome subunits to alter protein synthesis and cause cell death
- Changes in nucleic acid metabolism
- Blockage of specific essential metabolic steps by antimetabolites
- Inhibition of viral enzymes essential for DNA synthesis through nucleic acid analogs

Minimum Inhibitory Concentration (MIC)

The lowest concentration of an antimicrobial agent necessary to inhibit the growth of an organism.

Minimum Bactericidal Concentration (MBC)

The lowest concentration of an antimicrobial agent necessary to kill an organism.

Intracellular Bacteria

Retain the ability to reside and replicate within cells. Examples: *Salmonella typhi*, *Legionella* spp, mycobacteria, chlamydiae

H. Extracellular Bacteria

Reside and replicate outside cells.
Examples: *streptococci*, *staphylococci*, most gram (–) enteric rods and *Pseudomonas* spp

- Treat only if bacterial infection is present.
- Select according to most effective, narrowest spectrum, lowest toxicity, least potential for allergy, and most cost-effective.

Antibiotic resistance (GC and TB examples)

- Patterns of resistance differ from one community to the next and change rapidly.
- Consider patient's exposure and what the patient's treatment behavior has been.
- Culture and identify organism when possible.

- Monitor culture results and share information with colleagues.
- Mechanisms of resistance.
- Mutations occur in the gene that encodes the target proteins, so it no longer binds to the drug.
- Random events; does not require previous exposure to the drug.
- Examples of resistance through mutation:
  - *Mycobacterium tuberculosis, Escherichia coli, Staphylococcus aureus*
  - Transduction occurs when a virus that contains DNA infects bacteria that contain genes for various functions, including one that provides drug resistance
    - Incorporation of this bacterial DNA makes the newly infected bacterial cell resistant and capable of passing on the trait
    - Example: *Staphylococcus aureus*
  - Transformation involves transferring into the bacteria DNA that is free in the environment
    - Examples: Penicillin resistance in pneumococci and *Neisseria*
  - Conjugation is transfer of DNA from one organism to another during mating
    - Occurs predominantly among gram-negative bacilli
      - Examples: Enterobacteriaceae and *Shigella flexneri*

Methicillin-Resistant *Staphylococcus Aureus* (MRSA)

- First described in 1961
- Best prevention is HAND WASHING!
- Alteration of PBP-2A, a penicillin binding protein resulting in resistance to Beta Lactams
- Five major strains identified today
- Hospital-Acquired-MRSA vs. Community-Acquired-MRSA
- Transmission
- Mostly from hands of health care workers
- Contaminated environmental surfaces—Cultures of surfaces most often positive with UTI, wound infection, MRSA colitis
- Medical equipment (such as stethoscopes)
- Most commonly found in anterior nares

- Increases risk of future MRSA infection over the next year
- Routine use of bactroban nasally does not consistently clear MRSA
- Patients going for elective surgical procedures should consider bactroban to reduce chance of wound infection.
- Community-acquired MRSA
  - Most often skin and soft tissue infection in healthy young people without health care exposure
  - Sensitive to non-beta lactam drugs
  - Some have Panton-Valentine leukocidin cytotoxin, which causes enhanced virulence, with potential for necrotizing infections
- Risk factors include:
  - Skin trauma-lacerations, abrasions, tattoos, injections, body shaving
  - Incarceration
  - Sharing equipment not cleaned between uses
  - Physical contact with others infected or colonized
- Sites of infection:
  - Skin and soft tissue infection
  - Necrotizing fasciitis
  - Osteomyelitis
  - Urinary tract infection
  - Bacteremia
  - Sepsis
  - Pneumonia

Treatment Options

Trimethoprim-Sulfa 1–2 tabs bid or tetracycline or linezolid. May need to add beta lactam with trimethoprim-sulfa or tetracycline. Clindamycin 300–450 mg every 8 hours orally is another option (be wary of C. *diff*).

Review Questions

1. What is the number one infectious disease with the highest mortality worldwide?

   A. Tuberculosis

   B. Hepatitis B

   C. Influenza

   D. HIV/AIDS

2. Meningococcal meningitis is a bacterial infection that is spread by:

   A. Droplets of respiratory or throat secretions from carriers.

   B. Vector-borne transmission.

   C. Airborne contact within 20 feet.

   D. Non-contact transmission modes.

3. Infected mosquitoes can transmit the following diseases:

   A. Lyme disease, tularemia, and cholera.

   B. Chikungunya, malaria, and West Nile virus.

   C. *Yersinia pestis*, Rocky Mountain Spotted Fever, and echinococcosis.

   D. Cholera, *Yersinia pestis*, and tularemia.

4. A 22-year-old female tree worker was bitten by a raccoon that had been acting sluggish and frothing at the mouth. Upon arrival at the primary care office, the initial action of the nurse practitioner would be to:

   A. Send the young woman to the hospital Emergency Room.

   B. Call the Centers for Disease Control for direction.

   C. Report this to the local Department of Public Health.

   D. Wash the wound thoroughly with soap and water.

5. After cleaning the wound, the nurse practitioner notes that the raccoon bite has pierced the skin. The nurse practitioner realizes that the patient has never had a rabies vaccine and needs to get a rabies vaccination series started no later than:

   A. 48 hours.

   B. 72 hours.

   C. 36 hours.

   D. 24 hours.

6. Rabies vaccination series for those without prior vaccination are given after rabies immunoglobulin on days:

   A. 0, 3, 7, and 14.

   B. 0, 5, 12, and 21.

   C. 0, 1, 5, and 14.

   D. 0, 3, 14, and 21.

7. Signs and symptoms of measles (rubeola) include:

   A. Koplik's spots, high fever, cough.

   B. Parotitis, low-grade fever, vesicular lesions on the chest.

   C. High fever, confusion, and pustular lesions on arms and legs.

   D. Koplik's spots, headaches, and sore throat.

8. A 49-year-old male patient presents to the office upon returning from a trip to the Caribbean. His chief complaint is a high fever of 103°F and a headache. Related to his recent travel, the differential diagnosis will include:

    A. Rocky Mountain Spotted Fever, West Nile virus, meningitis.

    B. Dengue fever, malaria, and chikungunya.

    C. Dengue fever, West Nile virus, and variola.

    D. West Nile virus, bubonic plague, and malaria.

9. *Bartonella henselae* infection is most often caused by:

    A. Dog bites.

    B. Cat bites.

    C. Exposure to cat feces.

    D. Bites from rabid bats.

10. Signs and symptoms of *Bartonella henselae* infection include:

    A. Fever, headache, and swollen lymph nodes.

    B. Headache, cough, and runny nose.

    C. Fever, generalized rash, and cough.

    D. Generalized rash, headache, and pharyngitis.

11. Treatment of mild *Bartonella henselae* Infection includes:

    A. Broad spectrum cephalosporins.

    B. Tetanus vaccination.

    C. Antipyretics and analgesics as needed.

    D. Immunoglobulin.

12. Co-infection with Hepatitis D can occur with persons who are infected with:

    A. Hepatitis C.

    B. Hepatitis A.

    C. Hepatitis E.

    D. Hepatitis B.

13. Prevention of Hepatitis C includes:

    A. Vaccination of HCV.

    B. Twin-rix vaccination.

    C. Handwashing and avoiding contaminated foods.

    D. Not sharing injection drug paraphernalia.

14. A 28-year-old male comes to the clinic with complaints of watery diarrhea. He states he and his wife just returned from their honeymoon vacation deep-sea diving in Central America. An old wound is noted on his right lower leg. This raises suspicion for:

    A. Infectious mononucleosis.

    B. Malaria.

    C. Vibrio *parahaemolyticus*.

    D. Brucellosis.

15. A 33-year-old female patient with no significant past medical history arrives in the office with complaints of mild respiratory symptoms of cough, fever, and congestion. It is important for the nurse practitioner to be aware that:

    A. Patients with respiratory illness require antibacterial treatment most of the time.

    B. Patients with these symptoms often require inhaled corticosteroids.

    C. Approximately 90% of respiratory illnesses are viral.

    D. If the onset is insidious, it is most likely viral.

16. Due to drug resistance in gonococcal infections, which drug is no longer recommended for use in the United States?
    A. Ciprofloxacin
    B. Ceftriaxone
    C. Azithromycin
    D. Penicillin

17. Even though there is an effective vaccine, this childhood infectious disease remains one of the leading causes of death in young children. Which of the following is it?
    A. Rubeola
    B. Varicella
    C. Parotitis
    D. Erythema infectiosum

18. A 23-year-old male patients presents with complaints of "bumps" on his penis. Upon examination, raised lesions, which appear to be genital warts, are noted and a sample is sent for testing that returns positive for HPV. Treatment options include which of the following?
    A. Valcyclovir 500 mg bid for 5 days
    B. Imiquimod 3.75% to affected area once a day at bedtime for 8 weeks
    C. Corticosteroid cream 1% bid after showers for 2 weeks
    D. Azithromycin 1 gm orally once

19. Treatment for a positive Chlamydial infection is:
    A. Valcyclovir 500 mg bid for 5 days.
    B. Imiquimod 3.75% to affected area once a day at bedtime for 8 weeks.
    C. Corticosteroid cream 1% bid after showers for 2 weeks.
    D. Azithromycin 1 gm orally once.

20. Upon visualizing a wet mount for a patient complaining of greenish-colored vaginal discharge, trichomonads with 3 to 6 flagella are noted. Treatment for this patient will include:
    A. Valcyclovir 500 mg orally bid for 5 days.
    B. Imiquimod 3.75% to affected area once a day at bedtime for 8 weeks.
    C. Metronidazole 2 gm orally once.
    D. Doxycycline 100 mg orally bid for 7 days.

21. While infections are the most common cause of fever of unknown origin (FUO) in children, what are the most common causes of FUO in older persons?
    A. Neoplasms and connective tissue disorders
    B. Endocarditis and HIV
    C. Connective tissue disorders and hepatitis
    D. Long-term corticosteroid use and COPD

22. Persons who have varicella are advised that they may return to school or work:
    A. Seventy-two hours after blisters have erupted.
    B. Once they no longer have a fever.
    C. After 24 hours, as long as they keep the blisters covered tightly.
    D. After all the blisters have scabbed over.

23. Which patient should be started on opportunistic infection *Pneumocystis jiroveci* pneumonia prophylaxis?
    A. A 52-year-old male with an HIV viral load of 60,000 copies and a CD4 absolute count of 364
    B. A 22-year-old female with an HIV viral load of 325,000 copies and a CD4 absolute count of 325
    C. A 44-year-old female with an HIV viral load of 1,230 copies and a CD4 absolute count of 185
    D. An 18-year-old male with an HIV viral load that is undetectable and a CD4 absolute count of 255

24. A 24-year-old female patient asks the nurse practitioner about herpes infections since her new boyfriend told her he might have been exposed to it in a previous relationship. Which of the following statements is *not accurate* and therefore should not be the nurse practitioner's response?

    A. As long as your partner wears a condom, you do not have to worry about getting genital herpes.

    B. You and your partner can be tested for herpes type 1 and type 2 to check if you have been infected, since it could be asymptomatic.

    C. There is no cure for herpes infections.

    D. Genital herpes can be type 1 and/or type 2.

25. While working in the northeast, a 62-year-old gardener comes to the clinic with complaints of right knee pain and inflammation for a few weeks. Which of the following responses is the *best choice* to be included in the differential diagnosis?

    A. Multiple sclerosis

    B. Ankylosing spondylitis

    C. Lyme disease

    D. Tularemia

26. Patients should be encouraged to do which of the following to keep from becoming infected with West Nile Virus?

    A. Wear high socks and sturdy shoes when walking in the woods.

    B. Avoid contact with wild rabbits and deer.

    C. Apply permethrin onto exposed skin multiple times per day.

    D. Use insect repellants and empty outdoor water containers.

27. "Chandelier's sign" is associated with which condition?

    A. Inflammatory knee pain due to Lyme disease

    B. Cervical motion tenderness due to pelvic inflammatory disease

    C. A meningeal inflammation sign apparent during neurological examinations of arthritis.

    D. Optic nerve damage found upon assessment of cranial nerve II.

28. A patient with a penicillin allergy who needs antibiotics for an infection may safely be given any of the following EXCEPT:

    A. TMP-SMX.

    B. Doxycycline.

    C. Cephalexin.

    D. Azithromycin.

29. The nurse practitioner is on-call for the office and speaks by phone to an adult who complains of 48 hours of acute diarrhea consisting of 10 non-bloody loose stools per day. The patient states she has no fever but is asking for antibiotics. She denies any chronic medical diseases and takes no current daily medications. Which of the following is the best initial treatment plan for this patient?

    A. Encourage fluids, starches, and loperamide 4 mg initially, then 2 mg after each loose stool (not to exceed 16 mg per day)

    B. Flagyl 500 mg by mouth twice a day for 7 days, encourage hydration with electrolyte enhanced water drinks

    C. Ciprofloxacin 500 mg by mouth twice a day for 5 days, hydration, loperamide 2 mg (one tablet) every 4 hours (not to exceed 16 mg per day)

    D. Probiotics, hydration intravenously, triple antibiotic treatment for suspected parasite infection

30. A new patient tells the nurse practitioner that he has had a very bad allergy to peanuts in the past and carries an EpiPen wherever he goes. The nurse practitioner educates the patient by reinforcing the need to carry the EpiPen and that anaphylaxis is caused by:

    A. Chemicals released into the body system by mast cells and basophils.

    B. Mediators from IgG cells that are released into the blood stream.

    C. Histamines released into the alveoli by immunoglobulin M.

    D. Chemicals released into the major organs by eosinophils.

The next three questions relate to the following patient case study:

31. A 16-year-old male presents to the office with complaints of a wound on his left shoulder that has gotten "redder" and really sore over the past 3 days. Upon history intake, the patient states he needs to hurry because he has wrestling practice shortly and is afraid he will be unable to compete due to this wound. The physical examination reveals a temperature of 99.0 orally and a 3-cm abscess with surrounding erythema on the right posterior shoulder area, which is painful to the touch. The most appropriate next step would include:

    A. Incision and drainage of the abscess, including sending purulent discharge for culture and sensitivity.

    B. Applying an adhesive bandage to cover the entire abscess and sending the patient to the infectious disease specialist at the local hospital.

    C. Calling the wrestling coach to let him know that this student will be unable to compete in the next high school competition.

    D. Asking the patient about his current sexual partners.

32. The preceding case study patient tells the nurse practitioner (NP) that he is allergic to sulfa drugs. Based on the history and physical examination, as well as the correct action as an initial "next step," the NP writes a prescription. Which of the following would be the most appropriate medication to prescribe?

    A. Amoxicillin 250 mg twice a day orally for one week

    B. Keflex 250 mg twice a day orally for 5 days

    C. Azithromycin 500 mg orally once per day for 3 days

    D. Doxycycline 100 mg orally twice a day for one week

33. A new patient is candid during her history interview and admits her sexual partner is HIV+. She states they usually use condoms, but on occasion they take the risk and have unprotected intercourse. She also states they have talked about having a baby together at some point in the future since her partner is well controlled on his antiretroviral therapy. The nurse practitioner counsels the patient about pre-exposure prophylaxis (PreEp). Choose the most appropriate response from the following choices:

    A. It is never advisable to have unprotected intercourse with someone who is HIV-infected.

    B. We need to get you HIV-tested today.

    C. There are some options we can discuss.

    D. I can write you a prescription for antiretroviral therapy today so you don't get infected.

34. Post-exposure to HIV should commence within which timeframe?

    A. Less than 72 hours post-exposure

    B. Less than 4 days post-exposure

    C. Only if it has been less than 48 hours post-exposure

    D. Post-exposure treatment can begin within a week post-exposure

35. Complications of tertiary syphilis may include:

    A. Seizures and psychosis.

    B. Rashes and fevers.

    C. Shingles and pneumonia.

    D. Respiratory and renal failure.

36. Treatment of syphilis in pregnancy must be with:
    A. Doxycycline.
    B. Metronidazole.
    C. Keflex.
    D. Penicillin.

37. A 64-year-old patient comes to the office and states she found a tick on her abdomen a week or two ago which seemed engorged but she pulled it out and threw it in the garbage. She now has a circular rash that has the typical bull's-eye appearance. Treatment for this patient would be:
    A. Azithromycin 500 mg orally for 3 days.
    B. Keflex 500 mg orally for 7 days.
    C. Doxycycline 100 mg orally for 14–21 days.
    D. Ceftriaxone 1 gm IV daily for 3 days.

38. Vaccinations for HPV are:
    A. The same for males and females.
    B. Only indicated for females.
    C. Different in age ranges for men who have sex with men.
    D. Not indicated once the patient is 18 years of age.

39. The minimum inhibitory concentration (MIC) is important, because it indicates:
    A. The lowest dose of an antibiotic that is needed.
    B. The lowest concentration of an antimicrobial agent required to kill an organism.
    C. The smallest measurement of sensitivity of resistance.
    D. The method used to measure the peak dose of an antibiotic's effect.

40. What is the most commonly reported STD in the teenage and early adulthood years?
    A. HSV
    B. Syphilis
    C. Chlamydia
    D. Babesiosis

41. A patient presents to the NP's office and states that there was a deer tick crawling on her one month ago. She was sick with a cold recently and is concerned that perhaps she has contracted Lyme disease. The NP gets the following results from the serology studies:

    Lyme AB screen: 1.38 (a positive Lyme antibody screen is > or = to 1.10)

    A Western blot IGG and IGM is done. All bands are negative or non-reactive.

    The PCP correctly offers the following information:
    A. The patient has Lyme disease and should begin 21 days of therapy with doxycycline 100 mg bid.
    B. The patient does not have Lyme disease. No therapy is warranted.
    C. The patient has chronic Lyme disease and will need IV antibiotic therapy for 2–3 months.
    D. The patient should be treated prophylactically with a one-time dose of oral doxycycline.

42. All of the following statements regarding MRSA are true except:
    A. MRSA can be necrotizing to tissues.
    B. The transmission of MRSA infections can be reduced with good hand washing technique.
    C. MRSA is often transmitted from person to person during contact sports.
    D. Community-acquired MRSA is known to be more virulent than hospital-acquired MRSA.

43. The NP encounters a patient who is complaining of fever, headache, nausea, vomiting, cough, chills, and chest pain. The patient is hospitalized and is found to have multi lobar pneumonia due to a legionella infection. Which of the following teaching points is important for both the patient and the hospital staff?

    A. The patient should be placed on respiratory isolation with airborne precautions.

    B. The patient should be placed on contact and droplet precautions.

    C. Once symptoms appear, the patient is no longer contagious.

    D. Legionella is not transmitted from person to person.

44. The most common neurologic manifestation of Lyme disease is:

    A. Meningitis.

    B. Bell's palsy

    C. Guillain–Barré syndrome.

    D. Peripheral neuropathy.

45. A 17-year-old female comes in to the clinic with a chief complaint of vaginal discharge. Upon questioning, she says she has a new sexual partner and they often do not use condoms. The discharge is yellowish and the patient complains of dysuria. The nucleic acid amplification test (NAAT) is positive for Chlamydia. The nurse practitioner writes a prescription for which of the following medications?

    A. Flagyl 2 gm orally once

    B. Keflex 500 mg orally once

    C. Zithromax 1 gm orally once

    D. Levaquin 500 mg orally once

46. The nurse practitioner is aware that patient education is an important part of treating STDs. When treating a patient who has a positive Chlamydia test, which of the following statements should be discussed in addition to telling the patient that the sexual partner(s) should be treated as well? Choose the best answer.

    A. It is important that you abstain from sexual intercourse for 7 days and until your partner has gotten treated.

    B. It is not risky to have intercourse as long as your partner wears a condom.

    C. Once you have had Chlamydia, it is not possible to get re-infected.

    D. Getting tested for other STDs is not necessary once the medication has been taken.

47. For females, it is imperative to get tested and treated for STDs. Patient education should include which of the following? Choose the best answer.

    A. Sexually transmitted diseases in adolescents indicate a need for more parental supervision.

    B. Having Chlamydia or gonorrhea will cause difficulty when the patient is trying to conceive.

    C. Having an STD can cause pelvic inflammatory disease, which can cause infertility.

    D. Using sex "toys" will prevent the spread of STDs.

48. A bacteriostatic antibiotic can:

    A. Kill bacteria independent of the immune system.

    B. Inhibit the replication of bacteria.

    C. Typically cause diarrhea.

    D. Prevent mutations and resistance of a drug.

49. Most gram-negative rods:

    A. Live and replicate outside the cell.

    B. Live within the DNA of the cell.

    C. Do not cause illness.

    D. Are rarely resistant to medications.

50. An HIV-infected patient gets a diagnosis of AIDS when the CD4 cell count is below which of the following?

    A. 250 cells/mm^3

    B. 350 cells/mm^3

    C. 500 cells/mm^3

    D. 200 cells/mm^3

51. One option for decreasing an MRSA wound infection in a patient who has colonized MRSA and is scheduled for surgery is:

    A. Intravenous vancomycin daily for 3 days pre-operatively.

    B. There is no effective pre-treatment to decrease the wound infection.

    C. Applying Bactroban (mupirocin) nasally twice a day for 5 days pre-op.

    D. Routine screening during yearly physical examinations.

Answers and Rationales

1. D. The number one infectious disease with the highest mortality worldwide is HIV/AIDS. In 2013, there were 35 million people living with HIV globally. In the same year, 1.5 million people died from AIDS-associated illnesses.

2. A. Meningococcal meningitis is a bacterial infection that is spread by droplets of respiratory or throat secretions from carriers.

3. B. Infected mosquitoes can transmit chikungunya, malaria, and West Nile virus. Only malaria has prevention and treatment medications. Prevention measures include using insect repellent, wearing long-sleeve shirts and pants, and using windows and door screens.

4. D. In order to prevent infection and to promote optimal wound healing careful inspection and cleansing of wounds is required. Vaccinations for rabies, as well as tetanus, are also needed.

5. D. Rabies is transmitted by wild animals, with the bat being the most common vehicle in the United States. Vaccinations can begin after 24 hours post-bite; however, the more quickly a person seeks care the more quickly wound cleansing and the prevention of infections can begin, chiefly by starting the vaccination series. Rabies immune globulin should also be administered.

6. A. Rabies vaccinations for those who have received a prior series include one dose immediately, followed by a second dose on day 3. No rabies immune globulin is needed.

7. A. Signs and symptoms of measles (rubeola) include Koplik's spots, high fever, cough. These tiny white spots appear in the mouth 2–3 days after symptoms start.

8. B. All three of these illnesses are mosquito-borne and present with clinical symptoms of fever and headache, among other signs and symptoms. Recent travel to areas with endemic disease is a key factor to be assessed during the history portion of the exam.

9. B. *Bartonella* bacteria can cause three illnesses in humans, including cat-scratch fever. Trench fever is caused by *B. quintana*, and Carrión's disease is caused by *B. bacilliformis*.

10. A. Signs and symptoms of *Bartonella henselae* infection include fever, headache, and swollen lymph nodes.

11. C. Treatment of mild *Bartonella henselae* infection includes antipyretics and analgesics as needed. Moderate infection can be treated with azithromycin 500 mg orally on day one, followed by 250 mg orally daily for 4 days. Endocarditis requires antibiotic treatment and consulting with an infectious disease specialist.

12. D. Co-infection with hepatitis D can occur with persons who are infected with hepatitis B. Hepatitis D (delta virus) needs hepatitis B virus for replication. It can be acute or chronic.

13. D. Prevention of hepatitis C includes not sharing injection drug paraphernalia. Patient education regarding prevention of hepatitis C includes avoiding exposure to HCV-infected blood. The majority of transmission occurs from intravenous drug injection users who share needles and paraphernalia. Approximately 90% of IV drug users will become HCV infected within the first 5 years of use. Sharing toothbrushes, razors, etc. can transmit HCV due to blood exposure. Rarely is HCV transmitted by monogamous sexual partners, but there is higher risk in those with multiple sex partners and those whose sexual practices can cause the tearing of mucosa and exposure to blood.

14. C. This strain of Vibrio is not common, but can cause gastrointestinal illness in people, typically self-limiting over 3 days. However, in those with open wounds it can cause infection in the wound. Patients should be evaluated for septicemia, which would require rapid emergency treatment.

15. C. It is important for the nurse practitioner to be aware that approximately 90% of respiratory illnesses are viral. Viral respiratory illnesses typically improve within 7–10 days. If symptoms do not improve, or worsen, evaluation for bacterial infection from the weakened immune system should be initiated.

16. A. Fluoroquinolones used to be prescribed for gonorrhea; however, due to resistance, the CDC now recommends cephalosporins for treating gonorrhea.

17. A. Rubeola (measles) can have severe complications, including pneumonia, seizures, mental retardation, and death, but is preventable with vaccination.

18. B. Anogenital warts can spontaneously disappear within one year. Other treatment options include imiquimod, podofilox, sinecatechins, or cryotherapy, surgical removal, and TCA or BCA solutions.

19. D. Chlamydia is most common in persons 24 years of age and younger, and is the most common reportable STD. Other treatment options include doxycycline 100 mg orally twice a day for one week, and levofloxacin 500 mg orally once a day for one week, among other options, as noted in the STD Guidelines recommended by the CDC.

20. C. Trichamoniasis is the most common non-viral STD in the United States. Metronizadole can also be given 500 mg orally twice a day for one week. Tinadazole 2 gm orally once is another option.

21. A. In adults, FUO is defined as a temperature over 38.3 °C off and on for over three weeks duration, which has not been adequately diagnosed as an inpatient. Fevers associated with weight loss or other serious signs and symptoms suggest more dire illness, including cancers, HIV, and rheumatic and connective tissue diseases.

22. D. Persons who have varicella are advised that they may return to school or work after all the blisters have scabbed over.

23. C. HIV+ patients whose CD4 cell count falls below 200 cells/mm^3 need to start on Bactrim (TMP-SMX) or an alternative (dapsone, Mepron).

24. A. Because shedding of HSV can occur outside of the area that condoms cover, they may not be 100% effective.

25. C. This outdoor worker is at high risk for tick bites. Complications from untreated Lyme disease includes joint swelling, effusions, and arthritic symptoms.

26. D. Using these techniques can aid in reducing infection from mosquito-borne diseases.

27. B. During the pelvic examination, severe discomfort causes the patient to reach up toward the ceiling (where chandeliers hang).

28. C. Cross hypersensitivity can occur when using beta lactam antibiotics. Up to 10% can occur, in particular, with first-generation cephalosporins.

29. A. The best initial treatment plan for this patient is to encourage fluids, starches, and loperamide 4 mg initially, then 2 mg after each loose stool (not to exceed 16 mg per day).

30. A. Anaphylaxis is an acute, potentially life-threatening hypersensitivity reaction with the sudden onset of rapidly progressive urticaria and respiratory distress. Signs and symptoms occur between 5–30 minutes after contact with the allergen. Rashes, hives, pruritus, swelling of lips, throat, chest tightness, and a feeling of doom occur, and can be fatal. Treatment with epinephrine and transport to the emergency department is required.

31. A. The most appropriate next step would be incision and drainage of the abscess, including sending a purulent discharge culture and sensitivity. High suspicion for community-acquired MRSA should be on the differential diagnosis list. It is important to send a culture to identify the pathogen and to find out what antibiotics will work.

32. A. Doxycycline 100 mg orally twice a day for one week is correct. Children 8 years and younger, as well as pregnant women, should not use doxycycline. Clindamycin or linezolid may be options.

33. C. Developing a trusting relationship is essential in this scenario. Discussing the need for her partner to have his HIV well controlled with undetectable viral load is important. The need for this patient to understand the side effects of Truvada, as well as understand the need to take this medication every day, is vital for it to be efficacious. Encourage this patient to attend her partner's next medical visit with the HIV specialist to further discuss planning for preconception care.

34. C. Although post-exposure prophylaxis (PEP) will not guarantee that a person will not become infected with HIV, studies have shown that if treatment with the appropriate antiretrovirals is initiated within 72 hours, the risk of infection is significantly reduced. Treatment should continue for 28 days.

35. A. Complications of tertiary syphilis may include seizures and psychosis. Untreated syphilis can result in multisystem diseases, including severe neurological issues.

36. D. Most states require prenatal testing for syphilis to prevent congenital syphilis. Penicillin G is the only known effective treatment. Desensitization by a specialist is required.

37. C. If the patient had come to be seen immediately after noticing the engorged tick bite, a prophylactic one-time dose of doxycycline can be offered.

38. D. Vaccinations are indicated for 11–12 years through 26 years of age.

39. B. The minimum inhibitory concentration (MIC) is important because it indicates the lowest concentration of an antimicrobial agent required to kill an organism.

40. C. Highest in those 24 years of age and younger, Chlamydia should be a part of screening for sexually active young people, and those 25 years and older with risk factors.

41. B. The patient does not have Lyme disease, so no therapy is needed. The appropriate Western blot bands are required to qualify as a positive result. No positive or reactive bands means a negative result. In addition, the complaints of a cold are not consistent with more common symptoms of Lyme infection.

42. D. The genotype of the organisms varies and either community- or hospital-acquired MRSA can be more contagious and virulent depending on the particular organism.

43. D. Legionella is not transmitted from person to person. Transmission occurs when water mist or vapor contaminated with the bacteria is ingested.

44. B. The most common neurologic manifestation of Lyme disease is Bell's palsy.

45. C. The correct answer is Zithromax 1 gm orally once.

46. A. Reinfection can occur if both partners are not treated appropriately. The patient should be counseled on the benefits of condom use in decreasing the risk of STD acquisition.

47. C. Having an STD can cause pelvic inflammatory disease, which can cause infertility. Even subclinical PID can cause infertility; therefore, it is imperative to screen those at risk for STDs.

48. B. A bacteriostatic antibiotic can inhibit the replication of bacteria.

49. A. Most gram-negative rods live and replicate outside the cell.

50. D. An AIDS diagnosis is given when a patient has a low CD4 cell count (200 or less), and/or an AIDS defining condition, and/or CD4 cells are less than 14% of all lymphocytes.

51. C. Studies have shown a decrease in complications related to MRSA when patients are screened and treated pre-operatively.

• • • References

Bagaitkar, J., Demuth, R., & Scott, D. A. (2008). Tobacco use increases susceptibility to bacterial infection. *Tobacco Induced Diseases*, 4(1), 12. doi:10.1186/1617-9625-4-12

Blunt, E., & Reinsch, C. (2009). *Family nurse practitioner review manual, Volume 1 & 2*. ANA/ANCC Credentialing Center, Silver Springs, MD.

Centers for Disease Control and Prevention. (CDC). Emergency preparedness and response. Retrieved from http://emergency.cdc.gov/bioterrorism/factsheets.asp

Centers for Disease Control and Prevention. (CDC). Rocky Mountain Spotted Fever. Retrieved from http://www.cdc.gov/rmsf/symptoms/index.html

Centers for Disease Control and Prevention. (CDC). West Nile virus. Retrieved from http://www.cdc.gov/westnile/resourcepages/pubs.html

Molina, P., Happel, K., Shang, P., Kolls, J., & Nelson, S. (n.d.). Alcohol and the immune system. Retrieved from http://pubs.niaaa.nih.gov/publications/arh40/97-108.htm

Thomas, N., & Brook, I. (2011). Animal bite–associated infections. *Expert Rev Anti Infect Therapies*, 9(2), 215–226. Retrieved from: http://www.medscape.com/viewarticle/739023_4

World Health Organization. Global Health Observatory—HIV. Retrieved from http://www.who.int/gho/hiv/en/

15

Dermatology/Integumentary

Nancy L. Dennert, MS, MSN, FNP-BC, CDE, BC-ADM

Julie G. Stewart, DNP, MPH, MSN, FNP-BC, APRN

Approximately 49% of all adult outpatient/primary care visits are for skin conditions. Patients with chronic and common medical problems (obesity/diabetes) have increased the number of incidences, and these numbers are higher in the pediatric population.

The primary function of the skin is to protect underlying body structures from invasion by microorganisms, to control body heat, eliminate body waste through perspiration, and prevent injury to body structures.

There are three layers: epidermis, dermis, and subcutaneous fat (see Figure 15-1).

History

Obtain a history noting duration, rate of onset, location, and symptoms, as well as family history, allergies, medications, occupation, and previous treatments. The history is a vital component of the assessment.

The patient should be examined in appropriate lighting, and the skin viewed from a distance to seek patterns. Close inspection aids in diagnosis. Physical examination documentation should include:

- Primary lesion
- Type of lesion
- Shape of individual lesion
- Arrangement of multiple lesions
- Distribution of lesions
- Color
- Consistency and feel

Terminology

- Distribution: Localized, regional, generalized
- Lesion morphology: Wheals, macules, papules
- Secondary characteristics: Thick, silvery, scaly, thickening, lichenification
- Shape/Arrangement: Round/discoid, oval, annular, linear, stellate
- Border/Margin: Discrete, indistinct, active, irregular, advancing
- Pigmentation: Flesh, pink, erythematous, salmon, tan-brown, black, pearly, violaceous, yellow, etc.
- Atrophy: Thinning of skin
- Bulla: Vesicle or large blister filled with fluid; a bleb
- Crust: Dried serum, blood, or purulent exudate; slightly elevated, size/color may vary.
- Cyst: Closed sac or pouch with definite wall containing fluid, semifluid, or solid material
- Erosion: Loss of part of the epidermis, depressed
- Excoriation: Abrasion or loss of the epidermis by trauma, chemicals, burns, or other factors
- Fissure: Linear crack or break from the epidermis to the dermis; may be moist or dry
- Keloid: Scar formation in skin following trauma or surgical incision. Response out of proportion to amount of scar tissue required for normal repair

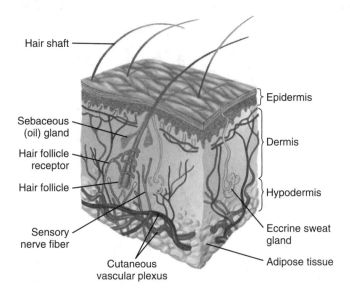

Figure 15-1 Epidermis, dermis, and subcutaneous fat

- Lichenification: Cutaneous thickening and hardening of epidermis, secondary to persistent rubbing, itching, skin irritation
- Macule: Flat, circumscribed area with change in color of skin; < 1 cm diameter
- Nodule: Elevated, firm, circumscribed, deeper in dermis than papule, 1–2 cm diameter
- Papule: Elevated, firm, circumscribed; < 1 cm diameter
- Patch: Flat, nonpalpable, irregular-shaped macule > 1 cm diameter
- Plaque: Elevated, firm, rough lesion; flat top surface; > 1 cm diameter
- Pustule: Elevated, superficial lesion; similar to vesicle but filled w/purulent fluid
- Scale: Heaped up keratinized cells; flaky skin, irregular, thick or thin, dry or oily, varies in size
- Scar: Thin to thick fibrous tissue that replaces normal skin following injury to dermis
- Telangiectasia: Dilated, superficial blood vessel
- Tumor: Elevated, solid, may/may not be clearly demarcated, deeper in dermis; > 2 cm diameter
- Ulcer: Loss of epidermis and dermis, concave, varies in size
- Vesicle: Elevated, circumscribed, superficial, not into dermis, filled w/fluid; < 1 cm diameter
- Wheal: Elevated, mostly round; solid, transient; variable diameter, white in center with pale red periphery

Actinic Keratosis

- Most common lesions seen in dermatology
- Characterized as precancerous
- Presents on sun-damaged skin
  - Head, neck, upper trunk, arms, also legs
- Macules or patches with mild erythema and a distinctive scale you can feel
- Described as scaly spot that won't go away or peels and comes back
- 10–20% can become an SCC (squamous cell carcinoma) if not treated.
- Tenderness and bleeding are concerning.
- Treatment:
  - LN2 most widely used modality
  - Topical 5FUs: carac, efudex
  - Topical imiquimod, also solaraze gel
- Prevention
  - Sunscreen, vitamin C, retinoids

Seborrheic Keratoses

- Benign skin lesion
- Sharply circumscribed
- Measures anywhere from 0.2 cm to 3 cm
- Colors vary from very dark brown, brown, tan
- Stuck on appearance
- Surface can be rough or smooth
- Genetic predisposition

- Treatment: usually cryosurgery, shave biopsy, electrosurgery, and curettage

Skin Cancers

- Most common cancer in both genders
- One in five Americans will develop a skin cancer in their lifetime
- 40–50% of Americans will have at least one skin cancer by age 65
- Treatment for NMSCs (non melanoma skin cancer) increased by 77% from 1992 to 2006
- 90% of NMSC caused by UV radiation
- Divided into NMSC and melanoma

Basal Cell

- Most common skin cancer
- 2.8 million diagnosed yearly
- Locally invasive, metastasis rare
- Commonly found on sun-exposed areas
- Fair skin most at risk, but all skin type as well
- History of sunburns, sun damage
- Arises from the basal epidermal layer
- Nodular
  - Accounts for 60% of BCCs (basal cell carcinoma)
  - Raised, translucent papule or nodule with telangiectasias
  - Ulcer may form.
  - Bleeding common
  - Can be pigmented and easily confused as a nodular melanoma
- Superficial BCC
  - Erythematous scaling patch
  - Can look like an AK (actinic keratosis)
  - Most common on trunk and extremities, but may present on face
- Morpheaform
  - Flat, slightly atrophic lesion, infiltrative
  - Can be white or pink; may appear similar to a scar
- Treatment
  - Mohs surgery if on face or morpheaform
  - Excision
  - Electrodessication and curettage (E, D & C)
  - Aldara (imiquimod): alone or in combo with E, D, & C
  - Very rarely LN2

Squamous Cell Carcinoma

- Second most common form of skin cancer
- Arises from sun-damaged skin
- Most common on sun-exposed areas
- Flat or thickened scaly lesion with erythematous base
- Many times tender to touch, described as bleeding or becoming larger
- Potential for metastasis is related to size, location, and depth of invasion
- Always have biopsied
- Immunocompromised patients at higher risk
- Can arise from actinic keratosis

Treatment
- Always excision or Mohs
- Radiation if lymph node involvement

Squamous Cell Carcinoma in Situ

- Also called Bowen's disease
- Slightly elevated, red, scaly plaques with surface fissures and some pigmentation
- Well-defined borders
- Can resemble psoriasis, superficial BCCs
- Slower growing and low chance to become invasive
- Treatment options include excision, E, D, & C, topical 5FUs, Aldara

Melanoma

- One person dies from melanoma every 57 minutes.
- The majority of melanoma diagnoses are white men over the age of 50.
- Majority of mutations found are caused by UV.
- One or more blistery sunburns doubles odds.
- Survivor has 9 times the chance of another melanoma.
- Caught early = 99% survival rate, but falls to 15% when more advanced
- Originates from melanocytes, the cells which produce the pigment melanin that colors our hair, skin, and eyes.
- Usually appears as black or brown, but can also be pink, white, purple, skin-colored
- Follow the ABCDE
  - Asymmetry, border, color, diameter, elevation

- Changing lesion or new lesion that is quickly enlarging
- Risk factors
  - Immediate family member diagnosed, fair skin, history of sunburns, many nevi, UV exposure, tanning booths
- High risk of distant metastasis, especially brain, lungs, liver, GI tract
- The most important prognostic factor is thickness and if ulceration is present
- Treatment depends on stage:
  - Surgery, immunotherapy, chemo/radiation

Acne Vulgaris

- Disease of pilosebaceous unit
- Appears near puberty
- Intensity and severity varies
- Psychosocial effects can be devastating
- Divided into inflammatory and non-inflammatory
- Treatment options dependent on type of acne
- Non-inflammatory
  - Open comedone: blackhead
  - Closed comedone: whitehead
- Treatment
  - Retinoids preferred
    - RAM, Differin, Tazorac
  - BPO as well, wash, topical
  - Exfoliation: scrubs OTC
- Inflammatory
  - Papulopustular or cystic
  - Mild, moderate, severe
  - Watch for scarring, more aggressive

Treatment

- Topical BPO/clindamycin (Duac, Acanya)
- Retinoids
- Oral doxycycline; Accutane if scarring

Rosacea

- Inflammatory disorder affecting central face, chin, forehead
- Rarely seen in people < 30 yrs of age
- More common in females
- Genetic predisposition and actinic damage
- Erythema and telangiectasis, superficial pustules

- Treatment:
  - Daily sunscreen, avoid triggers, metrogel, Finacea, or sodium sulfacetamide, and/or oral tetracycline. Laser for redness

Xerosis (Dry Skin)

- Most common on back and extremities
- Generalized fine scale, no erythema
- Seen more in winter months
- Moisturization important; stay away from fragrances
- If severe, test for hypothyroidism
- Occasionally need to use topical steroid

Cellulitis

- Acute inflammatory condition
- Deeper infection of skin
- Usually caused by *S. aureus* (though may be caused by many different bacteria) entering through a break in the skin
- Characterized by local pain, swelling, heat, erythema
- Occurs anywhere on body

Treatment

- Oral antibiotic: cephalosporin, doxycycline if concerned about MRSA, Hibiclens, topical steroid

Cysts

- Self-contained sacs of purulent material, bacteria, WBCs
- Commonly seen in women in axillae, groin, and legs (areas where shaving is common)

Treatment

- I+D most effective
- Oral antibiotics: tetracycline family, cephalosporin
- Kenalog injection

Folliculitis

- Blocked hair follicles result in small pustules
- Usually *S. aureus*
- Can occur in any hair-bearing area
- Treatment: BPO washes, clindamycin topical, oral doxycycline

Dermatitis

Types: contact, irritant, allergic

- Very common (plants, acids, metals, soaps, perfumes, lotions, etc.)

- Caused by hypersensitivity response
- Erythema, vesicles, urticarial lesions
- Complaints of burning, itching, redness

Treatment

- Topical steroid, antihistamines, oral prednisone tapering dose.
- Remember steroid use on face is not recommended for long periods or with higher potency steroids

Atopic Dermatitis: Eczema

- Consider personal, familial history of atopy, common in people with allergic disorders and/or asthma
- Cause: dysfunction in the epidermis
- Symptoms: intense itching, erythema, small bumps, skin flaking
- Scratching can cause skin inflammation which worsens with itching
- Affects infants' front of arms/legs/cheeks/scalp
- Affects adults' back of neck/elbow creases/posterior knees
- "The itch that rashes"
- Cutaneous expression of atopic state
- Thought to be a problem with immuno-regulatory abnormalities, including IgE, IL 4, and mast cell tryptase
- Can occur anywhere on body
- Consider personal, familial hx of atopy; common in people with allergic disorders and/or asthma
- Fragrance-free detergents, softeners, sheets
- Dove soap, cetaphil cleanser
- Daily moisturization
- Recommend lotion face, cream body
- Decrease heat in shower, house temp
- Topical corticosteriods prn (*pro re nata*)
- Antihistamines may help

Psoriasis

- Chronic inflammatory skin disorder
- Alteration in cell kinetics of keratinocytes; overabundance of T cells in affected cells; other immunologic factors
- Pink, sharply demarcated papules and plaques covered by silvery scale

- Lesions are variably pruritic
- Occurs equally in males and females
- Tends to run in families.
- Most common type is plaque type
- Most common areas are elbows, knees, and scalp. Also seen on hands, feet, nails
- Always ask about joint pain.

Treatment

- Topical steroids
- Topical vitamin D (dovonex)
- Coal tar (shampoos, especially)
- Phototherapy
- Methotrexate, cyclosporin, biologics

Seborrheic Dermatitis

- Common chronic disorder
- Characteristic greasy scales overlying erythematous patches or plaques
- Commonly seen in Parkinson's patients, people w/CVAs, HIV; vast majority have no underlying illness; evident in babies as "cradle cap," otherwise rare in children
- Most common location is scalp (dandruff); also face, eyebrows, lids, nasolabial folds.
- Usually causes itching, burning.

Treatment

- Ketoconazole, selenium sulfide, steroid shampoos

Pityriasis Rosea

- Cause unknown; thought to be viral trigger
- Herald patch appears first: large pink scaling patch on abdomen or thigh
- Will then develop smaller oval pink scaling macules on trunk, sometimes legs and arms
- Generally asymptomatic; mild itch at times
- Self-limiting up to 6–8 weeks

Warts: Verruca Vulgaris

- Cutaneous neoplasms caused by HPV (> 50 types identified)
- Appear anywhere on the body
- Many resolve spontaneously in 1–2 years
- Spread through contact

Treatment

- LN2, canthacur, salicylic acid, candida injection, laser

Skin Tags

- Very common
- Benign skin lesion
- Found on face, neck, axillae
- African Americans > Whites
- 1–2 mm outcroppings of skin
- Caused by friction, changes in weight
- Scissor removal

Impetigo

- Common superficial bacterial infection
- Caused by group A beta-hemolytic *streptococci* or *staph aureus*.
- Primary lesion is superficial pustule that ruptures and forms a characteristic honey-colored crust.
- Ecthyma is variant of impetigo that usually occurs on lower extremities.
  - Characterized by "punched out" ulcerative lesions

Treatment

- Bactroban, Keflex, doxycycline

Dermatophytosis

Tineas: Capitis, Corporis, Cruris, Pedis

- Usually caused by overgrowth of fungal organisms commonly found on skin
- Scaling erythematous lesions, annular on scalp, body. Moccasin on lateral feet
- Look for macerated skin between toes
- KOH if available, look for hyphae

Treatment

- Scalp: Griseofulvin since hair follicles are affected
- Body, feet: Naftin cream/gel bid (two times a day) for 2–4 weeks
  - Oral antifungal if severe enough
- Onychomycosis
- Fungal infection in nail/bed
- Common: toes > than fingers
- Yellowish, sometimes darker (brownish/bluish) discoloration of nail; white color is candida

Treatment

- Topicals first line due to liver toxicity with oral antifungal agents.

- Always use a gel or solution; penetrates better.
- Use urea gel in conjunction if nail thickened.
- Loprox gel, Naftin gel
- If oral, Diflucan; if candida, Lamisil fungal
- Tinea versicolor
- Overgrowth of yeast from sweating
- Pink velvety scaling patches on upper body
- Sun causes hypopigmentation

Treatment

- Selsun 2.5% shampoo, leave on 10 minutes, rinse off: use daily × 2 wks
- Loprox solution daily, potentially ongoing
- Diflucan weekly × 2 weeks for severe cases

Herpes Zoster (Shingles)

- Cutaneous viral infection involving a single dermatome, unilateral
- Reactivation of varicella virus that entered cutaneous nerves with chicken pox
- All ages inflicted
- Stress and sickness activate it
- Contagious to pregnant women, immunocompromised people and non-immunized children
- Best outcome if treated within 24–48 hours
- Complaints of itch, pain before rash appears
- Clustered vesicles on erythematous base
- Postherpetic neuralgia, can last months

Treatment

- Valacyclovir 1 gm tid (three times a day) × 7 days (or acyclovir)

Vitiligo

- Hypo-pigmented macular lesions 5 mm to 5 cm or more
- Occurs equally in males and females
- Appears in all races
- 1% of population
- Etiology unknown, three hypotheses: autoimmune, neurogenic, self-destruct
- Also can be related to immunotherapy treatment in cancer

Three General Patterns of Depigmentation

- Focal: lesions in single general area
- Segmental: lesions on one side of body
- Generalized: widespread distribution

Treatment

- Short-burst topical steroids
- Protopic 0.1 ointment bid (two times a day), short exposure to sun after application
- Sunscreen and sun protection education

Alopecia Areata

- Skin condition that causes sudden loss of patches of hair on scalp and other parts of body
- Non-scarring: no permanent damage to hair follicle
- Most people, hair eventually grows back, with 80% of people recovering in one year
- Occurs equally in men and women, all races equally, can develop at any age
- Not life threatening; no physical pain; cosmetic effect can be devastating
- Thought to be body attacking the pigment in hair follicle
- Stress can be a trigger
- Sometimes seen in correlation with vitiligo

Treatment

- High-potency topical steriod, kenalog injections

Urticaria (Hives)

- Distinct, raised areas of skin that itch intensely and are red with pale center
- Approximately 25% of people will experience at least once in their lifetime
- Acute, brief, or chronic
- Also physical urticarias: triggered by certain types of physical stimulation
- Dermatographism (skin writing)—skin welts when stroked firmly or scratched
- Angioedema can also develop with hives, occurs deeper in skin and causes puffiness of face, eyelids, ears, mouth, hands, feet, genitalia
- Triggers: Drugs, physical contact with allergens, insect stings, food allergies, infections
- Treatment: Antihistamines, avoid heat, oral steroids

Review Questions

1. When performing a skin assessment, what is the most vital component of the assessment?

    A. Assessing skin turgor for hydration status

    B. Visual examination of the skin surface

    C. A thorough history

    D. A biopsy of any unusual looking lesions

2. The NP is using the correct terminology to describe the *morphology* of a lesion. Which of the following is an appropriate description?

    A. "The lesion has irregular borders."

    B. "The lesion is a macule."

    C. "The lesion is erythematous."

    D. "The lesion is scaly."

3. A patch can be differentiated from a macule by observing that:

    A. A patch is less than 1 cm in diameter.

    B. A patch is elevated, firm, and circumscribed and less than 1 cm in diameter.

    C. A patch is an elevated, firm, rough lesion with a flat top surface and greater than 1 cm in diameter.

    D. A patch is a flat, non-palpable, irregular-shaped macule greater than 1 cm in diameter.

4. Vitiligo can be described as what?

    A. Distinct raised areas of the skin that are pruritic

    B. Hypo-pigmented macular lesions ranging in size from 5 mm to 5 cm or greater

    C. A loss of skin pigment and hair due to injury at the base of the hair follicle

    D. A progressive thickening and hardening of the epidermis

5. Treatment for vitiligo may include which of the following?

    A. Antihistamines

    B. Griseofulvin

    C. Topical steroids

    D. Lamisil cream

6. A patient presents to the office with concerns about sudden losses of patches of hair from her scalp. She denies any recent changes in use of hair products. She does not pull or tug at her hair. The NP diagnoses the patient with alopecia areata. Which of the following statements made by the NP would provide the most reassurance to the patient?

    A. "There is no treatment but it is always a benign condition."

    B. "If we can identify the causative agent, we may be able to prevent further hair loss."

    C. "A 1% topical naftifine cream (Naftin) applied bid for 2–4 weeks may help prevent further hair loss."

    D. "Eighty percent of all people with this condition will have spontaneous re-growth of hair within one year."

7. A 35 y.o. female patient is seen in the primary care office with concerns about multiple small, oval, pink, scaling macules that have appeared on her trunk. There is no associated pain or pruritus. There is one significantly larger scaly patch observed on the abdomen. The NP diagnoses the patient as having what?

    A. Roseola

    B. Pityriasis rosea

    C. Contact dermatitis

    D. Rosacea

8. An 8-year-old male child is seen in the clinic with a superficial pustule along his inner forearm that started as a mosquito bite. There is a characteristic honey-colored crust covering the entire lesion. The NP diagnoses the patient with which of the following?

    A. *Staph aureus* or Group A beta hemolytic *streptococcus* infection

    B. Group B: Beta hemolytic *streptococcus* infection

    C. Community-acquired Methicillin-resistant *staph aureus*

    D. Tinea corporis

9. A patient presents to the clinic with complaints of itching and flaking to bilateral feet. The NP observes that there is a characteristic macerated appearance between the toes. The NP diagnoses the patient with which of the following?

    A. Tinea pedis

    B. Onychomycosis

    C. Tinea versicolor

    D. Seborrheic dermatitis

10. A patient is seen in the primary care office. The patient has a maculo-papular rash with distinct vesicles on the lateral left trunk that follows along a dermatome. The patient states that the rash has been there for three days. Which of the following is important educational information that should be provided to the patient?

    A. The patient is experiencing a reactivation of the chicken pox virus and is not contagious.

    B. The patient is contagious and must avoid pregnant woman, immunocompromised individuals, and non-immunized children.

    C. The patient is only contagious for the first 48–72 hours that the rash is present.

    D. The patient is not contagious. The rash may remain for many months and there is no treatment.

11. Which of the following is the preferred treatment for herpes zoster (shingles)?

    A. Ketoconazole 200 mg tablet po daily × 10–14 days

    B. Lotrisome topical cream 0.5%; apply to affected area for two weeks

    C. Diflucan 150 mg one tablet po daily for 14 days

    D. Valcyclovir 1 gm tid × 7 days

12. Onychomycosis is:

    A. Caused by a viral infection.

    B. Caused by a fungal infection.

    C. Caused by a bacterial infection.

    D. There is no known etiology.

13. The preferred therapy for onychomycosis is topical agents. If the NP uses oral agents, the NP should first obtain lab work to determine what?

    A. The patient's renal function

    B. The patient's hepatic function

    C. The patient's coagulation factors

    D. The patient's immune-competency

14. Verruca vulgaris is more commonly known as warts. They are cutaneous neoplasms caused by which of the following?

    A. A fungal infection

    B. A bacterial infection

    C. HPV virus

    D. A dermatophyte

15. A patient is requesting more information about several warts that have appeared along his fingers on both hands. Which of the following is appropriate educational information for this patient?

    A. There is no known treatment, but generally most warts will resolve in 1–2 years.

    B. They are not spread through casual contact but rather through contact with an open area.

    C. They are usually confined to the hands or the feet.

    D. They are more common in women than in men.

16. Lichenification is a term used to describe which of the following?

    A. Scar tissue formation that is out of proportion to the healing process

    B. Thick fibrous tissue that replaces normal skin tissue

    C. A linear crack in the epidermis that has a scaly appearance

    D. A cutaneous thickening and hardening of the epidermis

17. The term *bulla* is used to describe a lesion that is:

    A. Elevated, firm, and circumscribed.

    B. A vesicle or large fluid-filled blister.

    C. An elevated firm rough lesion with a flat top surface.

    D. A large grouping of keritanized cells with thick oily walls.

18. The patient presents to the office with an apparent allergic reaction to an unknown antigen. The patient has pruritic hives on his arms, legs, trunk, and face. The patient has no difficulty breathing or swallowing, his lungs are clear, and there is no swelling of the lips or tongue. With this information, the NP should choose which of the following options for treatment?

    A. One-time dose of epinephrine via EpiPen stat in office

    B. Oral antihistamines, cool compresses, and oral corticosteroids

    C. Topical steroid cream to be applied to all affected areas × 1 week or until lesions disappear

    D. Using second-generation antihistamines and warm compresses to affected areas for 20 minutes tid

19. A patient presents to the office with complaints of skin inflammation, intense itching, and flaky skin on the elbows and knees. The NP diagnoses the patient with eczema. What would the NP expect to find when conducting the personal and family history?

    A. Mother has a history of asthma and COPD.

    B. Father had an MI at age 52.

    C. Sister has type 2 diabetes mellitus.

    D. The patient had a tonsillectomy at age 5.

20. A patient comes to the clinic concerned about non-pruritic lesions that are present on both of his elbows. The lesions are pink, sharply demarcated papular plaques covered with silvery scale. The NP diagnoses the patient with which of the following?

    A. Eczema

    B. Dermatitis

    C. Xerosis

    D. Psoriasis

21. A 35-year-old female with a past medical history that includes psoriasis presents to the office for an annual physical. While obtaining a detailed history, the NP recognizes that it would be important to inquire about any personal history of:

    A. Sexually transmitted diseases.

    B. Autoimmune disorders.

    C. Joint pains.

    D. Migraine headaches.

22. While performing a complete physical exam, the NP notes that the patient has very dry, scaly skin on all of the patient's extremities. The NP inquires about the use of moisturizers and fragrances and asks if there is a personal or family history of:

    A. Asthma.

    B. Rosacea.

    C. Diabetes.

    D. Hypothyroidism.

23. What is the most common lesion seen in dermatology?

    A. Basal cell skin cancer

    B. Squamous cell skin cancer

    C. Actinic keratosis

    D. NMSC (non-melanoma skin cancer)

24. What is the most common type of skin cancer?

    A. Basal cell carcinoma

    B. Squamous cell carcinoma

    C. Melanoma

    D. Seborrheic keratosis

25. An 18-year-old female patient presents to the office with complaints of papulopustular, cystic acne to her forehead, chin, and upper back areas. The NP is concerned with psychosocial affects as well as physiological long-term scarring. The NP decides to initiate therapy with which of the following?

    A. Exfoliation therapy

    B. Topical clindamycin

    C. Isotretinoin (Accutane)

    D. Retinoids

26. The NP prescribes Isotretinoin for an 18-year-old female patient with severe cystic acne. The pharmacist receives the prescription but refuses to fill it. What is the most likely reason for the pharmacist's refusal?

    A. The NP is not registered with the IPLEDGE program.

    B. The patient must first show a negative pregnancy test to the pharmacist.

    C. The pharmacist feels it is an inappropriate medication for an 18-year-old female patient.

    D. Female patients that are potentially fertile are not allowed to have Isotretinoin therapy due to its severe teratogenic effects.

27. A patient is diagnosed with alopecia areata. The nurse practitioner reassures the patient that there is no permanent scarring or damage to the hair follicle and that hair growth will likely return within one year. To prevent further episodes, the NP suggests that the patient do which of the following?

    A. Take 2000 international units of Vitamin D once daily.

    B. Use baby shampoo or shampoo that contains no perfumes or dyes.

    C. Consider practicing daily meditation, yoga, or guided imagery to reduce stress.

    D. Avoid tight hats and restrictive headbands.

28. The term dermatographism refers to what?

    A. Skin welts or redness that appears when the skin is scratched or stroked firmly

    B. The ability to correctly identify an item that is placed in the hand when the eyes are closed

    C. The visible burrows left by chiggers burrowing under the skin

    D. Areas of hypopigmentation that are the result of the presence of dermatophytes

29. A patient complains of a pruritic red rash that appeared on his body several days ago. The NP obtains a skin scraping, applies KOH, and visualizes multiple hyphae under the microscope. The nurse practitioner diagnoses the patient with which of the following?

    A. Herpes zoster

    B. Seborrheic dermatitis

    C. Tinea corporis

    D. Onychomycosis

30. A 19-year-old female college student is seen in the health center complaining of several pustules that have appeared in her groin area after shaving. The NP diagnoses the patient with folliculitis. The NP obtains a pregnancy test and then prescribes which of the following?

    A. Topical clindamycin and oral doxycycline

    B. Topical imiquimod lotion

    C. Azithromycin 250 mg; take 2 tabs on day one and then one tab for four days thereafter

    D. Medrol dosepak × 5 days

31. The nurse practitioner can expect to find more frequent skin conditions in which population?

    A. The African American population

    B. The diabetic population

    C. People who primarily work outdoors

    D. Health care workers

32. What is the first-line treatment for onychomycosis?

    A. Topical antifungal agents

    B. Oral antifungal agents

    C. Oral antibiotic agents

    D. Oral antiviral agents

33. The NP is evaluating a 57-year-old Caucasian female who is complaining of persistent facial erythema. The NP observes inflammatory papules and pustules on the periorificial area of the face. There is also dilated prominent telangiectasia evident over the cheekbones. The nurse practitioner diagnoses the patient with which of the following?

    A. Roseola

    B. Rubeola

    C. Acne

    D. Rosacea

34. The patient has been diagnosed with eczema and the nurse practitioner is providing educational recommendations for prevention of exacerbations. All of the following would be effective EXCEPT:

    A. Antihistamines prn to control pruritus.

    B. Topical steroids prn.

    C. Warm showers bid to open pores.

    D. Daily moisturizing to all affected areas.

35. What is the most effective treatment for cysts?

    A. Oral antibiotics

    B. Hibiclens scrub

    C. Incision and drainage

    D. Topical steroids

36. A patient has been told that he should have Mohs surgery on a cancerous lesion. The patient asks what Mohs surgery is. The nurse practitioner explains that:

    A. The cancerous lesion is removed, as well as the surrounding lymph nodes.

    B. The surface area of the lesion is excised and the underlying area is cauterized to prevent further growth.

    C. The lesion is excised and examined under a microscope to determine if wound edges are free from cancer or if further excision is required.

    D. A wide excision is performed to avoid having to do further surgery.

37. A patient's skin on his lower extremities is described by the NP as taut, shiny, and hairless. The nurse practitioner is aware that this skin appearance is consistent with which of the following?

    A. Aging skin

    B. Venous insufficiency

    C. Arterial insufficiency

    D. Chronic, long-term sun exposure

38. The patient presents with thin, friable skin with multiple bruised areas to the extremities. The nurse practitioner is aware that the patient's history may reveal which of the following?

    A. A history of insulin-dependent type 2 diabetes mellitus

    B. Hypothyroidism

    C. Long-term corticosteroid use

    D. Peripheral vascular disease

39. A patient presents to the clinic with complaints of pruritus of the left hand. The NP observes several erythematous papules and linear burrows in the interdigital web spaces of the left hand. The nurse practitioner diagnoses the patient with which of the following?

    A. Tinea corporis

    B. Scabies

    C. Lice

    D. Onychomycosis

40. A 45-year-old male patient presents to the clinic concerned about a mole on his upper back area. The nurse practitioner examines the mole and notes that it is well circumscribed, dark brown, circular, and 7 mm in diameter. The NP refers the patient to dermatology for excision and biopsy. Which of the following characteristics was most concerning to the NP?

    A. Location

    B. Size

    C. Color

    D. Border configuration

41. A patient presents to the primary care provider concerned about a distinct rash that has appeared on his lower leg. It is non-pruritic, 6 cm in diameter, with an annular homogenous erythema appearance, and central clearing. The NP inquires as to whether the patient:

    A. Has young children in the household with tinea corporis (ringworm).

    B. Is immunocompromised.

    C. Has been outdoors doing yard work, or has been camping or hiking in the past several weeks.

    D. Has had a rash that appeared like this in the past.

42. The nurse practitioner is documenting the appearance of a lesion. The NP writes that the lesion is "pearly" in appearance. What characteristic is the NP describing?

    A. Morphology

    B. Distribution

    C. Arrangement

    D. Pigmentation

43. Most cases of melanoma are seen in which of the following?

    A. Caucasian females over the age of 50

    B. Caucasian males over the age of 50

    C. Caucasian females with blue eyes and red or blond hair

    D. Any person of northern European descent

44. An important prognostic factor for a patient diagnosed with melanoma is which of the following?

    A. The number of blistering sunburns the patient has experienced over his lifetime.

    B. A family history of melanoma.

    C. The thickness of the lesion and if ulceration is present at the time of diagnosis.

    D. The diameter of the lesion.

45. A 35-year-old female patient presents to the nurse practitioner for a routine physical exam. During the skin assessment, the patient comments about a lesion that is present on the dorsal portion of her lower left leg. Which of the following statements made by the patient is the most concerning?

    A. "I think this mole is a different color than the other moles I have."

    B. "This mole seems like it grew overnight."

    C. "This mole is larger than the other moles I have on my body."

    D. "Sometimes this mole is itchy."

46. A patient's chances of developing a melanoma is closely related to which of the following?

    A. The number of melanocytes present in the dermis

    B. The number of blistering sunburns the patient has experienced in his or her lifetime

    C. The amount of time he/she has spent outdoors

    D. Chronic exposure to known carcinogens such as free radicals

47. An 18-year-old male of African American descent is traveling to a tropical area for vacation. He asks the nurse practitioner if it is necessary for him to wear a sunscreen higher than SPF 8. The NP makes her recommendation to the patient based on knowledge that:

    A. The large amount of deeply pigmented melanocytes will protect him from sun damage.

    B. The patient can sunburn and is still considered at risk for developing melanoma.

    C. The patient is not at risk for melanoma but should try to avoid sunburn to prevent skin damage.

    D. Protecting his skin now will prevent premature skin aging.

48. Actinic keratosis is often described by the patient as which of the following?

    A. A scaly spot that won't go away.

    B. A round, elevated lesion with a white center and a pale red border.

    C. A firm, elevated 1–2 cm nodule with distantly palpable borders.

    D. A birthmark or "beauty mark."

49. The nurse practitioner is describing lesions that are observed on a patient. The NP writes "The lesions are localized to the left lower extremity." The nurse practitioner is identifying the:

    A. Distribution.

    B. Morphology.

    C. Secondary characteristics.

    D. Arrangement.

50. Actinic keratosis is the most common lesion seen in dermatology. When providing education to the patient about actinic keratosis, the NP explains that:

    A. It is a form of skin cancer.

    B. It is a pre-cancerous lesion.

    C. It is an area of increased pigmentation.

    D. It is an area of hypopigmentation caused by sun damage.

Answers and Rationales

1. C. A thorough history is invaluable in identifying skin disorders. While the other answers are correct and may be considered, they are not as vital to the assessment.

2. B. Morphology is the term used to describe the shape of a lesion such as a macule, papule, or patch.

3. D. The primary difference between a macule and a patch is that the patch is > 1 cm in size.

4. B. By definition, vitiligo consists of hypopigmented lesions of varying size.

5. C. Although the etiology remains unknown, vitiligo may have an autoimmune component and, therefore, may respond to corticosteroid therapy.

6. D. Answer D is the best choice since it is the only answer that provides reassurance to the patient by providing information that hair growth is likely to reoccur spontaneously.

7. B. The significantly larger scaly patch that is seen on the patient's abdomen is known as a "herald patch" and is a classic sign seen with pityriasis rosea.

8. A. The patient is showing classic signs of impetigo which is consistent with a history of scratching a pruritic lesion such as a mosquito bite.

9. A. The macerated appearance between the toes is consistent with a tinea infection and is commonly called "athlete's foot."

10. B. This is a reactivation of the chicken pox virus and the patient is contagious. Precautions should be taken to avoid exposure to non-immune individuals.

11. D. Herpes zoster is a virus and therefore would respond best to antiviral treatment. The treatment should be started as early as possible to shorten the duration and intensity of the outbreak.

12. B. Onychomycosis, by definition, is a fungal infection of the nails. It is more commonly seen in the toenails but may be seen in the fingernails as well.

13. B. If an oral antifungal agent is used, the patient's hepatic function needs to be assessed first because the medication is metabolized extensively within the liver.

14. C. There are more than 50 different types of herpes virus responsible for the growth of warts.

15. A. There is no cure for warts, but most warts will resolve without any intervention. They are spread through contact and do not need to be in contact with an open skin area.

16. D. Lichenification can occur anywhere on the body. It is a thickening of the skin related to persistent rubbing or itching of an area that occurs over an extended period of time.

17. B. A bulla is a large fluid-filled blister. It is commonly seen in patients who have a severe allergy to poison ivy, poison oak, or poison sumac. Bullae can appear in response to any injury or allergic reaction.

18. B. The patient is having an allergic reaction but does not exhibit any signs or symptoms of impending anaphylaxis. For this reason, it is reasonable to treat the patient with oral antihistamines and corticosteroids. The patient should be prescribed an EpiPen because subsequent exposure to the antigen may cause a more severe reaction.

19. A. Patients with eczema often have a personal or family history of allergies, such as those commonly seen with patients who have asthma.

20. D. The patient has a classic presentation of psoriasis. The location and appearance are enough to diagnose the patient.

21. C. Psoriatic arthritis is commonly found in patients who have psoriasis. It is important to assess this early in the patient's history.

22. D. Many patients with dry scaly skin are found to have hypothyroidism. A patient with no other personal history that would explain the dry, scaly skin appearance should have a TSH level done.

23. C. Actinic keratosis is a pre-cancerous lesion and is the most common lesion seen in dermatology.

24. A. Basal cell carcinoma is the most common form of skin cancer. Squamous cell carcinoma is the second most common form.

25. C. Isotretinoin is the most effective of the treatments listed. It is a known teratogen and therefore is only used in severe cases of acne that interfere with the patient's quality of life.

26. A. The IPLEDGE program is designed to increase the awareness and accountability of both the health care provider (prescriber) and the pharmacist. These professionals are required to complete a program and be certified in the prescribing and dispensing of medications that are highly teratogenic.

27. C. Although there is no known etiology of alopecia areata, it is believed that stress may be a trigger. Practicing daily stress-relieving activities may decrease the chance of a reoccurrence.

28. A. Dermatographism is, by definition, the development of skin welts when the skin is scratched or stroked firmly.

29. C. The appearance of hyphae under the microscope is an indicator that yeast is present. Yeast is a fungus. Overgrowth of yeast on the skin is a common occurrence.

30. A. Folliculitis is treated with both topical and oral antibiotics. A pregnancy test should always be done first on a young female to avoid the risk of exposure to a known teratogen.

31. B. Diabetics are more prone to skin conditions due to the fact that both bacteria and fungi thrive in warm moist environments where large amounts of glucose may be present.

32. A. Although they may not be as effective as oral antifungal agents, topical antifungal agents are the preferred first-line treatment. Oral antifungal agents are hepatotoxic.

33. D. This is a classic presentation of rosacea, which is often seen in middle-aged men and women.

34. C. Patients with eczema should try to use cool moisture when possible and should try to avoid the drying effect that occurs with frequent showers or hot showers.

35. C. Cysts are self-contained pockets of bacteria and WBCs. The best treatment is to open the self-contained cyst and allow drainage to occur. Oral antibiotics or topical antibiotics may be prescribed after the I&D (incision and drainage).

36. C. The purpose of Mohs surgery is to minimize the amount of healthy skin tissue that is excised, while ensuring that all of the cancerous tissue is removed.

37. C. A patient with decreased arterial flow will often present with taut, shiny, and hairless lower extremities. The presence of hair on the lower extremities or on the toes is a good indicator of adequate blood flow.

38. C. Any patient chronically exposed to an abundance of cortisol will present with thin, friable skin that bruises easily. This can be from either exogenous sources (oral corticosteroids) or an endogenous source such as that seen with Cushing's syndrome.

39. B. Linear burrows are a classic sign of scabies. Scabies will often present in the interdigital areas of the hands, but are not limited to this area, and may appear anywhere on the body. The NP should examine all close family contacts because scabies is often found in crowded living conditions.

40. B. Using the ABCDE method, the NP would be aware that any mole that is > 6 mm in diameter should be excised and evaluated for possible melanoma.

41. C. The patient is presenting with erythema migrans, which is commonly called the "bull's-eye" rash. Inquiry should be made as to whether the patient has potentially been exposed to a deer tick in recent weeks.

42. D. When describing a lesion, it is important that the NP includes all characteristics of that lesion. Pearly is a descriptive term for the pigmentation.

43. B. Men over the age of 50 have the highest incidence of melanoma.

44. C. Characteristics such as thickening or ulceration at the time of diagnosis is the most important factor in the patient's prognosis. The other answers are indicative of the patient's risk for melanoma.

45. B. Any mole that has grown quickly must be immediately evaluated and biopsied because this is a typical characteristic of a malignant melanoma.

46. B. The number of blistering sunburns a person has had in their lifetime is a significant factor. A patient with one or more blistering sunburns doubles their chance of developing melanoma.

47. B. African Americans have a larger number of melanocytes but are still capable of burning their skin with UV rays. A sunscreen SPF of 30 is the standard recommendation for all persons exposed to the sun's rays.

48. A. Actinic keratosis is the most common lesion seen in dermatology. It may present as a persistent scaly area of skin or a distinct lesion.

49. A. The distribution of lesions can assist with assessment and diagnosis. Distribution refers to where the lesions are located on the body.

50. B. Although they are the most common lesion seen in dermatology, it is important for the patient who presents with actinic keratosis to understand that these are pre-cancerous lesions that need to be assessed and/or removed to prevent progression to skin cancer.

● ● ● **References**

IPLEDGE program. (2005). Retrieved from https://www.ipledgeprogram.com

Lau, G. S. (2014). *Dermatology in Primary Care*. Unpublished manuscript—PowerPoint, Dermatology Associates of Glastonbury, Connecticut.

Lyons, F. (2015). Solving skin rash in primary care. *Advance Healthcare Network for NPs and PAs*. Retrieved from http://nurse-practitioners-and-physician-assistants.advanceweb.com/Features/Articles/Solving-Skin-Rash-in-Primary-Care.aspx

The American Cancer Society. (2015). Melanoma. Retrieved from http://www.cancer.org/cancer/skincancer-melanoma/index?cancerTypeRedirect=/Cancer/index

16

Pediatrics

Julie G. Stewart, DNP, MPH, MSN, FNP-BC, APRN

Maryanne Davidson, DNSc, APRN, CPNP

Nancy L. Dennert, MS, MSN, FNP-BC, CDE, BC-ADM

Rebecca Smart, MPH, MSN, APRN, NNP-BC, FNP-BC

This chapter is not intended to be a comprehensive review of pediatrics. The chapter does review some of the more commonly tested items.

Growth and Development

Growth and development in children encompasses the physical, learning, language, and behavioral development of a child monitored at every well-child visit. The most recent statistics available estimate that one in six children, or about 15%, live with a developmental disability (CDC, 2015). It is imperative that nurse practitioners focus efforts on identifying children at risk, implementing early interventions, and providing up-to-date and comprehensive care for those children with disabilities and their families.

The American Academy of Pediatrics provides many screening tools and resources that identify core components of pediatric screening goals and measures. This following online tool is useful to identify key areas of wellness assessment for children from birth through twenty-one years of age (AAP, 2015).

Bright Futures/American Academy of Pediatrics (AAP) Periodicity Schedule

Bright Futures provides guidelines for clinicians, including all key areas of assessment for children:

https://brightfutures.aap.org/materials-and-tools/tool-and-resource-kit/Pages/default.aspx

Physical Growth and Development

Newborn and Infant Through 3 Months of Age

- Initial loss of 5–10% of birth weight is within normal limits, with expected regain within 10–14 days.
- Average expected weight gain = 0.5–1 ounce per day or about 2 pounds (1 kg) per month
- Average expected gain in length = 1.4 inches (3.5 cm) per month
- Average increase in head circumference = 0.8 inch (2 cm) per month

Infant 4–5 Months

- Birth weight should be doubled, and weight gain slows to approximately 5 ounces per week
- Average expected gain in length = 0.8 inches (2 cm) per month
- Average increase in head circumference = 0.4 inch (1 cm) per month

Infant 6–8 Months

- Average expected weight gain = 3–4 ounces per week or 1 pound per month

- Average expected gain in length = 0.5–0.6 inches (1.2–1.5 cm) per month
- Average increase in head circumference = 0.2 inch (0.5 cm) per month

Infant 9–12 Months

- Average expected weight gain = 1 pound (0.5 kg) per month
- Average expected gain in length = 0.5–0.6 inches (1.2–1.5 cm) per month
- Average increase in head circumference = 0.2 inch (0.5 cm) per month
- Birth weight triples by end of first year

Toddler to Preschool

- Birth weight quadruples by end of second year
- Average height increases by 5 inches in the second year
- Average height increases by 3–4 inches in the third year
- Average height increases 2–3 inches every year from year four until puberty

School-Age

- Average weight gain is 5 lbs per year
- Average height increases 2–3 inches every year from year four until puberty

Adolescent

- During adolescence for males and females weight doubles and height increases by 15–20%.
- Pubertal growth spurt begins, on average, 2 years earlier for females and lasts approximately two years for females and longer for males.
- Tanner staging assesses pubertal growth and maturation through the identification of the presence or absence of secondary sexual characteristics. In females, Tanner staging may be used to estimate the time of menarche. In the United States, the median age of menarche has been estimated at 12.43 years.

Table 16-1 illustrates the Tanner Stages of Development.

Gross Motor Development

- 1 Month—Turns head when prone
- 4 Months—Sits with support; able to roll over
- 6–7 Months—Sits independently; may rock on hands and knees

- 7–8 Months—Supports weight standing
- 7–9 Months—May begin to crawl
- 9–10 Months—Cruising
- 12 Months—Walks holding hand, stands alone
- 18 Months—Able to throw at a target, walks well independently
- 24 Months—Runs well, kicks a ball, walks up and down stairs
- 30 Months—Jumps with both feet off the ground
- 36 Months—May pedal a tricycle, hops on one foot, balances on one foot for a few seconds
- 60 Months—Skips, stands on one foot for 7–8 seconds, catches bounced ball
- School-age—Balance and coordination improve; skills continue to develop with practice

Fine Motor Development

- 4 Months—Reaching, ulnar/palmer grasp
- 7–8 Months—Digital grasp
- 12 Months—Pincer grasp
- 18 Months—Drinks well from a cup, scribbles, makes tower of 4 cubes
- 24 Months—Makes a tower of 7 cubes, unbuttons or unzips clothing
- 30 Months—Makes a tower of 9 cubes, imitates a circle, may hold fork
- 36 Months—Able to use scissors, starts to hold and use toothbrush, puts on shoes
- 48 Months—Dresses self, can string small beads
- 60 Months—May be able to print name, cuts out shapes, may pour from small pitcher
- School-age—Continued improvement in self-care skills, better control with handheld instruments, improvement in eye-hand coordination

Language Development

- 0–3 Months—Startles to sound, attends to voice
- 3–6 Months—Turns to sound, babbles, laughs
- 6–9 Months—Imitates sounds, may begin non-specific "mama" and "dada"
- 9–12 Months—May have one or two words with meaning, imitates sounds
- 12–18 Months—Approximately 10 words, names pictures and body parts
- 18–24 Months—Names self, begins to combine words

Table 16-1   Tanner Stages of Development

		Female				Male			
Stage	Age Range (Years)	Breast Growth	Pubic Hair Growth	Other Changes	Age Range (Years)	Testes Growth	Penis Growth	Pubic Hair Growth	Other Changes
I	0–15	Pre-adolescent	None	Pre-adolescent	0–15	Pre-adolescent testes (≤2.5 cm)	Pre-adolescent	None	Pre-adolescent
II	8–15	Breast budding (thelarche); areolar hyperplasia with small amount of breast tissue	Long downy pubic hair near the labia, often appearing with breast budding or several weeks or months Later	Peak growth velocity often occurs soon after stage II	10–15	Enlargement of testes; pigmentation of scrotal sac	Minimal or no enlargement	Long downy hair, often appearing several months after testicular growth; variable Pattern noted with pubarche	Not applicable
III	10–15	Further enlargement of breast tissue and areola, with no separation of their contours	Increase in amount and pigmentation of hair	Menarche occurs in 2% of girls late in stage III	1½–16.5	Further enlargement	Significant enlargement, especially in diameter	Increase in amount; curling	Not applicable
IV	10–17	Separation of contours; areola and nipple form secondary mound above breasts tissue	Adult in type but not in distribution	Menarche occurs in most girls in stage IV, 1–3 years after thelarche	Variable: 12–17	Further enlargement	Further enlargement, especially in diameter	Adult in type but not in distribution	Development of axillary hair and some facial hair
V	12.5–18	Large breast with single contour	Adult in distribution	Menarche occurs in 10% of girls in stage V.	13–18	Adult in size	Adult in size	Adult in distribution (medial aspects of thighs; linea alba)	Body hair continues to grow and muscles continue to increase in size for several months to years; 20% of boys reach peak growth velocity during this period

- 24–30 Months—Two- to three-word sentences
- 36–42 Months—Three- to four-word sentences
- 48–60 Months—Uses past and future tenses, asks "how" questions

Social and Emotional Development

- 0–3 Months—Turns to voice, smiles briefly, ability to quiet
- 3–6 Months—Smile to parental voice
- 6–9 Months—Enjoys social play, stranger anxiety may emerge
- 9–12 Months—Stranger anxiety, fears of new experiences, interactive social games
- Toddler and Pre-Schooler—Development of a strong sense of autonomy and independence
- School-Age—Development of social and emotional maturity. Peer group mastery
- Adolescence—Abstract thinking, judgment, self-discipline, ethical behavior, control of emotions

Social and Developmental Theorists

Freud, Kohlberg, Piaget, Maslow, Erikson

Erikson's Stages of Development for Children

0–12 months: Trust vs. mistrust

12–36 months: Autonomy vs. shame and doubt

3–6 years: Initiative vs. guilt

6–11 years: Industry vs. inferiority

12–17 years: Identity vs. role confusion

Body Mass Index

Body mass index (BMI) is the measure of a person's weight in kilograms divided by the square of height in meters. It is recommended that this measure be calculated at each well-child visit. The BMI for children and teens is both age- and gender-specific and is an indicator of body fat. The BMI allows for categorization of weight that may indicate potential health problems. BMI calculator and information may be accessed at: http://www.cdc.gov/healthyweight/assessing/bmi/childrens_bmi/about_childrens_bmi.html

Immunizations

Many factors influence the ability of the primary care provider to administer vaccines, such as shortages of vaccines, refusal, changing recommendations, complicated catch-up schedules. The website provided next is a direct link to clear guidelines, easy-to-read schedules, and is a resource to answer common questions. Please see the following for the current vaccine schedule and catch-up recommendations: http://www.cdc.gov/vaccines/schedules/hcp/child-adolescent.html#printable

Vital Signs

Normal heart rates, respiratory rates, and blood pressures are illustrated in Tables 16-2, 16-3, and 16-4 respectively.

(Reference: Pediatric Advanced Life Support Guidelines)

Heart Rate

Table 16-2	Normal Heart Rates by Age (beats/minute)	
Age	Awake Rate	Sleeping Rate
Newborn to 3 months	85–205	80–160
3 months to 2 years	100–190	75–160
2 to 10 years	60–140	60–90
>10 years	60–100	50–90

Respiratory Rate

Table 16-3	Normal Respiratory Rate by Age (breaths/minute)
Age	Normal Respiratory Rate
Infants (<12 months)	30–60
Toddler (1–3 years)	24–40
Preschool (4–5 years)	22–34
School age (6–12 years)	18–30
Adolescence (13–18 years)	12–16

Blood Pressure

Table 16-4	Hypotension Reference Ranges
Age	Systolic BP in mm Hg
Term Neonates (0–28 days)	< 60
Infants (1–12 months)	< 70
Children 1–10 years	< 70 + (age in years × 2)
Children >10 years	< 90

History

- Maternal history—Age, preexisting illness, medications, infertility, tobacco/drug/alcohol abuse, previous pregnancy outcome(s)
- Family History

Table 16-5	Assessment of the Newborn		
APGAR Score: Done at 1 and 5 Minutes After Birth. Each Area Scores 0, 1, or 2 Points			
	0	1	2
A – Appearance (Color)	blue/pale	acrocyanosis	pink
P – Pulse (Heart Rate)	absent	<100	>100
G – Grimace (Reflex/Irritability)	no response	grimaces	cries on stimulation
A – Activity (Tone)	none	some flexion	flexed arms and legs
R – Respirations	absent	weak, gasping	strong cry

- Obstetrical history—Screening tests, ultra-sounds, genetic testing, multiple gestation
- Labor and delivery—Abnormality of the fetal heart rate/rhythm, premature labor, maternal fever, meconium stained fluid, obstetrical anesthesia/analgesia, placental abnormalities (blood vessels, size)

Physical Exam

Should be done within the first 24 hours of birth. Maintain infant's body warmth. Use a systematic head-to-toe approach. See normal vital signs shown earlier.

Measurements: weight, length, head circumference, abdominal circumference

- Observe infant's overall appearance, posture, movements. Should be pink, no rashes, symmetrical, extremities flexed
- If quiet, assess heart and lungs

Heart

S1, louder at apex, S2 louder near base

- S3 may be heard near apex – considered normal
- S4 NEVER normal. Rapid HR, difficult to distinguish gallop sound

Lungs

Signs of distress—Flaring, grunting, retractions, assess chest wall symmetry

Skin

May find milia, Mongolian spots, jaundice, erythema toxicum, café au lait.

Head

Two fontanelles: Anterior and Posterior. There are 2 frontal bones, 2 parietal bones and 1 occipital bone. Sutures allow the bones to move during the birth process and the head to grow as the brain expands and these include the metopic, coronal, sagittal, and lambdoid. The Posterior closes the first few months to 1 year, the anterior by 18 months.

Cephalohematoma

1.5–2.5% of deliveries; injury to blood vessel in subperiosteal area. Does not cross suture lines. May take several days to weeks to resolve.

Caput Succedaneum

Edema due to pressure typically from vacuum-extraction, groggy, ill-defined, crosses sutures lines, resolves within 48 hours.

Primitive/Primary Reflexes

Immature nervous system

Moro Startle reflex (37 weeks–6 months)

Palmer Grasp 32 weeks–2 months)

Tonic neck 1 month–7 months)

Placing/Stepping (37 weeks–4 months)

Important Terms

Epstein pearls—Whitish-yellow cysts in roof of mouth and gums

Retinoblastoma—Most common malignant intraocular tumor in childhood 1/17,000 30% bilateral (*presents with leukocoria)

Nystagmus—Transient rapid, involuntary oscillating of eyes. Develops before 10 mo. Resolves by 12 months

Hypospadias—Urethral opening on underside of penis

Hydrocele—Fluid-filled sac around testes; common; usually resolves within first year without any intervention

Varicocele—Edema of veins in testes appearing as a bag of worms. Similar to varicose vein

Barlow maneuver (posterior displacement)—Gently move hips into mild adduction, then apply slight forward pressure to assess for hip dysplasia

Ortolani's test (anterior displacement)—The examiner puts hands on knees and places thumb on middle of thigh. With fingers, apply gentle upward stress on the hip and then slow abduction. A positive test will result in a "clunking" sound.

Wilm's tumor—Most common kidney cancer in children. Typically affects 3–4 years old. Prognosis good.

Talipes equinovarus—Clubfoot. Adduction, supination, and varus of the foot.

Genu varum—Bowed legs. Should resolve by age 3 or 4 years.

Breastfeeding

Gold standard (Baby Friendly Hospital Initiative) frequent sessions (8–12 times per day). Contraindications—galactosemia, HIV, cytotoxic drugs, radioactive compounds. Encourage exclusive breastfeeding for 4–6 months.

Anticipatory Guidance Topics

Car Seat

SIDS

Hepatitis B vaccine

Infection control measures (Flu vaccine – injection and mist*, Tdap)

Crib safety—Entrapment

"Babywearing"—Decrease in fussiness and increase in learning

Recall of "*Snugli*"—Suffocation deaths (three in 2009)

younger infants, < 4 months, late preterm especially vulnerable

- Follow-up appointment within 48 hours if hospital stay is less than 48 hours

Visiting nurse is an acceptable alternative.

Congenital Heart Defects

A congenital heart defect is a cardiac lesion present in neonates.

Acyanotic Defects—Left to Right Shunts

Results in increased pulmonary blood flow

1. **Atrial-Septal Defect (ASD):** 50% more common in females, accounts for 7–10% of congenital heart defects (CHD). Child may be asymptomatic or may fatigue easily. May get frequent URTIs and LRTIs. Small defect may close on its own. Large defects require intervention. Murmur grade I–III/VI is auscultated best in the pulmonic area. S2 is split widely and is fixed in relation to respirations.

2. **Ventricular-septal defect (VSD):** Most common congenital heart defect accounting for 25% of all CHD. Associated with Down syndrome. Up to 50% are very small and may close on their own by the time the child is four years of age. Murmur: Holosystolic murmur at LLSB. The murmur may be louder when the VSD is smaller since there will be more turbulent blood flow across the defect.

3. **Atrioventriculoseptal defect (AVSD):** Accounts for only 2% of congenital heart defects; however, up to 40% of patients with AVSD have Down syndrome. Children with complete canal defects may exhibit signs and symptoms of CHF—difficulty feeding, pale skin, poor weight gain, increased respiratory rate and effort. Murmur grade II–V/VI low-pitched, holosystolic at LLSB. Murmur may not be present until 2–8 weeks when pulmonary vascular resistance falls and blood is shunted across the ASD and VSD.

4. **Patent ductus arteriosis (PDA):** Normally, functional closure of the ductus arteriosis closes in 12–72 hours after birth. PDA accounts for 9–12% of all CHD. Females to males 2:1. Infant and children may be asymptomatic if the PDA is small. Large PDAs—child may manifest symptoms of CHF. Murmur is typically a grade II–V/VI harsh, rumbling continuous murmur heard in the pulmonic area.

Most infants with a small PDA are followed for two years to determine if there is spontaneous closure. Patients with larger PDAs may have their ductus ligated. Interventional radiologists may close a PDA by placing coils into the ductus in the cardiac catheterization lab.

Cyanotic Defects—Right to Left Shunts

1. **Transposition of the great arteries (TGA)—** Accounts for 5–8% of CHD. More common in males by 60–70%. With TGA, the aorta arises from the right ventricle and receives deoxygenated blood and returns it to the systemic circulation. The pulmonary artery arises from the left ventricle and sends oxygenated blood back through the pulmonic circulation. In order for the neonate or infant to survive, there must be another heart defect (either an ASD, VSD, or PDA) present to allow for mixing of the oxygenated and deoxygenated

blood. Without treatment, 90% mortality rate within the first year of life. Cyanosis is usually evident shortly after birth and CHF symptoms develop rapidly.

Tetralogy of Fallot (TOF)

Accounts for 10% of all CHD. Also referred to as TET, tetralogy of Fallot consists of four defects:

1. Pulmonic valve stenosis
2. Right ventricular hypertrophy
3. VSD
4. Overriding aorta that crosses the ventricular septum

TOF is the most common of the cyanotic defects, accounting for up to 9% of the cases of CHD. The severity of the cyanosis usually depends on the degree of right ventricular obstruction due to pulmonic stenosis. The child may present with dyspnea and cyanotic mucous membranes. Murmur: grade III–V/VI harsh systolic ejection murmur is heard at the left 2nd intercostal space. VSD murmur will be a holosystolic murmur at the LLSB.

Tricuspid Atresia

Accounts for less than 3% of all CHD. Results in no communication between the right atrium and the right ventricle. TGA also occurs in approximately 50% of these patients. The infant with tricuspid atresia presents with cyanosis, dyspnea, is easily fatigued, and exhibits poor growth. The right ventricle is usually hypoplastic (small).

Obstructive Lesions
Aortic Stenosis (AS)

AS accounts for 5% of all cases of CHD and is more common in males. Depending on the severity of the defect, growth may be normal or there may be activity intolerance, fatigue, chest pain, CHF, and syncope that may increase in severity as the child ages. The apical impulse may be pronounced. A grade II–IV/VI loud, harsh systolic ejection murmur in the heart at the upper right sternal border with radiation to the neck, LLSB, and apex. Treatment depends on the severity of the stenosis and may be unnecessary or may require valve replacement surgery.

Pulmonic Stenosis

Accounts for 6–8% of CHD. Due to the stenosis of the pulmonic valve, right ventricular pressure increases and RVH occurs. Murmur: A grade II–IV harsh mid-late systolic ejection murmur is heard over the upper-left sternal border in the pulmonic region and may radiate to neck and back regions.

Cyanosis and symptoms of right-sided CHF may occur with severe pulmonic stenosis.

Coarctation of the Aorta

Accounts for 5% of CHD. A narrowing of the portion of the aorta. The severity of the coarctation, location, and the degree of obstruction determines the manifestation of symptoms. Both systolic and diastolic pressures are high in the vessels that are above the narrowed area and hypotension exists in the vessels below the area of narrowing. Physical exam often reveals hypertension in the upper extremities and hypotension in the lower extremities. In severe cases, poor perfusion to the LEs may present with mottling or pallor. Bounding brachial, radial, and carotid pulses may be evident. Surgical resection of the constricted area and anastomosis of the upper and lower segments yields excellent prognosis.

Innocent Murmurs

Innocent heart murmurs, also known as functional or physiologic murmurs are harmless and can be common during infancy and childhood and often disappear by adulthood. Innocent murmurs usually are a grade I–II/VI and the murmur may change with position changes. The Valsalva maneuver may cause the innocent murmur to disappear. Typically, vital signs are normal, ECG is normal. Echocardiogram reveals no pathology.

Hypertrophic Obstructive Cardiomyopathy (HCOM)

Symptoms of hypertrophic cardiomyopathy may be any or all of the following: dyspnea, syncope, angina, palpitations, orthopnea, paroxysmal nocturnal dyspnea, congestive heart failure, dizziness, and sudden cardiac death. Sudden cardiac death has the highest incidence in preadolescent and adolescent children and is particularly related to extreme exertion. The risk of sudden death in children is as high as 6% per year. In more than 80% of cases, the arrhythmia that causes sudden death is ventricular fibrillation. The murmur is a systolic crescendo-decrescendo murmur best heard between the apex and left sternal border and radiating to the suprasternal notch. The murmur increases markedly with the Valsalva maneuver, and any increase in preload such as squatting.

Primary Care for Congenital Heart Defects

- Adequate nutrition
- Optimal psychosocial development
- Optimal preventive and primary care
- Prevention of complications (ensure good cardiology follow-up)

- Optimal fitness
- Optimal neurodevelopment

Chest Pain in Children

Two Types of Chest Pain:

1. Acute onset, severe chest pain
   - Most likely seen in Pedi ED
   - Only 4% due to cardiac
   - One-third idiopathic
2. Chronic and recurrent episodes of less severe chest pain
   - Most likely seen in the office
   - Patient unlikely to have pain at time of visit
   - Exam likely to be normal
   - Majority of "chest pain" complaints are not caused by cardiac disease
   - Most common cause of chest pain is costochondritis (20–75%).
   - Most common arrhythmia associated with chest pain is SVT.
   - 21–39% of children and adolescents with chest pain is thought to be idiopathic.
   - 30% is a result of musculoskeletal causes.
   - Anxiety and emotional causes account for 9–20% of chest pain in adolescents.

Associated Symptoms

- Fever
- Coughing
- Vomiting
- Lightheadness
- Syncope
- Palpitations
- Shortness of breath
- Diaphoresis

Common Causes of Chest Pain in Children (Cardiac and Non-cardiac)

Cardiac

Predisposing medical conditions: Marfan's syndrome, congenital heart disease, Kawasaki disease, mitral valve prolapse, pericarditis, endocarditis, juvenile rheumatoid arthritis, dysrhythmias (usually SVT)

All cardiac causes of chest pain need referral to pediatric cardiologist and/or emergency department

Non-Cardiac

Spontaneous pneumothorax (absent or decreased breath sounds, chest pain and splinting), pleural irritation, bacterial pneumonia/empyema, sickle cell crisis, pulmonary embolism, exercise-induced asthma/chronic asthma, hyperventilation syndrome, a "stitch," musculoskeletal inflammation, GERD, esophageal spasm, foreign body, achalasia, splenic or pancreatic pain, trauma, stress, depression

Pediatric Hypertension

Primary idiopathic or secondary (most common cause is renal disease)

5% of all children have hypertension; higher incidence in African Americans

Risk factors similar to adult hypertension

Treatment and Referral

- History and physical exam; diagnostic testing
- Diet
- Exercise
- Antihypertensive medications
- Diuretics
- ACE-inhibitors
- Beta-blockers
- Calcium channel blockers

Respiratory Conditions in the Pediatric Population

Asthma

A comprehensive review of the pathophysiology and treatment of asthma is found in the Respiratory chapter of this review book.

The Global Initiative for Asthma (GINA) has separate guidelines for managing asthma in children under 5 years of age. It is difficult to diagnose asthma in this age group because wheezing can occur from other causes. Diagnosis is based on symptom patterns and frequency of symptoms, in addition to history and physical examination findings. Full information on diagnosis and management of asthma in all age groups can be found at www.ginasthma.org.

- Close to 19 million American children (under 18 years old) have asthma according to the Centers for Disease Control (2015).
- It is the most common cause of missed school days and emergency department visits, and is the leading chronic disease of children.
- It is also more common in boys than girls.
- Factors that may aggravate asthma, causing increased or returning symptoms include exercise, stress, smoke, viral respiratory infections, and allergens such as dust mites, cockroaches, and pollens.

History—The patient (or parent) gives a history including symptoms such as wheezing, chest tightness, cough, and/or shortness of breath.

Physical examination—May be normal; may hear wheezing.

Diagnostic testing—FEV_1/FVC less than 0.90 in children, and after bronchodilator treatment the child's FEV_1 increased by more than 12% of the predicted value.

Description of Asthma Levels

Intermittent—Symptoms of wheezing and coughing no more than twice/week. Nighttime flares no more than twice a month.

Mild Persistent—Symptoms occur more than twice/week but not once/day. Symptoms may affect activity level. Nighttime flares more than twice/month but not weekly. Lung function approx. 80% of normal if not treated.

Moderate Persistent—Symptoms occur daily and flare-ups may last days. Activity affected due to coughing and wheezing. Sleep interrupted with nighttime symptoms. Lung function between 60–80% less than normal without treatment.

Severe Persistent—Wheezing and coughing occur daily and often. Activities and sleep disrupted. Lung function < 60% without treatment.

According to the Guidelines from the National Asthma Education and Prevention Program these steps should be followed:

Initial Visit: Diagnosis of asthma, assessment of the severity of asthma, prescription and education of medication and use, develop action plan in writing with patient and parent/guardian, and schedule follow-up.

Follow-up Visits: Assess how well controlled the asthma is, review how to use prescribed medications and assess adherence, as well as how well environmental factors are being controlled. Any changes in medication dosage (increased or decreased) should be reviewed; review the asthma action plan, and schedule a follow-up appointment.

Figure 16-1 illustrates the GINA assessment and step-wise guidelines for asthma.

Croup

- Syndrome of acute edema and obstruction of subglottal area
- *Etiology*—Viral parainfluenza, influenza A & B, respiratory syncytial virus (RSV), and can also be caused by allergies or acid reflux.

- *Occurrence*—Late fall to early spring
- *Manifestations*—URI for 3–5 days, brassy seal's bark sounding cough more apparent with recumbency at night, inspiratory stridor
  - Steeple sign (or wineglass) on X-ray—Tapering of the upper trachea on a frontal chest X-ray, which appears like that of a church steeple.

Treatment/Education

- Cool fluids/air
- Upright positioning
- Needs to run its course over several days
- Keep children calm
- Albuterol/Xopenex
- Systemic corticosteroids
- Hospitalization may be necessary—Danger signs: drooling, circumoral cyanosis, stridor, dyspnea
- Children with moderate to severe croup with labored breathing requiring hospitalization may need oxygen and racemic epinephrine

Bronchiolitis

- Acute inflammation of the bronchioles causing increased mucus secretion, bronchial constriction/obstruction, necrosis of the respiratory epithelium, air trapping, atelectasis
- Etiology
  - Viral, usually RSV or parainfluenza
- Occurrence
  - Late winter/early spring
  - Usually less than 2 years old but can range from 3 months to 3 years

Risk Factors

- Low birth weight
- Premature
- Crowded living conditions and/or daycare
- Parental smoking
- Congenital heart, respiratory, neurologic, or immune disease
  - **Manifestations**
    - Abrupt onset of fine wheezing and dyspnea
    - Tachycardia, tachypnea
    - Low-grade fever
    - Apnea
    - Poor feeding
    - Hypoxia
    - Retractions

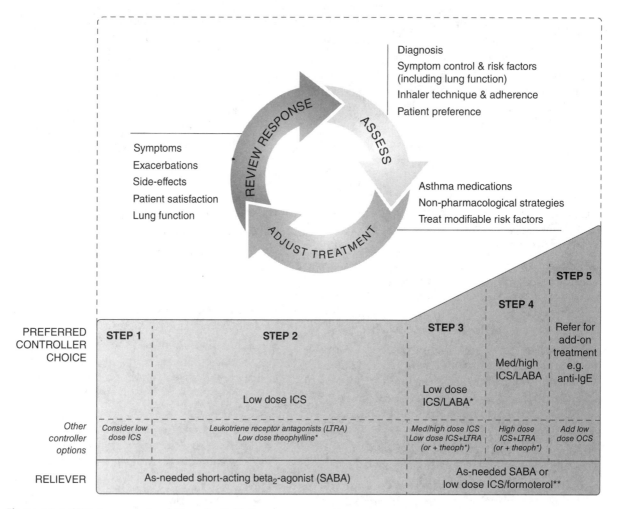

Figure 16-1 GINA Assessment and Step-wise Guidelines

Reproduced from Global Initiative for Asthma. (2011). At-a-glance asthma management reference. Retrieved from http://www.ginasthma.org/. From the Global Strategy for Diagnosis, Management and Prevention of COPD 2016 ©.

- **Treatment**
  - Primarily supportive therapy
  - Oxygen
  - Chest PT/cool mist therapy
  - Corticosteroids
  - Antivirals (ribavirin)
  - Nutrition/rest/electrolyte replacement
  - May require hospitalization with more serious signs and symptoms

Respiratory Syncytial Virus (RSV)

- Effects people of all ages, median age 3.3 months
- By age 2 years old, 80–90% of all children have had the illness, highly contagious
- 40% of those cases result in lower respiratory tract infections
- RSV accounts for >120,000 hospital admissions yearly
- Often occurs during November through April
- Long-term pulmonary sequelae/wheeze/asthma
- Complications
  - Respiratory failure, apnea, secondary bacterial infections
  - Subsequent wheezing
  - Respiratory failure, apnea, secondary bacterial infections
  - Subsequent wheezing
- Prevention—The American Academy of Pediatrics recommends vaccination with Palivizumab (a monoclonal antibody) monthly during fall, winter, and spring for those at highest risk for RSV hospitalizations. Details can be found at http://www.cdc.gov/rsv/clinical/.

Acute Bronchitis

- A temporary inflammatory condition that affects the distal trachea and the major bronchi.
  - Etiology
    - Usually occurs as a secondary infection while airways are vulnerable, causing thickened bronchial walls, mucous gland hypertrophy. Ninety percent are viral.
  - Occurrence
    - Winter and early spring
  - Manifestations
    - Primary symptom is cough.
      - Rhinitis
      - Wheezing
      - Low-grade fever
  - Differential Diagnoses: Asthma, bronchiectasis, bronchopulmonary dysplasia, chronic disease, heart murmur, poor feeding, GERD
  - Treatment/Follow-up for otherwise healthy children:
    - Supportive (fluids for fever, rest)
    - Bronchodilators for wheezing; if no improvement, may need to add oral corticosteroids.
    - Antibiotics for bacterial infection (secondary bacterial infections uncommon)
    - Chronic bronchitis is often actually asthma.

Pneumonia

Pneumonia is the leading infectious disease cause of death in children worldwide (WHO, 2014). Prevention by vaccines is available in developed countries; vaccines and antibiotics not available in many third-world countries. Spread by respiratory droplets person to person, as well as via fomites.

- Risk factors
  - Living in a home with smokers, wood-burning stoves, boys more commonly affected than girls
- Etiology
  - Viruses, bacteria (Chlamydia, mycoplasma, strep), fungi, chemicals, aspiration
  - Neonates more likely to have bacterial pneumonia, otherwise most are viral; children over age 5 most likely to have mycoplasma pneumonia

- Clinical manifestation
  - Sputum producing cough
  - Tachypnea, crackles
  - Pulse oximetry < 90%
  - Viral generally has a gradual onset, lower-grade fever, less acute symptoms, frequently preceded by upper respiratory infection
  - Bacterial has an acute onset, lethargy, green- or blood-tinged sputum.
  - The absence of wheezing is a positive predictor of pneumonia.
- Diagnostics
  - Clinical presentation
  - X-ray
  - Culture
- Treatment
  - Inpatient care if pulse oximetry < 92% and if younger than 3–6 months of age, concern for compliance and/or appropriate assessment of signs/symptoms, or other complicating factors
  - Antibiotics for outpatient: Amoxicillin, Augmentin for bacterial, azithromycin for atypical or alternatives per guidelines. Antibiotics for inpatient IV penicillin G, ampicillin, and IV azithromycin, or alternatives for atypical.
  - Supportive care, fluids, rest, oxygen
- Complications can include: pneumothorax, pleural effusion, abscess, acute respiratory failure, carditis, meningitis, sepsis

  *See HENT chapter for upper respiratory infections, including pharyngitis.

Sports Physical/Preparticipation Physical Evaluation

Sudden Death

- Males: Females = 3:1
- Activity-related:
  - 75% occur during mild physical activity
  - 10–15% during sleep
  - 10–15% during competitive athletics
- Most common symptoms prior to death:
  - Syncope
  - Chest pain

Causes

Myocarditis (20–40%), hypertrophic cardiomyopathy (25% and higher in AA), congenital coronary artery anomalies (18%), coronary artery disease (14%), conduction system abnormalities, mitral valve prolapse, aortic dissection, Marfan's syndrome.

The goal of the sports physical is to assess general health and detect potential life-threatening disorders. In addition, the screening aims to detect any medical issue and/or musculoskeletal issues that could cause injury. Each state determines what type of provider may perform this type of physical examination. Be sure to check this to be assured of practicing within the legal scope of practice.

History

A comprehensive personal and family history must be taken. Specific questions related to syncope, family history of cardiovascular problems, seizures, palpitations, and shortness of breath should be included.

Physical

A comprehensive full physical exam is essential. General appearance notes should include any indication of Marfan's syndrome, and the cardiac exam must include listening for murmurs while the patient is standing, sitting, and during the Valsalva maneuver. A robust musculoskeletal exam may indicate issues needing further evaluation.

The PPE 4 guidelines with monographs and forms for history and physical are available at https://www.aap.org/en-us/about-the-aap/Committees-Councils-Sections/Council-on-sports-medicine-and-fitness/Pages/PPE.aspx.

Pediatric Infectious Diseases Not Covered Elsewhere in Review Book

Parvovirus B19

Mode of transmission:

- Contact with Respiratory tract secretions
- Percutaneous exposure to blood or blood products
- Vertical transmission from Mother to Fetus
- Incubation period: 4 to 14 days, but can be as long as 21 days
- Shedding of the virus:
  - Fifth disease: once the rash appears the patient is no longer contagious
  - Aplastic crisis: 7 days (at risk children e.g. sickle cell)

This illness is also called erythema infectiosum. Symptoms are usually mild and include fever, coryza, and headache. After a few days, the child may get the "slapped cheek" appearance associated with Fifth disease. This can spread to the back, chest, rest of body, and last for 7–10 days. Women who are pregnant usually have mild disease, if at all, since approximately 50% are immune. However, there is a small risk that the fetus could develop severe anemia or the mother could miscarry.

Measles

- Incubation period: 7 to 21 days
- Contagious: 4 days before onset of rash through 4 days after
- Suspect Measles in patients with:
  - Fever + Rash
  - Hx of international travel in the past 3 weeks or contact with international visitors
  - A Hx OF 2 DOSES OF MMR DOES NOT EXCLUDE MEASLES

Transmission occurs when an infected patient coughs and sneezes. Infectious particles can remain in the air for up to 2 hours. Approximately 7–10 days after being infected, the patient will develop coryza, conjunctivitis, cough, and a high fever. Two to three days after symptoms begin, the patient may develop Koplik's spots in the mouth. Three to five days after symptoms start, the patient will develop a rash with flat red spots near the hairline, which spreads down the body. The flat spots may develop raised red bumps. The rash and symptoms disappear a few days later. Complications can include otitis media with potential hearing loss, and pneumonia. Less common severe complications include encephalitis and death. Premature delivery can occur in women who get infected, or babies may be born with low birth weights.

Impetigo

Caused by bacterial infections (usually strep or staph) via cuts and scrapes or other forms of skin breakdown. This infection usually occurs most often in the 2–5-year-old age group and is highly infectious. There are two forms: bullous and non-bullous. Typically, a honey-colored crust forms. The entire process usually lasts about 7 days.

Non-bullous impetigo can be caused by either strep or staph. Small red papules turn into blisters, which then become pustules.

Bullous impetigo is caused by staph infection. A toxin is produced that causes cell adhesion, which causes separation between the epidermis and dermis layers. A clear yellow-colored liquid fills the blisters, which break easily.

Gentle cleansing and application of Bactroban typically help resolve the infection and prevent secondary infections. If severe, oral antibiotics may be indicated such as amoxicillin or Augmentin.

Coxsackievirus (Hand, Foot, and Mouth Disease)

Incubation period: 2 to 6 days, *Transmission:* Fecal-oral and respiratory; *Shedding of the virus:* Several weeks (fecal-oral) and 1 week (respiratory). Manifestations include fever, malaise, rash, blisters (most commonly found in mouth and on soles of feet and palms of hands). Usually self-limiting. Treatment is symptomatic using acetaminophen, diphenhydramine, fluids (avoid citrus if oral ulcers). Complications are rare and include encephalitis and/or endocarditis.

Child Abuse

Abuse is defined as:

A non-accidental injury to a child which, regardless of motive, is inflicted or allowed to be inflicted by the person responsible for the child's care. It includes:

- Any injury which is at variance with the history given
- Maltreatment such as, but not limited to, malnutrition, sexual molestation, deprivation of necessities, emotional maltreatment or cruel punishment.

Statistics (U.S. Department of Health & Human Services, 2013)

- 1,520 children died from abuse and neglect in 2013.
- 74% were < 3 yrs old
- Boys have higher fatality rate.
- AA children have 3 × higher rates of fatality than Whites or Hispanics.
- 79% of perpetrators were parents acting alone, together, or with someone else.

Physical Abuse

is any physical injury inflicted other than by accidental means, any injury at variance with the history given of them, or a child's condition that is the result of maltreatment, such as malnutrition, deprivation of necessities, or cruel punishment.

Examples of Injuries That May Result from Physical Abuse

- Head injuries
- Bruises, cuts, or lacerations
- Internal injuries
- Burns, scalds
- Reddening or blistering of the tissue through application of heat by fire, chemical substances, cigarettes, matches, electricity, scalding water, friction, etc.
- Injuries to bone, muscle, cartilage, ligaments fractures, dislocations, sprains, strains, displacements, hematomas, etc.
- Death

Emotional Abuse

or maltreatment is the result of cruel or unconscionable acts and/or statements made, threatened to be made, or allowed to be made by the person responsible for the child's care that have a direct effect on the child. The observable and substantial impairment of the child's psychological, cognitive, emotional, and/or social well-being and functioning must be related to the behavior of the person responsible for the child's care.

The Role of the FNP

- Recognize signs and symptoms of abuse.
- Perform a thorough history and physical exam and DOCUMENT accurately (separate interviews for child and caregiver)
- Try not to be judgmental
- Ensure the child's safety as first priority
- Collect evidence
- REPORT suspicions in good faith.

  Remember that minor injuries are common and often witnessed by others.

  A child or adolescent needs an exam if:

  - There is any suspicion of abuse.
  - There is a suspicion of sexual abuse, even if it is sexual play.
  - There are physical signs and symptoms of genitourinary problems.
  - There is a history of pain, injury, or possible trauma.
  - The child/adolescent and family need reassurance.

Key Steps

- Gather and document pertinent information.
- Determine the safety and welfare of the child/adolescent.
- Determine who should examine the child/adolescent and when.
- Determine if you are mandated to report this situation.

TIPS

The injury/injuries do not "fit" with the explanation.

- Unexplained injuries, especially to protected body parts (buttocks, thighs, torso, frenulum, ears, neck, retina)
- Consider child's behavior and developmental ability.
  - Bruises are rare in infants who do not cruise.
  - Shape/pattern of injury (handprint, belt buckle, cord loops, glove or sock, etc.)
  - Transverse long-bone fracture in a 3-month-old is highly suspicious for abuse, yet may be unremarkable in an 8-year-old child.
  - A complete skeletal survey is needed in any child under 2 years of age when physical abuse is suspected.

Differential Diagnoses Include But Are Not Limited To

- Hematologic: Hemophilia, ITP, Von Willebrand's
- Dermatologic: Phytophotodermatitis, Mongolian spots, vascular malformations, s/c fat necrosis
- Infectious: Bullous impetigo, staph-scalded skin syndrome, petechia/purpura from systemic infections
- Metabolic: Osteogenesis imperfecta, rickets
- Insensitivity to pain disorders

Sexual Abuse

is any incident of sexual contact involving a child that is inflicted or allowed to be inflicted by the person responsible for the child's care.

Normal or Non-Specific Findings

- Hymenal tags, bumps, or mounds
- Labial adhesions

- Clefts or notches in the anterior half (between the 9- and 3-o'clock position) of the hymen
- Vaginal discharge
- Erythema of the genitalia or anus
- Perianal skin tags
- Anal fissures
- Anal dilatation with stool in the ampulla

Concerning But Not Diagnostic Findings

- Notches or clefts in the posterior half of the hymen
- Condylomata acuminata in a child older than two years who gives no history of sexual contact
- Immediate, marked anal dilatation
- Anal scarring

Diagnostic Positive Physical Findings

- Acute laceration or ecchymosis of the hymen
- Absence of hymenal tissue in the posterior half
- Healed hymenal transection or complete cleft
- Deep anal laceration
- Pregnancy without a history of consensual intercourse
- Most exams are "normal," with no signs of abuse due to a variety of reasons:
  - Nature of the abuse was not damaging.
  - Abuse may have occurred days or weeks before.
  - Complete healing may have occurred.
  - Children who have not been abused may have findings that seem "not normal," but actually are variations of normal.

Contact specialty team for evaluation, interview, and examination.

- **Emergency Care Required:**
  - Symptoms of head trauma: vomiting, headache, syncope, lethargy, visual disturbance
  - Symptoms of abdominal injury: vomiting, abdominal pain, bruising to the abdomen/flank/back, hematuria
  - Symptoms or history of recent traumatic sexual contact: bleeding from the vagina or rectum, genital pain, or other signs of injury

Review Questions

1. A well 12-year-old child recently arrived from South Africa presents for a school physical. She received BCG immunization shortly after birth and is up to date with required immunizations. A PPD is placed and read at 48 hours. Likely findings include which of the following?
   A. Negative PPD, no further follow-up
   B. Negative PPD, child requires a follow-up chest X-ray
   C. Positive PPD, no further follow-up
   D. Positive PPD, child requires a follow-up chest X-ray

2. What behavior in a 2-year-old would be considered worrisome?
   A. Ability to concentrate on a task for 2 minutes
   B. Carrying a favorite toy around the house
   C. Skipping pages in a book to find favorite shapes
   D. Unable to walk downstairs holding a rail

3. Baby Sabrina presents for her 6 month well child check-up. At 40 weeks gestation her documented birth weight was 6 lbs 6 oz, and length of 20 inches. Currently her weight is 10 lbs, 4 oz and length is 24 inches. The nurse practitioner concludes the following:
   A. The infant is failing to meet expected gains in weight only.
   B. The infant is failing to meet expected gains in both weight and length.
   C. All findings are within normal limits.
   D. The findings are acceptable since the mother is 5 feet in height.

4. During a sports physical for an 18-year-old male high school student, which finding would require further follow-up?
   A. Height of 5 feet, 11 inches, and weight of 175 lbs
   B. Tanner stage of 4
   C. Snellen eye chart vision screening results of 20/25 in both right and left eyes
   D. Scoliosis of the spine with a degree of curvature of approximately 10%

5. A 7-year-old male child is brought to the clinic by his parents for evaluation. The child has no significant PMH. Approximately seven days ago he developed a cold and since then has had a persistent cough and fever. His older sister was also ill with cold symptoms at the same time. The NP performs a physical exam and notes that the child has mild tachypnea, with crackles in both bases and a pulse oximeter of 90%. His temperature is 100.8 °F. There are no wheezes auscultated. The NP suspects that the child has which of the following?
   A. Bacterial pneumonia
   B. Viral pneumonia
   C. Bronchiolitis
   D. Bronchitis

6. For the 7-year-old child described in the previous question, what does the FNP expect to find on auscultation of the lungs?
   A. Crackles in a portion of a lung field, no wheezing
   B. Wheezing in most of the lung fields
   C. Rales and wheezing in the lower lung bases
   D. Normal breath sounds in all but one lung field, which will have decreased breath sounds

7. For the 7-year-old child described earlier, what will the FNP have as part of the plan of care?

   A. Supportive care, return to office in one week, call if worsening symptoms

   B. CXR now, hospitalization to pediatric unit

   C. Bronchodilator via nebulizer now, IV fluids in emergency department after nebulizer

   D. CXR now, supportive care at home; call in one day or if any worsening of symptoms; return to office in 2 days for follow-up evaluation

8. A 6-month-old male is being seen with his caretaker for a barking cough which is making the caretaker anxious. The baby seems to have mild respiratory distress and the oximetry reads at 94%. The FNP sends the baby for a CXR. What findings are likely to be reported?

   A. Ground glass appearance over affected lung field(s)

   B. Pneumothorax of an upper lung field

   C. Steeple-shaped appearance with narrowing in upper airway

   D. CXR will have normal markings

9. The most common organism responsible for otitis media is which of the following?

   A. *Haemophilus influenzae*

   B. Adenovirus

   C. *Streptococcus pneumonia*

   D. *Staphylococcus aureus*

10. A 19-year-old mother brings her 2½-month-old-boy to your clinic with a concern that the baby has become less interested in his feedings over the past 2 or 3 days, taking in only about half the normal amount of formula before becoming tired and falling asleep. His birth history is normal and he has normal development and weight gain. His temperature is 100.2 °F (axillary) now. He has no respiratory symptoms and your physical examination reveals no identifiable source of fever. Which of the following questions/observations would be MOST helpful in establishing a diagnosis?

    A. "Is anyone else at home ill at this time?"

    B. "How sick do you think he is?"

    C. "Has he ever had a temperature before?"

    D. "Did you have any infection or rash when you were pregnant?"

11. Which of the following infants are susceptible to respiratory syncytial virus (RSV) and bronchitis in the first year of life?

    A. Term infant with chronic rhinitis

    B. Very low birth weight infants

    C. Term infant with hypospadias

    D. 38-week gestation infant with feeding problems

12. A 4-week-old infant presents to the office in mid-January with a one-week history of nasal congestion and occasional cough. On the evening prior to this visit, she developed a temperature of 102 °F, refused to breast feed, had paroxysmal coughing, and noisy, labored breathing. Patient is an ill-appearing infant who is lethargic with tachypnea and intercostal retractions. She has a 4-year-old sibling who is in day care and who recently had a "cold." Considering the clinical presentation, what is the most likely cause of this infant's illness?

    A. Mycoplasma pneumonia

    B. RSV bronchiolitis

    C. Aspiration pneumonia

    D. Streptococcal infection of the pharynx

13. A 9-year-old child's symptoms occur four times a week during the day and three times during the night, with an FEV1 of 80%. What would be the severity classification per the National Asthma Education and Prevention Program?

    A. Severe persistent

    B. Moderate persistent

    C. Mild persistent

    D. Mild intermittent

14. An 8-year-old male has mild persistent asthma. Appropriate daily medication should include which of the following?

    A. An inhaled low-dose corticosteroid

    B. Short-acting beta2-agonists

    C. An oral systemic corticosteroid

    D. A cough suppressant

15. A 3-month-old female is brought to the office for a routine examination and numerous bruises in varying stages are noted on the infant's back and legs. The mother gets very upset when asked about the bruises and starts to cry. She refuses to talk any more about the bruises or how this may have happened. A necessary next step for this scenario is which of the following?

    A. Explain to the mother that she has to leave the baby with the office staff for Department of Children and Families to come and get her.

    B. Discuss with the mother that sometimes congenital bleeding issues can cause these types of bruises and make an appointment for her to return with the baby in 2 days for bloodwork.

    C. Explain to the mother that bruises such as these are uncommon in a 4-month-old, and further assessment, including a skeletal body scan, is required.

    D. Ask the mother to call the baby's father to come to the office so that the family can be interviewed regarding child abuse.

16. According to the developmental theory of Erikson, if the needs of the infant are met in a consistent manner, the infant will develop which of the following?

    A. Independence

    B. Responsibility

    C. Trust

    D. Love

17. The ability of an infant to turn his head to the side when lying prone occurs during the _____ month of life.

    A. first

    B. second

    C. fourth

    D. sixth

18. According to the vaccination schedule recommendations, the IPV (polio) vaccine, the DTaP (diptheria—tetanus-acellular pertussis), *Haemophilis influenzae* type B (HIB), Rotavirus (RSV1) pneumoccal vaccine (Prevnar-13), and second hepatitis B vaccine are given at _____ month(s) of age.

    A. 1

    B. 2

    C. 3

    D. 4

19. An infant would be expected to begin babbling and laughing by what age?
    A. 0–3 months of age
    B. 3–6 months of age
    C. 6–9 months of age
    D. 8 months of age

20. Most infants will begin to crawl around at _____.
    A. 4–6 months
    B. 7–9 months
    C. 8–10 months
    D. 10–12 months

21. The first solid food item that should be introduced into an infant's diet is _____.
    A. vegetables
    B. meat
    C. fruit
    D. cereal

22. The initial MMR (measles, mumps, rubella) vaccine is recommended at _____.
    A. 12 to 15 months of age
    B. 6 months of age
    C. birth
    D. 9 months of age

23. An infant develops increased coordination between his index finger and thumb and is now able to pick up small objects. This is known as what?
    A. Grasp reflex
    B. Moro reflex
    C. Pincer reflex
    D. Palmar reflex

24. The fine motor developmental ability that would be demonstrated first in the infant would be the ability to _____.
    A. pinch with the fingers
    B. grasp with the hands
    C. throw an object
    D. intentionally release an object

25. An infant's birth weight is 7 pounds. 5 ounces. What would the nurse practitioner expect the infant to weigh at 6 months of age?
    A. 12 pounds
    B. 15 pounds
    C. 18 pounds
    D. 22 pounds

26. A father brings his 2-year-old to the clinic. He verbalizes frustration with the child's willfulness and states that he would like to know what the best form of discipline would be for his child. The nurse practitioner responds that:

    A. A gentle spanking works best because it is the most effective.

    B. A 5-minute time-out is most effective.

    C. A 2-minute time-out is most effective.

    D. Discipline should be individualized to the child and family and based on social and cultural preferences.

27. One indication that the toddler is ready to toilet train is:

    A. The child has the ability to climb up on the toilet.

    B. The child has the ability to stay dry for one hour.

    C. The child is able to communicate that he or she is wet or needs to urinate or defecate.

    D. The child is willing to sit on the potty for at least 5 minutes.

28. Which type of play do 2-year-old toddlers most commonly exhibit?

    A. Associative play

    B. Team play

    C. Solitary play

    D. Parallel play

29. The nurse practitioner provides anticipatory guidance to the parents/guardians at every well-child visit. The NP is aware that the leading cause of death in infants and children is _____.

    A. accidents

    B. child abuse

    C. SIDS

    D. drowning

30. A parent is frustrated with her 2-year-old's inability to share her toys with siblings or playmates. The NP explains to the parent that a toddler has difficulty seeing anyone else's point of view and that this is a normal part of development and is referred to as _____.

    A. negativism

    B. ambivalence

    C. egocentric thinking

    D. autonomy

31. The stage that Erikson identified as a developmental stage for a toddler is the stage of:

    A. Trust versus mistrust.

    B. Autonomy versus shame and doubt.

    C. Initiative versus guilt.

    D. Industry versus inferiority.

32. A mother brings her child in for a well-child visit. She states that she is concerned that her child is exhibiting unusual behaviors. She states that her toddler insists on wearing his cowboy boots to bed and asks for the same bedtime story every night. The nurse practitioner reassures the parent that this is normal behavior for a toddler and that the behavior, which is known as "ritualism," helps the child to develop _____.

    A. control of his/her surroundings

    B. a sense of security and mastery of the world around him/her

    C. independent thinking and autonomy

    D. a feeling of love and belonging

33. The nurse practitioner provides anticipatory guidance as well as education to the parents at each well-child visit. The parents of a pre-school child verbalize that they are concerned because their child is still experiencing enuresis at night, although he has daytime dryness and control. The nurse practitioner tells the parents that the most effective way to manage this situation is for the parents to do which of the following?

   A. Be firm and consistent and provide immediate discipline each time this happens

   B. Teach the child to remove the sheets and put them in the hamper so that the child understands there are repercussions to this behavior.

   C. Tell the child that he is behaving like a baby and that he may need to return to wearing diapers at night.

   D. Recognize that it can be normal for a preschool child to experience enuresis.

34. When engaging in play, it is common for a 3-year-old to do which of the following?

   A. Play cooperatively with other children for extended period of time

   B. Play well with new friends

   C. Revert to parallel play if placed in a situation with children they do not know

   D. Share toys eagerly and willingly

35. The nurse practitioner observes that a three-year-old has amblyopia. The nurse practitioner recommends that the parents patch the stronger eye for 2–6 hours every day. The NP explains to the parents that patching the unaffected (stronger) eye will:

   A. Reinforce the connection between the brain and the weaker eye.

   B. Cause a gradual change in the structure and function of the lens of the weaker eye.

   C. Decrease abnormal eye muscle movement in the weaker eye.

   D. Decrease sensory input to the brain from both eyes.

36. Erikson believed that the school-age child is in which stage?

   A. Initiative versus guilt

   B. Identity versus role confusion

   C. Industry versus inferiority

   D. Autonomy versus shame and doubt

37. A 5-year-old female child is brought to the clinic by her mother. The mother verbalizes concern that the child has been sick for three days with a fever, malaise, and blisters in her mouth and on the palms of her hands. The NP performs a physical exam and notes a tympanic temperature of 101.2 °F and observes that the blisters are also observed on the soles of the child's feet. With this information, the NP diagnoses the child with which of the following?

   A. Coxsackie virus

   B. Impetigo

   C. Apthous ulcers

   D. Bronchitis

38. The nurse practitioner is evaluating a 3-month-old infant at the well-baby clinic. The NP places her hands on the infant's knees and her thumbs on the middle of the thigh. She applies gentle pressure on the hips and slowly abducts the hips simultaneously. The NP hears and feels a "clunking" sound when she does this. This is known as what?

   A. A positive Barlow maneuver

   B. A positive test for Genu-varum

   C. A positive Ortolani's test

   D. A positive test for Talipes equinovarus

39. A 16-year-old engages in a risky behavior such as driving while drunk. The parent asks the adolescent "Why would you do something that you know is so stupid?" The 16-year-old replies "I don't know." One possible explanation for this answer is that:

    A. Most adolescents do not think of the repercussion of getting caught.

    B. Most adolescents believe that bad things only happen to other people.

    C. Most adolescents have not formed the physiological connections within the brain that connects the prefrontal cortex with the limbic system.

    D. Most adolescents have not developed the ability to perform concrete operational thinking.

40. The mother of a 14-year-old female child verbalizes concern that her daughter is losing weight and exercising for several hours a day. The NP performs a complete history and physical exam on the 14-year-old adolescent. Which of the following is *not* a characteristic associated with anorexia nervosa?

    A. Amenorrhea that may last 3 months or longer

    B. Low self-esteem

    C. Improvement in body image as weight loss occurs

    D. Feelings of helplessness

41. The nurse practitioner is performing an assessment on a preterm neonate. The neonate was born at 34 weeks gestation. The NP observes the following: acrocyanosis, heart rate is 90, facial grimacing in response to stimulation, a weak cry, and mild flexion of the extremities. The assessment is done at both 1 minute and 5 minutes and remains unchanged during that time. The APGAR score for this neonate is which of the following?

    A. 3

    B. 5

    C. 7

    D. 9

42. The NP is performing a physical assessment on a 3-year-old child. The NP notes that there is a marked difference in blood pressure between the upper and lower extremities and observes that the lower extremities are slightly mottled in appearance. The NP suspects that the child may have which of the following?

    A. Patent ductus arteriosis

    B. Tetrology of Fallot

    C. Coarctation of the aorta

    D. Hypertrophic obstructive cardiomyopathy

43. A child with known tetralogy of Fallot may have hypercyanotic episodes, which are sometimes referred to as "TET" spells. During these spells, the child should be held or placed in a knee–chest position or squatting position. This maneuver will:

    A. Increase systemic resistance which will decrease the right to left shunting of blood across the VSD and thus increase pulmonary blood flow.

    B. Decrease systemic resistance and increase the right to left shunting, increasing pulmonary blood flow.

    C. Increase pulmonary blood flow by increasing venous return and decreasing afterload.

    D. Mimic the Valsalva maneuver, decrease the heart rate, and decrease pre-load.

44. A nurse practitioner is performing a sports physical on a 15-year-old male entering high school. The young male wants clearance to be allowed to play on the high school football JV team. The NP auscultates a systolic murmur in between the apex and the LLSB when he performs the Valsalva maneuver. The NP asks the patient to squat and then stand, when standing after squatting, the murmur becomes markedly louder. The NP suspects which of the following?

    A. An innocent murmur

    B. Hypertrophic obstructive cardiomyopathy

    C. Pulmonic stenosis

    D. Coarctation of the aorta

45. The NP is evaluating a 5-year-old female child that has been brought into the clinic by her mother for a sick visit. The mother states that the child has had a "cold" for approximately one week. The NP observes coryza, conjunctivitis, and the child's temperature is 103 °F. The NP performs an oral exam and observes Koplik's spots in the child's mouth. Which of the following questions will be most helpful to assist the NP in formulating a diagnosis?

    A. "What medications have you tried up to this point to treat the child?"

    B. "Can you supply me with your child's immunization records?"

    C. "Is there anyone else sick at home?"

    D. "Does the coughing awaken your child during the night?"

46. A 4-year-old African American female is brought in to the clinic by her mother. She has been complaining of intermittent abdominal pain around the right flank area. The NP performs an abdominal assessment and palpates a mass in the lower left quadrant. The NP suspects a Wilm's tumor. The NP stops any further palpation of the abdomen and orders imaging. The reason for this is because:

    A. Further palpation may interfere with the renal ultrasound results.

    B. Further palpation may illicit the abdominal pain and promote guarding.

    C. Further palpation may cause rupture of the mass into the peritoneal cavity.

    D. Further palpation may elicit rebound tenderness.

47. An acyanotic heart condition can be characterized as a condition where:

    A. There is a shunting of blood from the left side of the heart to the right side of the heart.

    B. Spontaneous closure of the congenital heart malformation will commonly occur.

    C. There is a shunting of blood from the right side of the heart to the left side of the heart.

    D. Open heart surgery is commonly performed after the child reaches the age of 1 year.

48. Transposition of the great arteries (TGA) is a cyanotic defect with a 90% mortality rate within the first year of life. Which of the following conditions will increase the infant's chances of survival?

    A. The infant was born at 42 weeks gestation.

    B. The infant has at least one other heart defect.

    C. The infant is female.

    D. The infant has no other congenitally acquired defects.

49. A 7-year-old child is brought in to the office for a sick visit evaluation by both of her parents. The child's parent's state that the child has had a cold for 4 days that has been associated with fever and a headache. The NP observes that the child's cheeks are reddened and appear as if the child was recently slapped on both sides of the face. With this information, the NP:

    A. Suspects child abuse and files a report in good faith with the Department of Family and Children's Services.

    B. Suspects meningitis and refers the child to neurology for further workup.

    C. Prescribes liquid Amoxicillin 30 mg/kg/day divided into Q12 hour doses for 7 days.

    D. Explains to the parents that only supportive therapy is necessary to treat her symptoms, and that the condition will resolve on its own.

50. The NP is performing a physical exam on a 4-year-old male child at a well-child visit. The child falls within the 80th percentile for height and weight. The NP auscultates a systolic murmur that is grade II/VI and is most clearly auscultated at the LLSB. There is no radiation. The murmur disappears when the child performs a Valsalva maneuver or changes position. VS and ECG are all WNL. Based on these clinical findings, the nurse practitioner:

   A. Suspects a ventricular-septal defect (VSD) and sends the child for a pediatric echocardiogram.

   B. Suspects hypertrophic obstructive cardiomyopathy (HCOM) and refers the child for an immediate cardiology workup.

   C. Suspects a physiologic murmur.

   D. Suspects patent ductus arteriosis (PDA) and refers the child to cardiology for follow-up with an interventional radiologist.

Answers and Rationales

1. D. The BCG, or bacilli Calmette–Guérin, is a vaccine for TB. Many foreign-born persons have been vaccinated with the BCG vaccine, especially in countries where there is a high incidence of TB. It is likely that this child will have a positive PPD test. It is not possible to determine in this case, however, if the child has active TB without a chest X-ray.

2. D. The nurse practitioner should always be aware of typical expected growth and development parameters. At two years of age, normal expected gross motor skills include having the ability to walk up and down stairs without difficulty. The child should be evaluated further for other delays in gross motor, fine motor, or language/social skills.

3. B. Infants age 0–3 months gain approximately 1.4 inches in height per month. Baby Sabrina would be expected to have achieved 24 inches in height by 3 months of age. At 5–6 months of age, infants have usually doubled their birth weight.

4. B. Typically, males age 13–18 will have developed to Tanner stage 5. An 18-year-old male that is in Tanner stage 4 should be evaluated for further growth and development deficits. Scoliosis of the spine of 10–15 degrees is generally not considered to be a problem unless the patient expressed concern or discomfort.

5. B. The child presents clinically with pneumonia. Viral pneumonia generally has a gradual onset with less acute symptoms and a low-grade fever. It is usually preceded by an upper respiratory infection. Wheezes are not present in children with pneumonia.

6. A. The absence of wheezing is a positive predictor for children with pneumonia.

7. D. All children with a diagnosis of pneumonia should be carefully monitored. The child has a classic viral pneumonia presentation, which tends to be less severe and can be cared for at home.

8. C. Children with croup will usually present with a brassy bark sounding cough, inspiratory stridor, and a steeple sign (or wineglass) appearance on a chest X-ray.

9. C. Streptococcus pneumonia is the most common organism responsible for otitis media. Amoxicillin remains the first choice of treatment for otitis media with a suspected bacterial etiology.

10. A. The child's symptoms are consistent with the prodromal phase of a viral or bacterial infection. Asking if there are sick contacts would provide the most valuable information at this point in time.

11. B. Although all infants are at risk for RSV, low birth weight infants, infants younger than 6 months of age, premature infants, and infants with an underlying condition such as heart or lung disease are at highest risk. By two years of age, almost all children will have had RSV.

12. B. The child has many risk factors associated with RSV, including a sibling in day care, along with the time of year. The child's clinical presentation is consistent with RSV bronchiolitis.

13. B. The child's symptoms are consistent with the diagnosis of moderate persistent asthma per the GINA (Global Initiative for Asthma) guidelines.

14. A. A child with mild persistent asthma should be using the stepwise approach to management. Per GINA guidelines, the child with mild persistent asthma should be using an inhaled low-dose corticosteroid to control symptoms.

15. C. Any child with unexplained bruises (especially in children who are not yet mobile) is required to have a full skeletal body scan.

16. C. According to the developmental theorist, Erikson, it is essential for an infant's needs to be met so they may develop trust in the world around them (Trust vs. Mistrust stage).

17. A. A neonate's normal gross motor skill development should include the ability to turn his/her head during the first month of life when placed in a prone position.

18. B. This is in accordance with the recommended vaccination schedule for children, as defined by the CDC.

19. B. Normal social development includes the ability for the infant to laugh and babble between the ages of 3 and 6 months. Infants that are not performing this behavior should be evaluated for further developmental delays.

20. B. This is the most common age for development of this gross motor skill.

21. D. Rice cereal is the least likely food to cause an allergic reaction in an infant and is generally considered to be the first recommended solid food.

22. A. Per CDC guidelines for childhood vaccinations.

23. C. Infants typically develop the pincer reflex at approximately 12 months of age. Anticipatory guidance includes teaching the parents that the child is at higher risk for choking/poisoning and putting foreign objects in their nares, mouth, or ears.

24. B. Grasping with the hands precedes the ability to perform more higher-level fine motor tasks such as throwing an object or intentionally releasing an object.

25. B. An infant is expected to double his/her body weight at 6 months of age.

26. C. The recommended form of discipline for a child is to use the "timeout" strategy. Most young children can sit in "timeout" for the same amount of minutes that is equal to what their age is in years.

27. C. Children are ready to toilet train when they are able to communicate their need and interest in doing so to their parents.

28. D. Young toddlers will often prefer to sit near other children when playing but typically their play is not associated with the other children.

29. A. Per U.S. national statistics, accidents remain the number one cause of death in children.

30. C. Egocentricity is commonly seen in toddlers as they develop a sense of self that is separate from their primary caregivers.

31. B. Erikson associated the second developmental stage to occur in toddlerhood and is closely tied to the child's ability to develop and accomplish tasks such as toilet training.

32. B. Most toddlers will prefer consistency and daily rituals to increase their sense of understanding of the world around them and promote a sense of security and belonging.

33. D. Children will often continue to have bed-wetting episodes during sleep for many months after they have achieved daytime dryness. Parents need to be educated that this is most likely not an intentional act by the child.

34. C. Three-year-olds may begin to demonstrate associative play. However, when placed in an unfamiliar environment, the child may revert to a more comfortable type of play, such as parallel play.

35. A. Patching the stronger eye reinforces connections between the brain and the weaker eye. Occlusion therapy has been the mainstay of treatment for amblyopia. The endpoint eye goal of occlusive therapy is equal visual acuity in both eyes. Once visual acuity has stabilized, patching may be decreased slowly and the child should be monitored for reoccurrence.

36. C. According to Erikson, the school-age child is in the industry versus inferiority stage. During this stage, children become capable of performing increasingly complex tasks. Children who are encouraged to complete tasks may develop feelings of self-confidence. Children that do not receive encouragement from parents, teachers, or peers will doubt their ability to be successful and will feel inferior to others their own age.

37. A. The child presents clinically with coxsackie virus. The mother should be reassured that the virus is self-limiting. Treatment is based on symptoms and the child should be monitored for any development of complications such as encephalitis.

38. C. The infant demonstrates a positive Ortolani's test and needs to be further evaluated for hip dysplasia.

39. C. Behavioral neuroscientists have speculated that the "pruning" of neurons that occurs in the prefrontal cortex occurs gradually over the period of time between childhood and adulthood. This "pruning" allows for greater control of behavior and less impulsivity and poor decision making.

40. C. Anorexia nervosa is a mental illness with a high mortality rate. The patient demonstrates an intense fear of weight gain, obsession with weight, and a persistent behavior to prevent weight gain. Most patients are unable to recognize or appreciate the severity of the situation even in the presence of severe starvation and impending death.

41. B. Using the APGAR rating scale, each of the five characteristics the neonate is demonstrating is assigned 1 point each. Therefore, the neonate would receive a score of 5.

42. C. A child with coarctation of the aorta will exhibit a higher blood pressure above the area of coarctation and a lower pressure below the area of coarctation. Occasionally, the arterial flow to the lower extremities can be severe enough to cause mottling.

43. A. In the case of tetralogy of Fallot, increasing systemic resistance will allow for increased blood flow through the pulmonary artery. A characteristic of infants and children with tetralogy of Fallot is to place themselves in a squatting position. Frequent squatting is a compensatory mechanism of diagnostic significance.

44. B. It is essential that the nurse practitioner can distinguish an innocent or functional murmur from the murmur of hypertrophic obstructive cardiomyopathy. While many of the characteristics are similar, a person with HCM will have an increase in the intensity of the murmur during both the Valsalva maneuver and when standing after squatting.

45. B. The child presents with symptoms of the measles. It would be essential for the NP to ascertain if the child has received the MMR and if the child missed any doses of the recommended schedule for vaccinations.

46. C. Physical exam often will reveal a palpable abdominal mass. The abdominal mass should be carefully examined. Palpating a mass too vigorously could lead to rupture of the Wilm's tumor into the peritoneal cavity.

47. A. The shunting of blood from an area of high pressure (left side of the heart) to an area of lower pressure (right side of the heart) occurs when there is an opening between the two sides that allows for a mixing of deoxygenated and oxygenated blood.

48. B. Transposition of the great arteries (TGA) is a cyanotic defect that is not conducive to survival unless the infant has at least one other heart defect that would allow for the mixing of oxygenated and deoxygenated blood.

49. D. The child has a classic presentation of parvovirus B19 (Fifth disease). The parents should be educated that it is a viral disease that requires only supportive therapy, while allowing the virus to run its course. The parents should also be told that the child may develop a rash on the trunk or back within a few days. Most adults are immune to the disease. However, pregnant woman should be cautioned to avoid exposure to a child with known parvovirus as it has been associated with spontaneous abortion in pregnant women that do not have immunity.

50. C. The child exhibits symptoms of a physiologic murmur with a classic presentation. The NP would continue to assess the murmur at each visit and could expect that the child will remain asymptomatic and eventually outgrow the condition.

● ● ● References

American Academy of Pediatrics (AAP) (2015). Bright futures. Accessed 11/15/15 at https://brightfutures.aap.org/materials-and-tools/tool-and-resource-kit/Pages/default.aspx

Botash, A. (2015). Child abuse evaluation and treatment for medical providers. Retrieved from http://www.childabusemd.com

Burns, C. E., Dunn, A. M., Brady, M. A., Starr, N. B., & Blosser, C. G. (2013). *Pediatric Primary Care* (5th ed.). Philadelphia, PA: Elsevier.

Carolan, P. (April, 2015). Pediatric bronchitis. *Medscape*. Retrieved from http://emedicine.medscape.com/article/1001332-medication#showall

CDC. (2015). Facts about developmental disabilities. Retrieved from http://www.cdc.gov/ncbddd/developmental disabilities/facts.html

CDC. (2015). About child and teen BMI. Retrieved from http://www.cdc.gov/healthyweight/assessing/bmi/childrens_bmi/about_childrens_bmi.html

CDC. (2015). Birth–18 years and "catch-up" immunization schedules, United States, 2015. Retrieved from http://www.cdc.gov/vaccines/schedules/hcp/child-adolescent.html#printable

CDC. (2015). Parvovirus B19 and Fifth disease. Retrieved from http://www.cdc.gov/parvovirusb19/fifth-disease.html

CDC. (2015). Respiratory syncytial virus: For health professionals. Retrieved from http://www.cdc.gov/rsv/clinical/

Chumlea, W. C., Schubert, C. M., Roche A. F., Kulin, H. E., Lee, P. A., Himes, J. H., & Sun, S. S. (2003). Age at menarche and racial comparisons in U.S. girls. *Pediatrics*, *111*(1), 110–113.

Global Initiative for Asthma. (2015). A Guide for Healthcare Professionals: Based on the Global Strategy for Asthma Management and Prevention.

Haines, C., Soon, A., & Mercurio, D. (2013). Community acquired pneumonia in pediatric populations. *Emergency Medicine Reports*, *34*(17), 197–207.

Seto, C. (2011). The preparticipation physical exam. *Clinical Sports Medicine, 30*, 491–501. doi:10.1016/j.csm.2011.03.008

U.S. Department of Health and Human Services; Administration for Children and Families; Administration on Children, Youth and Families; Children's Bureau. (2013). *Child maltreatment 2013*. Retrieved from http://www.acf.hhs.gov/programs/cb/research-data-technology/statistics-research/child-maltreatment

World Health Organization (WHO). (2014). *Pneumonia fact sheet*. Retrieved from http://www.who.int/mediacentre/factsheets/fs331/en/

CHAPTER

17

Women's Health

Pennie Sessler Branden, PhD, CNM, RN

Definition of Women's Health

The absence of illness and the presence of physical and mental well-being in women from puberty to menopause.

GYN Issues/Conditions

Intimate Partner Violence (IPV)

- Intimate partner violence is the cause of the highest number of female homicides in the United States.
- Women are most frequently assaulted by someone they know, such as a spouse/partner, family member, or friend.
- IPV frequently escalates with a pregnancy.
- IPV is the cause of multiple short- and long-term health issues, therefore causing undue suffering of women in physical and emotional ways.

  Sexual preferences and identification must be recognized and the woman must be counseled about her sexual identity and preferences in order to completely and accurately address any health issues frequently seen in those groups. Careful assessment of each woman is integral to good health care.

Sexual Behaviors

Each woman needs to be assessed for risk-taking behaviors, multiple partners, and partners who have multiple partners, all of which can put the woman at higher risk for acute and chronic health problems.

- Heterosexual women may have issues regarding STIs, IPV, etc.
- Lesbian women have higher numbers of alcohol and drug abuse, as well as depression, than do heterosexual women.

Contraception/Family Planning

In GYN and postpartum

- Accurate and complete assessment of what the woman desires to use as a contraceptive method must be done.
- Does she have other risk factors that may preclude her from using a certain type of contraceptive method?

Hormonal Methods

- Advantages: many woman prefer this to reduce their menstrual flow each month; relieves PMS symptoms; can resume ovulation within one month of discontinuing use of hormanal method
- Disadvantages: does not protect a woman from STIs; may have side effects such as severe headache and hypertension, increased risk of DVT, and stroke if woman smokes or has a history of DVT
- Depo-Provera is an injectable hormonal contraceptive. It is given intramuscularly every three months.

- Oral contraceptive pills (OCs) are to be taken each day at the same time in order to effect the best possible coverage to reduce ovulation activity. The type of OCP is to be evaluated based on the woman's history and previous use if applicable.

- A transdermal contraceptive patch (Ortho-Evra) is a thin, flexible patch that is effective for 7 days, and the woman will use each patch for 7 days and replace it weekly for three weeks. In the fourth week of her cycle, she goes without a patch for 7 days and her menses occurs.

- Vaginal contraceptive ring (NuvaRing) is a transparent, flexible ring of a polymer that is infused with etonogestrol. The ring is inserted vaginally for 21 days and removed for a one week ring-free period, when the woman will have her menses.

Barrier Methods

- Condoms: male and female
  - Advantages: convenient; relatively inexpensive; able to purchase without a health care practitioner's prescription; offers protection from STIs
  - Disadvantages: may interrupt foreplay; can cause irritation if have a latex allergy; must be applied and removed correctly to prevent spilling of semen into vagina

- Diaphragm, Cervical cap, Sponges: devices inserted into the woman's vagina before intercourse that may be left in with multiple incidents of intercourse if more spermicide is applied.
  - Advantages: only used with intercourse; no hormones involved; more effective if used with spermicide; can offer protection from STIs
  - Disadvantages: need to be fitted by an HCP and refitted if patient loses or gains >10–15 pounds; FNP needs to assess the proper insertion of each of these in the office before the patient begins using it; need to insert more spermicide with repeated intercourse up to 24 hours; need to leave in place for at least 6 hours after last intercourse; cannot be used by women with poor vaginal tone

Intrauterine Device (IUD)

A small device inserted into the uterus through the cervix by a trained HCP. A negative pregnancy test and the absence of STIs must all be confirmed before this insertion.

- Advantages: long-term protection from pregnancy; immediate return to fertility upon removal of the IUD

- Disadvantages: needs to be inserted by an HCP; increased risk of STIs if woman has multiple partners or her partner has multiple partners; possible unintentional expulsion of IUD; potential perforation of uterus when inserted

Abstinence

Not having sexual intercourse.

- Total abstinence will reduce the occurrence of STIs and pregnancy if abstaining all the time.

- Natural family planning is abstinence when the woman ovulates, which is also called *family awareness-based* methods. There are a number of different types of this method when the woman checks her cervical mucus, her temperature each day before rising, and abstains when these things point to her ovulation time. Counseling about the 72-hour viability of the sperm is important to teach the woman because if she is sexually active 2–3 days before she ovulates, she could become pregnant.

Sterilization

Sterilization of the woman or her male partner(s) is a surgical procedure rendering the woman or man incapable of getting pregnant or assisting a woman to get pregnant. These procedures—bilateral tubal ligation for the woman and a vasectomy for a man—are permanent surgical procedures. Careful education and counseling must be done by the FNP in order to make sure the woman and her partner are absolutely certain they want this permanent procedure. Referral to a physician who does these procedures must be done

Menses and Menstrual Cycle Conditions

Amenorrhea is the absence of menstrual bleeding. Accurate history taking is vital to a complete picture of what is happening with the woman and her menstrual cycles. She should be encouraged to keep a journal of her menstrual cycles, their onset, length, and amount of bleeding. Depending on the type and timing of the amenorrhea, counseling and education are important for the woman to better understand what is happening with her body.

- Primary amenorrhea "is the failure of menses to occur by age 16 years, in the presence of normal growth and secondary sexual characteristics. If by age 13, menses has not occurred and the onset of puberty, such as breast development, is absent, a workup for **primary amenorrhea** should start."

- Secondary amenorrhea "is defined as the cessation of menses sometime after menarche has occurred."

Uterine Bleeding

Normal bleeding occurs with menses every 26–40 days and the woman generally knows her cycle length and amount of bleeding. No two women are alike and each has a unique picture of her cycles.

Abnormal bleeding can occur from a number of things. Again, it is important to get a complete and accurate assessment and history of the bleeding and its timing, amount, etc. This bleeding can be between menses, excessive bleeding, or postmenopausal bleeding.

- Post-coital bleeding may indicate a friable cervix secondary to vaginal infections and/or STIs. A Pap test and cervical cultures must be done to rule out STIs, cervical inflammation.

- Bleeding after a positive pregnancy test could indicate a spontaneous abortion (a.k.a., miscarriage). The FNP needs to evaluate this by testing the woman's blood with serial Beta-hCGs to see if the level is increasing and doubling every 48 hours. If it is not, it could indicate a spontaneous loss (SAB) or ectopic pregnancy. (See B-hCG under pregnancy diagnosis.)

- Bleeding after menopause could indicate endometrial cancer and needs to be followed up with an endometrial biopsy to rule out abnormalities.

Puberty "is the period of human development during which physical growth and sexual maturation occurs."

Perimenopause is the "time in a woman's life when physiological changes occur that begin the transition to menopause." Anticipatory guidance for the changes that will occur are necessary.

Menopause "is the time when there have been no menstrual periods for 12 consecutive months". Clearly this is assessed retrospectively after the woman has not had a menstrual cycle for a full year. Hormone replacement therapy that includes estrogen only, progesterone only, or estrogen/progesterone combined, may be indicated and/or desired for and by the woman to relieve discomforts accompanying menopause, such as vaginal dryness and decreased vaginal stretching with intercourse. HRT may be contraindicated in women with heart disease or diabetes. The FNP needs to do a complete risk assessment on these women.

Breast Abnormalities/Conditions

Nipple discharge can be from physiologic or pharmacologic causes. Physiologic include breastfeeding, combined oral contraceptive use, nipple piercing, or cloudy appearance in premenopausal women. Pharmacologic causes include estrogen products, metoclopramide, SSRIs, TCAs. Diagnosis: prolactin levels, CBC, TSH, cytology of breast discharge, mammogram. Refer as needed for surgery and educate patient about breast care.

Fibrocystic breast changes a common noncancerous breast condition occurring in one or both breasts and generally occurring in women of childbearing age. Diagnosis breast exam for lumpy, slightly painful breasts one to two weeks before menses; diagnostic mammogram or breast ultrasound; refer for needle biopsy as appropriate. Treatment is symptomatic with NSAIDs for discomfort, supportive bra, and decreased caffeine intake; use OCPs with low estrogen content and activity.

Breast Infections

Mastitis is a painful localized inflammation of the breast generally from a clogged duct or a bacterial infection such as *staphylococcus*. It presents with a streak of redness, pain and localized tenderness in the breast, with fever, chills, and malaise. If nursing, do not stop breastfeeding; apply warmth and hand express the area to increase passing of milk and decreasing clogged ducts. Treated with antibiotics such as cephalexin 500 mg po tid (by mouth three times day) or dicloxacillin 500 mg po qid (by mouth four times a day) for 10 days. Ibuprofen for pain and antipyretic effects every 4–6 hours.

Mammography as per the American Cancer Society should be offered to women 40–44 years of age to begin annual mammography; women ages 45–54 should have annual mammograms; women 55 and older should switch to every 1–2 years. Screenings should continue on this schedule as long as woman is healthy. However, if she has a personal history or a family history of breast abnormalities, she should be encouraged to continue annual mammograms. Education from and discussion with the FNP is an invaluable resource for women.

Vulva, Vagina, and Cervix Conditions

- **Atrophic vaginitis** is an inflammation, drying, and thinning of the vaginal walls caused by decreased estrogen levels. Happens most frequently after menopause and at times during breastfeeding. Symptoms include dyspareunia, vaginal burning, dryness, and discharge; decreased vaginal lubrication. Treat with a vaginal moisturizer such as Vagisil or Replens.

- **Vulvitis** is an allergic or inflammatory reaction of vulvar tissue. Symptoms include vulvar itching and/or burning; excoriation of vulva, scaly thickened white patches. Treatment is to discourage tight clothing, urge sitz baths to decrease itching, apply topical estrogen cream and water-based vaginal lubricants.

Uterine and Ovarian Abnormalities

- **Ovarian cyst** is a follicular sac that does not open or dissolve after ovulation. The cyst accumulates fluid, forming the cyst. Symptoms may include dyspareunia, breast tenderness, lower back pain, pelvic pain during menses. Treatment can include oral contraceptives that will stop ovulation and decrease incidence of cysts forming or possible laparoscopy to remove the cyst.
- **Uterine fibroids** are non-cancerous growths of uterus that cause the uterus to be irregularly shaped. They will not convert to cancerous tumors.
- **Polycystic Ovarian Syndrome (PCOS)** is a hormonal disorder in which the estrogen and progesterone level are imbalanced. This condition decreases fertility and menses, can increase potential cardiac disorders, and causes problems with appearance being more masculine due to overproduction of androgen.
- Diagnosis includes thyroid function tests, fasting glucose tests, and lipid level assessments. Treatment is determined by the various levels of hormonal differences and whether or not the woman wants to become pregnant.

Group B-Streptococcus (GBS)

Can be considered normal vaginal flora of a woman when she is not pregnant. However, in pregnancy a positive GBS is correlated with poor outcomes because they can increase the neonatal morbidity and mortality. In pregnancy, a woman is tested for GBS sometime after 35 weeks gestation. If she is positive, she will be treated with antibiotics at the onset of her labor. This treatment has been found to reduce the incidence of neonatal respiratory distress syndrome.

Patient education is specific to the condition and the medication being used. It is important to empower the woman to increase self-care as needed and desired.

OB Care Specific to the FNP

Frequently, pregnancy is the woman's entry into the health care system. She may also bring her children and family to the health care system at this time. Therefore, timely, accurate, and compassionate care are integral to facilitating their entry into, and their desire to remain in, the health care system.

Goals of Prenatal Care

1. Accurate dating of gestational age
2. Education about pregnancy and infant care
3. Advice on how to reduce risks; screening and risk assessment
4. Treatment of medical conditions throughout pregnancy
5. Ultimately, the delivery of a healthy infant and having a healthy mother

Barriers to Prenatal Care

1. Poor socioeconomic status with cost of health care; transportation to see FNP; loss of work time and income due to appointments
2. Poor health behaviors
3. Poor attitudes of health care provider with biases and prejudices
4. Maternal barriers including lack of understanding of need for prenatal care; no assistance with other children; poor accessibility to clinic and its hours of operation
5. Lack of support of woman by partner and family

Initial Antepartum Visit
History

- ID Information (make sure you have current address and way to contact woman)
- Chief complaint
- History of present illness (HPI) if any, and general review of systems (ROS)
- Cultural considerations
- Family history
- Client medical history
- Client surgical history
- Gynecologic history
- Obstetric history with number of pregnancies using G-TPAL system
- History of habits and risk-taking behavior(s)
- Vaccination history
- Occupational history

- Intimate partner violence (IPV): Does she feel safe in her home? It may take multiple encounters with a woman for her to trust the FNP sufficiently enough to divulge this information.

The **first prenatal physical exam** should include a complete physical assessment including vital signs, height, weight, cardiac, lung and abdominal exams, pelvic and rectal exams, and assessment of extremities for varicosities, Homan's sign, and edema.

Diagnosis of Pregnancy

Diagnosis of pregnancy is generally done with a set of data or compilation of signs and symptoms of pregnancy that assist the practitioner in concluding the woman is pregnant. These include the following:

- Last menstrual period (LMP) is determined by the first day of the last normal menses.

- Naegele's rule is a simple calculation by which the practitioner can determine the woman's estimated date of delivery (EDD). This calculation is: First day of LMP + 7 days − three months + one year = EDD: OR first day of LMP + 7 days + 9 months.

- Uterine sizing as described in table in the next page.

- Ultrasonography is most accurate the earlier in the pregnancy it is performed. The later in the pregnancy it is done, it can be less accurate as a starting point. However, serial ultrasounds can assist the practitioner in more closely watching the fetal growth.

- There are maternal signs and symptoms that can assist the practitioner in diagnosing a pregnancy as well. Please see "Signs and Symptoms of Pregnancy" later in this text.

- Pregnancy tests: There are a number of accurate home pregnancy urine tests that a woman can use to determine if she is pregnant. These ELISA (enzyme linked immunosorbent assays) can detect pregnancy 1 week after fertilization of ovum. These need to be done accurately and following the instructions closely because there can be false positives and negatives depending upon how they were performed.

- Beta-Human Chorionic Gonadotropin (Beta-hCG) is the hormone that is the earliest biologic marker measured in pregnancy blood tests. Its presence is due to the placenta producing it.

- The hCG concentration doubles every 29 to 53 hours during the first 30 days after conception in a viable, intrauterine pregnancy.

- Serum hCG reaches peak concentrations of 100,000 IU/L at 8 to 10 weeks after the last menstrual period.

- Concentrations start to decrease after week 12 and stay fairly constant at approximately 30,000 IU/L from about the 20th week until term.

Prenatal Care Visit Schedule

Pre-conceptual care is very important, especially if the woman has concurrent health and social issues. Optimally, all women should have pre-conceptual care in order to assess the potential problems and challenges that they may have in pregnancy and to stabilize any medical conditions they may have before conceiving. Referral to other health care professionals should be made in an interprofessional collaborative manner.

Prenatal Care Visits

First prenatal visit should be done as soon as possible after woman suspects she may be pregnant.

Return prenatal visits*:

Every 4 weeks until 28–30 weeks gestation
Every 2 weeks until 36 weeks gestation
Every 1 week until delivery

*These return visits can be adjusted and changed at the discretion of the FNP based on maternal and fetal needs.

Normal Pregnancy Findings

Maternal

Weight Gain and BMI

Weight gain in pregnancy is determined by the starting weight of a woman when she becomes pregnant and her Basal Metabolic Index (BMI). If the woman is underweight with a BMI of < 18.5, she may gain 28–40 lbs. Conversely, if the woman is overweight (BMI of 25.0–29.9) or obese as determined by weight and BMI ≥ 30.0, she may lose weight if she is eating more healthily in pregnancy.

Generally speaking, the recommended weight gain for a women of a normal weight is 25–35 depending on pre-pregnant weight and a BMI of 18.5–24.9. These calculations are done assuming a 1.1–4.4 lbs. (0.5 to 2 kg) weight gain in the first trimester.

Nutritional requirements during pregnancy range from 2200–2900 kcal/day and protein intake increases of 60–75 g/day.

This weight gain can be achieved with the following simple guidelines for increases in a daily healthy diet:

- An extra 300 calories/day (during the second and third trimesters)

- A minimum of 60 g of protein/day (For a teen: 75–80)

- 4 servings of calcium daily (1000 mg)
- Limit artificial sweeteners to 1–2/day
- Limit caffeine: This includes coffee, black tea, caffeinated beverages (e.g., soda, energy drinks, etc.)
- Increase water intake

Vital Signs

Vital signs do change throughout pregnancy depending on the woman's health status and her pre-pregnant vital signs. It is important to note for each visit how the woman's vital signs trend and to assess if there is a change in the pattern at any given time.

Temperature may be a high normal of 99.2 to 99.6.

Pulse may be elevated by 10–15 bpm.

Respiratory rate increases up to 15% later in pregnancy due to pressure of uterus on diaphragm.

Blood pressure decreases in second trimester, then returns to pre-pregnancy levels.

Signs and Symptoms of Pregnancy: Presumptive, Probable, Positive

Presumptive are those subjective symptoms reported by the woman:

Nausea, vomiting, amenorrhea, breast tenderness and enlargement, fatigue, quickening, urinary frequency

Probable are those objective physiologic and anatomic changes noted by the practitioner:

Abdominal enlargement, ballottement, Braxton–Hicks contractions, Chadwick's sign, Hegar's sign, palpation of fetal parts, positive pregnancy test, uterine enlargement, skin hyperpigmentation (e.g., chloasma, linea nigra)

Positive signs and symptoms are those attributed to the presence of the fetus

Fetal outline and/or movement felt by practitioner

Fetal heart rate heard: at 10–12 weeks with a Doppler, at 20 weeks with a fetascope

Embryo/fetus seen on ultrasound

Uterine Sizing

There are landmarks for uterine growth that can be used to assess gestational age, gestational size, and adequate vs. inadequate uterine growth. What is important is that the woman has consistent and steady growth throughout her pregnancy.

Before 12 weeks gestation, the uterus needs to be assessed for size and position by doing a bimanual pelvic exam. At 12 weeks gestation, the fundus can be felt at the rim of the symphysis pubis. After 12 weeks gestation, the uterus can be measured from the symphysis pubis to the fundus. Sufficient growth is equal to one cm of growth for each week of gestation (e.g., for a 25-week gestation, the fundus would measure 25 cm).

Gestational Age in Weeks	Uterine Shape	Uterine Size
6 weeks	Slightly globular shape with isthmus softening	Lime
8 weeks	Globular shape with some irregularity	Lemon
10 weeks	Globular shape	Orange
12 weeks	Uterine fundus at pelvic brim above symphysis pubis	Medium grapefruit
16 weeks	16 cm, fundus midway between symphysis pubis and umbilicus	
20 weeks	20 cm, fundus approx. at umbilicus	
24 weeks	24 cm, fundus 2 FB above umbilicus	
28–30 weeks	Fundus 1/3 way between umbilicus and xyphoid process	
36–38 weeks	Fundus 1 FB below xyphoid process	
40 weeks	40 cm, at or 2–3 FB below xyphoid process	

Laboratory Tests at First Prenatal Visit

- Pap smear and wet smear
- Vaginal/cervical cultures: GC, Chlamydia, GBS
- Blood type/Rh
- CBC with differential and red cell indices to assess for types of anemias.
- Antibody screen/antibody titer at initial visit and 28 weeks gestation visit
- Sickle Cell prep
- VDRL, RPR, or STS
- Hepatitis B surface antigen
- Rubella titer
- Varicella antibody screen (if woman denies previous infection)
- U/A, C and S

Laboratory Tests to Be Offered to All Women

- HIV testing and counseling at first prenatal visit and at 35–37 weeks as indicated
- TB screening indicated for high-risk populations
- Quad Screen at 15–20 weeks: measures maternal serum Alpha-Fetoprotein (AFP), hCG, unconjugated estriol, and inhibin A
- Screening ultrasound after first prenatal visit
- GCT, 1 hour at 26–28 wks
- GBS, GC, Chlamydia screening at 35–37 wks
- Repeat H/H at 28 wks and as needed at 35–37 wks
- Other labs depending on practice and needs for pt (patient)-specific situation

Laboratory Tests to Consider as Appropriate

- Urine culture if signs and symptoms of UTI, cystitis, pyelonephritis
- Herpes culture
- Urine drug screen(s) if history of drug use
- GTT, 3 hr if GCT is elevated, history of GDM, BMI > 35 or baby 1 lb larger than previous one
- Pre-eclampsia labs:
  - Blood tests: H/H, platelets, creatinine, uric acid, AST
  - Urine for 24-hour protein
- Genetic testing as indicated by maternal history, maternal age, or maternal family history. May include quad-screening, chorionic villus sampling (CVS) at 10–13 weeks, or amniocentesis at 15–18 weeks.

Group B-Streptococcus (GBS)

All pregnant women should be screened for group B-streptococcus colonization with swabs of both the lower vagina and rectum at 35 to 37 weeks of gestation. If this culture is positive or if patient has GBS bacteria in the urine during pregnancy, she will be treated with antibiotics in labor to prevent the potential for neonatal pneumonia.

Common complaints by the mother include body changes that occur with pregnancy and can be generally attributed to hormonal or physical changes. They include but may not be limited to: fatigue, constipation, leukorrhea, nausea and vomiting, pigmentation changes of skin, supine hypotension, food cravings, heartburn, constipation, varicose veins, headaches, shortness of breath, ankle edema, and leg cramps. Treatment of these is to identify the maternal concerns and educate her about the normalcy of these things. Give her information to address each of these things on her own.

Embryo/Fetus

- Fetal heart rate (FHR) at 12 weeks with Doppler; FHR at 20 weeks with fetascope
- Quickening at 16 weeks in multigravida and 20 weeks in primigravida

Teratogenicity affects the embryo and fetus most dramatically during the periods of rapid cell division, especially during weeks 3–16 gestation. Avoidance of these substances and environments will decrease the chances of teratogenic activities affecting the fetus.

Drug use and its implications: Any medications taken as prescribed, over the counter, or illegally, need to be assessed and addressed appropriately. Teratogenic activity while using any medication or drug needs to be considered and assessed via ultrasound testing. Certain street drugs can cause the fetus to be dependent upon the drug, meaning the infant may need to be detoxed after birth.

Education for initial prenatal visit should include: anticipatory teaching of what to expect with pregnancy, visits, etc.; nutritional guidance, sexuality, and contraceptive methods; choice of newborn nutrition. Also, appropriate follow-up and referrals must be made as appropriate.

Return prenatal visits are done as described to follow the woman's course of pregnancy and the fetus's growth pattern. Woman to take one prenatal vitamin daily with the addition of folic acid 400–800 mg by mouth daily to reduce neural tube abnormalities of the fetus.

At each return visit, evaluate vital signs, urine for protein, ketones and glucose, weight, fetal heart rate, fetal presentation and activity, fundal height measurement. At 36, 38, and 40 weeks, depending on the practice, a cervical exam may be indicated.

Education for return prenatal visits is generally personalized for the woman based on her weeks of gestation (e.g., fetal growth, maternal weight gain, etc.), normal signs and symptoms of pregnancy, any questions she and/or partner might have concerning findings from the labs, etc. Discussion of course of normal pregnancy and community resources available.

Abnormal Pregnancy Findings

GDM diagnosis and treatment: Screening GCT with 50 gram glucose load at 24–28 weeks → if > 95, then do a GTT for three hours after 100 grams glucose load → two or more values elevated = GDM.

Large for gestational age (LGA) vs. small for gestational age (SGA): diagnosis and findings, then testing and follow-up

LGA

Incorrect dates, polyhydramnios, multiple fetuses, full maternal bladder, LGA infant secondary to maternal GDM. LGA requires referral to MD for confirmation of and management of woman's prenatal care.

SGA

Incorrect dates, oligohydramnios, placental insufficiency, poor maternal weight gain/malnourishment; SROM, maternal illicit drug abuse. SGA requires referral to MD for confirmation of and management of woman's prenatal care.

Testing and diagnosis include using the data collected with the woman's exams and her trending. Ultrasounds can be done to assess fetal growth, fluid volume, and fetal movement. Biophysical profile can be done to assess; includes ultrasound assessment of fetal tone, fetal breathing movements, fetal movements, amniotic fluid index, in conjunction with a non-stress test. Each category is scored with a 2 or a 0. Any score of 6 or below is suspect of chronic asphyxia and needs further follow-up.

- **Abnormal lab values:** diagnosis, treatment and follow-up: CBC, type and Rh, AFP, anemia, positive urine C&S, proteinuria/glucosuria/ketonuria, ultrasound
- Vaginal bleeding and differential diagnoses: placenta previa vs. placental abruption vs. friable cervix
- Woman reports decreased fetal movement after doing daily fetal movement counts; check fetal heart rate and do a non-stress test to evaluate fetal heart rate patterns. Want a reactive test. If non-reactive, then do a contraction stress test (CST). With a CST, look for negative results, indicating no late decelerations are seen.

Diagnosis of Spontaneous Abortion/Miscarriage (SAB)

Bloodwork of B-hCG not doubling every 48 hours; visualization of cervix and vagina to note any fetal tissue seen; patient reports passing a sac-like material after having lower back ache and/or cramping and bleeding.

Labor Diagnosis

True vs. False labor: The FNP needs to be able to determine true versus false labor.

- **False:** Contractions are irregular and may stop with walking; felt in back or abdomen; can often be stopped using comfort measures. Cervix does not dilate or efface.

- **True:** Contractions are regular and get stronger and closer together; increasingly strong with walking; felt in lower back that extend around to the front of the abdomen; do not abate with comfort measures. Cervix shows progressive dilation and effacement.

Term after 37 weeks 6 days to delivery.

Preterm before the completion of 37 weeks gestation.

Medical Issues Complicating Pregnancy

Any medical illness can complicate pregnancy and should be managed with an interprofessional team. All medications used prior to pregnancy need to be assessed for levels of teratogenicity and safety to the fetus. However, a risk/benefits assessment must be utilized to ensure maternal health while using various medications.

FDA Classification System of Medication Use during Pregnancy

A: Safe after multiple studies that failed to show a risk to the fetus in the first trimester

B: Caution advised because no adequate studies have been done in pregnant women (e.g., prenatal vitamins, Tylenol)

C: Animal studies show adverse fetal effects but no controlled human studies OR no controlled human or animal studies. To be used only if benefits outweigh the risks.

D: Positive evidence that human fetal risk/maternal benefit may outweigh fetal risk in serious or life-threatening situations; some significant risks associated.

X: Always contraindicated unless using the medication outweighs the risks because animal or human studies have found evidence of human fetal risk.

Hypertension Has a Number of Different Classifications in Pregnancy

Chronic hypertension is defined as hypertension that occurred before pregnancy.

Gestational hypertension begins with pregnancy and is *without* proteinuria. Hypertension is > 140 systolic and/or > 90 mm Hg diastolic.

Pre-eclampsia is pregnancy specific, where hypertension and proteinuria develop after 20 weeks gestation. Cure of pre-eclampsia is delivery of fetus.

Diabetes is the most common endocrine disorder associated with pregnancy. Pregnancy will complicate the need for insulin and make the pregnancy high risk. These women should be cared for by an interdisciplinary professional team.

Asthma causing inadequate oxygenation of mother and fetus. Some women have an improvement of asthma when pregnant, while others have increased severity and frequency of asthma attacks.

Medications used for asthma can cause maternal tachycardia and irritability.

Patient Education

Warning signs, normal expectations, plans for delivery/adoption/etc.

Review Questions

1. A woman at 38 weeks gestation has been setting up her baby's nursery over the weekend. This was done with a lot of bending and lifting. Today, which is Tuesday, she calls the FNP's office to get clearance to use ibuprofen for body aches. She denies fever or chills but "complains of sore muscles." The FNP advises her against using ibuprofen because ibuprofen is what?

   A. Pregnancy category A drug

   B. Pregnancy category B drug

   C. Pregnancy category C drug

   D. Pregnancy category X drug

2. A 15-year-old adolescent who is 12 weeks pregnant with her first child comes for a prenatal visit. The FNP notes that the adolescent had been taking Ortho Tri-cyclen 28 for acne. Upon questioning, the adolescent reports that "I only took the medication when my acne was really bad. I want to continue it because my skin has had a bad breakout for the past month." The FNP's best response is:

   A. "Feel free to continue the Ortho Tri-cyclen 28 as it will help your acne."

   B. "Do not continue the Ortho Tri-cyclen because it won't help reduce your acne during pregnancy."

   C. "Ortho Tri-cyclen 28 should not be taken during pregnancy because it can affect the baby's development."

   D. "Ortho Tri-cyclen 28 should not be taken during pregnancy because it can increase your incidence of morning sickness."

3. A woman reports having her last menstrual period on August 13. The FNP knows that using Naegele's rule will give this woman an estimated due date of which of the following?

   A. May 20

   B. May 6

   C. November 20

   D. November 6

4. A woman comes to the FNP for her second prenatal exam. The FNP knows that the woman, by her dates, is 16 weeks gestation. When the FNP measures the fundal height, she gets 16 cm. This is which of the following?

   A. Too small for dates

   B. Too large for dates

   C. Exactly correct size for dates

   D. Possible sign of more than one fetus

5. A woman at 25 weeks gestation reports to the FNP that after intercourse she had bright red bleeding that lasted for a few hours, soaking one peripad. She denies pain, cramps, or other problems. The FNP knows that this is an indication for what type of testing?

   A. Ultrasound

   B. CBC

   C. Estimated fetal weight

   D. Cervical culture

6. A woman at 25 weeks gestation reports to the FNP that after intercourse she had bright red bleeding that lasted for a few hours soaking one peripad. She denies pain, cramps, or other problems and asks what could have caused this bleeding. The FNP's best response is which of the following?

   A. "Bleeding after intercourse is a normal finding. Don't worry about it."

   B. "Vaginal bleeding occurs during transition in labor."

C. "Having painless vaginal bleeding can be a troublesome sign."

D. "Having painless vaginal bleeding is a sign that labor is imminent."

7. A woman at 25 weeks gestation reports to the FNP that after intercourse she had bright red bleeding that lasted for a few hours, soaking one peripad. She denies pain, cramps, or other problems. The FNP knows that these are signs of which of the following?

A. A placental abruption

B. A friable cervix

C. A placenta previa

D. A sexually transmitted infection

8. A woman at 25 weeks gestation reports to the FNP that after intercourse she had bright red bleeding that lasted for a few hours, soaking one peripad. She denies pain, cramps, or other problems. The FNP knows that management of this situation includes which of the following? (Choose all that apply.)

A. Putting the woman on bedrest as appropriate

B. Assessing fetal well-being

C. Allowing the woman to continue sexual intercourse

D. Having an ultrasound done to assess the placental abruption

E. Having an ultrasound done to assess the placental location

9. A woman comes to the FNP for her fifth prenatal visit and is 34 weeks by dates and size. She shares with the FNP that she is afraid to be alone at home with her partner. The best response from the FNP would be which of the following?

A. "He doesn't hit you does he?"

B. "Many women feel that way at this point in their pregnancies."

C. "Would you like to tell me more about this?"

D. "That is silly since he is the father of your baby."

10. A woman comes for her first prenatal visit and reports she has a three-year-old with spina bifida. The FNP knows that this is a neural tube problem and decides to put the woman on folic acid daily. This is done to:

A. Reduce the chances of a neural tube defect in this pregnancy.

B. Increase the risk of neural tube defects.

C. Increase the woman's hematocrit.

D. Decrease the woman's hematocrit.

11. A woman comes to her prenatal visit at 38 weeks gestation reporting regular fetal movement until this morning. She reports that she has not felt the baby move since last night. She reports having a full breakfast today as well. The FNP's priority action is to do which of the following?

A. Calm the woman with soothing words.

B. Take the woman's vital signs.

C. Listen to the fetal heart rate with a Doppler.

D. Measure the woman's fundal height.

12. An adolescent girl comes to the FNP with vesicular lesions around her vaginal introitus that burn and hurt. She reports having intercourse with her boyfriend two weeks before. The FNP knows that this is a primary case of which of the following?

A. Genital Chlamydia

B. Genital herpes

C. Vulvovaginitis

D. Monilia

13. A 57-year-old woman who went through menopause 6 years ago comes to see the FNP today. She tells the FNP that she has been having vaginal bleeding for the last 5 days. She denies intercourse in the past few weeks. The FNP decides to look into this further by ordering which of the following tests?

    A. Uterine ultrasound

    B. Complete blood count to rule out anemia

    C. An endometrial biopsy

    D. A mammogram

14. A woman comes to the FNP for her first prenatal appointment. By her dates and LMP, the FNP believes her to be 12 weeks gestation. The FNP is able to assess the uterine size and finds it to be consistent with the woman's dates at what size/location?

    A. Uterine size of a lemon

    B. Uterine size of a baseball

    C. Uterine fundus at umbilicus

    D. Uterine fundus at symphysis pubis

15. The best time for the genetic assessment of an Alpha-fetoprotein (AFP) screening test is which of the following?

    A. 12–14 weeks gestation

    B. 16–18 weeks gestation

    C. 22–24 weeks gestation

    D. 28–30 weeks gestation

16. The FNP is caring for a pregnant women who reports her obstetric history as having three children, all of whom are living. One was born at 39 weeks gestation, another at 34 weeks gestation, and another at 35 weeks gestation. How will the FNP document the patient's gravity and parity using the G-TPAL system?

    A. G3 1-2-0-3

    B. G3 0-3-0-3

    C. G4 1-1-1-3

    D. G4 1-2-0-3

17. The FNP is caring for a woman in the prenatal clinical who is in her sixth week of pregnancy. The patient reports urinary frequency and asks if this will continue throughout the pregnancy. Which response by the FNP is MOST accurate?

    A. "If you decrease your fluid intake, the problem will be less bothersome."

    B. "Urinary frequency persists until the 12th week, but it may continue if you have poor bladder tone."

    C. "It is difficult to predict how long this will last for individuals."

    D. "This may last until the 12th week of your pregnancy but will be alleviated as your due date approaches."

18. A 28-year-old woman who is eight weeks pregnant comes to see the FNP with complaints of nausea, vomiting, and frequent urination. Based on this information, the FNP knows these are most indicative of which signs of pregnancy?

    A. Presumptive signs of pregnancy

    B. Positive signs of pregnancy

    C. Probable signs of pregnancy

    D. Signs of a urinary tract infection

19. A woman returns for her second prenatal visit at 14 weeks gestation. The FNP measures her fundal height at the woman's umbilicus. The FNP will order which diagnostic test to assess the situation?

    A. Amniocentesis to assess for fetal genetic abnormality

    B. GCT to assess for gestational diabetes

    C. Maternal serum AFP to assess for Down syndrome

    D. Ultrasound to assess for number of fetuses

20. The nurse practitioner is working in an outpatient obstetric office and assesses four primigravida clients. Which of the following client findings would the nurse prioritize for a potential referral?

    A. 17 weeks gestation; denies feeling fetal movement

    B. 24 weeks gestation; fundal height at umbilicus

    C. 27 weeks gestation; complaints of excessive salivation

    D. 34 weeks gestation; complaints of hemorrhoid pain

21. Susan comes to the FNP for her first prenatal appointment with this pregnancy. Using Naegele's rule and the woman's last menstrual period date, the FNP determines she is 12 weeks gestation. Susan reports previous pregnancies, and the FNP documents them as G3 T-1, P-1, A-0, L-1. She reports having a fetal demise at 34 weeks gestation during her second pregnancy and states the autopsy revealed a male infant, weighing 4300 grams with no evident cause of death. Upon questioning, the woman reports "I think they told me my sugar testing was high but they never did anything about it. What does the FNP know that could have contributed to Susan's fetal demise?

    A. A second pregnancy

    B. A small-for-gestational age fetus

    C. A normal-sized fetus

    D. An elevated blood sugar level

22. With Susan's case in the earlier question, what will the FNP do to rule out a potential for gestational diabetes mellitus? (Select all that apply.)

    A. Order an ultrasound for gestational dating.

    B. Have the patient do fetal movements counts every day.

    C. Have the patient go for a glucose challenge test.

    D. Check her urine for ketones and glucose.

    E. Check her urine for protein.

    F. Do a history just from the last pregnancy.

23. The FNP is caring for a patient at 24 weeks gestation, complaining of low back pain and increased vaginal secretions. She denies flu-like symptoms or other problems. What is the most likely diagnosis for this patient?

    A. Vaginal infection

    B. Premature rupture of membranes

    C. Preterm labor

    D. Back strain due to heavy lifting

24. A 22-year-old woman comes to the FNP to discuss her menstrual cycle. She reports irregular menses with light vaginal bleeding every 30–40 days. She also reports facial hair and an increase in her weight. Based on this information, the FNP suspects what diagnosis for this patient?

    A. Premenstrual syndrome (PMS)

    B. Polycystic ovarian syndrome (PCOS)

    C. Pregnancy

    D. Perimenopause at an early age

25. The FNP knows there are a number of risk factors for breast cancer. Of the following conditions, which of them put the woman at higher risk for breast cancer? (Choose all that apply.)

    A. Polycystic ovarian syndrome

    B. Pregnancy

    C. Family history of breast cancer

    D. Positive genetic workup for breast cancer

    E. Long-term use of oral contraceptive pills

    F. History of late menarche

26. A teenage girl at 13 years old is brought to the FNP for a discussion about preventing cancers. What things might the FNP suggest to protect the girl from various cancers? (Choose all that apply.)

    A. Do monthly breast self-exams.

    B. Get the series of injections to reduce the chances of getting herpes.

    C. Get the series of injections to reduce the incidence of HPV.

    D. Take an MVI each day.

    E. Avoid getting sunburned while on the beach.

27. The FNP knows that giving a teenager the three-injection vaccine series of Gardasil will reduce the teen's chances of contracting what?

    A. Breast cancer

    B. Rubella

    C. Human papilloma virus

    D. Syphilis

28. The menopausal woman has many hormonal changes that may cause her to have dyspareunia. The FNP knows that, in order to reduce dyspareunia, the woman could be put on hormone replacement therapy (HRT). What is an absolute contraindication to doing this?

    A. History of hirsutism

    B. History of fibrocystic disease

    C. History of a mastectomy

    D. History of mood changes

29. A patient who is 27 weeks gestation comes for her fourth prenatal appointment with the FNP. She reports no issues but asks "Is it okay for me to use peripads to keep my panties dry? I continue to have wet panties since last week." What is the best response from the FNP?

    A. "Peripads are fine to use. Just don't use tampons."

    B. "Tell me more about this wetness that you are describing."

    C. "Any wetness in your panties during pregnancy is due to what we call leukorrhea. It is normal in pregnancy."

    D. "Don't worry about anything. I will make sure everything is okay with your pregnancy."

30. A woman who is 32 weeks gestation comes to the FNP's office reporting leaking of clear, odorless fluid since two days ago. The woman denies fever, chills, or reduced fetal movement. What test will give the FNP the best information to address this issue and form a diagnosis?

    A. Doing the first sonogram

    B. Doing a ferning test

    C. Doing a Leopold's maneuver

    D. Doing a HA1C

Answers and Rationales

1. D. Ibuprofen is considered a Pregnancy category X drug and should not be given in the third trimester.

2. C. Ortho Tri-cyclen 28 should not be taken during pregnancy because it can affect the baby's development and is a pregnancy category X medication.

3. A. Naegele's rule is used to determine an EDD based on the woman's reported LMP. To calculate the EDD, take the first day of the LMP + 7 days – 3 months + one year.

4. C. For each week gestation after 12 weeks, the normal growth pattern of a single-fetus uterus is 1 cm per week of gestation.

5. A. The woman is describing a potential for a placenta previa with bright red bleeding after intercourse. The course of action is to ascertain if this is the diagnosis; an ultrasound would clarify this. If there is no partial or complete placenta previa, then the FNP will rule out other potential causes, such as a friable cervix. A CBC would not ascertain the cause of the blood loss. Measuring estimated fetal weight has no connection to the woman's reported signs and symptoms. A cervical culture or vaginal exam would never be done before ascertaining if the bleeding is from a placenta previa first.

6. C. The most accurate and therapeutic answer is C. Vaginal bleeding after intercourse is never normal. In regard to bleeding with labor, the woman is 25 weeks gestation and if the bleeding is a sign of labor there are usually other signs such as low back pain or cramping that accompany the bleeding, which is generally dark red in color. Further, if the woman was in preterm labor, that would be a troubling sign and answer C fits this as well.

7. C. A placenta previa presents with the classic signs of painless, bright red, vaginal bleeding, especially in the second trimester. A placental abruption presents with abdominal pain, dark red bleeding, and is not generally related to intercourse. A friable cervix would generally not present with bleeding that lasted a few hours and soaked a peripad. An STI could potentially cause cervical friability, but not this heavy vaginal bleeding.

8. A, B, and E. The rationale for the previous four questions: Painless, bright red, vaginal bleeding at 25 weeks gestation is a classic sign of a placenta previa. Management for this includes auscultating the FHR and listening for at least one minute; a sonogram to assess the fetal well-being and the placental location. Management is watchful waiting/expectant with the woman on bedrest, and nothing in her vagina. Education about danger signs is integral to keeping the woman and fetus healthy. Accurate documentation of all these steps is very important. Referral to an OB MD is needed.

9. C. In a pattern of IPV, the woman needs to understand she can tell someone whom she trusts about her violent situation. The best way for the FNP to react is to open the door for the woman to discuss it more.

10. A. Giving the woman oral folic acid has been shown to reduce the risk of neural tube defects, especially with those woman who have had an infant with such a defect in the past.

11. C. The priority action is to assess the fetal heart rate and the fetal well-being. Once a fetal heart rate has been auscultated, then other things can be done.

12. B. The most likely diagnosis is genital herpes that occurs 2–7 days after exposure and presents with painful, burning vesicles.

13. C. A woman who has been postmenopausal and presents with vaginal bleeding needs to have an endometrial biopsy to rule out endometrial cancer.

14. D. The normal uterine size and location for 12 weeks gestation is just above the symphysis pubis. Eight weeks gestation is the size of a lemon; 10 weeks is the size of a baseball; uterine fundus at the umbilicus is 20–22 weeks gestation.

15. B. The best time to get the most accurate reading of an AFP test is at 16–18 weeks gestation. Alpha-Fetoprotein is produced by the fetal liver and can be tested for via the maternal blood. It is a screening test to assess the risk for Neural Tube Defects (NTD) in each pregnancy. This test is best performed between 16 and 18 weeks gestation for increased reliability. If the test is abnormal, follow-up procedures to rule out NTD include genetic counseling for families with history of NTD, repeated AFP, high resolution ultrasound, and potentially an amniocentesis.

16. B. The pregnant woman is now experiencing her fourth pregnancy, which is documented as G4. One child was full term and two children were born prematurely at less than 38 weeks. All three children are living. She is a G4, P = 1 FT, 2 (premature), 0 abortions, and 3 living.

17. D. Urinary frequency usually disappears around week 12 of gestation (the fetus takes up more space higher in the uterus with less pressure on the bladder), but as the enlarging uterus puts pressure on the bladder, the problem returns near the due date.

18. A. Presumptive signs of pregnancy are breast changes, amenorrhea, nausea, vomiting, and urinary frequency and quickening. Signs of a urinary tract infection are burning and pain on urination, strong malodorous urine. Positive signs of pregnancy are visualization of the fetus via ultrasound and the auscultation of fetal heart tones. Probable signs include a positive pregnancy test; Goodell's, Hegar's, and Chadwick signs; and ballottement.

19. D. At approximately 16 weeks gestation, the maternal uterine size will be greater than dates if there is more than one fetus. An ultrasound will assist in the determination of the number of fetuses in the woman's uterus. An amniocentesis, GCT, or AFP test does not address the larger-than-normal uterus.

20. B. A normal fundal height for 24 weeks gestation is 1–2 fingerbreadths above the umbilicus/24 cm from the symphysis pubis to the uterine fundus. Since this is smaller than expected, the FNP will consider a referral to an OB/GYN. The other findings are normal changes that happen with pregnancy.

21. D. A woman who has "high sugar" levels is possibly a gestational diabetic. With these pregnancies, the woman will have a large-for-gestational-age infant, with the potential for a fetal demise due to uncontrolled maternal blood sugar levels. A second pregnancy has nothing to do with the fetal demise. The fetus was a large-for-gestational-age fetus, being over 4000 g.

22. A, C, and D. The FNP is considering that Susan has gestational diabetes (GDM). The initial screenings need to be done ASAP to rule this out and to ascertain the correct gestational age. Checking her urine for ketones and glucose assist the FNP to further evaluate for GDM. Daily fetal movement counts cannot be done until the fetus is able to be felt moving around 16–18 weeks gestation for a multigravida. The history taking should be a complete history since this is the first prenatal appointment for this woman and this pregnancy.

23. C. A 24-week gestation pregnancy with these symptoms should alert the FNP to potential signs of pre-term labor. The other answers do not fit this scenario. The FNP will need to do a thorough history and vaginal exam to rule all of this out or to confirm the diagnosis.

24. B. These symptoms reported by this woman are consistent with PCOS. The symptoms that support this diagnosis are light, irregular periods, weight gain, and androgenic changes. The symptoms are not consistent with the other choices.

25. C, D, and F. These things have been correlated to increased risk of breast cancer in women. The other three things are not correlated to increased breast cancer risk.

26. A, C, and E. Doing monthly BSE empowers the teen to be aware of the potential breast changes that can occur as her body matures. Gardasil is a recombinant human papillomavirus vaccine [types 6, 11, 16, 18] used in the prevention of certain strains of human papillomavirus, specifically HPV types 6, 11, 16, and 18. It also reduces the potential for getting cervical cancers by reducing HPV that is correlated to cervical cancer. Avoiding the sun and/or using sunscreen will reduce the potential for skin cancers in her future. There is no Herpes vaccine. Taking an MVI daily can add to her health but will not protect her from cancers.

27. C. Gardasil is a recombinant human papillomavirus vaccine [types 6, 11, 16, 18] used in the prevention of certain strains of human papillomavirus, specifically HPV types 6, 11, 16, and 18. It also reduces the potential for getting cervical cancers by reducing HPV that is correlated to cervical cancer. There is no vaccine for the prevention of breast cancer or syphilis. Rubella occurrences are reduced by giving a single-dose vaccine against that virus.

28. C. A history of breast cancers for which a mastectomy was done is an absolute contraindication to HRT. History of hirsutism and fibrocystic disease are not contraindications for HRT. Mood changes are potential side effects of HRT but are not absolute contraindications.

29. B. The best response is this therapeutic one. The others are not accurate or helpful.

30. B. The ferning test will evaluate whether the woman has spontaneous rupture of membranes (SROM). An initial sonogram cannot be compared to anything to assess if amniotic fluid volume is reduced. A Leopold's maneuver or hA1C do not evaluate for SROM.

• • • References

Books and Articles

Akkerman, D., Cleland, L., Croft, G., Eskuchen, K., Heim, C., Levine, A., . . . Westby, E. (2012). Routine prenatal care. *Institute for Clinical Systems Improvement.* http://bit.ly.Prenatal0712. Updated July 2012.

Hatcher, R. A., Trussell, J., Nelson, A. L., Cates, W., Stewart, F. H. & Kowal, D. (2012). *Contraceptive technology,* 20th ed. New York, Ardent Media Group.

Hodgson, B. B., & Kizour, R. J. (2014). *Saunders nursing drug handbook, 2014.* St. Louis, MO. Elsevier Saunders Publishers.

Lowdermilk, D. L., Perry, S. E., Cashion, K., & Alden, K. R. (2016). *Maternity & women's health care,* 11th *ed.* Elsevier Publishers, USA.

Manning, F. A., Harman, C. R., Morrison, I., Menticoglou, S. M., Lange, I. R., & Johnson, J. M. (1990). Fetal assessment based on fetal biophysical profile scoring. *American Journal of Obstetrics and Gynecology, 162(3),* 703–710.

Web References

http://www.cancer.org/healthy/findcancerearly/cancer screeningguidelines/american-cancer-society-guidelines-for-the-early-detection-of-cancer

http://emedicine.medscape.com/article/252928-overview

http://www.healthline.com/health/ovarian-cysts#Diagnosis5

http://www.healthline.com/health/polycystic-ovary-disease#Complications6

http://www.iom.edu/en/Reports/2009/Weight-Gain-During-Pregnancy-Reexamining-the-Guidelines.aspx

http://www.mayoclinic.org/diseases-conditions/vaginal-atrophy/basics/definition/con-20025768

http://www.mayoclinic.org/diseases-conditions/uterine-fibroids/basics/definition/con-20037901

http://medical-dictionary.thefreedictionary.com

http://www.medicinenet.com/script/main/art.asp?articlekey=8943

http://www.medscape.com/viewarticle/842786

http://www.webmd.com/women/guide/fibrocystic-breast-changes-symptoms-treatments-causes

http://www.webmd.com/women/tc/polycystic-ovary-syndrome-pcos-topic-overview

18

Geriatrics

Stacie Zibel, DNP, APRN-BC, CDE

Considerations for the Geriatric Patient

Advances in medicine and technology have enabled older adults to live longer and healthier lives. Since the start of the 20th century, the average life expectancy in the United States has increased considerably. In fact, the United States Census Bureau (2012) reports that during the last decade life expectancy has risen by approximately 2 years.

Family nurse practitioners must be prepared to provide comprehensive care to older adults across the continuum of health care delivery services (e.g., primary care, subacute rehabilitation care, long-term care, assisted living facilities, etc.), including the management of geriatric syndromes and health maintenance, as well as have a solid foundation and understanding of the physiology of aging based on scientific underpinnings. Table 18-1 describes the physiologic changes and its clinical implications in older adults. They must also be well-informed about reimbursement and regulatory issues that guide advanced practice nursing.

Geriatric Fast Facts: A Profile of Older Adults

Older adults are often divided into groups:
- Young-old, 65–75 years
- Middle-old, 75–84 years
- Old-old, 85 plus
- Centenarians, 100+

Oldest Old Is Fastest Growing Segment of Older Adults

Population growth for the 85+ population is projected to increase from 5.5 million in 2010 to 6.6 million by 2020, and is projected to surpass 9 million by 2030 with an estimated 20 million by 2050 (AoA, 2011).

Multiple Chronic Care Needs

Older adults—four out of five—live with one or more chronic conditions (e.g., diabetes, hypertension, chronic obstructive pulmonary disease [COPD], congestive heart failure [CHF], etc.).

Continued Growth of Minority Populations

(i.e., ethnic and racial) from 5.7 million in 2000 (16.3% of the older adult population) to 8.1 million in 2010 (20% of the older adult population). Projected increase to 13.1 million in 2020 (24% of the older adult population).

Women outnumber men at 23.0 million to 17.5 million.

Marital Status

- Men are more likely to be married than women; 72% of men are married, compared to 42% of women.
- 40% of older women are widows.

Living Arrangements

- As of 2014, over 57% of older adults lived in the community with their spouse.
- An estimated 72% of older men and 46% of older women lived with their significant other.
- Proportion decreased with age (e.g., approximately 32% of older women > 75 years old lived with their significant other.
- Institutionalized older adults account for 1.5 million for those 65+. Increases with age.

Leading Causes of Death

- Heart disease
- Cancer
- Chronic lower respiratory disease

Income

- Income—Almost 15.9% of older adults were below the poverty level as a result of out-of-pocket medical expenses in 2011.

Major Source of Income Is Derived from

- Social Security
- Private pensions
- Assets
- Earnings
- Government-related pensions

Prescription, Over-the-Counter (OTC), and Alternative Therapy Use

- Many take multiple medicines at the same time. A recent survey of 17,000 Medicare beneficiaries found that 2 out of 5 patients reported taking five or more prescription medicines.
- Account for 30% of total OTC usage and 34% of prescription drug consumption.
- Older adults are at increased risk of serious adverse drug events, including falls, depression, confusion, hallucinations, and malnutrition, which are an important cause of illness, hospitalization, and death among these patients.
- Drug-related complications have been attributed to the use of multiple medicines and associated drug interactions, age-related changes, human error, and poor medical management (e.g., incorrect medicines prescribed, inappropriate doses, lack of communication, and monitoring).

- Almost 40% of seniors are unable to read prescription labels, and 67% are unable to understand the information given to them.

Goals of Geriatric Care

The goal of geriatric care is to provide safe, comprehensive, and cost-effective quality health care based on evidence-based practice (EBP) to maintain and/or optimize function and improve the quality of life. To this aim, the family nurse practitioner must create an environment that provides for a private and quiet face-to face encounter away from noise and other distractions in a well-lighted and ventilated area. The face-to-face interaction (interview) between the family nurse practitioner and patient is key to obtaining a thorough and comprehensive health history that will guide the plan of care and formulate a differential diagnosis.

Key elements essential to the health history include all of the components in the adult health history, with an additional focus on the following:

- **Family history**—Review of parent and sibling health history, including the cause of death if appropriate
- **Work history**—To include previous exposures to occupational or environmental toxins
- **Medication use**—Over-the-counter, prescription, herbals, alternative modalities, as well as medications prescribed for family or friends
- **Allergies or sensitivities**—To foods, medication, latex
- **Smoking status**—Including present and past smoking history
- **Substance abuse**—Alcohol use or abuse and history of illicit drug use
- **Nutritional assessment**—Includes ability to shop for and prepare food, change in appetite, alteration in taste, and attitude toward eating. A sudden weight loss of 5% total body weight is a red flag and warrants further assessment and evaluation.

Note: The Mini-Nutritional Assessment Short Form is a 6-question screening tool used to identify older adults (65+) who are at risk of malnutrition or who are malnourished. The test takes about 5 minutes to complete and can be integrated into the comprehensive geriatric assessment.

Table 18-1	Age-Related Changes	
Organ/System	**Physiologic Change**	**Clinical Implications**
Body	Decrease in lean body mass Decrease in skeletal mass Decrease in total body H_2O Increase in adipose tissue until age 60, then decreases	Increased risk of dehydration Decrease strength Alteration in drug levels
Ears	Hearing loss (high frequency) Sensorineural/conductive	Presbycusis Inability to understand speech and tone
Eyes	Increase in cataracts Pupil reflex—increased time Decrease in lens flexibility Decrease in tear production Increase in intraocular pressure Cell breakdown in macula of the retina— loss of central vision	Changes in visual acuity Difficulty adjusting to light Increased glare Presbyopia Dry eyes Glaucoma Macular degeneration
Olfactory	Alterations in smell	Decrease in appetite Varied taste sensation
Oropharyngeal	Decrease in salivation Decrease in muscle strength for mastication	Dry mouth (xerostomia) Dysphagia
Cardiac	Change in intrinsic heart rate Diminished baroreflex in response to change in blood pressure	Increase in syncopal events Increase in atrial fibrillation Decrease in ejection fraction Rise in diastolic heart failure and dysfunction
Pulmonary	Increase in residual volume Decrease in vital capacity Decrease in FEV1	Increased incidence of pneumonia Complications related to chronic lung disease Increased shortness of breath
Gastrointestinal	Changes in motility Alteration in splanchnic blood flow	Constipation or diarrhea
Musculoskeletal	Decrease in bone density Demineralization Fibrosis Cartilage degeneration Compression of spine	Increased risk of fractures Progression to osteoarthritis Joint tightening Loss of height
Renal	Decrease in glomerular filtration Decrease in renal mass Renal blood flow decrease Decrease in reabsorption and secretion of renal tubular	Increased risk of dehydration Alterations in drug levels Risk of adverse effects
Hepatic	Activity decrease of P-450 system Decrease in hepatic mass	Alterations in drug levels
Integumentary	Decrease in elasticity Decrease in collagen and subcutaneous fat tissue	Shearing and skin tears Prolonged wound healing
Immune System	Decrease in T-cells Atrophy of thymus	Risk of developing infections
Central Nervous System	Slowdown in cognitive processing Decrease in dopamine receptors	Parkinson's disease

- **Sleep hygiene**—Hours of sleep? Need for non-pharmacological or pharmacological sleep aids. Sleep patterns. Naps? Location where sleep takes place.

  Note: The Epsworth Physical Activity—Including exercise (e.g., walking, swimming, dancing, etc.)
- **Health maintenance**—Screenings (e.g., mammograms, prostate specific antigen, colonoscopy, ophthalmology exams, etc.), dental exams, and immunizations
- **Past medical history**—A compilation of information relevant to the patient's past health and illness. The information obtained will provide the family nurse practitioner with vital clues related to contributing factors or underlying etiology pertinent to the patient's current health status and includes the following:
- **Childhood and adult illnesses**—Document date of diagnosis, treatment, and whether ongoing or resolved.
- **Immunizations**—Document dates of last immunizations (e.g., influenza, pneumovax, Varicella, Prevnar 13, tetanus, diphtheria, pertussis, etc.). Documentation of Mantoux tuberculin skin test or Bacilli Calmette-Guerin (BCG).
- **Hospitalizations** (medical, surgical, and mental health)—Record basis for admission, course of treatment, and resulting complications.
- **Accidents, injuries, or falls**
- **Religious beliefs and health practices**

Health Maintenance

The U.S. Preventive Services Task Force [USPSTF] (2014) recommends clinical services for adults 65 and over. The evidence-based practice guidelines target preventive health services pertinent to older adults. They include:

- Abdominal Aortic Aneurysm
- Breast Cancer Screening
- Carotid Artery Stenosis Screening
- Cervical Cancer Screening
- Colorectal Cancer Screening
- Coronary Heart Disease Screening
- Dementia Screening
- Fall Prevention in Older Adults
- Hearing Loss in Older Adults
- Hormone Replacement in Older Adults
- Immunizations (Adult)
- Osteoporosis Screening
- Ovarian Cancer Screening

- Peripheral Artery Disease Screening
- Prostate Cancer Screening
- Thyroid Disease Screening
- Vision Screening in Older Adults

The decision to screen for any or all of the recommended preventive services should be individualized to the patient and circumstance. The USPSTF has assigned a letter grade to each of the recommendations which reflects the certainty and strength of the evidence in support of the provision for a specific preventive service and guides the health care provider and patient in clinical decision making. Only services with a letter grade of "A" or "B" should be discussed with appropriate patients.

Communication Techniques

- Sit face to face, maintain eye contact. Do not stand over the patient.
- Be an attentive listener.
- Show genuine concern for the patient
- Do not shout. Speak slowly.
- Know your personal biases.
- Be cognizant of ethnic and cultural differences
- Observe for signs of distress (e.g., exhaustion, anxiety, confusion, etc.)
- Ask specific open-ended questions to illicit important health care information
- Address one issue at a time

Creating the Relationship

- Recognize communication barriers and make appropriate changes.
- Be cognizant of cultural and ethnic diversities.

Eliciting the Health History

The primary objective—If patient is unable to provide history, it may be necessary to gather history from another responsible individual (e.g., family member, friend, conservator, or Power of Attorney for the person). Key elements essential to the health history include, but are not limited to, the following:

- Biographical Data
  - Similar to other populations. Be sure to include emergency contact information.
- Family History
  - Provide family history for parents and siblings. If applicable and available include cause of death.
  - List history of any major medical problems (e.g., mental health issues, cancer, diabetes, substance abuse, cardiac disease, neurocognitive disorders, etc.)

Geriatric Health Maintenance

Health maintenance initiatives, including implementation of preventive measures, are key to promoting the optimal health and well-being of older adults. As with other populations (e.g., pediatrics, adolescents, adults, etc.), optimizing the management of acute and chronic morbidities in older adults will result in an overall improvement in quality of life and physical function. In addition to scheduled follow-up or interval visits, which are determined by the family nurse practitioner and is multifactorial dependent on presenting symptomatology and management of the underlying disease, the Centers for Medicare and Medicaid (CMS), as a result of the Affordable Care Act signed into law in 2010, has implemented:

Welcome to Medicare Preventive Visit (Initial Preventive Physical Examination) [IPPE]

- Goals of IPPE—health promotion, disease prevention, and detection
- Medicare allows for one IPPE during the beneficiary's lifetime.
- Provided within first 12 months of enrollment of beneficiary to Medicare Part B.

The Seven Components Required Are

- **Review of medical and social history** (e.g., past medical and surgical history, medication and supplement use, family history, use of alcohol or other substance abuse, tobacco use, diet, and physical activity)
- **Review potential risk factors for depression and other mood disorders.**
- **Review safety and functional ability** (e.g., fall risk, activities of daily living, hearing acuity, home safety) utilizing standardized questionnaires or screening tools
- **Exam** includes height, weight, body mass index (BMI), blood pressure, visual acuity screening, additional elements pertinent to the beneficiary's medical and social history, congruent with current standards of practice
- **End-of-life planning**—To include written or verbal information relevant to the beneficiary's ability to prepare an advance directive in the event of an injury or illness that impacts the beneficiary's capacity to make health care decisions, as well as whether the health care provider is willing to follow the wishes of the beneficiary as stated in the advance directive.
- **Educate, counsel, and refer**—Based on the previous five components

- **Educate, counsel, and refer for other preventive services**—To include written plan of care (e.g., appropriate **screenings** and Medicare-covered preventive services), as well as once-in-a-lifetime screening, and electrocardiogram, as appropriate

Medicare Annual Wellness Visit

- Review of medical and family history
- Recent medical events (i.e., siblings, children, etc.)
- Personal medical and surgical history
- Illness and hospital stays
- Medication use, including non-prescription medications (i.e., over the counter (OTC) or herbals)

Role of Family Nurse Practitioner (FNP)

- Routine body measurements and assessments
- Height, weight, body mass index (Note significant weight loss (5%) or significant weight gain in past year because this may indicate underlying comorbidities.)
- Vital signs including blood pressure, pulse, and temperature
- Detection of cognitive impairment (Note: Centers for Medicare Services [CMS] does not specify tool or test to be used. Examples include: Mini Mental Status Exam [MMSE], Saint Louis University Mental Status Exam [SLUMS], Mini-Cog.)
- Depression screening (only during initial Annual Wellness Visit). Note: There is no specified tool or instrument. (Examples of tools include: Geriatric Depressions Scale [GDS], Patient Health Questionnaire 9 [PHQ-9], Patient Health Questionnaire 2 [PHQ-2].) Document alterations in sleep or appetite, expressed feelings of social isolation, anhedonia (loss of ability to experience pleasure), suicidal thoughts, etc.
- Functional capacity and level of safety at home (Timed Get Up and Go test), risk of falls
- Assess hearing and vision.
- Assess ability to perform Activities of Daily Living (ADLs). Examples of instruments: Katz Index of Independence in Activities of Daily Living (Katz), Instrumental Activities of Daily Living (Lawton and Brody).
- Assess identified risk factors and maladies.
- Establish individual screenings and preventive services (5–10 years, as appropriate).
- Develop personalized health advice and referrals as indicated.

Medicare Basics

Medicare was signed into law by President Lyndon B. Johnson on July 30, 1965. The initial intent of this program was to provide basic health coverage for those who did not have health insurance. Medicare continues to provide coverage to older adults and individuals that are disabled. Enrollment and eligibility requirements for Medicare services is not based on income level. Medicare has evolved from the cost and charge reimbursement fee for service toward value-based payment. At this time, Medicare has four distinct entities that cover different services.

They are:

Medicare Part A—Referred to as hospital insurance

- Covers *most* medically necessary hospital, skilled nursing, home health care, or hospice services.
- Individuals who are 65 and older who are eligible for Social Security are automatically enrolled whether retired or not.
- Criteria—Must have worked and paid Social Security taxes for at least 40 calendar quarters (10 years), or if worked less, will be required to pay a monthly fee.
- Individuals who are younger than 65 and are permanently and totally disabled may enroll in Medicare Part A upon receiving disability benefits from Social Security for two years.
- **Note: Advanced practice nurses who are employed in the hospital setting will not be paid directly for their services rendered.**

Medicare Part B—Referred to as medical insurance (supplemental)

- Requires monthly premium payment by beneficiary
- May be covered by Medicaid for low-income individuals meeting criteria for eligibility.
- Covers **most** medical services to 80% of approved services when annual deductible is met, including: preventive (e.g., mammograms, influenza, pneumococcal, hepatitis), physician services, X-rays, laboratory services, durable medical equipment, physical therapy, speech therapy, occupational therapy

Medicare Part C—Referred to as Medicare Advantage Plans

- Not a separate benefit
- Allows private insurance companies to provide Medicare benefits
- Provided through Health Maintenance Organizations (HMOs) and Preferred Provider Organizations (PPOs)

- Additional services and screenings may be provided
- Beneficiary pays monthly premium

Medicare Part D—Outpatient prescription drug coverage

- Provided by private insurance companies who have contracts with the government
- Not included in "original" Medicare
- Allows older adults to receive prescriptions at lower out-of-pocket expenditures
- Each plan has its own formulary of covered drugs
- Changes in formulary may occur; beneficiary must receive written notice within 60 days prior
- Deductibles vary in drug plans—No Medicare drug plans can have a deductible of more than $320 in 2015 and $360 in 2016
- Some plans have coverage gap (donut hole)—temporary limit on what the drug plan will cover.
- Not applicable to all
- In 2015, when beneficiary and plan has spent $2960 on covered drugs, beneficiary is covered.
- Will change annually

Advanced Beneficiary Notice (ABN)—A standardized notice that must be issued to a beneficiary prior to providing certain outpatient services under Plan B (e.g., electrocardiogram being done after initial IPPE with no medical diagnosis or documentation to support the need for it) or Part A (e.g., hospice, home health)

- Allows beneficiary to make informed decisions about whether to accept financial responsibility and receive services that may not be covered by Medicare
- Note—If ABN is not completed and Medicare requires it for payment, the patient cannot be billed and it is the financial responsibility of the family nurse practitioner or practice.

Prescribing Practices in Older Adults

Polypharmacy is a common problem among older adults regardless of where they reside. The use of multiple medications is common due to multiple comorbidities. Age-related physiological changes place older adults at increased risk for adverse events and poor outcomes. Polypharmacy becomes problematic when multiple providers are prescribing medications without the knowledge of other health care providers. Family nurse practitioners must have a thorough understanding of pharmacodynamics (what the drug does to the body), pharmacokinetics (what the body does to the drug), drug interactions, adverse effects, etc., to ensure safe and effective practice when prescribing for older adults.

Pharmacokinetics

Every drug has a specific pharmacokinetic profile based on given parameters (sex, age, body mass index, renal and hepatic function). Based on the pharmacokinetic profile, proper dosing can be established for each individual.

Pharmacodynamics

Absorption

Gastrointestinal changes can occur in aging and impact drug absorption.

- Aging can decrease gastric motility
- Gastric acid secretion reduced causing increase in gastric pH
- Decreased gastric blood flow and increased pH can result in reduced drug absorption; whereas decreased gastric motility may result in increased drug absorption.
- Absorptive changes may be influenced by concurrent use of medications and fluctuating pH
- Use of proton pump inhibitors (PPIs) and antacids can alter gastric pH
- Drugs that utilize first-pass metabolism may be affected (e.g., lipophilic beta-blockers, propranolol, and nitrates)
- **Note**—Absorption of drugs can be influenced by other factors (e.g., use of feeding tubes, dysphagia, and nutritional status)

Distribution

Begins after the drug enters the bloodstream (e.g., into brain after crossing blood brain barrier, body fluids, or tissues)

Factors influencing distribution include:
- Molecular size
- pH
- Protein binding of drug (only unbound drug is distributed)
- Solubility of drug (hydrophilic or lipophilic)
  - Example—Dilantin (phenytoin); highly protein bound; can lead to adverse effects in older adults with reduced albumin levels (check free Dilantin and pre-albumin levels to monitor for toxicity)
- Decrease in muscle mass, along with increased proportion of body fat, resulting in greater volume of distribution in older adults

- For drugs distributed in muscle tissue, the volume of distribution may be decreased.
- Example—Valium (diazepam) dosing changes may be required until desired outcome is achieved. Not frequently used in older adults.
- Other factors to consider—reduction in total body water

Metabolism

The primary organ responsible for metabolism is the liver.

- Alteration in the normal metabolic process can significantly impact the pharmacokinetics of the drug.
- Significant adverse events are increased if the metabolic process is slowed, thereby
- prolonging the half-life of the drug. In contrast, if the process is sped up, the half-life of the drug is reduced and the efficacy of the drug is changed.
- Other factors impacting drug metabolism include genetics, nutritional status, diet, sex, and alcohol consumption.

Excretion

The elimination of drugs primarily occurs in the renal system. Renal function decreases with age, which may increase the half-life of a drug.

- Physiological changes (e.g., decrease in kidney mass, reduced blood flow to the kidneys reduction in number and size of nephrons)
- Renal changes can be predictive to some degree
- Several tools available to calculate (e.g., Cockgroft–Gault)

Adverse Drug Events in the Geriatric Patient

Adverse drug events (ADEs) occur in 15% or more of older adults seen in primary care, extended care facilities, and hospital settings, and are the result of inappropriate prescribing practices, medication errors, drug-to-drug interactions, drug-to-disease interaction and poor compliance. Physiological changes of aging in older adults increase the probability of an ADE. The annual cost associated with ADEs is reported to be 70 to 80 billion dollars annually. An estimated 35% of ambulatory older adults experience an adverse drug event; 29% of these reactions require intervention from a health care provider or hospital admission. Many of them can be prevented.

Serious adverse drug events include:

- Delirium
- Falls
- Orthostatic hypotension
- Heart failure
- Gastrointestinal hemorrhage
- Intracranial bleed
- Renal failure
- Death

Common adverse drug reactions attributed to older adults include:

- Anorexia
- Dizziness
- Gastrointestinal complaints (e.g., nausea, vomiting, constipation, diarrhea)
- Edema
- Urinary incontinence

Commonly Prescribed Drug Categories for Older Adults Resulting in Potential Side Effects

- Cardiovascular agents
- Antibiotics
- Diuretics
- Anticoagulants
- Hypoglycemics
- Steroids
- Opioids
- Anticholinergics
- Non-steroidals
- Benzodiazepines

Associated Problems with Medication Use

- Visual impairment—Difficulty reading labels and instructions may result in improper medication use
- Manual dexterity—Physical changes (e.g., osteoarthritis, gout, hemiplegia), unable to open bottles, difficulty handling small pills, administer injectables or use of an inhaler
- Insufficient knowledge—Inadequate health information provided by health care provider, language barrier illiteracy, hearing deficit
- Costs—Prescription not filled due to costs and limited financial resources

- Cognitive deficit—May forget to take med or take more than actual dose; may not understand the rationale for taking
- Multiple health care providers—Prescribing additional meds or duplication of current meds (generic/brand names), using both local and mail-order pharmacies

Assessment Tools to Reduce Medication Risks in Older Adults

- The Beers Criteria for Potentially Inappropriate Medication Use in Older Adults
- Indexes medications that cause side effects in older adults due to physiologic changes of aging
- Used by health care providers for older adults residing in community, hospitalized older adults, those residing in long-term care (e.g., assisted)
- Living and skilled nursing facilities, and post-acute settings
- Medications to be used cautiously in older adults include:
  - Tertiary tricyclic antidepressants
  - First-generation antihistamines
  - Muscle relaxants
  - Benzodiazepines
  - Digoxin > 0.125 mg, etc.

STOPP/START Tool

(Screening Tool of Older Person's Potentially Inappropriate Prescriptions)

- Medication review to identify risks versus benefits of prescription drugs
- Criteria is organized by system
- Emphasis on drug–drug interaction and duplicate drug class prescriptions

(Screening Tool to Alert doctors to the Right Treatment)

- Focus on prescribing omissions and identifying under treatment in older adults

Psychiatric

Delirium

- Incidence in elderly: 14–56% of hospitalized older adults
- Present in 10–22% of older adults at time of hospital admission
- 10–30% develop after admission to hospital for other causes

- Postoperative delirium accounts for 5–10% following general surgery. Orthopedic surgery highest risk: up to 42%.

There is no specific laboratory test to diagnose delirium. The diagnosis is based on clinical assessment. According to *The Diagnostic and Statistical Manual of Mental Disorders*, 5th edition (DSM-5), diagnostic criteria for delirium includes:

- A disturbance in attention (i.e., reduced ability to focus, direct, sustain, or shift attention) and awareness (a reduced orientation to the environment)
- Alteration in cognition (e.g., disorientation, memory deficit, language, and/or perceptual disturbance that is not founded upon pre-existing, established, or evolving dementia.
- Acute in onset. Develops over a short interval of time (hours to days). It is a change from one's baseline behavior and varies in severity during the course of the day.
- Supporting evidence from patient history, physical examination, or laboratory findings that the disturbance is triggered by a direct physiological consequence of an underlying medical condition, medication use (e.g., initiation of drug therapy or withdrawal; see Beers Criteria for inappropriate drug use in older adults), exposure to a toxin, as well as multiple etiologies.
- Goal of treatment—Determine underlying cause and reverse or stop symptoms. Avoid physical restraints. Maintain stable, quiet, and well-lighted environment.
- Correct sensory deficits with use of hearing aids and eye glasses.

Neurocognitive Disorders

Family nurse practitioners play a critical role in the treatment, management, and care for patients diagnosed with Alzheimer's disease and other related dementias. Currently, there is no treatment intervention (e.g., pharmacological or non-pharmacological) available to reverse the process. The goal is to preserve functional and cognitive ability, minimize associated behavioral issues, and to impede disease progression. Failure to diagnose and inadequate treatment lead to rapid deterioration for the patient and severely impacts the lives of the patient and family.

Replaces dementia in DSM-5. Diagnostic criteria is as follows:

- **Mild**—Cognitive impairment in one or more cognitive domains (moderate decline; e.g., language, judgment, abstract thinking, and executive functioning). Deficits do not impair the ability to live independently.
- **Major**—Presents with significant cognitive decline in one or more cognitive domains. Impairs ability to live independently. Documented by standard neuropsychological testing.

Neurocognitive Disorders include:

- Alzheimer's disease
- Frontotemporal Lobar Degeneration
- Lewy Body
- Parkinson's disease
- Vascular Dementia
- Other Neurocognitive (e.g., Huntington's disease, traumatic brain injury, human immunodeficiency virus (HIV)

Classify: Mild, Moderate, or Severe

Document with or without behavioral disturbance.

Neurocognitive Domains

- **Language**—Naming, word finding, expressive language
- **Social cognition**—Recognition of emotions, inappropriate social behavior
- **Perception**—Visual-motor, praxis
- **Learning and memory**—Long-term memory, short-term memory, and recent memory
- **Executive Functioning**—Planning and decision making
- **Complex attention**—Sustained attention, divided attention, selective attention

Treatment Interventions

- Non-pharmacologic: complementary therapies, aromatherapy, creative arts expression (e.g., art therapy, music therapy, etc.), behavioral therapy, reality orientation, reminiscence, pet therapy
- Goal of therapy: Patient-centered focus to improve the patient's quality of life
- Pharmacologic: Cholinesterase inhibitors are utilized as first-line therapy in patients diagnosed with mild to moderate dementia.
- In patients diagnosed with moderate to severe dementia, a glutamate antagonist is used.
- Other treatment modalities are in development at this time.

Treatment Options

Cholinesterase Inhibitors

Aricept (Donepezil)—Approved for mild to moderate dementia

Side effects—Nausea, vomiting, diarrhea, increase in agitation; resolves after several weeks

Note: Gastrointestinal reported complaints may be reduced if taken with food.

Razadyne (Galantamine)—Approved for mild to moderate dementia

Side effects—Gastrointestinal complaints (e.g., nausea, vomiting, or diarrhea)

Note: Gastrointestinal effects can be reduced by taking with meals and gradual dose titration.

Exelon (Rivastigmine)—Approved for mild to moderate dementia

Available in capsule and patch

Side effects—Abdominal pain, weight loss, headaches, nausea, vomiting, diarrhea

Note: Gastrointestinal effects are less likely to occur with use of patch

NMDA Antagonist

Namenda (Memantine)—Approved for moderate to severe dementia

Available in short-acting oral tablets, extended-release tablets, and oral suspension

Side effects—Dizziness, fatigue, somnolence, back pain, headache, constipation, hypertension

Combination Pill

Namzaric (donepezil/memantine)

Available in tablet

Side effects—Similar to profile for donepezil and memantine

Not indicated for first-line therapy

Goal of therapy: To preserve cognitive and functional ability, maintain patients' and caregivers' quality of life, slow disease progression, and decrease behavioral disturbances.

Additional pharmacological modalities may be necessary to target specific behaviors and symptoms.

Depression

Depression is a medical condition that impacts the lives of many older adults and can be treated successfully. It is estimated that up to 5% of community dwelling older adults meet the diagnostic criteria for major depression, while the prevalence of a major depressive episode for older adults residing in long-term care is approximately 12.4%. An additional 30% of older adults residing in long-term care present with significant depressive symptoms. This is in contrast to a reported 15% of community dwellers with symptomatology indicative of significant depression. It is important to note that depression is not a normal process of aging.

Symptoms of Depression

- Depressed mood or change in affect
- Feelings of worthlessness
- Difficulty concentrating or making decisions
- Changes in sleep patterns
- Weight gain or loss
- Talk of hurting oneself
- Lack of energy
- Loss of interest in activities once enjoyed

Risk Factors for Depression

- Unresolved grief
- Loss of independence
- Chronic pain
- Chronic medical issues
- Past episodes of depression
- Cognitive changes
- Medications
- Financial and social stressors
- Progressive sensory losses

Criteria for Diagnosis of Depression in Long-Term Care

- **Major Depressive Disorder**—Individual must present with at least 5 of 9 depressive symptoms for at least 2 weeks, along with impaired social function
  - **Psychotic Depression**—A subtype of major depression more commonly found in older adults residing in long-term care.
  - Characterized by major depressive symptoms, along with delusions and/or hallucinations
  - Delusions are persecutory and somatic.
- **Minor Depression**—Not meeting the preceding criteria for presence of subthreshold symptoms (e.g., poor self-reported health, impaired physical functioning, marital status, etc.)

- **Dysthymia**—Low-grade depression symptoms that are chronic > 2 years
- **Depression in Alzheimer's Disease**—Must present with three symptoms specific to criteria.
- Irritability is a qualifying symptom.
- Additional symptomatology includes:
  - Anhedonia (inability to experience pleasure)
  - Poor sleep
  - Poor appetite
  - Social isolation (not a symptom of major depressive disorder
  - Fatigue
  - Feelings of worthlessness

Workup for Depression in Long-Term Care

- Screening for depression with Geriatric Depression Scale
- Past medical history, including past trial of antidepressant medications
- Present illness history, including medications and report of suicidal ideation
- Cognitive evaluation—Mini Mental Status Exam or other tool
- Laboratory tests (e.g., basic metabolic profile, thyroid profile, complete blood count, serum B12, and albumin if poor nutritional status is suspected)
- Additional workup may include electrocardiogram, sleep studies, or MRI of brain
- Treatment modalities include:
  - **Non-pharmacological treatment** (e.g., cognitive behavioral therapy, light therapy, etc.)
  - Electroconvulsive therapy (ECT) used only in severe cases when medication therapies have failed or rapid deterioration of patient is evident.

Pharmacological treatment includes:

- Selective Serotonin Reuptake Inhibitors [SSRI]:
  - Lexapro (escitalopram)
  - Celexa (citalopram)
- Serotonin norepinephrine reuptake inhibitors [SNRI]:
  - Effexor (venlafaxine)
  - Cymbalta (duloxetine)
  - Tricyclic antidepressants
  - Dopamine norepinephrine reuptake inhibitor (buproprion)
  - Serotonin modulator (trazadone)
  - Norepinephrine serotonin modulator (mirtazapine)
  - Psychostimulants
  - Treatment strategies and pharmacological treatment choices based on provider selection and targeting symptoms
  - Start low, go slow

Adverse effects associated with pharmacological treatment—Class-dependent

SSRIs include: decreased appetite, may cause hyponatremia in older adults, agitation, insomnia, initial weight loss, and somnolence.

- Tricyclic antidepressants—constipation, urinary retention, dry mouth, orthostatic hypotension, delirium, change in cognition, blurred vision, dry mouth arrhythmia
- Buproprion—hypertension, dry mouth, seizures (do not stop abruptly)
- SNRIs—dry mouth, increased risk of hypertension at higher doses (> 150 mg to 225mg/day), including adverse events similar to SSRIs
- Serotonin modulator (Trazadone)—Priaprism (rare but reported), sedation, postural hypotension at increased doses
- Psychostimulants—anorexia, insomnia, elevated blood pressure, arrhythmias, anxiety, and weight loss

Clinical Pearl

It may be necessary for the health care provider to adjust doses of other medications due to the potential for interactions and possible adverse effects of antidepressant medications in order to achieve therapeutic success.

Contraindications associated with particular drug classes should be considered prior to initiation.

Chronic Disease and Older Adults

Older adults account for the fastest-growing population in this country. Between the years 2003 and 2013, it is estimated that for individuals 60+ there was a 30.7% increase from 48.1 million to 62.8 million older adults. These numbers will continue to rise over the next several decades. Older adults are more vulnerable to chronic disease than other populations.

The likelihood of developing one or more chronic illnesses continues to escalate as one ages.

The consequences of living and/or caring for an older adult with a chronic illness impacts not only health care services and expenditures, it places undue burdens on the patient and their family support system, which manifests in myriad somatic, physical, and psychological complaints, in addition to an enhanced likelihood of social isolation as a result.

Stats at a Glance

- More than 50% of older adults live with one chronic condition.
- It is estimated that 11 million older adults live with five or more chronic conditions.
- Older adults with a diagnosis of hypertension is projected to be at greater than 40%.
- Dyslipidemia accounts for 1 out of 4 older adults.
- Mental illness of varying degrees impacts almost 20% of older adults.
- Diabetes is a growing concern in older adults, with an approximate 15% living with the diagnosis.
- Other chronic illnesses include: osteoarthritis, osteoporosis, hypothyroidism, etc.

Hypertension

Recommendations from the Joint National Committee (JNC8) include a blood pressure (BP) goal of:

- A systolic blood pressure (SBP) of < 150 mmHg or a diastolic blood pressure (DBP) in patients 60+ without chronic kidney disease (CKD) or diabetes
- Patients diagnosed with diabetes should have, as their goal, a SBP < 140 or a DBP < 90 mmHG.
- Older adults with CKD and a glomerular filtration rate (GFR) of greater than or equal to 60 mL/min/1.73m² should have as their goal a SBP of < 140 or a DBP < 90.
- For older adults > 70 years of age with CKD and a GFR of < 60, there is little data available.
- Pharmacological treatment should be initiated if BP goal has not been achieved using non-pharmacological interventions (e.g., diet, exercise, meditation, etc.).
- First-line treatment modalities for older adults include:
  - Thiazide diuretics
  - Calcium channel blockers
  - ACE or ARBs

  Caution when initiating therapy due to increased risk of orthostatic BP

  Close follow-up until target BP is achieved

Renal artery stenosis should be considered if a new onset of diastolic hypertension in a previously well-controlled patient, despite pharmacological treatment with three or more anti-hypertensive agents at maximum doses.

Treatment goals should be individualized for each patient and the family nurse. Practitioner should consider underlying comorbidities.

Diabetes

Criteria for diagnosis discussed in previous chapter.

Goals of treatment developed by the American Diabetes Association and American Geriatrics Society:

- Hospitalized—Older adults who have a significant life expectancy and have maintained cognition and physical function should have similar goals to other populations.
- Older adults residing in long-term care/skilled nursing facilities should not use a sliding-scale insulin regimen for diabetes management.
- **Healthy** older adults should have an HgbA$_{1c}$ goal of 7.0–7.5
  - Fasting or post prandial goals: 90–130
  - Bedtime goal of 90–130
  - Consider BP target of < 140/80 and statin therapy
- **Complex** older adults should achieve an HgbA$_{1c}$ goal of 7.5–8.0
  - Fasting or post-prandial goals: 90–150
  - Bedtime goal of 90–150
  - Use of statin and target BP goal as discussed.
  - Complex patients may have multiple comorbidities, a diagnosis of mild-to-moderate cognitive impairment or a deficit in 2+ Instrumental activities of daily living
  - **Older adults who are very complex or in poor health** should achieve an HgbA$_{1c}$ of 8.5–9.0.
- Fasting or post-prandial of 100–180
- Bedtime goal of 110–200
- BP goal < 150/90
- These patients have multiple comorbidities and often reside in long-term care.
- Careful consideration must be given when choosing treatment. Sulfonylureas, although inexpensive, can increase mortality.
  - Treatment modalities should be individualized based on other comorbidities and goals of treatment.

– Annual recommendations and frequency of visits for community-dwelling older adults should be based on evidence based practice guidelines.

Osteoarthritis (OA)

Can include:

- Inflammatory—Morning stiffness of more than 30 minutes, and complaints of night pain
- Findings from diagnostic X-rays, may reveal a joint effusion
- Non-inflammatory—General findings include crepitus, joint tenderness, and bony prominence. Complaints of pain and disability.

Physical Examination Includes:

- Gait—Difficulties in maintaining balance or any other gait abnormalities should be further evaluated.
- Range of motion—Should be performed effortlessly
- Evaluation of joint pain

Osteoarthritis of knee may present with crepitus, knee locking, and unsteadiness of gait.

Patients with suspected OA of hip may present with a limp to avoid pain on the affected side. This is known as an antalgic gait.

Diagnosis can be made with or without X-rays. Findings include subchondral cyst formation, osteophytosis, and joint space narrowing.

Treatment Modalities Include Pharmacologic and Non-Pharmacologic Therapies

- Non-pharmacologic therapies—aqua therapy and walking
- Pharmacology treatment modalities—Acetaminophen is the drug of choice. Risk of toxicity.
- Limit to < 3000 mg/day. Educate patients about risks; found in many over-the-counter products.
- Use of COX 2 inhibitors (e.g., Celebrex [celecoxib]). Contraindicated for some.
- Lidocaine patches
- Capsaicin cream
- Diclofenac (e.g., gel, patch, or tablet)
- Corticosteroid injections

Osteoporosis

Definition by the National Osteoporosis Foundation

- Progressive, chronic disease characterized by bone fragility, a microarchitecture.

Black men and women have a lower risk of developing the ailment. Those diagnosed have a similar risk of fractures compared to other groups.

Risk of developing osteoporosis in Caucasian women over a lifetime is 50%; Caucasian men 70%.

- USPSTF recommends screening for all women > 65+
- USPSTF reports insufficient evidence to screen all men > 70
- Workups for newly diagnosed older adults with osteoporosis should include:
  - Thyroid stimulating hormone
  - Vitamin D 25 hydroxyl
  - Creatinine
  - Evaluation for secondary osteoporosis (e.g., epilepsy, Parkinson's disease, COPD, celiac, etc.)

FRAX WHO Fracture Risk Assessment Tool

Treatment interventions should include:

- Smoking cessation
- Fall risk assessment
- Exercise
- Moderation of alcohol intake
- Consideration of over the counter pharmacological interventions
- Initiation of bisphosphonate therapy (careful consideration should be given to previous osteonecrosis of jaw)
- Other treatment modalities—Hormone replacement therapy; use of denosumab or teriparatide

The continuation of bisphosphonate therapy after 5 years should be weighed considering benefits versus risks.

Falls

It is estimated that one third of community-dwelling older adults and nearly 60% of nursing home residents fall each year. Falls account for multiple emergency room visits and hospitalizations, annually resulting in expenditures of nearly 30 billion dollars, and possibly resulting in brain injuries, hip fractures, physical decline, social isolation, and death. Falls are not a normal expectation of aging.

Risk Factors

- History of previous falls
- Parkinson's disease

- Gait deficit
- Vertigo
- Balance deficit
- Depression
- Medication use (e.g., benzodiazepines, anti-psychotics, antiarrhythmics, antihypertensives, diuretics, muscular skeletal relaxants, SSRIs, MAOIs, TCAs, etc.)
- Cognitive impairment
- Pain
- Visual or sensory deficits, etc.

USPSTF recommends assessing the risk of falling annually and at episodic visits. Three factors to be considered:

- Poor performance on the Timed Get up and Go Test
- History of mobility issues
- Prior history of falls

Multidisciplinary approach should be utilized.
    Home safety should be evaluated.

Atypical Presentation of Disease in Older Adults

Atypical presentation of acute illness in older adults is complicated by underlying comorbidities, along with the physical changes of aging. It is essential the family nurse practitioner recognizes the more common atypical presentations seen in this population. Subtle changes from an individual's baseline (physical or cognitive) may be the first sign of illness. These may include: increased confusion, a decrease in appetite, weakness, etc. Older adults greater than 85+ and on multiple medications and with multiple comorbidities are at increased risk, as well as other older adults who have underlying physical and cognitive impairments.

The family nurse practitioner must incorporate strategies to assess for atypical presentation of illness in older adults. The ability to differentiate between true pathology and age-related changes is key.

Urinary Tract Infections

- Use of McGeer's Criteria
- Worsening or new onset of incontinence
- Increased urgency or frequency

- Falls
- Increased confusion

Acute Abdomen

- Vague respiratory symptoms
- Mild discomfort
- Complaint of diarrhea or constipation
- Absence of symptomatology

Pneumonia

- No fever
- General malaise or weakness
- Nausea or vomiting
- Minimal cough
- Symptom of new cardiac arrhythmia
- No leukocytosis on CBC

Other Atypical Presentations Include

- Myocardial infarction
- Malignancy
- Diabetes
- Hypothyroidism

End-of-Life Care/Advance Care Planning

Family nurse practitioners have long established the capacity to provide quality, safe, and cost-effective health care to patients in multiple health care environments. Advance care planning is essential to both primary care, and acute and long-term care institutions. Advance care planning encourages the patient, family, and loved ones to reflect on their personal values and beliefs when considering end-of-life care. It is a process that requires the family nurse practitioner to have an open and honest discussion with the patient and family regarding end-of-life preferences should the time come when the patient is not able to speak for themselves or can no longer make medical decisions. It is not simply about completing an advance directive; it is a very sensitive matter that has the potential to impact the patient and family on multiple levels. Advance care planning needs to begin in the primary care setting and, at minimum, be discussed annually or any time there is a change in the patient's condition.

Review Questions

Questions 1–3 relate to the following scenario.

1. Mr. Jones, an 89-year-old man, has recently relocated from the West Coast to be closer to his daughter who is also a patient in your office. He wants to establish a new PCP. His daughter reports that he has multiple comorbidities and is on seven prescribed medications. What medications should be assessed?

   A. His prescription drugs only

   B. Whatever he decides to bring to the office

   C. All of his medications, including prescription drugs, OTCs, and nutritional and herbal supplements

   D. Only his OTCs, because these can contribute to adverse events

2. His medication list includes Digoxin (Lanoxin) 0.25 mg by mouth daily, which was prescribed by his previous PCP for control of his CHF and atrial fibrillation. As the new PCP, what would you exclude from your plan?

   A. Measure a digoxin level.

   B. Do nothing because he looks fine.

   C. Consider decreasing his dose.

   D. Discuss with his previous HCP.

3. His daughter, who was not present for the exam, calls at the end of the day to discuss his visit. She is concerned that her father did not provide her with all of the details. What should be the next step?

   A. Provide her with a summary of the visit.

   B. Ask her to come into your office to discuss it.

   C. Tell her that the information can only be discussed with the patient.

   D. Request a copy of his advanced directives.

4. When should the medication reconciliation be done?

   A. Upon request of the patient's health care plan

   B. Upon discharge from the hospital or post-acute rehab center

   C. During each visit

   D. Annually

5. All of the following are covered under Medicare Part A EXCEPT:

   A. Inpatient hospital care.

   B. Hospice services.

   C. Durable medical equipment.

   D. Short-term rehab.

6. Delirium in the elderly is associated with functional decline, increased use of chemical and physical restraints, prolonged delirium post hospitalization, and increased mortality. Predisposing risk factors for delirium include older age, multiple comorbidities, a recent severe illness, past ETOH abuse, hearing or vision impairments, and a past history of delirium. Which of the following is the best tool to assess a patient for delirium?

   A. Geriatric Depression Scale

   B. MMSE (Mini Mental State Exam)

   C. CAGE Test

   D. CAM (Confusion Assessment Method)

7. Mrs. White is 85 years old and lives in her own house. Her husband died about 3 years ago. Mrs. White has two daughters who live about 30 minutes from her. Although she talks to them daily, she has not seen them in over 2 weeks. On her most recent visit to the office, she reports that she continues to experience considerable pain from her left hip and has been more and more disabled by this for the past

6 months. She states that she is on a waiting list for a hip replacement. In general, she states, "I feel miserable and I no longer enjoy reading or gardening. I have no energy and everything is an effort."

   A. Tell her that the symptoms she is experiencing are likely due to old age.

   B. Check a UA if positive C and S.

   C. Perform a Geriatric Depression Scale.

   D. Recommend that she move to an assisted living facility because there will be staff that can assist her with her ADLs.

8. Mr. Sanchez is a 76-year-old Hispanic male hospitalized for a right total knee replacement. Prior to his discharge, he was diagnosed with a deep vein thrombosis (DVT) in his right lower extremity. His nurse reports increased confusion in the past 13 hours. Mr. Sanchez has been trying to climb out of bed, is agitated, tugging on his Foley catheter, pushing at the staff, calling out for his family, and has not responded to redirection. His labs are reported "within normal limits." His vital signs are stable. The most likely cause is:

   A. Mr. Sanchez is agitated that he can't go home as promised.

   B. He developed an infection post-surgery.

   C. Depression, which he should be screened for.

   D. Hospital-acquired delirium.

9. Which of the following statements is the most accurate description of Alzheimer's disease (AD)?

   A. The disease is reversible with pharmacological treatment modalities, including Aricept (donepezil) and Namenda.

   B. The disease is progressive.

   C. The disease is characterized by remissions and exacerbations.

   D. Over 50% of older adults will develop AD at some time.

10. The Geriatric Comprehensive Assessment (GCA) includes all of the following EXCEPT:

   A. Functional health.

   B. Physical health.

   C. Quality of life measures.

   D. Exercise regimen.

11. The *only* acetyl cholinesterase inhibitor (ACHI) approved to treat moderate to severe dementia is:

   A. Exelon (rivastigmine).

   B. Aricept (donepezil).

   C. Namenda (memantine).

   D. Razadyne (galantamine).

12. JNC 8 recommends:

   A. lowering BP < 120/80.

   B. SBP < 150 mmHG or DBP < 90 mmHG in adults 60+ without chronic kidney disease or diabetes.

   C. ETOH intake at 2 ounces/day.

   D. Anaerobic exercise of up to 30 minutes most days.

13. The FNP is preparing to do a round on hospital patients in the a.m., prior to going to your office. Which of these hospitalized patients should be checked on first?

   A. A 67-year-old male who had a Right BKA yesterday, following a motor vehicle accident who is complaining of phantom pain

   B. A 76-year-old female, who is less than 24 hours post, complaining of back pain with a new onset of urinary incontinence

   C. An 80-year-old male who received 2 units of packed red blood cells (PRBCs) the previous day for a suspected upper gastrointestinal bleed (GI)

   D. A 90-year-old nursing home patient who is scheduled for an endoscopy later in the day, who demands that she have her breakfast

14. The FNP has just seen Mr. Lyons, an elderly patient in the practice with suspected osteoarthritis of the hip. What is the most distinguishing characteristic of the physical examination?

    A. Gait abnormality

    B. Pain with external or internal rotation

    C. Joint instability

    D. Crepitus

15. Recommended immunizations for adults 65+ include:

    A. An annual influenza vaccine, TDAP vaccine every 5 years, shingles vaccination, pneumococcal vaccine(s) 13 and 23

    B. TDAP vaccine every 10 years, annual influenza vaccine, shingles vaccine after age 60, pneumococcal vaccine(s) 13 and 23

    C. An annual influenza vaccine, annual pneumococcal vaccines, TDAP every 10 years, and shingles vaccine after age 60

    D. Shingles vaccine—2 doses given 6 months apart, TDAP every 10 years, annual influenza vaccine, pneumococcal vaccines 13 and 23

16. A patient presents to the office who has multiple comorbidities and is taking multiple prescription medications to manage his chronic diseases. He is concerned about the rising cost of his medications. He will soon be enrolling in Medicare. Which Medicare Plan would help cover his prescription drugs?

    A. Medicare A

    B. Medicare B

    C. Medicare C

    D. Medicare D

17. The prevalence of elder abuse in this country is estimated to be approximately _____, according to epidemiological studies.

    A. 50–60%

    B. less than 1%

    C. 2–10%

    D. 12–35%

18. Which of the following is NOT included in the definition of elder abuse, according to the National Center of Elder Abuse?

    A. Physical abuse

    B. Abandonment

    C. Financial exploitation

    D. All of the above can be considered in the definition.

19. Therapeutic communication with older adults include:

    A. Talking to family members who are present to elicit a comprehensive health history.

    B. Speaking slowly in a deep tone and addressing your questions to the patient.

    C. Standing close to ensure they will hear you.

    D. Addressing the patient by their first name to create a "friendly atmosphere."

20. Goals of geriatric care include:

    A. Maintaining function and quality of life.

    B. Having a signed advance directive.

    C. An aggressive plan of care that is curative.

    D. Complying with the family's requests.

21. When prescribing for an older adult, all should be considered EXCEPT:
    A. Beer's Criteria.
    B. Pharmacodynamics.
    C. McGeer's Criteria.
    D. Pharmacokinetics.

22. Anatomical and physiological changes occur as a result of the aging process. Which is a normal, non-pathological change related to the respiratory system?
    A. Improved coughing reflex
    B. Increase in A/P chest diameter
    C. Decreased residual volume
    D. Tissue elasticity increased

23. Screening instruments used to evaluate cognition include all of the following EXCEPT:
    A. Clock drawing test.
    B. MRI of brain.
    C. MMSE.
    D. SLUMS.

24. According to the American Geriatrics Society, the hemoglobin A_{1C} (HgbA$_{1C}$) goal for an older adult with 3 multiple comorbidities or mild to moderate cognitive impairment should be:
    A. Individualized for each patient.
    B. HgbA$_{1C}$ < 6.0.
    C. HgbA$_{1C}$ between 6.5–7.0.
    D. HgbA$_{1C}$ between 7.5–8.0.

25. Which class of drug should be used cautiously in older adults with diabetes, due to the increased risk of hypoglycemia?
    A. Biguanides
    B. Sulfonylureas
    C. DPP- IV
    D. SGLT2

26. The USPSTF recommends primary, secondary, and tertiary preventive services. Which of the following is not considered a primary preventive service?
    A. Smoking cessation
    B. Mammogram
    C. Immunizations
    D. Physical activity

27. Visible signs of intrinsic aging related to the integumentary system include all of the following EXCEPT:
    A. Increased melanin production.
    B. Decreased pigmentation.
    C. Ridging of nail.
    D. Loss or increase of subcutaneous fat deposition.

28. Older adults are at increased risk for abuse. Risk factors for elder abuse do NOT include:
    A. Substandard living arrangements to meet the needs of older adults.
    B. The education level of caregivers.
    C. Social isolation.
    D. Family stressors.

29. Which of the following is the most common form of anemia diagnosed in older adults?

   A. Iron (Fe) deficiency anemia

   B. Cooley's anemia

   C. Anemia of chronic kidney disease

   D. Vitamin B12 deficiency

30. Which of the following statements is true regarding suicide rates?

   A. Non-married women are more at risk.

   B. Caucasian men 85 and older are more at risk.

   C. Hispanic men of any age are more at risk.

   D. African American widowers are more at risk.

31. The FNP is seeing Mr. Larson, a 65-year-old male, for the "Welcome to Medicare" exam. As required by Medicare guidelines, the FNP begins the discussion regarding end-of-life planning. Mr. Larson becomes visibly shaken and states, "I plan on being around for a while. Look at me. I am as fit as a teenager." Which of the following responses is best?

   A. End-of-life care planning is mandatory in all 50 states once you go on Medicare.

   B. You are right, Mr. Larson, you are a healthy man. Therefore, there is no further need for discussion at this time.

   C. Once they are written, they cannot be changed.

   D. End-of-life care planning, which includes designating a Health Care Proxy and Advance Directives, ensures that your preferences for end-of-life care are specified if you are unable to make medical decisions or speak for yourself.

32. The family nurse practitioner is seeing Mrs. Watson, an elderly woman who appears much older than her stated age. Mrs. Watson is accompanied by her son, John. Over the past few weeks, Mrs. Watson has been seen in the ER multiple times after falling and using her Life Alert to call for help. The discharge planner recommended she be seen for a follow-up after her recent admission for a subdural hematoma. The FNP reviews her discharge summary, including consults, labs, and other diagnostics. Her visit today is not significantly different from her baseline, with the exception of bilateral lower extremity weakness. The next step is:

   A. Instruct the patient to keep a "fall diary."

   B. Order durable medical equipment (e.g., bedside commode, walker).

   C. Perform the "get up and go test."

   D. Report her to Social Services because she is not able to care for herself.

33. Which of the following statements is correct? By the year 2040,

   A. There will be about 100 million older people, twice the number seen in 2000.

   B. There will be a decrease in ethnic and minority populations.

   C. The number of people who are 85+ is projected to triple from 6 million in 2013 to 14.6 million in 2040.

   D. There will be no significant changes.

34. The major sources of income for older adults include all of the following EXCEPT:

   A. "Gifting" by family members, as allowed by the Internal Revenue Service.

   B. Social Security.

   C. Assets.

   D. Pensions.

35. The underlying characteristics of Alzheimer's disease includes:

   A. Atrophy of the brain.

   B. Atherosclerotic changes in the cerebral and carotid arteries.

   C. Amyloid plaques and neurofibrillary tangles.

   D. Multi-microvascular infarcts of the cerebellum.

36. Which of the following is NOT a concern when caring for the elderly?
    A. Visual changes
    B. Increased sensitivity to heat or pain
    C. Gait or balance instability
    D. Diminished reaction time when behind the wheel of a car

37. Which of the following is a common skin condition seen in older adults?
    A. Contact dermatitis
    B. Pressure ulcers
    C. Stasis dermatitis
    D. Fifth Disease

38. Contributing factors associated with an increased risk of falls in older adults include all of the following EXCEPT:
    A. Osteoporosis.
    B. Auditory changes.
    C. Urinary incontinence.
    D. Cardiovascular disease.

39. Which of the following statements is correct? In a patient with diabetes, the JNC 8 recommends a BP goal of:
    A. Systolic < 130 or diastolic < 80.
    B. Systolic < 140 or diastolic < 90.
    C. Systolic < 120 or diastolic < 80.
    D. There are no set goals and they are individualized for the patient based on comorbidities.

40. The first-line drugs for treating hypertension in older adults includes all of the following EXCEPT:
    A. ACEI or ARB.
    B. Thiazide diuretic.
    C. Beta-blockers.
    D. Calcium channel blockers.

41. Health care providers working with older adults refer to activities of daily living (ADLs) and instrumental activities of daily living (IADLs) to assess independent living skills. Which of the following is NOT considered to be an activity of daily living (ADL)?
    A. Feeding
    B. Medication management
    C. Dressing
    D. Bathing

42. Osteoporosis is a disease in which decreased bone mass results in an increased risk for bone fracture and bone frailty. What is the most common fracture associated with osteoporosis?
    A. Hip fracture
    B. Vertebral fracture
    C. Distal radial fracture (Colles fracture)
    D. All of the above have the same incidence of occurrence.

43. What is the leading cause of blindness in older adults?
    A. Cataracts
    B. Detached retina
    C. Glaucoma
    D. Macular degeneration

44. Hearing loss impacts an estimated one-third of older adults between the ages of 61 and 74 and continues to rise as one ages. Which of the following is presbycusis most commonly associated with?

    A. Cholesteatoma

    B. Ototoxic drugs

    C. Cerumen impaction

    D. Loss of high-frequency sounds

45. Which of the following is characterized by a waxy papule with a stuck-on appearance?

    A. Basal cell carcinoma

    B. Sebaceous cyst

    C. Seborrheic keratosis

    D. Squamous cell carcinoma

46. Which of the following drugs is least likely to cause ototoxicity (resulting in hearing loss)?

    A. Sildenafil (Viagra)

    B. Salicylates

    C. Loop diuretics (e.g., Lasix [furosemide])

    D. Acetyl cholinesterase inhibitors (e.g., Aricept, Exelon, Rivastigmine)

47. Physiological and anatomical changes related to normal aging can present atypically with symptomatology not observed in other populations. Older adults with a UTI may exhibit:

    A. Urinary incontinence and dehydration.

    B. A change in mental status, falls, and dehydration.

    C. Complaints of pain, urinary incontinence, and a change in appetite.

    D. Dementia, weight gain, and a change in appetite.

48. The guiding principles that define the decision "to treat or not to treat" a suspected UTI in an older adult residing in a skilled nursing facility is based on multiple factors. Using McGeer's criteria for a voided urine, which of the following should not be considered?

    A. New or increased incontinence

    B. Characteristic changes of urine

    C. Single oral temperature of >100 degrees Fahrenheit

    D. Dysuria

49. Which of the following statements is true?

    A. The USPSTF recommends that colorectal screening continue to age 85.

    B. The use of computed tomographic colonography is preferred over colonoscopy and yields better results in older adults.

    C. The USPSTF recommends against routine screening for colorectal cancer in older adults age 76 to 85 years old.

    D. Screening for colorectal cancer should continue throughout one's lifetime, beginning at age 50.

50. The components of a nutritional assessment for an older adult includes all the following EXCEPT:

    A. A food intake diary of 1 to 3 days.

    B. A physical assessment including anthropometric measures.

    C. A meal preparation assessment.

    D. Use of a valid nutritional screening tool.

Answers and Rationales

....

1. C. Medication review of all OTC (e.g., nutritional supplements, herbals, vitamins, etc.) and prescription medications at each patient encounter is fundamental to health maintenance. In addition to the family nurse practitioner, older adults may see additional providers.

2. A. The best response is to measure his digoxin level. All of the other responses should also be considered with the exception of response B. Older adults are at increased risk for digoxin toxicity, with dosages of > 0.125 mg/day.

3. C. The Health Insurance Portability and Accountability Act (HIPPA) provides health care consumers with protection with respect to their private health information. A patient who has the mental capacity to make his/her medical decisions is not required to agree to sharing personal/medical information with family members.

4. C. Medication reconciliation should be done at each visit. Older adults, on average, take six prescription drugs in addition to over-the-counter remedies. Also, older adults may have additional health care providers who prescribe medications. Therefore, it is essential that the family nurse practitioner reconcile medications at each visit.

5. C. Durable medical equipment is covered under Medicare Part B.

6. D. The best way to assess for delirium is the CAM (Confusion Assessment Method). The CAGE is used to assess ETOH abuse. The MMSE is used to assess cognition in older adults.

7. C. The Geriatric Depression Scale is a valid and reliable assessment tool to screen for depression in the clinical setting. It is available in a short and long form. It does not assess for suicide risk.

8. D. Hospital-acquired delirium is the most likely cause. Elderly patients who are hospitalized are at increased risk of delirium. Precipitating factors include medications, psychological stressors, sensory overload, nutritional deficiencies, etc.

9. B. Alzheimer's disease is a progressive disease. There is no cure available at this time.

10. D. The domains of the Geriatric Comprehensive Assessment include physical health, functional health, physiological health, socio-environmental supports, and quality of life measures.

11. B. The only acetyl cholinesterase inhibitor approved to treat moderate to severe dementia is Aricept (donepezil).

12. B. The JNC 8 recommends that older adults 60+ without chronic kidney disease or diabetes should have a SBP < 150 mmHg or DBP < 90 mmHg.

13. B. The patient that should be evaluated first is the 76-year-old female who is less than 24 hours post op, complaining of back pain with a new onset of urinary incontinence. This is a red flag and should be further evaluated. All of the other responses, although important, are secondary to this scenario.

14. A. The most distinguishing characteristic of the physical examination for suspected osteoarthritis of the hip is gait abnormality. Patients with osteoarthritis of the hip routinely present with an antalgic gait to avoid pain in the affected hip.

15. B. Recommended immunizations for adults 65+ include TDAP every 10 years, an annual influenza vaccine, a shingles vaccine after the age of 60, and pneumococcal vaccines 13 and 23. The other responses are not correct.

16. D. Medicare Part D is referred to as the Medicare prescription drug benefit and helps to offset the costs associated with outpatient drug coverage. Medicare Part A covers hospitalization, skilled nursing services, and hospice care. There is no cost to enroll if the beneficiary has worked and paid Social Security taxes for a minimum of 40 calendar quarters. If the beneficiary has not contributed, there may be a monthly premium required. Medicare Part B covers outpatient services (e.g., diagnostics, visits to health care providers, etc.) and durable medical equipment. Medicare Part C allows private insurance companies to provide health benefits (e.g., Medicare Advantage plans).

17. C. The prevalence of elder abuse in this country is estimated to be 2 to 10%. Unfortunately, this is a fraction of the cases that should be reported to Protective Services for the elderly. The family nurse practitioner should be aware of mandated reporting of elder abuse in the state of practice.

18. D. All of the responses can be considered in the definition of elder abuse.

19. B. The most appropriate response is to speak slowly in a deep tone and address your questions to the patient. When interviewing the patient, the family nurse practitioner should be seated face to face with the patient. Do not assume that the patient wants to be called by his/her first name. It is important to ask how they wish to be addressed.

20. A. The goals of geriatric care are to maintain function and quality of life.

21. C. McGeer's criteria utilizes guiding principles that define infections (e.g., UTIs) in the long-term care setting using specific benchmarks. All of the other responses should be considered.

22. B. Increase in A/P chest diameter is a normal, non-pathological change related to the respiratory system.

23. B. The use of an MRI of the brain for screening is not supported. All of the other responses can be done by the family nurse practitioner and are considered to be an important part of the screening process.

24. D. The American Geriatric Society supports the HgbA$_{1c}$ recommendation of the American Diabetes Association for older adults with 3 or more multiple comorbidities or mild to moderate cognitive impairment. The final decision for each patient should involve patient and provider goals.

25. B. Sulfonyureas should not be used as a first choice for treating diabetes. The first-generation sulfonylureas have been shown to increase the risk of hypoglycemia in older adults. The second-generation sulfonylureas, which include glipizide, are a better choice, in addition to other treatment options.

26. B. A mammogram is a secondary form of prevention. The intent of primary prevention is to implement measures to avert the onset of disease or illness. Secondary preventive practices include those activities aimed at early detection to prevent or slow down the disease process, as well as disability.

27. A. Increased melanin production is an extrinsic cause of aging. Decreased pigmentation, ridging of nails, and the loss or increase of subcutaneous fat deposits are all related to intrinsic aging changes that occur in the integumentary system.

28. C. The education level of caregivers is not considered. The family nurse practitioner must understand that elder abuse does not discriminate by level of education. The increased risk for elder abuse is multifactorial and includes societal, relational, community, as well as individual factors that lead to abuse.

29. C. Anemia of chronic disease is the most common anemia found in older adults. Cooley's anemia is the most severe type of beta thalassemia, often requiring blood transfusions. Iron deficiency anemia can be found in older adults. It is a microcytic anemia which can be the result of acute blood loss due to malignancy or gastrointestinal pathology. Vitamin B12 deficiency is a macrocytic anemia. It is treatable and usually presents with another underlying medical illness.

30. B. The greatest suicide rate occurs in Caucasian males 85+.

31. D. Advance care planning is an ongoing process that should begin in the primary care setting and be addressed periodically whether the patient is young and healthy, is managing a chronic disease, or is living with a terminal illness. Advance care planning, or end-of-life care planning ensures that the patients' preferences for end-of-life care treatment are specified and followed if the patient is no longer able to make health care decisions or speak for themselves. Although the signing of an Advance Directive is encouraged, the role of the family nurse practitioner should include providing education to ensure a clearer understanding of the process.

32. C. The best response is to perform the "Get up and Go Test." The purpose of the test is to check mobility. A patient that scores a 3 or more is at increased risk for falls.

33. C. It is estimated that the population growth for those 85+ will triple from 6 million in 2013 to 14.6 million by 2040. Ethnic and minority populations will continue too grow.

34. A. Gifting is not a major source of income for older adults. Social Security, pensions, and assets provide income for older adults.

35. C. Amyloid plaques and neurofibrillary tangles are the hallmark characteristics of Alzheimer's disease.

36. B. Older adults often present with a *decreased* sensitivity to heat or pain due to physiological changes secondary to normal aging that affect the structure and function of the nervous system.

37. C. Stasis dermatitis is a common skin condition in older adults. It is characterized by pruritus, discoloration or hyperpigmentation of lower extremities, and edema. Contact dermatitis is a rash that occurs when the skin comes in contact with a foreign substance. Fifth Disease is a virus that is more common in children than older adults.

38. B. Auditory changes do not increase the risk for falls. The risk for falls increases in older adults due to underlying comorbidities, medications, and contributing risk factors.

39. B. According to the JNC 8, a BP goal of < 140/90 is recommended for a patient with diabetes.

40. D. Beta-blockers are not typically used for first-line treatment of hypertension in older adults, unless they have ischemic heart disease or heart failure.

41. B. Medication management is an example of an IADL. ADLs include bathing, continence, dressing, eating, toileting, and transfer. IADLs include the ability to use a phone, shopping, food preparation, housekeeping, laundry, transportation, medication management, and the ability to manage one's finances.

42. B. The most common fracture associated with osteoporosis is a vertebral fracture. It is estimated that more than 700,000 new vertebral fractures occur in this country, accounting for expenditures close to 1.5 billion dollars annually, as well as an increase in hospital admissions.

43. D. Macular degeneration is the leading cause of vision loss in adults 65 and over. It causes vision loss in the center of the vision field.

44. D. Presbycusis is a hearing loss in older adults. It is associated with a failure to hear high-frequency sounds.

45. C. A seborrheic keratosis is a benign finding and can appear anywhere on the body. It can vary in color and has a stuck-on appearance. Basal cell carcinoma is a malignant finding that appears as a pearly white, dome-shaped papule with a bleeding, crusted ulcerative center. A sebaceous cyst is a circumscribed dermal lesion with overlying punctum. Squamous cell carcinoma is found on the head, neck, hands, and sun-exposed areas. It is red on a poorly defined base with a necrotic crusted center.

46. D. Acetyl cholinesterase inhibitors do not cause ototoxicity. Commonly used prescription and non-prescription medications can cause ototoxicity. The list includes non-steroidal, salicylates, acetaminophen, sildenafil, macrolides, aminoglycosides, topical preparations containing neomycin/polymixin B, and some chemotherapeutic drugs.

47. B. Atypical presentations of acute illness in older adults is common given the physiological changes of aging complicated by underlying comorbidities. Changes in cognition and/or physical function provide the family nurse practitioner with "clues" of an acute illness. Atypical symptoms associated with a UTI in an older adult can include increased confusion, falls, lethargy, cough, weakness, abdominal pain, anorexia, and dehydration.

48. B. Characteristic changes in the urine are no longer included. The McGeer criteria, developed in 1991 and updated in 2012, defines the guiding principles "to treat or not to treat" a suspected UTI in an older adult residing in a skilled nursing facility. It includes fever (e.g., single temperature greater than 100 degrees Fahrenheit or repeated temperatures greater than 99 degrees Fahrenheit), leukocytosis (>14,000 wbc/mm^3, shift to the left > or = to 1500 bands/mm^3), an acute change in mental status from the baseline, and acute functional decline.

49. C. The USPSTF recommends against routine screening for colorectal cancer in older adults age 76 to 85 years old. The decision to screen should be individualized to the patient.

50. C. Meal preparation assessment may be included with an occupational therapy evaluation. The components of a nutritional assessment include: a food intake diary, the use of a valid screening tool, physical assessment including anthropometric measures, and biomarkers.

• • • References

Administration on Aging. (2012). Older Americans behavioral health issue brief 4: Preventing suicide in older adults. Retrieved from http://www.aoa.gov/AoA_Programs/HPW/Behavioral/docs2/Issue%20Brief%204%20Preventing%20Suicide.pdf

Administration on Aging. (2013). Older Americans behavioral health issue brief 6: Depression and anxiety: Screening and intervention. Retrieved from http://www.aoa.acl.gov/AoA_Programs/HPW/Behavioral/docs2/Issue%20Brief%206%20Depression%20and%20Anxiety.pdf

Administration on Aging. (2014). A profile of older Americans: 2014. Retrieved from http://www.aoa.acl.gov/Aging_Statistics/Profile/2014/docs/2014-Profile.pdf

Administration on Aging. (n.d.). Aging statistics. Retrieved from http://www.aoa.acl.gov/Aging_Statistics/index.aspx

Administration on Aging. (n.d.). Living arrangements. Retrieved from http://www.aoa.acl.gov/Aging_Statistics/Profile/2014/6.aspx

Alagiakrishnan, K., & Ahmed, I. (2014). Delirium. Retrieved from http://emedicine.medscape.com/article/288890-overview

American Diabetes Association. (2015). Standards of medical care in diabetes. Retrieved from http://care.diabetesjournals.org/content/38/Supplement_1

American Geriatrics Society Core Writing Group of the Task Force on the Future of Geriatic Medicine. (2005). Caring for older Americans: The future of geriatric medicine. Retrieved from http://www.caretransitions.org/documents/Caring%20for%20older%20Americans%20-%20JAGS.pdf

American Geriatric Society. (2012). Identifying medications that older adults should avoid or use with caution: The 2012 American geriatrics updated Beers criteria. Retrieved from http://www.americangeriatrics.org/files/documents/beers/BeersCriteriaPublicTranslation.pdf

American Geriatric Society. (2014). *Geriatrics at Your Fingertips*. New York, NY: American Geriatric Society.

Berkow, R., & Beers, M. H. (2000). *Merck manual of geriatrics* (3rd ed.), Whitehouse Station, NJ: Merck Research Laboratories.

Boult, C., Counsell, S., Leipzig, R., & Berenson, R. (2010). The urgency of preparing primary care physicians to care for older people with chronic illnesses. *Health Affairs, 29*(5), 811–815. Retrieved from http://content.healthaffairs.org/content/29/5/811.full

Centers for Disease Control and Prevention. (2013). The state of aging and health in America. Atlanta, GA: Centers for Disease Control and Prevention, U.S. Dept. of Health and Human Services. Retrieved from http://www.cdc.gov/features/agingandhealth/state_of_aging_and_health_in_america_2013.pdf

Centers for Disease Control and Prevention. (2015). Older adult falls: Get the facts. Retrieved from http://www.cdc.gov/homeandrecreationalsafety/falls/adultfalls.html

Centers for Disease Control and Prevention, Administration on Aging, Agency for Healthcare Research and Quality, and Centers for Medicare and Medicaid Services. (2011). Enhancing use of clinical preventive services among older adults. Washington, DC: AARP. Retrieved from http://www.cdc.gov/aging/pdf/clinical_preventive_services_closing_the_gap_report.pdf

Federal Interagency Forum on Aging Related Statistics. (2012). Older Americans 2012: Key indicators of well-being. Washington, DC: U.S. Government Printing Office. Retrieved from http://www.agingstats.gov/agingstatsdotnet/Main_Site/Data/2012_Documents/Docs/EntireChartbook.pdf

Golan, D. E., Tashjiaaaaan, A. H., Armstrong, E. J. & Armstrong, A. (2012). *Principles of Pharmacology: The Pathophysiologic Basis of Drug Therapy* (3rd ed.). Philadelphia, PA: Wolters Kluwer/Lipincott Willliams & Wilkins.

Halloran, L. (2013). Prescribing for the elderly. *Medscape Medical Students.* Retrieved from http://www.medscape.com/viewarticle/779494

James, P., Oparil, S., Carter, B., Cushman, W., Dennison-Himmelfarb, C., Handler, J., . . . Ortiz, E. (2014). 2014 Evidence-based guideline for the management of high blood pressure in adults: Report from the panel members appointed to the eighth joint national committee (JNC 8). *JAMA, 311*(5), 507–520. Retrieved from jama.jamanetwork.com/article.aspx?articleid=1791497

Jeremiah, M., Unwin, B., Greenawald, M., & Casiano, V. (2015). Diagnosis and management of osteoporosis. *American Family Physician ,92*(4), 261–268.

Kennedy–Malone, L., Fletcher, K., & Plank, L. (2014). *Advanced practice nursing care in the older adults.* F. A. Davis Company: Philadelphia, PA.

Na, C. R., Wang, S., Kirsner, R. S., & Federman, D. G. (2012). Elderly adults and skin disorders: Common problems for nondermatologists. *Southern Medical Journal, 105*(11), 600–606. Retrieved from www.medscape.com/viewarticle/774527_2

Namzaric. (2015). Drug monograph. Retrieved from http://www.empr.com/search/NAMZARIC/

National Council on Aging. (2015). Falls prevention. Retrieved from https://www.ncoa.org/resources/falls-prevention-fact-sheet/

National Osteoporosis Foundation. (2014). *Clinician's guide to prevention and treatment of osteoporosis.* Washington, DC: National Osteoporosis Foundation

Nelson, J., & Good, E. (2015). Urinary tract infections and asymptomatic bacteriuria in older adults. *The Nurse Practitioner, 40*(8), 43–50.

Nestle's Nutrition Institute. (n.d.). MNA-Mini Nutrional Assessment. Retrieved from http://www.mna-elderly.com/

Office of Disease Prevention and Health Promotion (n.d.). Older adults. Retrieved from http://www.healthypeople .gov/2020/topics-objectives/topic/older-adults

Rhoads, J., & Petersen, S. W. (2014). *Advanced health assessment and diagnostic reasoning* (2nd ed.). Jones and Bartlett: Burington, MA.

Rounds, L., Rappaport, B. A., & Mallary. L. L. (2013). Polypharmacy in senior adults. *Journal for Nurse Practitioners, 17,* 7–14.

Sadowsky, C., & Galvin, J. (2012). Guidelines for the management of cognitive and behavioral problems in dementia. *JAFBM, 25*(3), 350–366.

Taylor, W. (2014, Sepember 25). Depression in the elderly. *NEJM, 371,* 1228–1236. Retrieved from http://www.nejm .org/doi/full/10.1056/NEJMcp1402180

U.S. Preventive Services Task Force (2012). Falls prevention in older adults: Counseling and preventive medication. Retrieved from http://www.uspreventiveservicestaskforce .org/Page/Document/UpdateSummaryFinal/falls-prevention-in-older-adults-counseling-and-preventive-medication,

Wolff, K., & Johnson, R. A., & Saavedra, A. (2013). *Fitzpatrick's color atlas and synopis of clinical dermatology* (7th ed.). New York, NY: McGraw-Hill

Ward, K. T., & Ruben, D. B. (2013). Comprehensive geriatric assessment. *UpToDate.* Retreived from http://www.upto date.com/contents/comprehensive-geriatric-assessment

Zagaria, M. A. E. (2012). Potentially inappropriate medications for seniors: Focus on the 2012 Beers criteria. *American Journal for Nurse Practitioners, 16,* 26–28.

Zibel, S. (2011). Advance care planning in primary care: An interventional approach to enhance patient understanding of treatment preferences at the end-of-life. (unpublished doctoral capstone). Chatham University: Pittsburgh, PA.

19

Mental Health in Primary Care

Tina Walde, DNP, PMHNP

Brandi Parker Cotton, PhD, MSN, PMHNP

Primary care providers have an important role in identifying and managing mental health disorders, including:

- Screening for and eliciting mental health and substance abuse concerns
- Facilitating referral to psychiatric care
- Initiating treatment pending transition to psychiatric care
- Managing patients who are stable on medication with a confirmed diagnosis

Mood Disorders

Mood disorders are a group of diagnoses characterized by either prolonged periods of sadness, periods of excessive energy, or both. Some are chronic and lifelong disorders, such as bipolar disorder, while others, like major depressive disorder, may be a single episode or chronic.

Major Depressive Disorder and Persistent Depressive Disorder

According to the National Institute of Mental Health, major depressive disorder affects more than a million Americans every year (n.d.). It is one of the leading causes of death and disability in the world. More than a quarter of young adults will experience depression before age 24 years (Kessler et al., 2007). Further,

more than two-thirds of adults with depression will not seek treatment (Wang, Lane, Pincus, Wells & Kessler, 2005). Primary care providers are well positioned to recognize and respond to symptoms of depression, which often present as unexplained physical problems, such as fatigue, pain, or vague symptoms that result in frequent medical visits.

Screening

Since 2002, the United States Preventive Services Task Force (USPSTF) has recommended routine screening for depression in primary care, along with adequate treatment and follow-up care (2009). There are several available screening tools to help identify and manage depression. One of the most commonly used in the primary care setting is the PHQ-9 (Kroenke, Spitzer, & Williams, 2001).

Assessment

A mnemonic, SIGECAPS (Carlat, 1998), may assist in remembering the symptoms of major depression and persistent depressive disorder:

Sleep disorder (increased or decreased)

Interest deficit (anhedonia)

Guilt (worthlessness, hopelessness, regret)

Energy deficit

Concentration deficit

Appetite disorder (increased or decreased)

Psychomotor retardation or agitation

Suicidality

PATIENT HEALTH QUESTIONNAIRE (PHQ-9)

NAME:_____ DATE:_____

Over the last *2 weeks*, how often have you been
bothered by any of the following problems?
(use "✓" to indicate your answer)

	Not at all	Several days	More than half the days	Nearly every day
1. Little interest or pleasure in doing things	0	1	2	3
2. Feeling down, depressed, or hopeless	0	1	2	3
3. Trouble falling or staying asleep, or sleeping too much	0	1	2	3
4. Feeling tired or having little energy	0	1	2	3
5. Poor appetite or overeating	0	1	2	3
6. Feeling bad about yourself—or that you are a failure or have let yourself or your family down	0	1	2	3
7. Trouble concentrating on things, such as reading the newspaper or watching television	0	1	2	3
8. Moving or speaking so slowly that other people could have noticed. Or the opposite — being so figety or restless that you have been moving around a lot more than usual	0	1	2	3
9. Thoughts that you would be better off dead, or of hurting yourself	0	1	2	3

add columns   [ ] + [ ] + [ ]

(Healthcare professional: For interpretation of TOTAL, please refer to accompanying scoring card).   TOTAL: [ ]

10. If you checked off *any problems*, how *difficult* have these problems made it for you to do your work, take care of things at home, or get along with other people?	Not difficult at all _____ Somewhat difficult _____ Very difficult _____ Extremely difficult _____

Figure 19-1 Patient Health Questionnaire

PHQ-9 Patient Depression Questionnaire

For initial diagnosis:

1. Patient completes PHQ-9 Quick Depression Assessment.
2. If there are at least 4 ✓s in the shaded section (including Questions #1 and #2), consider a depressive disorder. Add score to determine severity.

Consider Major Depressive Disorder

- if there are at least 5 ✓s in the shaded section (one of which corresponds to Question #1 or #2)

Consider Other Depressive Disorder

- if there are 2-4 ✓s in the shaded section (one of which corresponds to Question #1 or #2)

Note: Since the questionnaire relies on patient self-report, all responses should be verified by the clinician, and a definitive diagnosis is made on clinical grounds taking into account how well the patient understood the questionnaire, as well as other relevant information from the patient.
Diagnoses of Major Depressive Disorder or Other Depressive Disorder also require impairment of social, occupational, or other important areas of functioning (Question #10) and ruling out normal bereavement, a history of a Manic Episode (Bipolar Disorder), and a physical disorder, medication, or other drug as the biological cause of the depressive symptoms.

To monitor severity over time for newly diagnosed patients or patients in current treatment for depression:

1. Patients may complete questionnaires at baseline and at regular intervals (eg, every 2 weeks) at home and bring them in at their next appointment for scoring or they may complete the questionnaire during each scheduled appointment.

2. Add up ✓s by column. For every ✓: Several days = 1 More than half the days = 2 Nearly every day = 3

3. Add together column scores to get a TOTAL score.

4. Refer to the accompanying **PHQ-9 Scoring Box** to interpret the TOTAL score.

5. Results may be included in patient files to assist you in setting up a treatment goal, determining degree of response, as well as guiding treatment intervention.

Scoring: add up all checked boxes on PHQ-9

For every ✓ Not at all = 0; Several days = 1;
More than half the days = 2; Nearly every day = 3

Interpretation of Total Score

Total Score	Depression Severity
1-4	Minimal depression
5-9	Mild depression
10-14	Moderate depression
15-19	Moderately severe depression
20-27	Severe depression

Figure 19-1 Patient Health Questionnaire (Continued)

For Major Depressive Disorder, *symptoms must be present nearly every day* for at least a two-week period. For Persistent Depressive Disorder, symptoms are continuous for at least a two-year period of time. Clinical judgment is needed to tell apart depression from a normal response to loss.

In certain populations, depressive symptoms may vary. In children and teenagers, depression may manifest as increased clinginess, increased physical complaints, poor attendance or school refusal, and avoidance of social interactions or loss of friendships. In older adults, depression may manifest as problems with memory, changes in personality, or social isolation. The experience of depression across different cultures and ethnicities may lead to differing presentations as well, commonly presenting as increased physical health complaints.

Management

Nonpharmacologic

Treatment plans made in coordination with the patient must consider:

- Symptom severity
- Level of functioning
- Psychosocial stressors
- Degree of support
- Patient motivation
- Patient preferences

Psychotherapy is the treatment of choice for mild to moderate depressive symptoms, while pharmacologic intervention and psychotherapy combined are first-line treatments for severe symptoms. Nonpharmacologic treatment includes evidence-based therapeutic modalities such as Cognitive Behavioral Therapy (CBT), Interpersonal Therapy (IPT), and Problem-Solving Treatment (PST). Other strategies include mindfulness, behavioral activation, healthy sleep habits, stress management, and increased physical activity.

Pharmacologic

Generally, the second-generation antidepressants are considered first-line treatment for depression. These include the selective serotonin reuptake inhibitors (SSRIs), such as citalopram, escitalopram, fluoxetine, and sertraline, selective norepinephrine reuptake inhibitors (SNRIs), such as venlafaxine and duloxetine, and buproprion. These medications have fewer side effects than their earlier cousins and are safer in overdose. Common side effects include headache, agitation, insomnia, and sexual side effects.

Tricyclic antidepressants, including nortriptyline and amitriptyline, should be monitored closely in patients with heart problems, risk of drug-drug interactions, or high risk of suicide. Monoamine oxidase inhibitors (MAOIs), such as imipramine, phenelzine, and selegeline, are typically restricted to patients who do not respond to other options. This is because of the MAOIs' many side effects and the risk of dangerously elevated blood pressure in the patient when taken with certain foods or medications. Consider prescribing these medications in consultation with a psychiatric provider.

Clinical Pearls for SSRIs, SNRIs, and Buproprion

- Typically take two weeks or longer until response is titrated to the appropriate dosage.
- Continue for 6–12 months after symptom remission.
- Side effects are common and are likely to remit after a few weeks of treatment.
- For patients who do not respond to the maximum dosage or who have intolerable side effects, consider switching agents.
- Consider CBC, CMP, and TSH on initiation to rule out general medical conditions.
- Consider maintenance therapy if a patient has experienced multiple episodes of depression, rapid recurrences, severe episodes, residual symptoms, or has a significant family history.

Warning about Serotonin Syndrome

Serotonin Syndrome is a potentially life-threatening condition associated with an increase in serotonin in the central nervous system—a risk when initiating or adjusting serotonergic medications. This is a medical emergency and requires prompt treatment.

It may include:

- Confusion
- Agitation
- Dilated pupils
- Nausea/vomiting/diarrhea
- Shivering
- Fever
- Seizures
- Irregular or rapid heart rate

Postpartum Depression

While postpartum depression affects up to 22% of women, most women are not screened properly (Gaynes et al., 2005). A commonly used screening tool is the Patient Health Questionnaire (PHQ-9 or abbreviated PHQ-2), which takes very little time and is easily administered during routine office visits (see Figure 19-1). Pediatric providers treating infants during routine well-child visits are in an optimal position to screen women for postpartum depression given the frequency of visits during the infant's first year of life.

Management

- For mild to moderate PPD, psychotherapy is considered first-line treatment.
- For moderate to severe PPD, pharmacotherapy should be considered.
- For women who are breast-feeding, antidepressants in general, including fluoxetine, sertraline, and tricyclics, are considered relatively safe treatment considering low transmission in breast milk and minimal adverse effects in neonates.
- Infants should be monitored for adverse effects or changes in behavior.
- Medication, when effective, should be continued for at least 6 months and likely longer in women who have a history of depression.

Bipolar Disorder

Bipolar Disorder affects 2.6% of the American population aged 18 years and older (NIMH, n.d.). With a median age of onset of 25 years, it can affect people as young as early childhood and as old as in their late 40s and 50s (Kessler, Chiu, Demler, & Walters, 2005). It is characterized by intense shifts in mood, energy, and activity that impacts day-to-day functioning.

Screening

While routine screening for Bipolar Disorder is not generally recommended, there are a number of tools that may help identify symptoms and encourage further evaluation. One of these tools is the Mood Disorder Questionnaire (MDQ). It is a brief self-report tool that takes approximately five minutes to complete (Hirschfield et al., 2003).

Assessment

Bipolar Disorder is typified by periods of mania or hypomania, or elevated, expansive, or irritable mood. Mania and hypomania are differentiated by degree of impairment, with mania being severely impairing and hypomania being mild to moderately impairing.

Bipolar Disorder includes a history of mania, whereas Bipolar II Disorder includes a history of hypomania only. While many people also experience episodes of depression with Bipolar Disorder, it is mania that is diagnostic.

A mnemonic that facilitates recalling the symptoms of hypomania/mania is DIG FAST:

Distractibility

Indiscretion

Grandiosity

Flight of ideas

Activity increase

Sleep deficit

Talkativeness

Psychosis may or may not be present during episodes of severe mania. As many patients in the acute phase of mania or hypomania have poor insight into their symptoms, involving family members in their care may provide helpful collaborative information.

Cyclothymic Disorder

Cyclothymic Disorder is a rare mood disorder in which a person experiences ups and downs in mood that are impairing but not as extreme as Bipolar I or II Disorder. Symptoms must occur persistently for two or more years with no more than two symptom-free months. Treatment management is consistent with those used for Bipolar I and II Disorder.

Disruptive Mood Dysregulation Disorder

While some children meet the full criteria for Bipolar Disorder, many children with chronic irritability may experience significant impairment but do not meet full criteria for Bipolar Disorder. This subset of children may be more likely to go on to develop Major Depressive Disorder or Generalized Anxiety Disorder in adulthood. The DSM-V defines Disruptive Mood Dysregulation Disorder as severe and recurrent temper outbursts in excess of what is considered developmentally appropriate and out of proportion to the situation at hand. These tantrums must occur at least *three times a week for a minimum of one year*.

As this is a new diagnosis, there is not yet clinical evidence regarding the most effective treatment. Treatment may include a combination of psychotherapy and pharmacologic management, with agents such as stimulant medication, antidepressants, and/or mood stabilizers.

Management

Nonpharmacologic

A presentation of mania, particularly when accompanied by psychosis, is a medical emergency and often necessitates hospitalization. Pharmacologic management is indicated for Bipolar Disorder and Bipolar II Disorder as a first-line treatment. However, studies have also shown that therapy in conjunction with medication, particularly during a period of residual mood symptoms, may help reduce the risk of recurrence (Perlis, et al., 2006).

Pharmacologic

There is no evidence to support antidepressant monotherapy for Bipolar Disorder and, in fact, antidepressants may exacerbate manic symptoms and/or lead to relapse in stable patients. There are several classes of medication used to treat Bipolar Disorder, including lithium, anticonvulsants, and atypical antipsychotics. Often, multiple medications must be used to target the symptoms of depression and mania equally, as well as other presenting problems such as poor sleep.

Lithium

- Only medication that has a known protective mechanism against suicide
- Effects should occur in 1–3 weeks
- Requires frequent tests to monitor trough lithium plasma levels (should be between 0.5–1.2 mEq/L)
- Caution with use of drugs that have renal clearance
- Potential side effects: ataxia, tremor, polyuria and polydipsia (nephrogenic diabetes), sedation, weight gain, diarrhea, nausea, goiter
- Drug monitoring: kidney function tests (creatinine and urine specific gravity), TSH, and EKG over 50 years on initiation; repeat 1–2 times a year

Anticonvulsants

- Drug monitoring: CBC, LFTs, kidney function tests (creatinine and urine specific gravity), and TSH
- Potential side effects: Sedation, weight gain, dizziness, headache, nausea, vomiting, diarrhea, blurred vision
- Effects should occur within a few weeks but may take several weeks to months to stabilize

Carbamazepine (Tegretol)

- Rare aplastic anemia or agranulocytosis may occur (unusual bleeding or bruising, mouth sores, infections, fever, sore throat)

- Rare Syndrome of Inappropriate Antidiuretic Hormone Secretion with hyponatremia may occur
- Risk Category D pregnancy

Valproate (Depakote)

- Rarely causes alopecia
- Requires frequent tests to monitor trough plasma levels (50–125 ug/ml)
- Risk Category D pregnancy—may cause neural tube defects particularly when used in the first trimester

Lamotrigine (Lamictal)

- Generally tolerated well
- No monitoring of plasma levels
- Titration often takes 6 or more weeks due to risk of Stevens–Johnson Syndrome

Atypical Antipsychotics

Refer to section on psychotic disorders.

A Warning about Neuroleptic Malignant Syndrome

NMS is a potentially life-threatening situation that arises within two weeks of initiating or modifying a neuroleptic medication (i.e., typical or atypical antipsychotic medication). It requires immediate evaluation and treatment. It includes:

- Severe muscle rigidity
- Fever
- Autonomic instability
- Changes in level of consciousness

Attention-Deficit/Hyperactivity Disorder

ADHD affects about 5% of school-age children. For adults, the prevalence decreases to 2.5 percent (American Psychiatric Association, 2013). The disorder is characterized by functionally impairing symptoms of impulsivity, hyperactivity, and inattention across settings such as home, school, and work. The disorder is described as one of the following: ADHD predominately inattentive presentation, ADHD predominately hyperactive and impulsive presentation, or combined presentation. Of the following symptoms of each subcategory, *symptoms must have been observed* before age 12 and present for at least 6 months.

Assessment of ADHD for children requires a report from a parent and teacher. Routine collaboration in the form of standardized assessment tools, such as the Vanderbilt (Wolraich, Feurer, Hannah, Pinnock, & Baumgaertel, 1998) or Conners Rating Scale (Conners, 2001) is critical for treatment management.

Inattention

- Easily distracted
- Difficulty with follow-through on work or activities
- Difficulty with organizational skills
- Avoidance of activities that require sustained attention
- Often forgetful
- Difficulty listening when spoken to
- Trouble sustaining attention

Hyperactivity and Impulsivity

- Fidgets with hands and feet
- Difficulty remaining seated
- Excessive running, climbing
- Difficulty enjoying or participating in quiet activities
- Excessive talking
- Behavior appears that person is "driven by a motor"
- Interrupts, intrudes on others
- Has difficulty waiting for turn
- Blurts out answers before questions are finished

Nonpharmacologic

- Recommended as first-line therapy for children under 6
- Includes parent training and recommendations for classroom
- Used adjunctively with medications when appropriate and especially if comorbid psychiatric disorder is present

Pharmacologic

Recommended for children ages 6 to 11

Stimulant Medications

- Methylphendiate (Ritalin, Concerta, Daytrana, Metadate CD, Methylin)
- Dexmethylphenidate (Focalin)
- Dextroamphetamine (Dexedrine, Dextroamphetamine)
- Mixed Amphetamine Salts (Adderall, Adderall XR)
- Lisdexamphetamine—Vyvanse

- – Controlled substances (C-II) with high abuse potential
- – Monitor growth, including weight and height
- – Avoid if there is family history of cardiac disease.
- – Side effects include insomnia, loss of appetite (weight loss), tics, hypertension, and tachycardia.

Non-stimulant Medications

- Atomoxetine (Strattera)—SNRI, once daily dosing
- Monitor for mood changes, GI complaints, including decreased appetite
- All antidepressants carry black box warning for increased suicidal ideation.

Clonidine (Catapres) and guanfacine (Tenex, Intunive)—alpha-agonists

- Helpful with impulsive and hyperactive behaviors.
- Especially helpful if patients presents with comorbid Tourette's Syndrome or other tic disorders.
- Monitor blood pressure, pulse, and potential sedation.

Desipramine (Norpramin) and imipramine (Tofranil)—tricyclics

- For use when alternative therapies are ineffective or intolerable
- Recommended ECG at baseline and with increased dosage
- Blood levels helpful in determining optimal dosing
- Monitor for anticholinergic effects, suicidal ideation (FDA Black Box Warning)

Bupropion (Wellbutrin)—NDRI

- Monitor for decreased appetite, sleeping difficulties
- Potential for lowered seizure threshold

Psychotic Disorders

Psychosis includes a range of abnormalities in thought from many possible causes. Psychosis is a potential result of illicit drugs, a psychiatric disorder such as schizophrenia, or an adverse effect of medication. Patients experiencing psychosis may be difficult to engage or are disorganized, making communication difficult. The following categories outline psychotic disorders:

Schizophrenia is one of the most debilitating psychiatric illnesses. Symptoms are conceptualized as either *positive* or *negative* symptoms. Positive symptoms are characterized by delusions, hallucinations (either auditory and/or visual), speech that is disorganized and/or nonsensical, and disorganized behavior. Negative symptoms refer to poverty of speech, lack of motivation, lack of emotional expression and feelings of pleasure, and impairments in cognitive functioning.

Other Psychotic Disorders

- Major Depression with Psychotic Features—psychosis present during mood disorder. Symptoms must be present for 2 weeks.
- Mania with Psychosis—psychosis present during manic episode of Bipolar Disorder.
- Brief Psychotic Disorder—symptoms present for at least 2 weeks, but with complete remission in 1 to 3 months. Often preceded by significant psychosocial stressors.

Pharmacological Treatment

Antipsychotic medications are the treatment of choice for schizophrenia.

First-Generation Antipsychotics

- Medications such as haloperidol, fluphenazine, and chlorpromazine
- High risk of extra pyramidal symptoms or movement-related symptoms, such as tardive dyskinesia
- Effects up to 75% of patients, prescribed for first-generation psychotics
- In some cases, the adverse effects are irreversible.

Second-Generation Antipsychotics (Atypical Antipsychotics)

- Olanzapine, risperidone, ziprasidone, aripiprazole, quetiapine, paliperidone, and clozapine
- Adverse effects include weight gain, metabolic syndrome, and hypercholesteremia
- Requires routine monitoring of weight, lipid profile, glucose, LFTs, and prolactin levels on initiation, at least annually, and more frequently as indicated
- Clozapine requires ongoing blood monitoring for potential agranulocytosis, and in rare cases can cause myocarditis

The Abnormal Involuntary Movement Scale (AIMS) should be administered to patients prescribed first- and second-generation antipsychotics to aid in the early detection of tardive dyskinesia as well as for ongoing maintenance (see Figure 19-2).

Anxiety Disorders

Anxiety Disorders are collectively the most common mental health problem in the United States, effecting over 40 million people each year (NIMH, n.d.). While many people experience normal reactions to stress, people with anxiety disorders experience excessive worry that is difficult to control and contributes to a range of physical, psychological, and social impairments.

Screening

Given the prevalence of anxiety in the primary care population, screening may help identify patients at risk of these disorders. A commonly used screening tool is the GAD-7, or the abbreviated GAD-2, a seven- or two-question instrument, respectively, designed for use in primary care. While developed to recognize symptoms of Generalized Anxiety Disorder, this tool has also been shown to be effective in detecting symptoms of social anxiety, panic, and posttraumatic stress disorders.

Assessment
Physical Symptoms

Heart palpitations, shortness of breath, shakiness, trembling, chest pain, nausea, dizziness, choking sensation, dry mouth, numbness, decreased sexual desire, sleep disturbance

Psychological Symptoms

Worried thoughts that are difficult to control, derealization (feeling of being detached from oneself), restlessness, difficulty concentrating, irritability, and distressing memories

Social Symptoms

Avoidance of activities, changes in routines, fear of leaving home, distorted blame of self or others, poor performance in work or school settings

There are many different types of anxiety disorders and often they may occur together. The most common include:

Generalized Anxiety Disorder: Excessive worry and anxiety more days than not for at least 6 months (see Figure 19-3)

AIMS Examination Procedure

Should be completed before entering the ratings on the AIMS form.

Either before or after completing the Examination Procedure, observe the patient unobtrusively at rest (eg, in waiting room).

The chair to be used in this examination should be a hard, firm one without arms.

1: Ask patient whether there is anything in his/her mouth (ie, gum, candy, etc) and if there is, to remove it.

2: Ask patient about the current condition of his/her teeth. Ask patient if he/she wears dentures. Do teeth or dentures bother patient now?

3: Ask patient whether he/she notices any movements in mouth, face, hands, or feet. If yes, ask to describe and to what extent they currently bother patient or interfere with his/her activities.

4: Have patient sit in chair with hands on knees, legs slightly apart, and feet flat on floor. (Look at entire body for movements while in this position).

5: Ask patient to sit with hands hanging unsupported. If male, between legs, if female, and wearing a dress, hanging over knees. (Observe hands and other body areas.)

6: Ask patient to open mouth. (Observe tongue at rest within mouth.) Do this twice.

7: Ask patient to protrude tongue. (Observe abnormalities of tongue movement.)

*8: Ask patient to tap thumb, with each finger, as rapidly as possible for 10-15 seconds: separately with right hand, then with left hand. (Observe facial and leg movements.)

9: Flex and extend patient's left and right arms, one at a time. (Note any rigidity and rate it.)

10: Ask patient to stand up. (Observe in profile. Observe all body areas again, hips included.)

*11: Ask patient to extend both arms outstretched in front with palms down. (Observe trunk, legs, and mouth.)

*12: Have patient walk a few paces, turn, and walk back to chair. (Observe hands and gait.) Do this twice.

Figure 19-2 AIMS Scale

William Guy, Ph.D.: ECDEU Assessment Manual for Psychopharmacology - Revised (DHEW Publ No ADM 76-338), US Department of Health, Education, and Welfare, 1976.

ABNORMAL INVOLUNTARY MOVEMENT SCALE (AIMS)

Patient's Name (Please print) _____ Patient's ID information _____

Examiner's Name _____

CURRENT MEDICATIONS AND TOTAL MG/DAY

Medication #1 _____ Total mg/Day _____ Medication #2 _____ Total mg/Day _____

INSTRUCTIONS: COMPLETE THE EXAMINATION PROCEDURE BEFORE ENTERING THESE RATINGS.

	None, Normal	Minimal (may be extreme normal)	Mild	Moderate	Severe
Facial and Oral Movements					
1. Muscles of Facial Expression e.g., movements of forehead, eyebrows, periorbital area, cheeks; include frowning, blinking, smiling, grimacing	☐0	☐1	☐2	☐3	☐4
2. Lips and Perioral Area e.g., puckering, pouting, smacking	☐0	☐1	☐2	☐3	☐4
3. Jaw e.g., biting, clenching, chewing, mouth opening, lateral movement	☐0	☐1	☐2	☐3	☐4
4. Tongue Rate only increases in movement both in and out of mouth, NOT inability to sustain movement	☐0	☐1	☐2	☐3	☐4
Extremity Movements					
5. Upper (arms, wrists, hands, fingers) Include choreic movements (i.e., rapid, objectively purposeless, irregular, spontaneous); athetoid movements (i.e., slow, irregular, complex, serpentine). DO NOT include tremor (i.e., repetitive, regular, rhythmic).	☐0	☐1	☐2	☐3	☐4
6. Lower (legs, knees, ankles, toes) e.g., lateral knee movement, foot tapping, heel dropping, foot squirming, inversion and eversion of foot	☐0	☐1	☐2	☐3	☐4
Trunk Movements					
7. Neck, shoulders, hips e.g., rocking, twisting, squirming, pelvic gyrations	☐0	☐1	☐2	☐3	☐4

SCORING:
- Score the highest amplitude or frequency in a movement on the 0-4 scale, not the average;
- Score Activated Movements the same way; do not lower those numbers as was proposed at one time;
- A POSITIVE AIMS EXAMINATION IS A SCORE OF 2 IN TWO OR MORE MOVEMENTS or a SCORE OF 3 OR 4 IN A SINGLE MOVEMENT
- Do not sum the scores: e.g., a patient who has scores 1 in four movements DOES NOT have a positive AIMS score of 4.

Overall Severity
	None, Normal	Minimal	Mild	Moderate	Severe
8. Severity of abnormal movements	☐0	☐1	☐2	☐3	☐4
9. Incapacitation due to abnormal movements	☐0	☐1	☐2	☐3	☐4

	No Awareness	Aware, No Distress	Aware, Mild Distress	Aware, Moderate Distress	Aware, Severe Distress
10. Patient's awareness of abnormal movements (rate only patient's report)	☐0	☐1	☐2	☐3	☐4

Dental Status
11. Current problems with teeth and/or dentures?   ☐Yes ☐No
12. Does patient usually wear dentures?   ☐Yes ☐No

Comments: _____

Examiner's Signature _____ Next Exam Date _____

Figure 19-2 AIMS Scale (Continued)

William Guy, Ph.D.: ECDEU Assessment Manual for Psychopharmacology - Revised (DHEW Publ No ADM 76-338), US Department of Health, Education, and Welfare, 1976.

GAD-7

Over the <u>last 2 weeks</u>, how often have you been bothered by the following problems? *(Use "✔" to indicate your answer)*	Not at all	Several days	More than half the days	Nearly every day
1. Feeling nervous, anxious or on edge	0	1	2	3
2. Not being able to stop or control worrying	0	1	2	3
3. Worrying too much about different things	0	1	2	3
4. Trouble relaxing	0	1	2	3
5. Being so restless that it is hard to sit still	0	1	2	3
6. Becoming easily annoyed or irritable	0	1	2	3
7. Feeling afraid as if something awful might happen	0	1	2	3

(For office coding: Total Score T____ = ____ + ____ + ____)

Figure 19-3 GAD-7 and GAD 2

Reproduced from Pfizer. (n.d.). GAD-7. Retrieved from phqscreeners.com.

Social Anxiety Disorder: Intense anxiety and distress around a feared situation (i.e., being in groups of people) that is unreasonable or excessive and continues for at least 6 months.

Specific Phobia: An intense fear reaction to a specific object or situation (i.e., flying, heights, animals, blood, injections) that causes an immediate anxiety response, and the avoidance of which impairs a person's normal routine.

Panic Disorder: Sudden and intense fear that typically peaks in less than 10 minutes from onset with a range of physical and psychological symptoms.

Agoraphobia: Fear of being in a situation where leaving would be difficult or embarrassing, including places such as home, transportation, standing in line, or being in a crowd.

Somatic Symptom Disorder: Excessive fear or worry about health that occurs for greater than six months and which is disproportionate to either a diagnosed medical disorder or medically unexplained symptoms.

Separation Anxiety Disorder: Intense fear of separating from parents, caregivers, or home that may develop in childhood or adulthood and leads to severe anxiety and agitation even when anticipating a separation.

Selective Mutism: A childhood disorder that begins prior to age 5 in which a child experiences a lack of speech that is not due to knowledge of comfort of speech in at least one social situation.

Management

Nonpharmacologic

As with depressive disorders, treatment plans are made in coordination with the patient and must consider symptom severity, level of functioning, psychosocial stressors, degree of support, patient motivation, and patient preferences. Therapeutic modalities may include CBT or exposure therapy. Patients often benefit from developing stress management and relaxation skills as well.

Pharmacologic

As with the depressive disorders, SSRIs, SNRIs, and buproprion are considered first-line medication options.

Additional classes of medication that may be helpful, particularly for panic attacks and short-term management, include buspirone and benzodiazepines.

Buspirone

- Generally well tolerated
- Typically prescribed in 2–3 divided doses
- Does not cause dependence or withdrawal symptoms
- May take for 2–4 weeks to achieve efficacy

Benzodiazepines

- May be short, intermediate or long-acting
- Often provides immediate relief
- Are not indicated for chronic management given high abuse and dependency potential
- Caution should be used in the older adult population due to the increased risk of cognitive impairment

Post-Traumatic Stress Disorder

Post-Traumatic Stress Disorder (PTSD) affects 6.8% in the general population of adults in America (Kessler et al., 2005). The disorder is characterized by three main symptom categories: intrusive thoughts, hyperarousal, and avoidance in response to real or perceived threat of death, injury, or sexual violence. Patients often present with flashbacks, nightmares, increased startle response, and avoidance of speaking about the trauma, as well as persons or places that remind them of the traumatic experience.

Screening for PTSD

A commonly used screening tool in primary care is the PC-PTSD (Prins et al., 2003). An answer "yes" to three or more questions warrants follow-up and referral.

---

1. Have had nightmares about it or thought about it when you did not want to?
   YES/NO

2. Tried hard not to think about it or went out of your way to avoid situations that reminded you of it?
   YES/NO

3. Were constantly on guard, watchful, or easily startled?
   YES/NO

4. Felt numb or detached from others, activities, or your surroundings?
   YES/NO

Nonpharmacologic Treatment

There are several effective and evidence-based therapies for PTSD, including Cognitive Behavioral Therapy (CBT), Exposure Therapy, and Eye Movement Desensitization and Reprocessing Therapy (EMDR). People have varying and complex responses to trauma, and the main goal of trauma-informed therapy is to reduce distress related to the event and to help the person cope with reminders of the trauma.

Pharmacologic Treatment

SSRIs are frequently used to alleviate symptoms of PTSD. Paroxetine and sertraline are both FDA-approved for treating the disorder. Prazosin (Minipress) and propranolol (Inderal) are often used to help alleviate nightmares and improve sleep. Anxiolytics such as benzodiazapines may be used in appropriate patients for short-term symptom improvement only.

Pediatrics: Post-Traumatic Stress Disorder in Children

PTSD often presents differently in children than adults. The following symptoms are more common in children 6 years of age and older:

- Intrusive thoughts—distressing nightmares (content not required), flashbacks, physiological reactions
- Persistent avoidance of stimuli
- Negative alterations in cognitions—negative emotional states, loss of interest, withdrawn behavior

- Persistent reduction in expression and positive emotions
- Alterations in arousal and reactivity
- Irritable, hypervigilant, exaggerated startle response, sleep disturbance

Substance Abuse

Addiction is frequently encountered within primary care. Abuse of illicit and prescription drugs are dangerous and rarely reported by patients without prompting. The following are several classes of commonly abused substances:

- *Alcohol*—Alcohol use is common and defining alcohol abuse or misuse is often difficult. Guidelines have been developed to assist with definitions.
- *Low-risk drinking*—Defined for women as no more than 3 drinks per day and less than 7 per week; for men, defined as no more than 4 drinks per day and less than 14 per week.
- *At-risk drinking*—Alcohol intake above the recommended guidelines.
- *Harmful drinking*—Alcohol use that creates physical, social, and relational problems.

The following screening tool is common for screening for alcohol use or misuse within the primary care setting:

CAGE Questionnaire

Have you ever felt you should **Cut** down on your drinking?

Have people **Annoyed** you by criticizing your drinking?

Have you ever felt bad or **Guilty** about your drinking?

Have you ever had a drink first thing in the morning to steady your nerves or to get rid of a hangover (**Eye opener**)?

Reproduced from Dhalla, S., & Kopec, J. A. (2007). The CAGE questionnaire for alcohol misuse: A review of reliability and validity studies. *Clinical and Investigative Medicine*, *30*(1), 33–41.

- *Opioids*—Heroin, morphine, and opioid analgesics act on mu, kappa, and gamma. This produces euphoria and analgesia. Commonly abused prescription drugs include oxycodone, morphine, and other medications within this class.
- *Cannabinoids*—Marijuana acts on the cannabinoid receptors (CB1 and CB2) and inhibit

adenaylate cyclase. Dopamine and opioid mechanisms likely play a role in the reward pathways of cannabinoid use.

- *Psychostimulants*—Drugs such as cocaine and amphetamine act on dopamine, serotonin, and noradrenaline receptors, blocking reuptake. Amphetamines and methylphenidate are commonly abused prescription medications within this class.
- *Sedative or Anxiolytics*—Benzodiazepines and barbiturates act on GABA receptors and are CNS depressants. These drugs are frequently abused, given their highly addictive properties; can impair memory and cognition, and cause autonomic depression. Muscle relaxers are also in this category of potentially abused prescription drugs.
- *Hallucinogens*—Drugs such as PCP, LSD (lysergic acid diethylamide), ecstasy, and psilocybin (magic mushrooms, shrooms, etc.) often cause disassociation and altered perceptions.

Screening for substance abuse is essential during primary care visits. The following acronym is useful for assessing and screening for potential abuse for drugs and/or alcohol (The Center for Adolescent Substance Abuse Research, n.d.).

C—Have you ever ridden in a CAR driven by someone (including yourself) who was "high" or had been using alcohol or drugs?

R—Do you ever use alcohol or drugs to RELAX, feel better about you, or fit in?

A—Do you ever use alcohol/drugs while you are by yourself, ALONE?

F—Do you ever FORGET things you did while using alcohol or drugs?

F—Do your family or FRIENDS ever tell you that you should cut down on your drinking or drug use?

T—Have you gotten into TROUBLE while you were using alcohol or drugs?

Opioid Substitution Therapy

Buprenorphine and methadone maintenance are both treatments offered to patients struggling with opioid addiction. There are different risks, benefits, and considerations for each medication. Treatment options should be discussed with patients, including access, insurance considerations, risk of diversion, feasibility of treatment, and the patient's treatment goals.

Suicide Risk and Prevention

Assessing for suicide is imperative when a provider feels that a patient is at risk. Using the acronym "SAL" assists providers in conducting a risk assessment:

Specificity—Is there a plan for suicide? How detailed is this plan (time, place, means, intention to write suicide letter, saying goodbye to family and friends)?

Availability—If there is a plan, are the means readily available (access to weapon, medication, etc.)?

Lethality—Is the plan intended to be lethal? What degree is the lethality (firearm, medication, jumping from high building)?

Risk Factors

- Race and Ethnicity—white males are at greatest risk; minorities and immigrants also at risk
- Age—over 65 greatest risk for suicide
- Psychiatric diagnoses
- History of psychiatric hospitalizations
- Previous suicide attempt
- Family history of suicide
- Substance abuse disorders
- Chronic pain or illness
- Loss or bereavement

Warning Signs

- Impulsive behaviors
- Acute anxiety
- Social isolation
- Changes in sleep patterns
- Lack of future-oriented thinking

- Suicidal planning or gesturing
- Anger, rage

Patient Education and Safety Measures

- Emergency referral when patient is at risk to him/herself
- A contract between provider and patient that commits to not harming oneself and seeking immediate attention if suicidal thoughts/urges increase
- Barring access to firearms, sharp objects, and medication (prescribed and over-the-counter) if patient is at imminent risk
- Limiting prescription to 7-day supply if there is a potential danger of overdose
- Providing emergency contact numbers in case suicidal symptoms increase
- Following up within 24 hours of appointment

Domestic Violence and Intimate Partner Violence

Intimate partner violence (IPV) crosses all lines of ethnicities, age, and class. The Centers for Disease Control and Prevention defines IPV as physical violence, sexual violence, stalking, and psychological aggression (including coercive acts) by a current or former intimate partner. Screening for IPV is paramount within the trusting alliance of the nurse practitioner–patient relationship to avoid potential death, injury, and long-term physical and emotional health consequences (see Box 19-1).

BOX 19-1   HITS Tool for Intimate Partner Violence Screening

HITS Tool for Intimate Partner Violence Screening: Please read each of the following activities and fill in the circle that best indicates the frequency with which your partner acts in the way depicted.

How often does your partner?

	Never	Rarely	Sometimes	Fairly often	Frequently
1. Physically hurt you?	O	O	O	O	O
2. Insult or talk down to you?	O	O	O	O	O
3. Threaten you with harm?	O	O	O	O	O
4. Scream or curse at you?	O	O	O	O	O
	1	2	3	4	5

Each item is scored from 1-5. Thus, scores for this inventory range from 4-20. A score of greater than 10 is considered positive.

Reproduced from Clinical Research and Methods (Fam Med 1998;30(7):508-12.) HITS is copyrighted in 2003 by Kevin Sherin MD, MPH. For permission to use HITS, email kevin_sherin@doh.state.fl.us. *HITS is used globally in multiple languages, 2006.

Personality Disorders

Personality disorders are characterized by maladaptive, inflexible relational patterns that impair a person's global functioning. Genetic, social, environmental, and psychological domains typically influence personality disorders. Personality Disorders are commonly encountered in primary care. Symptoms may elicit strong feelings in the primary care provider and may make it challenging to diagnose and treat medical and other psychiatric illnesses. Table 19-1 provides descriptions of personality disorders.

Antisocial—Patterns of exploiting others without regard to the boundaries, needs, or feelings of others. Often manipulative, with tendencies toward violence and aggressive behaviors.

Avoidant—Patterns of intense social anxiety and concern about how others perceive them. Fear of rejection and social anxiety impair typical social relationships.

Borderline—Marked by feelings of emptiness and fears of separation. Often impulsive and reckless. Characterized by "splitting," or fluctuating between idealistic adoration of others to intense anger and rage.

Dependent—Self-sacrificing to atypical degree, often submissive, afraid to be alone.

Histrionic—Patterns of overly flirtatious, seductive behaviors meant to draw attention. Often experiences suicidality.

Narcissistic Personality Disorder—Patterns of behaviors marked by grandiosity, feeling like one is superior to others. As a result, often exploitive and extremely sensitive to criticism.

Obsessive-Compulsive—Patterns of rigid, inflexible need for correctness and perfectionism. As a result, can be very critical of self and others.

Paranoid—Mistrusting and suspicious of others. As a result, can become violent and aggressive to others.

Schizoid—Avoidant and asocial. Tends to keep to self and extremely reclusive.

Schizotypal—Often possesses odd beliefs, superstitions, and ideas of reference. Struggles socially, with perceptual disorders common.

Neurodevelopmental Disorders

The neurodevelopmental disorders begin in early childhood and may have a wide-ranging impact on brain function. Disorders in this group include intellectual disability, communication disorders, autism spectrum disorder, attention deficit hyperactivity disorder, specific learning disorder, and motor disorders. There is much comorbidity amongst these disorders, with a focus on targeted symptom management.

Tourette's Syndrome

A tic is described as a sudden, rapid, and non-rhythmic motor movement or vocalization.

Table 19-1	Descriptions of Personality Disorders	
Cluster A—odd or eccentric	**Cluster B—dramatic, emotional, or erratic**	**Cluster C—anxious or fearful**

Paranoid
  Pervasive pattern of mistrust and suspiciousness
  Begins in early adulthood
  Presents in a variety of contexts
	Antisocial
	  Disregard for rights of others
	  Violation of rights of others
	  Lack of remorse for wrongdoing
	  Lack of empathy
		Avoidant
		  Social inhibition
		  Feelings of inadequacy
		  Hypersensitivity to criticism

Schizoid
  Detachment from social relationships
  Restricted range of emotional expressions
	Borderline
	  Instability of interpersonal relationships, self-image, and affects
	  Marked impulsivity
		Dependent
		  Excessive need to be taken care of
		  Submissive behavior
		  Fear of separation

Schizotypal
  Social and interpersonal deficits
  Cognitive or perceptual distortions and eccentricities
	Histrionic
	  Excessive emotionality
	  Attention-seeking behavior
		Obsessive-compulsive
		  Preoccupation with orderliness and perfectionism
		  Mental and interpersonal control

	Narcissistic
	  Grandiosity
	  Need for admiration	

From Randy Ward, Assessment and Management of Personality Disorders, American Family Physician 70(8), October 15, 2004, Table 2. Used by permission of American Academy of Family Physicians.

For a diagnosis of Tourette's syndrome, multiple motor tics and one or more vocal tics must be present at some point (though not necessarily at the same time) *for greater than 1 year*. Tics often wax and wane, but have persisted in patient for more than 1 year since onset.

Nonpharmacologic

Habit Reversal Therapy is usually first-line treatment for those who experience an urge or sensation prior to tics.

Pharmacologic

Typical and atypical antipsychotics can be used to alleviate symptoms.

- Alpha-adrenergic agonists also used—less effective than antipsychotics but have safer side-effect profile

Autistic Spectrum Disorder

According to the CDC, ASD affects one in 68 children with a higher risk in males as well as siblings, especially twins (CDC, n.d.).

Screening

The CDC recommends screening specifically for ASD at ages 18 and 24 months, with additional screening if behavioral symptoms are present or if there is high risk (i.e. prematurity, sibling with ASD).

In children 16–30 months, the recommended screening tool is the Modified Checklist for Autism in Toddlers (M-CHAT). This tool, as is true with all rating scales, is not diagnostic (see Figure 19-4). While a significant number of children may score as high risk, many will not meet diagnostic criteria following a comprehensive evaluation.

Assessment

Diagnosis of ASD requires a multidisciplinary assessment, including referrals to genetics, neurology, audiology, developmental pediatrics or child psychiatry, and speech therapy. Many urban areas have specialized teams that help assess for ASD.

Physical exam and differential diagnosis for ASD should include evaluations for dysmorphology, seizures, family history, infections (encephalopathy or meningitis), endocrine (hypothyroidism), metabolic (homocystinuria), traumatic (head injury), toxic (fetal alcohol syndrome), and genetic (chromosomal abnormality). Genetic screening should include a G-banded karyotype, Fragile X, and chromosomal microarray.

- *Social communication:* Deficits in reciprocity, nonverbal communication, and developing and understanding relationships
- *Restrictive/repetitive interests:* Stereotyped or repetitive movements, use of objects, or speech, insistence on sameness, inflexible routines, ritualized patterns or behavior, fixated interests, hyper- or hyporeactivity to sensory input

Management

Nonpharmacologic

Comprehensive and early interventions that address core deficits, including social communication, play skills, and maladaptive behavior, lead to the most promising outcomes in treating ASD. Unfortunately, there is a lack of evidence from randomized control trials regarding nonpharmacologic approaches to treatment, with no approach being found superior, and very limited research on children younger than age 2 or adolescents. Different modalities include Applied Behavioral Analysis, the Early Start Denver Model, and social skills programs (Volkmar et al., 2014).

Pharmacologic

There is no pharmacologic treatment for ASD itself. Medications are selected on a case-by-case basis for target symptom improvement. Target symptoms may include hyperactivity and inattention, maladaptive behaviors, or sleep. Medications for these symptoms are mostly prescribed off-label. Only risperidone and aripiprazole are FDA-approved for treatment of irritability in ASD, including tantrums and self-injurious behavior.

1. If you point at something across the room, does your child look at it? (FOR EXAMPLE, if you point at a toy or an animal, does your child look at the toy or animal?)

   ❍ Yes ❍ No

2. Have you ever wondered if your child might be deaf?

   ❍ Yes ❍ No

3. Does your child play pretend or make-believe? (FOR EXAMPLE, pretend to drink from an empty cup, pretend to talk on a phone, or pretend to feed a doll or stuffed animal?)

   ❍ Yes ❍ No

4. Does your child like climbing on things? (FOR EXAMPLE, furniture, playground equipment, or stairs)

   ❍ Yes ❍ No

5. Does your child make unusual finger movements near his or her eyes? (FOR EXAMPLE, does your child wiggle his or her fingers close to his or her eyes?)

   ❍ Yes ❍ No

6. Does your child point with one finger to ask for something or to get help? (FOR EXAMPLE, pointing to a snack or toy that is out of reach)

   ❍ Yes ❍ No

7. Does your child point with one finger to show you something interesting? (FOR EXAMPLE, pointing to an airplane in the sky or a big truck in the road. This is different from your child pointing to ASK for something [Question #6.])

   ❍ Yes ❍ No

8. Is your child interested in other children? (FOR EXAMPLE, does your child watch other children, smile at them, or go to them?)

   ❍ Yes ❍ No

9. Does your child show you things by bringing them to you or holding them up for you to see - not to get help, but just to share? (FOR EXAMPLE, showing you a flower, a stuffed animal, or a toy truck)

   ❍ Yes ❍ No

10. Does your child respond when you call his or her name? (FOR EXAMPLE, does he or she look up, talk or babble, or stop what he or she is doing when you call his or her name?)

   ❍ Yes ❍ No

Figure 19-4 M-CHAT

Reproduced from M-CHAT. (2009). Retrieved from https://www.m-chat.org/mchat.php.

11. When you smile at your child, does he or she smile back at you?

    ○ Yes   ○ No

12. Does your child get upset by everyday noises? (FOR EXAMPLE, does your child scream or cry to noise such as a vacuum cleaner or loud music?)

    ○ Yes   ○ No

13. Does your child walk?

    ○ Yes   ○ No

14. Does your child look you in the eye when you are talking to him or her, playing with him or her, or dressing him or her?

    ○ Yes   ○ No

15. Does your child try to copy what you do? (FOR EXAMPLE, wave bye-bye, clap, or make a funny noise when you do)

    ○ Yes   ○ No

16. If you turn your head to look at something, does your child look around to see what you are looking at?

    ○ Yes   ○ No

17. Does your child try to get you to watch him or her? (FOR EXAMPLE, does your child look at you for praise, or say "look" or "watch me"?)

    ○ Yes   ○ No

18. Does your child understand when you tell him or her to do something? (FOR EXAMPLE, if you don't point, can your child understand "put the book on the chair" or "bring me the blanket"?)

    ○ Yes   ○ No

19. If something new happens, does your child look at your face to see how you feel about it? (FOR EXAMPLE, if he or she hears a strange or funny noise, or sees a new toy, will he or she look at your face?)

    ○ Yes   ○ No

20. Does your child like movement activities? (FOR EXAMPLE, being swung or bounced on your knee)

    ○ Yes   ○ No

Figure 19-4 M-CHAT (Continued)

Review Questions

1. Which of the following patients is not appropriate for management in the primary care setting?
   A. A 27-year-old female with new onset depressive symptoms and a scheduled psychiatric intake in 6 weeks
   B. A 27-year-old male with new onset inattentive symptoms and no history of psychiatric evaluation
   C. A 32-year-old female who is acutely manic and suicidal and currently has no psychiatric provider
   D. A 32-year-old male who has been psychiatrically stable on lithium for a year

2. By 2020, the World Health Organization estimates which of the following illnesses will be the number two cause of "lost years of healthy life" worldwide?
   A. Bipolar Disorder
   B. Schizophrenia
   C. Major Depressive Disorder
   D. Generalized Anxiety Disorder

3. According to the National Institute of Mental Health, half of all mental illness begins by which age?
   A. 8 years old
   B. 14 years old
   C. 24 years old
   D. 32 years old

4. A 70-year-old male patient comes to see his family nurse practitioner complaining of vague aches and pains and forgetfulness over the past 3 months. His wife shares with the nurse practitioner that he is snapping at family members, no longer likes to go out for weekly family dinners, and is not interested in sex. He has a history of diabetes but his labs are normal. He scores a 28/30 on his Folstein Mini Mental Status Exam (MMSE). What does the family nurse practitioner suspect?
   A. Major Depressive Disorder
   B. Alzheimer's disease
   C. Major Neurocognitive Disorder
   D. Complications of diabetes

5. A 37-year-old female patient requests a prescription for antidepressant medication. She reports low energy, poor self-esteem, overeating behaviors, difficulty making decisions, and feeling hopeless. When asked how long her symptoms have been occurring, she states, "I've always been this way." The nurse practitioner suspects which of the following?
   A. Borderline Personality Disorder
   B. Major Depressive Disorder
   C. Persistent Depressive Disorder
   D. Bipolar Disorder

6. A family nurse practitioner is seeing a 33-year-old patient for a follow-up visit for her depression. The patient began sertraline (Zoloft) 50 mg four weeks ago and reports a partial response. The nurse practitioner does which of the following?
   A. Increases the dosage
   B. Advises switching to a different medication
   C. Considers augmenting with another agent
   D. Refers to a psychiatric provider

7. A 55-year-old male patient returns for follow-up after starting an antidepressant after one week. He reports occasional headaches and worries it is not working. The family nurse practitioner advises all *but* which of the following?

   A. "Side effects are common but often go away in a couple of weeks."

   B. "Successful treatment often involves a dose adjustment."

   C. "Patients typically show improvement in the first week, so it is time to consider a switch."

   D. "Do not stop taking the medication without calling me."

8. A 61-year-old male patient is following up 6 months after discharge from the hospital after having a heart attack. The family nurse practitioner would like to begin an SSRI for his symptoms of depression. He is also taking clopidogrel (Plavix). The nurse practitioner proceeds cautiously recognizing which of the following risks?

   A. Sleep disturbance

   B. Serotonin Syndrome

   C. Increased risk of bleeding

   D. Akathesia

9. A 27-year-old female patient follows up with her family nurse practitioner after having her first baby. Her nurse midwife began escitalopram (Lexapro) during pregnancy for symptoms of depression and the patient is concerned about the risks to the baby of continuing this medication while breast-feeding. Which of the following is the best advice the nurse practitioner can give?

   A. The patient should stop this medication because it can cause withdrawal symptoms in the baby.

   B. The patient should switch to a tricyclic antidepressant that has lower risk to the baby.

   C. This medication is relatively safe and the amount of the drug to the nursing infant is low.

   D. The patient should stop the medication and begin psychotherapy instead.

10. A patient who is being treated with lithium 600 mg twice daily has a trough lithium level of 0.9 mEq/L. The patient is currently euthymic. The nurse practitioner does which of the following?

    A. Decreases the medication to prevent toxicity

    B. Discontinues the medication to prevent toxicity

    C. Maintains the current dosage because the plasma level is within range

    D. Maintains the current dosage because the benefit outweighs the risk

11. The family nurse practitioner orders all but the following lab work for an annual follow-up visit of her patient on lithium treatment.

    A. Thyroid function tests

    B. Urine creatinine

    C. Urine specific gravity

    D. Lipid panel

12. A 28-year-old new mom returns four weeks after being prescribed escitalopram for postpartum depression by her family nurse practitioner. She reports that she feels better than she has ever felt, does not feel tired after several sleepless nights up with the baby, and has re-connected with previous friends to chat in her free time. She notes that her husband thinks she's doing well, too, because she has been so sensual. The family nurse practitioner does which of the following?

    A. Continues the current dosage of escitalopram

    B. Decreases the dosage of escitalopram

    C. Advises the new mom that she is responding to oxytocin and should pace herself as hormone levels readjust

    D. Suspects Bipolar Disorder and discontinues the medication

13. A 19-year-old male college student expresses concerns about being unable to talk to others, avoidance of joining activities he likes, fear of speaking in class, and avoiding approaching professors. His grades are poor due to concentration and lack of participation. His diagnosis is which of the following?

    A. Generalized Anxiety Disorder

    B. Social Anxiety Disorder

    C. Attention Deficit Hyperactivity Disorder

    D. Antisocial Personality Disorder

14. Which nonpharmacologic modality is most recommended for the treatment of Generalized Anxiety Disorder?

    A. Psychoanalytic Therapy

    B. Prolonged Exposure Therapy

    C. Cognitive Behavioral Therapy

    D. Social Rhythm Therapy

15. Which of the following stress-relieving activities would be difficult for a patient with agoraphobia?

    A. Listening to relaxing music

    B. Going to a friend's house

    C. Deep breathing

    D. Caring for a pet

16. A 42-year-old female presents for follow-up after two emergency room visits for shortness of breath, heart palpitations, sweating, and fear of dying. A comprehensive workup shows no cause of medical illness. A urine drug screen prior to the office visit is positive for marijuana. The patient states, "Ativan really helped in the emergency room. Will you continue it?" What does the FNP advise?

    A. "Ativan is a safe and effective treatment for your panic attacks."

    B. "SSRIs are a better option for the long-term management of your panic disorder."

    C. "Psychotherapy can help you cope with feelings of panic."

    D. "Marijuana may be causing your anxiety or making it worse. Let's talk more about your use."

17. A 51-year-old newly established female patient has changed providers three times in the past year due to feelings that her medical care is inadequate. She has been in to see the family nurse practitioner twice in the past month. At each visit, she shares that she has spent long hours researching her health concerns and is very anxious about her undiagnosed illness, despite reassurances from the FNP that her medical workup is normal. The FNP does which of the following?

    A. Schedules regular, noninvasive visits

    B. Schedules the patient with a specialist for further evaluation

    C. Begins antidepressant medication

    D. Encourages the patient to limit stressful daily activities

18. A family nurse practitioner prescribes Imitrex to a 39-year-old female patient with a history of migraines who is also taking Cymbalta 60 mg daily for anxiety. After taking the first dosage of Imitrex, the patient returns for a same-day visit and reports that she is shivering, has diarrhea, and muscle aches. She is afebrile and her heart rate is normal. The nurse practitioner:

    A. Suspects a panic attack and advises the patient to continue her medications.

    B. Suspects Serotonin Syndrome and discontinues the Imitrex.

    C. Suspects Serotonin Syndrome and discontinues the Cymbalta.

    D. Advises the patient to go to the emergency department for cardiovascular assessment.

19. Elderly adults are at increased risk from impaired cognition and falls due to which of the following medications?

    A. Fluoxetine

    B. Duloxetine

    C. Lorazepam

    D. Buspirone

20. During a well-child visit, the mother of a 17-month-old shares concerns that her daughter is not yet pointing to objects to ask for what she wants and is very difficult to comfort. The family nurse practitioner takes which of the following as the next step?

    A. Assures the mother that this is typical for a child of her age

    B. Administers the M-CHAT

    C. Administers the ASQ

    D. Schedules a visit in 6 months to see if the child has improved communication

21. A 12-year-old male who has been diagnosed with Autistic Spectrum Disorder comes to see the family nurse practitioner because he is experiencing increased anxiety since beginning middle school. Previously, he liked school and was earning average grades. He is in a general education classroom with a good support system for social skills and transitions. The FNP finds that his heightened anxiety impacts his functioning in which of the following ways?

    A. He has started hitting his classmates.

    B. He refuses to go to class.

    C. He feels hopeless about his ability to complete his assignments.

    D. He believes his teachers are out to get him.

22. A 42-year-old nonverbal male with Autism Spectrum Disorder who lives in adult foster care presents with symptoms of increased aggression following recent changes in staffing at the home. Despite modifications to his behavior plan, for the past two months he has been hitting other residents and staff members. He is at risk of losing his placement. The family nurse practitioner initiates which of the following?

    A. Risperdal 0.5 mg

    B. Prozac 40 mg

    C. Clonzepam 1 mg

    D. Haldol 5 mg

23. A 7-year-old female comes in to see the family nurse practitioner because she is having problems in school. Her father is concerned that she has Attention Deficit Hyperactivity Disorder because she has trouble concentrating and sitting still in class. The family nurse practitioner does what as an initial step?

    A. Observes and documents how the child interacts in the exam room

    B. Sends a validated rating scale to the teacher to obtain collateral information

    C. Prescribes a stimulant medication

    D. Refers the child to a psychiatrist for additional evaluation

24. A 12-year-old male was recently suspended from school for having a bad attitude and deliberately annoying other students in the hallway between classes. His mother schedules an appointment to request stimulant medication so he can go back to class. The family nurse practitioner does which of the following?

    A. Sends a Vanderbilt ADHD Rating Scale to his teacher for collaborative information

    B. Provides guidance to his mother on positive and negative reinforcement of behaviors

    C. Refers the child and family to a behavioral therapist

    D. Initiates treatment with Concerta 18 mg

25. A 20-year-old college student is home for the summer and schedules an appointment to see his family nurse practitioner because he is concerned about ADHD. He was previously an A student in high school but notices that lately he is unmotivated, has trouble concentrating, and has experienced a decline in grades. The family nurse practitioner:

    A. Suspects depression and requests the student complete a PHQ-9.

    B. Suspects depression and prescribes an antidepressant.

    C. Suspects malingering and calls his mother.

    D. Suspects malingering and orders a random urine drug screen.

26. You are interviewing a 10-year-old female with a recent history of physical abuse. Which of the following symptoms is seen primarily in adults with PTSD but not with children?

    A. Sense of foreshortened future

    B. Unwillingness to speak about the traumatic event

    C. Nightmares

    D. Increased startle response

27. The parents of a 14-year-old child with a history of Tourette's syndrome are asking about his prognosis? Which is the most appropriate response?

    A. This is a chronic disorder that you will likely experience throughout your lifetime.

    B. Tics typically wax and wane so you are likely to experience tics throughout your lifetime during stressful periods.

    C. Most commonly, tics begin to decrease in adolescence. Most people are symptom-free in adulthood, although other people will experience tics throughout their lifetime.

    D. Tics will improve considerably with medication that is both safe and effective.

28. The FNP is seeing a 24-year-old patient who is requesting another prescription for hydrocodone since she lost the previous one. The FNP is concerned about potential abuse. Which of the following is an important *first step* in the intervention?

    A. Request that the patient complete a urine drug screen to test levels of opioid in the urine. Inform her that she cannot receive another prescription today.

    B. Explain to the patient that this is a highly addictive drug and ask if she believes she is beginning to struggle with a dependence on hydrocodone.

    C. Discontinue the medication and offer her an alternative therapy without abuse potential.

    D. Complete the CRAFFT questionnaire.

29. Which of the following patients most urgently requires a follow-up suicide risk screening?

    A. A 30-year-old female who is grieving the loss of her father. She is diagnosed with major depressive disorder.

    B. A 30-year-old male who has a history of multiple psychiatric hospitalizations and who reports he has not attended work for 2 weeks and has avoided friends and family.

    C. A 54-year-old woman who is in the middle of a divorce and involved in an intense custody battle. She is experiencing intense rage at her children's father.

    D. A 20-year-old male with a history of substance abuse who reports sleep disturbances after beginning sobriety 30 days ago.

30. The nurse practitioner who is employed at the VA hospital is seeing a 24-year-old male returning from overseas who reports intense nightmares. He is afraid to sleep at night and feels he is functioning poorly both at home and at work. Which of the following is the most appropriate response by the nurse practitioner?

    A. "I would like to recommend sertraline for your symptoms. Sleep should improve as your symptoms improve."

    B. "I would like to recommend Ativan for sleep since it is a fast-acting medication."

    C. "I would like to refer you to a therapist to help you with your symptoms. In the meantime, I would like to start prazosin to improve sleep and decrease nightmares."

    D. "Cognitive Behavioral Therapy (CBT) is the best treatment for the symptoms you are describing. I would like to refer you to a therapist."

31. Which of the following patients is most appropriate for treatment with sertraline?
    A. A pregnant female who was treated several years ago with an SSRI for depression
    B. A woman breast-feeding her infant who is reporting sleeplessness and difficulty finding time to socialize since the birth of her baby
    C. A woman with a history of depression who reports poor attachment to the infant and feeling over-whelmed and helpless most of the time
    D. A woman presenting with severe mood lability that has increased since the birth of her baby

32. The NP is working with a 45-year-old patient with a 3-year history of heroin and cocaine dependence who expresses readiness to begin opioid substation therapy. He has an extensive legal history involving drug trafficking. The patient asks for advice on which opioid substitution therapy "is better." Which is the most appropriate response?
    A. "Buprenorphine is more dangerous during the induction phase, so methadone is a better choice."
    B. "Methadone is administered at the clinic daily and is more effective when someone is experiencing dependence to both heroin and cocaine."
    C. "Each has its own risks and benefits. Methadone is more stigmatized, so buprenorphine is a better choice."
    D. "Either way, because of your history of trafficking, you will have to be monitored closely with weekly urine drug screens."

33. A patient treated with clozapine would need to be aware of which fact?
    A. Clozapine requires laboratory monitoring in the beginning of treatment because of the potential risk of agranulocytosis.
    B. Clozapine requires blood work monthly for the potential risk of agranulocytosis.
    C. Clozapine requires blood monitoring if the patient has a family history significant for heart disease due to the potential risk of myocarditis.
    D. Clozapine requires blood monitoring weekly during the first 6 months of treatment, biweekly for the following 6 months, and then once a month for the entire duration of therapy.

34. The NP has a 30-year-old patient with elevated prolactin levels who is receiving risperidone for schizophrenia. What action should the NP take?
    A. Continue therapy if patient is tolerating medication with no reported side effects and continue to monitor both prolactin levels and potential adverse effects.
    B. Discontinue therapy given the potential risks for hyperprolactinemia.
    C. Immediately lower the dose of risperidone.
    D. Risperidone is the only atypical antipsychotic that does not require monitoring prolactin levels.

35. Which of the following patients presenting with psychosis would warrant further screening for schizophrenia?
    A. A 19-year-old male presenting with grossly disorganized speech, flat affect, and who appears suddenly suspicious of family and friends.
    B. A 20-year-old male with a history of severe mood disturbances, presenting with rapid speech and grandiosity, telling the office personnel that he has been appointed to solve the country's immigration problem.
    C. A 44-year-old female who is suspicious that her coworkers are trying to sabotage her employment after discovering a hand-written note in her employer's office.
    D. A 35-year-old male with treatment-resistant depression who has begun to experience auditory hallucinations.

36. Which information is accurate regarding screening for intimate personal violence (IPV)?
    A. Typically, IPV occurs in heterosexual relationships.
    B. Poverty is stressful, so providers should monitor for IPV more carefully when working with low-income families.
    C. IPV occurs in all ages and ethnicities, without regard to socioeconomic status.
    D. IPV is particularly problematic in same-sex relationships.

37. The NP is seeing a 23-year-old female with Borderline Personality Disorder who reports that she wishes she were dead because her boyfriend just ended a short but intense relationship with her. What is the most appropriate response?

    A. Perform a careful risk assessment even if it appears that she is trying to gain attention and has no plan or intention to harm herself.

    B. Recognize that suicidal ideation and impulsivity are very common in patients diagnosed with Borderline Personality Disorder. Validate her feelings and screen her carefully for intention, plan, and other self-injurious behavior.

    C. Acknowledge her feelings but give little attention to her "acting out" and suicidal threats.

    D. Inform her family of her threats so she can be monitored at home. Give emergency numbers in case suicidality increases.

38. Which of the following laboratory tests is NOT required when a patient is receiving therapy with an atypical antipsychotic?

    A. Prolactin

    B. Oral glucose tolerance test

    C. Hepatic panel

    D. Weight

39. A 30-year-old female reports that she enjoys a "couple of drinks" when she goes out with friends. This occurs 3 or 4 times a week. She states that she has missed work a few times due to hangovers and her girlfriend ended their relationship because she didn't like her "partying so much." What is the most appropriate action by the nurse practitioner?

    A. Explain to her that this behavior is considered at-risk drinking because she is above the recommended limit for alcohol intake for females.

    B. Realize that she has to recognize harmful drinking on her own.

    C. Ask her if she believes the drinking is getting in the way of her job and relationships. Explain to her what harmful drinking means. Perform the CRAFFT and CAGE questionnaire. Screen for other potential substance abuse.

    D. Refer her for substance abuse treatment.

40. A patient presents for his follow-up appointment. He has a stable job as a software programmer, is well groomed with proper hygiene with no symptoms of psychosis. The patient reports that he is suspicious that the office staff has been reading his medical chart. You ask him why he believes this and he responds with, "The HIPAA Confidentiality stuff is just a smoke screen for the government to know our business." When the nurse practitioner attempts to refute this, he becomes angry and hostile. The nurse practitioner would screen for which of the following personality disorders?

    A. Paranoid Personality Disorder

    B. Social Anxiety Disorder

    C. Schizophrenia

    D. Schizoid Personality Disorder

41. The "SAL" for suicide risk assessment screens for which three important domains?

    A. Safety, Access, and Lethality

    B. Security, Accessibility, and Lethality

    C. Specificity, Accessibility, and Legitimacy

    D. Specificity, Availability, and Lethality

42. Which of the following is the most appropriate action to take for a 21-year-old female with a history of overdoses?

    A. Do not prescribe any medication until safety is established.

    B. Refer to visiting nurse services so medication can be administered directly by home health care staff.

    C. Prescribe only a 7-day supply of medication.

    D. Avoid medication that is the most lethal in overdose.

43. The NP at the VA is treating a 24 year-old male recently deployed to the Middle East who returned home last month. Which of the following should the nurse practitioner prioritize?

    A. Validating patient's feelings and experiences

    B. Sleep quality and content and startle response

    C. Risk of hypertension and DM Type II

    D. Infectious disease

44. A 13-year-old female presents to the NP's office and reports she has been "hearing voices." The NP screens for psychosis. Which of the following descriptions of the "voice" would most concern the treating nurse practitioner?

    A. "It's like a voice telling me that I am ugly and stupid."

    B. "I hear it a lot. It sounds like a whisper, but then it tells me that I should hurt people."

    C. "I only hear the voice when I'm really sad but it sounds like my mom's voice trying to cheer me up."

    D. "It's the "inner voice" that helps me do the right thing."

45. The NP is seeing a 14-year-old male with recent onset of both motor and vocal tics who is requesting a medication to "make the tics go away." What is the most appropriate response?

    A. "I can see that the tics are really bothering you. The best thing we can do is start a form of therapy known as "habit reversal therapy." If that doesn't work, then we can try a medication."

    B. "I can see that the tics are really bothering you. Let's try a therapy known as Habit Reversal Therapy and a medication called risperidone, which will help decrease the tics."

    C. "I know the tics are bothering you, but there is a really good chance they will go away on their own and we won't need medication."

    D. "Tics are not really a big problem. You can learn how to control it."

46. The NP is treating a patient with a diagnosis of ADHD who reports he is doing well in school but is experiencing poor attention in the afternoon. This has become increasingly problematic since his schoolwork consists of several hours of homework each night. He is currently prescribed Concerta 36 mg. Which is the next best step?

    A. Suggest an increase in Concerta.

    B. Suggest stopping Concerta and beginning an alternative long-acting stimulant.

    C. Add methylphenidate 5 mg at 3 pm.

    D. Add a second dose of Concerta at noon.

47. Which of the following medications should be avoided when treating a patient with a diagnosis of ADHD and a history of opiate abuse?

    A. Lorazepam

    B. Percocet

    C. Adderall

    D. Lexapro

48. The NP initiates Lamictal for a patient. Which of the following is critical information that should be shared with the patient?

    A. "We have to monitor routine blood levels for this medication."

    B. "This medication has to be titrated slowly because it can cause agranulocytosis."

    C. "This medication has to be titrated slowly and you should monitor for signs of a rash."

    D. "This medication can cause infertility."

49. A patient presents with confusion and is complaining of "muscles feeling weird." Which of the following is the most likely cause?

    A. Patient recently started on valproic acid.

    B. Patient recently increased dosage of haloperidol.

    C. Patient recently discontinued lithium.

    D. Patient recently began methylphenidate for ADHD.

50. Which of the following classes of medications would the nurse practitioner avoid if a patient makes the following statement: "I'll take the pills as long as it doesn't interfere with my life too much. I'm not great at following rules."

    A. SNRI

    B. SSRI

    C. Second-generation antipsychotics

    D. MAOI

Answers and Rationales

1. B. Patients with newly identified symptoms who do not present imminent risk should be referred for a mental health evaluation.

2. C. Major Depressive Disorder will soon be the second worldwide cause of disability-adjust life years lost due to ill-health, disability, or early death.

3. B. Fifty percent of all mental illness begins by age 14.

4. A. In older adults, symptoms of depression often include physical aches and pains not caused by a medical condition, memory difficulties or personality changes, and social withdrawal. Dementia would be considered if the patient showed signs of cognitive decline, such as a low score on the MMSE. A score of 23 or lower indicates cognitive impairment.

5. C. The symptoms of persistent depressive disorder occur for at least two years, with no more than 2 months without symptoms.

6. A. The next step would be to increase the dosage until full response.

7. C. It generally takes at least 2 weeks to show a response, though for many patients it takes at least 4–6 weeks.

8. C. Patients taking an SSRI along with an antiplatelet agent are at increased risk of bleeding. While they are not absolute contraindications to be taken together, the nurse should weigh the risks of bleeding and untreated depression, monitor INR, and ask the patient to report signs of bleeding promptly.

9. C. When clinically warranted, antidepressants in breast-feeding are considered relatively safe for use. SSRIs are the best studied. While they are secreted in breast milk, there is no evidence that they pose a significant risk to the nursing infant. Tricyclic antidepressants are also considered relatively safe during breast-feeding. However, there is no known benefit of one antidepressant over another, and switching may put the mother at risk of relapse.

10. C. The recommended therapeutic range of lithium is between 0.5–1.2 mEq/L.

11. D. Lithium alters sodium transport across cell membranes and increases risk for acute and chronic kidney disease. Urine creatinine and urine specific gravity should be checked on initiation, at least annually, and if symptomatic. Furthermore, lithium increases the secretion of intrathyroidal iodine, inhibiting the release of T3 and T4 and increasing the risk for hypothyroidism. A thyroid function panel should be checked upon initiation, at least annually, and if symptomatic. A lipid panel is not indicated for lithium initiation or maintenance. However, lithium is associated with weight gain and it is prudent to screen for dyslipidemia in overweight or obese patients.

12. D. Symptoms of mania include increased energy, decreased need for sleep, more talkative than usual, and excessive interest in pleasurable activities. Antidepressants may trigger symptoms of mania when underlying mood disorders are present. While oxytocin increases in the immediate postpartum period, as it drops off, new moms are more likely to experience symptoms of depression.

13. B. Social Anxiety Disorder is characterized by intense anxiety and distress around the fear situation, recognition that the fear is unreasonable or excessive, and social, academic, or occupational impairment related to avoidance of activities associated with the fear.

14. C. Cognitive Behavioral Therapy (CBT) has been proven effective for a range of anxiety disorders, including Generalized Anxiety Disorder. It is a structured, problem-focused, and goal-oriented approach that helps modify negative thinking and beliefs in order to change behavior.

15. B. People with agoraphobia fear being in situations where escape can be difficult or embarrassing and they often avoid leaving home.

16. D. Substances, such as marijuana, may cause symptoms of anxiety and panic. A timeline of psychiatric symptoms and substance use is needed to differentiate psychiatric disorders from substance-induced symptoms.

17. A. The patient is experiencing Somatic Symptom Disorder, characterized by disproportionate or excessive health anxiety and body vigilance that continues for 6 or more months. Treatment should include regular noninvasive medical assessments, acceptance of physical symptoms rather than a goal

of symptom resolution, and encouraging the patient to remain active and limit the effect of the target symptom on daily functioning.

18. B. Serotonin Syndrome is a serious adverse drug reaction caused by medications with direct and indirect serotonergic effects. Mild cases are typically self-limiting and respond to discontinuation of the offending agent. However, in the case of severe symptoms, including fever, irregular heart rate, and/or seizures, the patient may require hospitalization and supportive care to prevent life-threatening complications.

19. C. Elder adults are at increased risk of adverse effects, including cognitive impairment, from benzodiazepines.

20. B. Early signs of Autistic Disorder may include deficits and social and communication skills, including not being comforted by others and not pointing or responding to pointing. The M-CHAT may be utilized for toddlers aged 16–30 months. While the FNP may call the child back in 6 months, early intervention is of primary importance and a referral is indicated if a child scores high on developmental screening.

21. B. Anxiety in a child with Autistic Disorder may lead to school avoidance, a drop in grades, or increased social isolation.

22. A. Risperdal is FDA-approved for the treatment of irritability, including aggression, self-injurious behavior, and temper tantrums, in both adults and children with Autistic Disorder.

23. A. A physical exam noting behavioral observations is the initial step in diagnosing ADHD. However, symptoms may not be present in a brief office visit. Further steps include a caregiver interview and obtaining caregiver and teacher rating scales, such as the Conners or Vanderbilt Rating Scales.

24. C. Behavioral therapy is indicated for this child, given the degree of functional impairment related to school performance. Medication is generally not indicated for managing oppositional behaviors.

25. A. While a person with ADHD may have difficulty initiating work and completing tasks, a person with depression is more likely to experience decreased motivation and related functional impairment.

26. A. Children often do not present with a sense of foreshortened future. The developmental context of the perspective of the child is important to consider. Symptoms listed in choices B, C, and D are typical of children presenting with PTSD.

27. C. Tics typically begin to decrease in adolescence. This is important to inform both children and parents of the prognosis and that there is a chance the child will not experience tics in adulthood.

28. B. The therapeutic alliance is important, and exploring the issue in an honest, non-threatening context is the most effective approach. While a urine toxicology screen and follow-up regarding other potential problems with substance abuse or misuse is important, the first step is exploring the situational context with the patient.

29. B. Both social isolation and past psychiatric hospitalization is a warning sign of suicide risk. While the other patients warrant additional assessment in the context of safety and suicide risk, the clinical scenario of choice B is most worrisome.

30. C. Referring to a therapist is important given that the patient will need ongoing follow-up care. However, initiating prazosin is the best choice given the patient's report of debilitating nightmares. Sertraline is prescribed for PTSD, but a thorough assessment of PTSD symptoms is warranted before sertraline should be initiated. Ativan is highly addictive and not the best choice for this clinical situation.

31. C. The risk of depression is high in this scenario and the consequences of untreated depression in this context carry serious risks for both mother and child. D is incorrect because "mood lability" warrants a more comprehensive investigation into the symptoms, and an antidepressant might not be the appropriate medication. B is incorrect because sleep disruption and changes in sociality are typical for mothers with newborns.

32. B. Choice B contains correct information for the patient and empowers the patient with knowledge to make the best choice for her/himself. While choice D is true—a patient with a legal history might be required to comply with a urine drug screen—this would not be a therapeutic response.

33. D. This is the FDA requirement for patients prescribed clozapine.

34. A. Elevated prolactin levels are common with risperidone. Monitoring for side effects is important, but elevated levels alone do not necessarily require discontinuing.

35. A. This patient is presenting with both positive and negative symptoms typical of schizophrenia. Choice B more accurately reflects a patient experiencing a manic episode of bipolar. Choice C requires further investigation but does not necessarily reflect paranoid ideation. Choice D requires further follow-up, but because psychosis is a symptom of severe depression, depression with psychotic features is more likely.

36. C. Choice C is the only correct response. IPV is present in all ages, sexual orientation, and ethnicities.

37. B. Choice B is the most appropriate therapeutic response. It is important to validate the patient's feelings while also screening for suicidality. Choices A and C assume that the patient is not at risk, which is a potentially false assumption. Choice D is important, but only after responding therapeutically to the patient and then assessing for risk.

38. B. Monitoring glucose is required, but an oral glucose tolerance test is not specifically indicated.

39. C. Assessing where the patient is regarding at-risk substance abuse behavior is important. The first step should be an honest, non-threatening conversation, and then an assessment to determine the risk of substance abuse or misuse. While A and D are reasonable choices, the first step is building the therapeutic alliance and assessment. Choice B is not correct because the patient has opened a dialogue regarding the effects of her drinking, and ignoring this would be inappropriate and potentially harmful.

40. A. This patient is presenting with signs of paranoid personality disorder, including suspicion, anger, and hostility.

41. D. This is the only correct choice for utilizing the SAL acronym for suicide risk assessment.

42. C. A 7-day supply and asking the patient to return in one week is safer than prescribing an entire month's supply of medication. Choice A is incorrect because medication may be indicated, and discontinuing prescriptions is potentially harmful. Choice B is possible but not always feasible. Choice D is an important guideline to guide prescription management, but not always possible given the individual complexities of a patient's treatment needs.

43. B. Poor sleep, nightmares, and an exaggerated startle response are common symptoms of PTSD. Although it is always important to validate patients' feelings and experiences, this is patient is at high risk for PTSD and should be screened appropriately.

44. B. Auditory hallucinations that are commanding in nature and involve voices instructing the person to harm oneself or another are most concerning and require further assessment and management. Choice A is also concerning and warrants further assessment, but command hallucinations with dangerous content are most concerning. Choices C and D are likely not auditory hallucinations.

45. A. Habit Reversal Therapy (HRT) is first-line therapy. If this fails to result in adequate progress, medication can be considered. Choice B assumes concomitant therapy, which is appropriate only after HRT has failed to produce an adequate response. Choice C is not appropriate considering the patient finds the tics distressing. Choice D is invalidating of the patient's feelings and therefore not appropriate.

46. C. C is correct because the attention problems are occurring during a time when the Concerta is unlikely to have therapeutic effects. Since many children take their morning stimulant early in the day, rebound inattention can occur at the end of the day when homework assignments pose a challenge. Increasing the Concerta is not necessary since the patient is reportedly doing well in school. Administering a second dose of Concerta at noon is also incorrect.

47. C. The potential for abuse with Adderall and other stimulants is high and should be avoided when possible for patients who have a history of substance abuse or misuse. Lorazepam, Percocet, and Lexapro are not medications used to treat ADHD.

48. C. Lamotrigine (Lamictal) has been known to cause Stevens–Johnson syndrome, a serious and potentially fatal rash. Lamotrigine does not cause agranulocytosis or infertility. In general, no laboratory monitoring is required.

49. B. Neuroleptic Malignant Syndrome (NMS) is characterized by confusion, fever, muscle rigidity, and autonomic instability. This is a dangerous potential side effect of haloperidol. Neither valproic acid, lithium, nor adderall are known to cause NMS.

50. D. MAOIs require that patients avoid foods high in tyramine. This includes some cheeses, meats, and soy-based products. Failure to avoid these guidelines can result in a hypertensive crisis.

• • • References

American Psychiatric Association. (2013). *Diagnostic and Statistical Manual of Mental Disorders* (5th ed.). DSM-5. Washington, DC: Author.

Autism spectrum disorder. (n.d.). Retrieved December 12, 2015, from http://www.cdc.gov/ncbddd/autism/data.html

Bonhomme, J., Shim, R. S., Gooden, R., Tyus, D., & Rust, G. (2012). Opioid addiction and abuse in primary care practice: A comparison of methadone and buprenorphine as treatment options. *Journal of the National Medical Association, 104*(0), 342–350.

Carlat, D. J. (1998). The psychiatric review of symptoms: A screening tool for family physicians. *American Family Physician, 58*(7):1617–1624.

Conners, C. K. (2001). Development of the CRS-R. In Conners, C. K. (Ed.). *Conners' Rating Scales-Revised.* North Tonawanda, NY: Multi-Health Systems: 83–98.

Dhalla, S., & Kopec, J. A. (2007). The CAGE questionnaire for alcohol misuse: A review of reliability and validity studies. *Clinical and Investigative Medicine, 30*(1), 33–41.

Gaynes, B. N., Gavin, N., Meltzer-Brody, S., Lohr, K. N., Swinson, T., . . . Miller, W. C. (2005). Perinatal depression: Prevalence, screening accuracy, and screening outcomes. Evidence report/Technology assessment No. 119. Rockville, MD: Agency for Healthcare Research and Quality, February. AHRQ Publication No: 05-E006-2.

Hirschfeld, R. M., Holzer, C., Calabrese, J. R., Weissman, M., Reed, M., . . . Hazard, E. (2003). Validity of the mood disorder questionnaire: A general population study. *American Journal of Psychiatry, 160*(1), 178–180.

Kessler, R. C., Amminger, G. P., Aguilar-Gaxiola, S., Alonso, J., Lee, S., & Berirhan Ustun, T. (2007). Age of onset of mental disorders: A review of recent literature. *Current Opinions in Psychiatry, 20*(4), 359–364.

Kessler, R. C., Berglund, P., Delmer, O., Jin, R., Merikangas, K. R., & Walters, E. E. (2005). Lifetime prevalence and age-of-onset distributions of DSM-IV disorders in the National Comorbidity Survey Replication. *Archives of General Psychiatry, 62*(6), 593–602.

Kessler, R. C., Chiu, W. T., Demler, O., & Walters, E. E. (2005). Prevalence, severity, and comorbidity of twelve-month DSM-IV disorders in the National Comorbidity Survey Replication (NCS-R). *Archives of General Psychiatry, 62*(6), 617–627.

Kroenke, K., Spitzer, R. L., & Williams, J. B. W. (2001). The PHQ-9: Validity of a brief depression severity measure. *Journal of General Internal Medicine, 16*(9), 606–613.

Lowe, B., Decker, O., Muller, S., Brahler, E., Schellberg, D., Herzog, W., & Herzberg, P.Y. (2008). Validation and standardization of the Gneralized Anxiety Disorder Screener (GAD-7) in the general population. *Medical Care, 46*(3), 266–274.

National Institute of Mental Health. (n.d). Any anxiety disorder among adults. Retrieved December 12, 2015, from http://www.nimh.nih.gov/health/statistics/prevalence/any-anxiety-disorder-among-adults.shtml

National Institute of Mental Health. (n.d). Bipolar disorder among adults. Retrieved December 12, 2015, from http://www.nimh.nih.gov/health/statistics/prevalence/bipolar-disorder-among-adults.shtml

National Institute of Mental Health. (n.d). Major depression among adults. Retrieved from http://www.nimh.nih.gov/health/statistics/prevalence/major-depression-among-adults.shtml

Perlis, R. H., Ostracher, M. J., Patel, J. K., et al. (2006). Predictors of recurrence in bipolar disorder: Primary outcomes from the Systematic Treatment Enhancement Program (STEP-BD). *The American Journal of Psychiatry, 163*(2), 217–224.

Prins, A., Ouimette, P., Kimerling, R., Cameron, R. P., Hugelshofer, D. S., Shaw-Hegwer, J., . . . Sheikh, J. I. (2003). The Primary Care PTSD Screen (PC-PTSD): Development and operating characteristics (PDF). *Primary Care Psychiatry, 9*, 9–14. doi:10.1185/135525703125002360 PILOTS ID: 26676

Prins, A., Ouimette, P., Kimerling, R., Cameron, R. P., Hugelshofer, D. S., Shaw-Hegwer, J., . . . Sheikh, J. I. (2004). The Primary Care PTSD Screen (PC-PTSD): Corrigendum (PDF). *Primary Care Psychiatry, 9*, 151.

U.S. Preventive Services Task Force. (2009). Screening for depression in adults: U.S. Preventive Services Task Force Recommendation Statement. *Annals of Internal Medicine, 151*(11), 784–792.

Volkmar, F., Siegel, M., Woodbury-Smith, M., King, B., McCracken, J., & State, M. (2014). Practice parameter for the assessment and treatment of children and adolescents with autism spectrum disorder. *Journal of the American Academy of Child and Adolescent Psychiatry, 53*(2), 237–257.

Wang, P. S., Lane, O. M., Pincus, H. A., Wells, K. B., & Kessler, R. C. (2005). Twelve-month use of mental health services in the United States. *Archives of General Psychiatry, 62*(2), 629–640.

Wolraich, M. L., Feurer, I., Hannah, J. N., Pinnock, T. Y., & Baumgaertel, A. (1998). Obtaining systematic teacher reports of disruptive behavior disorders utilizing DSM-IV. *Journal of Abnormal Child Psychology, 26*, 141–152.

CHAPTER

20

Professional Issues

Julie G. Stewart, DNP, MPH, MSN, FNP-BC, APRN

Nurse practitioners must graduate from entry-level master's, post-master's, or doctoral degree programs. The National Organization for Nurse Practitioner Faculties (NONPF) and the American Association of Colleges of Nursing (AACN) define the competency statements for nurse practitioners. There are basic core competencies, and there are population-focused competencies for the various areas depending on the educational program (FNP, PNP, etc.) available on the NONPF and AACN websites. In order to take one of the certification exams, it is required that the graduate have attended a program that is accredited by either the Commission on Collegiate Nursing Education (CCNE) or the Accreditation Commission for Education in Nursing (ACEN) (formerly NLNAC | National League for Nursing Accrediting Commission). In addition, graduates who are family nurse practitioners (FNPs) must have accumulated at least 500 hours in direct patient clinical care in preparation for their profession as a primary care provider.

Scope of Practice

At this time, nurse practitioners have the authority to diagnose, treat, and prescribe medications without the requirement for physician collaboration or oversight in 21 states and the District of Columbia. In the remaining 29 states, there is some form of physician collaboration or supervision required, despite the IOM's recommendations to allow nurses to practice to the full extent of their education and training. The scope of practice for nurse

practitioners can be found on the AANP website, although each state can define the scope of practice in statutes, some of which are detailed and others more general. It is essential that NPs review the most current scope of practice legislated by the state where she/he practices (Stewart & DeNisco, 2015).

The Consensus Model was developed by the APRN Joint Dialogue Group Report (APRN Consensus Work Group & the National Council of State Boards of Nursing APRN Advisory Committee) in an effort to reach an agreement for the regulation of APRNs (see Figure 20-1). As a review, the title Advanced Practice Registered Nurse (APRN) includes certified registered nurse anesthetists (CRNAs), certified nurse-midwives (CNMs), clinical nurse specialists (CNSs), and certified nurse practitioners (CNPs). To date, each state has been able to define the legal scope of practice for each, recognize the roles and titles of each, as well as define the criteria for entry in practice, and the certification examinations that are acceptable. The APRN Regulatory Model's goal is to have consistency in licensure, accreditation, certification, and education (LACE) in all states. APRNs can specialize in an area such as diabetes or palliative care, but must be licensed in one of the four roles with a population focus. All of the advanced practice educational programs must be accredited and provide the core courses, including advanced pathophysiology, advanced pharmacology, and advanced health assessment (the 3 P's). Certification must meet the standards given by the LACE guidelines, which would assure entry-level competency of the APRN role and population focus (Stewart & DeNisco, 2015, pp 268–270).

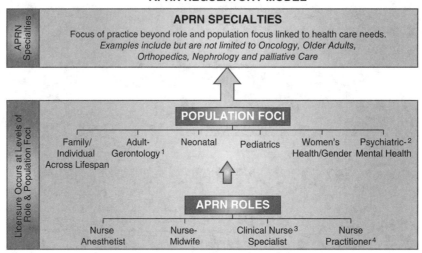

Figure 20-1 APRN Concensus Regulatory Practice Model

Reproduced from American Nurses Association. (2008). *Consensus Model for APRN Regulation: Licensure, Accreditation, Certification & Education.* (July 7, 2008). p. 10.

Advanced Practice State Licensure

Once the certification exam has been passed successfully, the graduate sends required documentation to the state in which they are applying to practice in for advanced practice nurse licensure. Most states require the following: successfully completed thirty (30) hours of education in pharmacology for advanced nursing practice; holds a master's degree in nursing or in a related field recognized for certification as a nurse practitioner, a clinical nurse specialist, or a nurse anesthetist by one of the above-recognized certifying bodies. Most states will want the application to be notarized and have photo identification. The Pearson Report is an excellent reference for all nurse practitioners. It provides an annual state-by-state national overview of nurse practitioner legislation and health care issues. The Pearson report will provide the NP with the definition of the legal scope of practice for each individual state. Again, it is important that the FNP understand the specific functions included in their states definition of FNP scope of practice related to diagnosing, treatment, prescribing practices, hospital admission privileges, referrals, education, and ordering diagnosis tests. Each state's scope of practice also delineates what the legal role and requirements' are of physician involvement in the NP practice. Language such as collaboration, supervision, independent practice, and consultation are examples of varying forms of physician involvement with the NP (Stewart & DeNisco, 2015, p 344). One excellent reference for practice authority in the United States is the Pearson Report.

Drug Enforcement Agency (DEA) Licensure

In addition, the NP must apply for the State Controlled Substances licensure and the DEA (Drug Enforcement Administration) licensure. Through the Department of Justice and Drug Enforcement Administration, the NP must apply for a DEA number pursuant to Title 21, Code of Federal Regulations, Section 1300.01(b28), which states "the term *mid-level practitioner* means an individual practitioner, other than a physician, dentist, veterinarian, or podiatrist, who is licensed, registered, or otherwise permitted by the United States or the jurisdiction in which he/she practices, to dispense a controlled substance in the course of professional practice" (Mid-Level Practitioners Authorization by State, 2012). Examples of "mid-level" practitioners include, but are not limited to, health care providers such as nurse practitioners, nurse midwives, nurse anesthetists, clinical nurse specialists, and physician assistants who are authorized to dispense controlled substances by the state in which they practice (Stewart & DeNisco, 2015, p 345).

National Provider Identification (NPI)

The Health Insurance Portability and Accountability Act of 1996 (HIPAA) mandated the adoption of a standard unique identifier for health care providers.

This is particularly important for reimbursement of health care services that the NP provides. In 2004, the Center for Medicare/Medicaid (CMS) adopted the National Provider Number (NPI) as the standard unique identifier number for all health care providers to use when filing and processing health care claims (Stanley, 2010). All nurse practitioners (NPs) are required to apply for a National Provider Number (NPI) and be assigned only one number, which will follow the NP wherever they practice. The application must be completed by the nurse practitioner to avoid any potential error that could delay billing and reimbursement (Stewart & DeNisco, 2015, p 345).

Health Policy

In March of 2010, the Affordable Care Act (ACA) became law. The ACA and the Health Care and Education Reconciliation Act have had the greatest impact on the United States health care system since Medicaid and Medicare were put into law in the 1960s. The intent of the ACA was to get more Americans quality health care insurance, lower the number of uninsured people, and also lower the cost of health care insurance. In addition, it was to encourage hospitals and primary care practices to improve technology and clinical outcomes with the goal of increased access to care, lower costs, and improved health outcomes. States cannot be forced to expand Medicaid and will not lose Medicaid funding if they choose not to. Since 2010, it is estimated that there are over 11 million people less who are uninsured.

In 2010, the legendary report from the Institutes of Medicine (IOM), *The Future of Nursing: Leading Change, Advancing Health*, was released, which recommended:

- Nurses should practice to the full extent of their education and training.
- Nurses should achieve higher levels of education and training through an improved education system that promotes seamless academic progression.
- Nurses should be full partners, with physicians and other health care professionals, in redesigning health care in the United States.
- Effective workforce planning and policy making require better data collection and information infrastructure.

(IOM (Institute of Medicine). (2011). The Future of Nursing: Leading Change, Advancing Health. Washington, DC: The National Academies Press.)

Nurse practitioners have the opportunity to put these recommendations into effect and have positive impacts on the nation's health, as well as the scope of practice issues for NPs. To this end, the National Organization for Nurse Practitioner Faculties (NONPF) has a set of competencies for all student nurse practitioners related to health policy, which have been recently updated and reflect the competencies listed in the DNP Essentials. These are listed next.

NONPF NP Policy Competencies

1. Demonstrates an understanding of the interdependence of policy and practice.
2. Advocates for ethical policies that promote access, equity, quality, and cost.
3. Analyzes ethical, legal, and social factors influencing policy development.
4. Contributes in the development of health policy.
5. Analyzes the implications of health policy across disciplines.
6. Evaluates the impact of globalization on health care policy development.

(Data from National Organization of Nurse Practitioner Faculties. (Amended 2012). Nurse Practitioner Core Competencies April 2010. Washington, D.C.: NONPF. Stewart., J., and DeNisco, S. (2015). Role development for the nurse practitioner. Jones & Bartlett: Burlington, MA.)

American Association of Nurse Practitioners: Position on Terms such as Mid-level Provider and Physician Extender

The use of terms such as "mid-level provider" and "physician extender" in reference to nurse practitioners (NPs) individually or to an aggregate inclusive of NPs is inaccurate and misleading. The American Association of Nurse Practitioners opposes the use of these terms and calls on employers, policy-makers, health care professionals and other parties to refer to NPs by their title. In 2010, the IOM developed a blueprint for the future of nursing. A key recommendation of this report is that NPs should be full partners with physicians and other health care professionals. Achieving this recommendation requires the use of clear and accurate nomenclature of the nursing profession.

NPs are licensed, independent practitioners. Nurse practitioners work throughout the entirety of health care from health promotion and disease prevention to diagnosis that prevents and limits disability. These inaccurate terms originated decades ago in bureaucracies and/or organized medicine; they are not interchangeable with use of the NP title. The terms fail to recognize the established national scope of practice for the NP role and authority of NPs to practice according to the full extent of their education. Further, these terms confuse health care consumers and the general public due to their vague nature and are not a true reflection of the role of the NP.

The term "mid-level provider" implies an inaccurate hierarchy within clinical practice. Nurse practitioners practice at the highest level of professional nursing practice. It is well established that patient outcomes for NPs are comparable or better than that of physicians. NPs provide high-quality and cost-effective care.

The term "physician extender" originated in the physician community and was related to the extension of physician services by other providers. The NP role, however, evolved in response to identified health care needs across populations. NPs continue to meet the current and evolving future needs within a complex health care system. NPs are independently licensed, and their scope of practice is not designed to be dependent on or an extension of care rendered by a physician.

In addition to the terms cited above, other terms that should be avoided in reference to NPs include "limited-license providers," "non-physician providers," and "allied health providers." As it would be inappropriate to call physicians non-nurse providers, it is similarly inappropriate to call all providers by something that they are not. Similarly, the usage of the term "allied health provider" has no clear definition or purpose in today's environment.

When it is necessary to group providers for policymaking or other purposes, more appropriate terms may instead be: primary care providers; health care providers; health care professionals; advanced practice providers; clinicians; and/or prescribers. AANP stands with the IOM, the National Council of State Boards of Nursing and other nursing associations to recognize nursing's role in the health care system and only endorses the term nurse practitioner. Best practices call for clearly informing patients and referring to each health care provider by their individual title to recognize their unique but overlapping roles. Now is the time to eliminate outdated terms to ensure clarity and public understanding of the title of nurse practitioner.

(Reproduced from AANP. (2009). (Revised 2015). AANP White Paper: Use of Terms Such as Mid-Level Provider and Physician Extender. Retrieved from http://www.aanp.org/images/documents/publications/useofterms.pdf)

Responsibility to Patients/Care Priorities

The FNP has a variety of responsibilities, roles, and priorities for care. As a primary care provider, educator, mentor, researcher, administrator, and advocate for the NP profession, the FNP has multiple responsibilities. The American Association of Nurse Practitioners (2013) lists the various priorities for the NP's practice model. These include patient and family education, assisting the patient to participate in care, promoting optimal health, providing culturally competent care, assisting patients to access health care, and promoting an environment that is safe.

Ethics

Autonomy—the patient has the right to self-determine choices and actions.

Beneficence—doing good/helping others.

Confidentiality—keeping patient information private unless sharing is required by legal need to share and/or to protect children and elders from domestic violence, psychiatric violence, etc.

Non-maleficence—doing no harm. The benefit(s) outweigh the risk(s).

Fidelity—developing and maintaining trust in the patient-provider relationship based on truthfulness.

Justice—a complex term that basically means equals should be treated equally.

Paternalism—in the case of the health care provider, it means the provider knows better than the patient and therefore would make decisions for the patient. This directly contradicts the concept of autonomy.

Minors

A minor is a person under the age of 18 years. There are federal and state laws that pertain to the provision of health care to a minor without parental/guardian consent. Of note, any person who is going to receive health care must provide informed consent; meaning the patient needs to understand his/her condition and the options being offered for treatment, as well as the risks for declining treatment. Many states allow for adolescents to obtain care without parental consent. The American Academy of Pediatrics has valuable information regarding confidential health care services for minors. It is vital for the FNP to be aware of the laws pertaining to minors and health care in the state in which he/she practices.

Review Questions

1. The term "LACE" stands for which of the following?

    A. Licensure, accommodation, consensus, and education

    B. Licensure, accreditation, certification, and education

    C. Liberation, accommodation, consensus, and education

    D. Liberation, accreditation, certification, and education

2. An FNP sees a patient, Mr. A, who is HIV+. After the patient is gone, the next patient to be seen mentions she knows Mr. A, and is aware he is HIV+ and is in an intimate relationship with someone who is unaware of Mr. S's status. Of the available choices below, choose the best response for the FNP:

    A. Mr. A is not HIV+, and I am not sure where you got that information.

    B. Please report your concerns to the local public health department who can follow up on Mr. A's inappropriate behavior.

    C. Patient confidentiality and privacy are the basis for our clinical practice, therefore I do not discuss your or any other patient's information unless it is necessary for your health care.

    D. Thank you for the information. I will follow up on this.

3. Ms. J is being seen for a variety of vague complaints, including malaise and mild body aches that have not gone away for several weeks. The initial workup included a complete blood count, comprehensive metabolic panel, mono-spot, and Lyme antibody. All tests were negative and/or within normal limits. Ms. J wants a full-body magnetic resonance imaging test ordered, and a prescription for an antibiotic "just in case." While formulating an appropriate response, the FNP is aware that balancing the basis for her response will depend on which of the following ethical concepts?

    A. Non-maleficence and beneficence

    B. Virtue and action

    C. Justice and altruism

    D. Ecocentrism and procedural justice

4. A 15-year-old female patient is seen in the office. She discloses she has been having unprotected sexual intercourse with a 15-year-old male she has known for many years. She would like to discuss contraceptive options but she is afraid to tell her mother. The best next step for the FNP is:

    A. Let the minor know the FNP cannot discuss contraception with her unless one parent or guardian is present.

    B. Make an appointment for the girl to go to an STD clinic.

    C. Assure the girl that the discussion will be confidential and review contraceptive options as well as possible STD testing.

    D. Make a separate appointment in 2 weeks for the girl to return and have a full gynecological examination and discussion of options at that time.

5. Ms. K is a 28-year-old female patient who is very shy and can be indecisive. She has a small non-tender lump on her right breast. When the FNP recommends an ultrasound and possible mammogram, Ms. K is tearful and says she needs time to decide. After a few days of not being able to make a decision, the FNP calls her and says she made the appointments for her so she has to go for testing. This concept is best described as which of the following?

    A. Aggressive medicine

    B. Non-maleficence

    C. Paternalism

    D. Distributive justice

6. The Health Insurance Portability and Accountability Act of 1996 (HIPAA) mandated the use of which of the following to improve the efficiency and effectiveness of electronic records' transmissions.

   A. National Provider Identification

   B. Medicare Provider Unique Number

   C. Healthcare Privacy Identifier

   D. Unique Insurance and Portability Number

7. An FNP is moving from Maine to Ohio. In addition to applying for a license in the new state, he is aware of the need to know which of the following?

   A. The Consensus Model enforces each state to provide the same licensing and scope of practice for all APRNs.

   B. Although many states have incorporated portions of the Consensus Model, there are varying requirements and practice acts among states.

   C. His license from Maine will be honored in most other states.

   D. All states have some form of physician supervision in the practice act.

8. A local medical center is advertising for an APRN. The FNP requests further information prior to applying for a position. The need to ask about the role for this position is important because:

   A. APRNs are not just NPs, but also certified nurse midwives (CNMs), nurse anesthetists (CRNAs), and clinical nurse specialists (CNSs).

   B. APRNs include NPs, as well as clinical nurse leaders (CNLs).

   C. APRNs are specifically identified in each state, which may vary.

   D. APRNs are all nurses with masters' degrees.

9. In most states, adolescents (under age 18 years) would not have the right to refuse medical treatment if a parent decided it was necessary for that teenager to be healthy. Which one of the following scenarios is true?

   A. All states allow a female adolescent to obtain abortion services if desired.

   B. Fifty states require an adolescent to co-sign medical treatment forms.

   C. At least one state allows adolescents to request abortion services without parental permission but has not allowed refusal of chemotherapy for a curable cancer.

   D. The majority of states do not allow adolescents to get treated for sexually transmitted diseases without parental or guardian approval.

10. A 45-year-old male and a 52-year-old male are seeking treatment options for increased prostate-specific antigen levels. One of these men has no health insurance and the other has very comprehensive coverage. The FNP knows that they must both be offered the same options/recommendations based on which ethical principle?

    A. Maternalism

    B. Non-maleficence

    C. Deontology

    D. Justice

11. A newly graduated, certified, and licensed FNP has taken a position in a large medical practice. The physicians repeatedly refer to him as a "mid-level provider" when introducing him to patients and the office staff. What is an appropriate next step to help inform the physicians and staff about the use of the term "mid-level"?

    A. Make copies of the position paper on the use of the term "mid-level" from AANP and leave it on the physicians' desks.

    B. Ask for a meeting with the lead physician of the practice to discuss some positive feedback about the role and also discuss the negative use of the term "mid-level" and offer other terms that would reflect a more positive image to patients and staff, such as "primary care or health care provider" and/or "clinician."

C. Plan to discuss this at the next full staff meeting with the intention of letting everyone know how insulting this has been and threaten to quit if it continues.

D. Since this is the FNP's first job, it would be better to let them continue calling him a mid-level and address this in a year or so when they realize how competent he is.

12. Two examples of the FNP role as it relates to health policy and practice would be:

A. Joining the local community center's board of directors.

B. Serving as a leader in the local Girl Scout troop.

C. Volunteering to work on increasing access to care for the local homeless shelter.

D. Advocating for concussion evaluations and best-fit helmets for the local youth football league.

13. The newly licensed FNP is seeing a patient who has acute pain related to a severe ankle strain. The collaborating physician recommends that she write the patient a prescription for Tylenol #3 (acetaminophen with codeine). The FNP is aware of her state's law that she needs which of the following to be able to prescribe this medication?

A. A state controlled-substances license and a DEA registration certificate for schedule III drugs

B. A state license and NPI registration number

C. A federal license to practice and a state license allowing her to prescribe Schedule 1 and II drugs.

D. A state controlled-substances license and a state registration license for Schedule II–IV drugs.

14. An FNP is deciding what state to move to in an effort to expand her practice. The easiest and best option is to look up the latest:

A. Pearson Report.

B. LACE Report.

C. Consensus Report.

D. Federal Scope of Practice Report.

15. An FNP is completing paperwork for a new position in a large hospital-based outpatient center. Forms to be signed include strict guidelines about physician supervision of the FNP and patient care. Which of the following statements is true?

A. The institution can dictate whatever restrictions on physician oversight they prefer, even if FNPs are allowed to practice without supervision in that state.

B. The institution cannot dictate that the FNP must be supervised when providing care in an outpatient setting if that state allows full unsupervised practice.

C. The FNP will need to report to the supervising physician on each patient seen prior to the end of the patient medical visit.

D. The FNP can sign the forms and then make an agreement with the chief medical officer about which patients can be seen without any supervision.

Answers and Rationales

1. B. The term "LACE" stands for: licensure, accreditation, certification, and education.

2. C. Of the available choices, the FNP should respond "Patient confidentiality and privacy are the basis for our clinical practice, therefore I do not discuss your or any other patient's information unless it is necessary for your health care."

3. A. The FNP is balancing the ethical concepts of non-maleficence and beneficence.

4. C. The FNP should assure the girl that the discussion will be confidential and then review contraceptive options, as well as possible STD testing.

5. C. The concept is best described as paternalism.

6. A. The Health Insurance Portability and Accountability Act of 1996 (HIPAA) mandated the use of National Provider Identification to improve the efficiency and effectiveness of electronic records' transmissions.

7. B. Although many states have incorporated portions of the Consensus Model, there are varying requirements and practice acts among states.

8. A. APRNs are not just NPs, but also certified nurse midwives (CNMs), nurse anesthetists (CRNAs), and clinical nurse specialists (CNSs).

9. C. At least one state allows adolescents to request abortion services without parental permission but has not allowed refusal of chemotherapy for a curable cancer.

10. D. The correct answer is justice.

11. B. The FNP should ask for a meeting with the lead physician of the practice to discuss some positive feedback about the role and also discuss the negative use of the term "mid-level" and offer other terms that would reflect a more positive image to patients, and staff such as "primary care or health care provider" and/or "clinician."

12. C. Two examples of the FNP role as it relates to health policy and practice would be: volunteering to work on increasing access to care for the local homeless shelter; and advocating for concussion evaluations and best-fit helmets for the local youth football league.

13. A. The following would be needed: a state controlled-substances license and a DEA registration certificate for schedule III drugs.

14. A. The Pearson Report.

15. A. The institution can dictate whatever restrictions on physician oversight that they prefer, even if FNPs are allowed to practice without supervision in that state.

● ● ● References

American Association of Nurse Practitioners. (2013). Use of Terms Such as Mid-Level Provider and Physician Extender. AANP: Austin, TX.

Drug Enforcement. (2012). *Mid-level practitioners authorization by state*. October 31. Retrieved from the Office of Diversion Control at http://www.deadiversion.usdoj.gov/drugreg/practioners/index.html

Institute of Medicine. (2010). *The future of nursing: Leading change, advancing health*. Retrieved from http://books.nap.edu/openbook.php?record_id=12956&page=R1

National Council of State Boards of Nursing. (n.d.). *The Consensus Model for APRN regulation: A guide for advanced practice registered nurses (APRNs)*. Retrieved from https://www.ncsbn.org/2010APRNbookletforAPRNsweb.pdf

National Organization of Nurse Practitioner Faculties. (amended 2012). *Nurse practitioner core competencies April 2010*. Washington, D.C.: NONPF. Retrieved from http://www.nonpf.com/displaycommon.cfm?an=1&subarticlenbr=14

Stewart., J., & DeNisco, S. (2015). *Role development for the nurse practitioner*. Jones & Bartlett: Burlington, MA.

Reimbursement for Nurse Practitioner Services

Adapted from Role Development for the Nurse Practitioner
Lynn Rapsilber, MSN, ANP-BC, APRN, FAANP, DNP(c)

Introduction

Fiscal responsibility is paramount for nurse practitioners (NPs) to understand. Correct coding can increase revenue and decrease liability. The 1997 Balanced Budget Act (BBA) liberalized Medicare coverage of nurse practitioner (NP) services. Effective January 1, 1998, NPs and Clinical Nurse Specialists (CNSs) became authorized to bill directly for their professional services and be reimbursed at 85% of the physician rate for services provided to a patient (Department of Health & Human Services, 2007). Understanding proper medical record documentation and billing procedures for an office visit can maximize reimbursement for services, affecting both the practice's and the nurse practitioners' bottom line. This chapter will inform the nurse practitioner of the tools for reimbursement and how to utilize the key components of evaluation and management to select the most appropriate code for the service provided and recognize potential audit triggers. Lastly, "incident to" billing will be reviewed so the nurse practitioner will be able to identify and protect from unintentional fraudulent billing and legal issues because the NP is accountable for all the services billed by a practice.

Important Steps in Reimbursement Eligibility

National Provider Number

In order for a nurse practitioner to be eligible for reimbursement, he/she must hold a minimum of a master's degree in nursing and successfully pass the national certification exam given by AANP (American Association of Nurse Practitioners) or the ANCC (American Nurses Credentialing Center). The Health Insurance Portability and Accountability Act of 1996 (HIPAA) mandated the adoption of a standard unique identifier for health care providers. In 2004, the Center for Medicare/Medicaid (CMS) adopted the National Provider Number (NPI) as the standard unique identifier number for all health care providers to use when filing and processing health care claims (Stanley, 2010). All nurse practitioners (NPs) are required to apply for a National Provider Number (NPI) and be assigned only one number, which will follow the NP wherever they practice. The application must be completed by the nurse practitioner to avoid any potential error that could delay billing and reimbursement (National Provider Identifier, 2012).

Employer Provider Number

Once employed by a practice, the nurse practitioner will be assigned a provider number by the employer. This number reflects where the services will be provided to a patient. If the medical practice has two office locations, there will be a different provider number for both the practice settings. Before billing a third-party payer, whether Medicare, Medicaid, or a private insurer, the patient service must have the national provider number who provided the service and the provider number where the service occurred in order to bill.

Third-Party Credentialing

Lastly, the nurse practitioner must receive credentialing by the third-party payer in order to bill insurance companies for their services. While this is usually completed by the practice manager, the nurse practitioner should become familiar with the rules and policies of the third-party payer. A provider application form is filled out which is also known as the "credentialing form." The nurse practitioner will be required to complete an attestation form to verify that the information submitted is correct. Once the nurse practitioner has obtained an NPI number, employer provider number, and third-party credentialing or insurance company membership, he/she is ready to begin billing for services.

Practice Authority

The NP practice authority is determined by the state. The level of practice authority is defined by the American Association of Nurse Practitioners as full, reduced, or restricted practice as determined by the ability to assess, diagnose, treat, and prescribe. Full practice authority allows the NP to provide unencumbered patient care. Reduced practice authority requires a collaborative agreement with an outside health discipline to provide patient care. Some states allow a physician or NP to be a collaborator. Restricted practice authority requires supervision, delegation, or team-management by an outside health discipline in order for the NP to provide patient care. Consult the AANP website (www.AANP.org) for the latest map of the state practice environment.

Coding and Billing Resources

Before billing for services rendered, the nurse practitioner needs to identify appropriate diagnoses for the patient, the type of patient encounter either new or established, and what procedures were performed during the patient encounter. Other reportable, billable services would be what medications were administered, if any, and what supplies were used to provide care. Lastly, the nurse practitioner must provide clear and accurate documentation validating the reported diagnoses and procedural codes reported for billing purposes. An understanding of medical coding and resources to support these activities are the responsibility of the nurse practitioner.

Definition of Medical Coding

Medical coding is best defined as the translation of the original medical record documentation regarding patient diagnoses and procedures into a series of code numbers that describe the information in a standard manner. Coded medical information is used for patient care, research, reimbursement, and evaluation of services (Aalseth, 2006). International Classification of Diseases (ICD) codes, developed by the World Health Organization, are used to identify the patient's diagnoses or reasons for seeking care. These codes cover specific illnesses or diseases as well as signs and symptoms that would result in the patient encounter (Centers for Disease Control and Prevention, 2011). ICD codes are also useful for classifying morbidity and mortality data from inpatient and outpatient records and most National Center for Health Statistics (NCHS) surveys. Another component of medical billing is the Current Procedural Terminology (CPT), published by the American Medical Association, which describes the services or procedures and/or procedures for which reimbursement is sought.

This publication was initiated in 1966 as a way of standardizing terms for medical procedures used for documentation purposes (Phillipsen, 2008). CPT codes are used for specific types of patient encounters and innumerable procedures and diagnostic studies that will be described in more detail later in this chapter.

The CPT and ICD 10 Books

There are several resources the nurse practitioner needs to be aware of regarding medical coding and billing for services. As previously mentioned, the first publication is called CPT (Current Procedural Terminology). Only nurse practitioners, physician assistants, and physicians can use these codes and they are updated annually. CPT reflects "what was done" (e.g., types of visits, consultations, referrals, procedures, diagnostic studies, treatment regimens). Obtaining a copy of this book is very important because the information presented in this chapter is found in the beginning sections of this book.

The next book is called ICD-10 (International Classification of Diseases, 10th edition). This reflects "why it was done." This book classifies diseases with numeric codes. The NP must select a code for the disease or symptom by "what you know," being as specific as possible. If you have not yet determined or confirmed the patient's diagnosis, you will list or code for the presenting symptoms. For example, if the patient has "heartburn" and you have not completed your evaluation, do not choose the ICD-10 code for gastroesophageal reflux disease with esophagitis (K210). Instead, designate "heartburn" as the diagnostic code (R12) until you have the results of an endoscopic biopsy.

The ICD-10 classification system is widely used in Europe and was not released in the United States until October 1, 2015 (Classification of Diseases, Functioning, and Disability: International Classification of Diseases, Tenth Revision, Clinical Modification, 2012).

Medical Necessity

When you have the "what" was done with the "why" it was done, this equals medical necessity: CPT + ICD-10 = Medical Necessity. Medical Necessity is defined as: medical items and services that are "reasonable and necessary" for a variety of purposes. By statute, Medicare may only pay for items and services that are "reasonable and necessary for the diagnosis or treatment of illness or injury or to improve the functioning of a malformed body member," unless there is another statutory authorization for payment. Determination of medical necessity involves comparing the procedure being billed to the diagnosis being submitted. If the NP receives a denial notification from the payer for a particular procedure, it means that the payer does not think the procedure was justified for the diagnosis given (Aalseth, 2006).

There is an additional resource called HCPCS (Healthcare Common Procedure Coding System). For Medicare and other health insurance programs to ensure health care claims are processed in an orderly and consistent manner, standardized coding systems are essential. The HCPCS Level II code set is one of the standard code sets used by medical coders and billers for services such as medical supplies, durable medical goods, non-physician services, and services not represented in the Level I code set determined by CPT (e.g., ambulance, prosthetics, orthotics, etc.) (AAPC, 2012). With the utilization of electronic health records, all these codes are recorded and the information is submitted electronically to the insurance company for reimbursement.

Medical Record Documentation

The medical record is the most important document in the reimbursement process. Any information provided to the patient on a particular date of service must be recorded in the record. If it was not documented, it was not done. The medical record clearly should state what was done and why it was done. The Centers for Medicare and Medicaid Services (CMS) has specific documentation criteria. The medical record should be complete and legible. It should include a chief complaint, why the patient presents to the office, relevant history, assessment, physical exam, diagnostic testing, and a treatment plan, signed by the provider of record (the one who performed the service). Rationale for testing must be apparent. Health risks must be identified. Responses to treatment and follow-up must be clear. CPT and ICD-10 must be supported in the documentation. The data must sequential. If something is inadvertently omitted from a previous date of service (DOS), it can be entered using today's date and state "addenda to DOS on date" and add your note. If something is erroneously entered, an addendum to the chart is made detailing the reason for the error and the correction. CMS recognizes that the electronic health record should not replace the need for good documentation by the provider.

Payment for Services

The current system for reimbursement is based upon the resource-based relative value scale (RBRVS). This system replaced the fee for service. The system was developed based upon data acquired by Dr. Hsaio and a multidisciplinary team of researchers from Harvard University in 1988 (Goodson, 2007). Three separate factors were used to calculate physician value: (1) work effort (52%), (2) practice expense (44%), and (3) malpractice expense (4%). Provider work effort is defined by a relative value unit. The Geographic Practice Cost Index (GPCI) refers to the cost of service applied to the geographic location in the country. In New York and California, it costs more to deliver care than in Tennessee or Mississippi. The conversion factor is the variable that changes from year to year.

Evaluation and Management Documentation Guidelines

Evaluation and management (E&M) documentation guidelines are the foundation of fiscal responsibility and were developed by the American Medical Association (AMA) and Health Care Financing Administration (HCFA) (Aalseth, 2006). Understanding this system will insure proper coding of visits and maximize reimbursement; these guidelines are used by Medicare and other third-party payers when making reimbursement decisions. There are three key components to E&M documentation: (1) history, (2) examination, and (3) medical decision making. These variables are broken down into their own set of levels. This will be discussed further in the "key components" section of this chapter. Additionally, the NP needs to identify who is a new patient versus an established patient. A new patient is defined as an individual new to the practice (seeing any provider in the practice for the first time) or someone who has not been seen in three years. The new patient can also be a hospital patient who is being referred for care and not previously seen by any provider in the practice. An established patient is one who has an ongoing relationship with a practice. The hospital patient can be an established patient if a provider from the practice has seen the patient in the hospital and is returning for a follow-up visit. Specialty providers for this discussion will be defined as a health care provider and as part of a group and is considered a specialist; the provider must have received special training and is board certified in that specialty.

General Coding Guidelines

The next step is to know which ICD-10 codes you will use to bill for the office visit. Coding takes the words the NP used as the diagnosis or symptom and converts this into a category code. Codes for valid diagnoses may have up to 7 digits. Codes that describe symptoms as opposed to diagnoses are acceptable if the NP has not yet established a diagnosis responsible for the symptomatology of the patient.

Structure of the ICD-10 Diagnoses Codes

The diagnosis system is contained in three volumes: Tabular List, Instruction Manual, and Alphabetical Index.

1. Tabular List: Disease and health-related problems. It contains 22 chapters and over 11,000 codes.
2. The Instruction Manual provides data for morbidity (hospital statistics) and mortality (causes of death).
3. The Alphabetical Index

Within each of these major areas are categories that are logically sequenced by body system, site, or by etiology. Combination codes are available for certain diseases. The use of "other" NOS (not otherwise specified) or NEC (not elsewhere classified) is no longer permitted in ICD-10. The HCFA 1500 insurance claim form allows unlimited diagnostic codes to be used and each is linked to a CPT or procedural code. A word of caution: Use only the codes you intend to do something about, otherwise it can trigger an audit.

Structure of the CPT Procedure Codes

CPT codes are categorized into six main sections with five numbers representing a service:

1. Anesthesia (00100–01999)
2. Surgery (10040–69990)
3. Radiology (70010–79999)
4. Pathology & Laboratory (80048–89399)
5. Medicine (90281–99199)
6. Evaluation and Management (99201–99499)

The categories of the codes don't mean that a primary care provider cannot utilize a code in the surgery section—for example, CPT code 10060 Incision and Drainage of abscess (cutaneous or subcutaneous abscess, cyst, or paronychia); simple or single may be used by the NP in the outpatient setting. The categorization of the codes is set up for the expediency and the provider and billing personnel may also use the index to look up specific items.

Location of Patient Encounter

Knowing where your feet are planted and using specific patient encounter locations will result in a different code for billing purposes. If the NP is in the office, the following CPT codes will be used: (1) new patient codes 99201–99205 and (2) established patient codes 99211–99215. Care will be provided in the inpatient, outpatient settings or in the home or extended care facility. Consult the CPT book for the specific criteria for each code.

Levels of Patient Encounter

The NP will bill for a level of office visit based upon the amount of work involved with history, physical exam, and medical decision making. There are five levels of codes to bill for new and established office patients. The level one visit code is for a nurse visit and is not listed in the discussion. Problem focused is a level 2. Expanded problem focused is a level 3. Detailed is a level 4. Comprehensive is a level 5. Billing a higher level of the office visit requires more work involving history, physical exam, and medical decision making. This will be discussed in the section that follows.

Key Components of Reimbursement

The history, physical examination, and medical decision-making level are the key components that determine reimbursement for the patient encounter. Counseling, coordination of care, the nature of the presenting problem, and time also weigh into the evaluation of a patient visit.

The History and Reimbursement Decisions

The history is the first key component of the reimbursement process. There are four components of the history that are considered in determining the level of the visit.

1. The history includes the chief complaint: what brought the patient to the office that day or it can also include chronic disease management and follow-up care.

2. The nurse practitioner gathers the history of present illness (HPI). This includes: location, quality, severity and timing, context, modifying factors, and associated signs and symptoms.

3. The review of systems (ROS) is performed, which is conducted systematically to gather information, including constitutional signs such as weight loss and overall condition, as well as ears, eyes, nose, mouth, throat, respiratory, cardiovascular, gastrointestinal, genitourinary, musculoskeletal, skin, neurological, psychiatric, hematologic and lymphatic, and immune and allergy.

4. The last component—past history, family and social history (PFSH)—is considered. Past medical history includes: illnesses, surgeries, injuries, treatment, and current medications. Family history includes: hereditary diseases that increase the patient's risk factors for those conditions. The components of history are placed into a table by the amount of work done by the provider.

Problem focused is a level 2, which includes only a brief HPI. Expanded problem focused is a level 3, which includes a brief HPI and problem focused ROS, but no PFSH is done. Detailed visits are coded at level 4, which includes an extensive HPI, ROS, and pertinent PFSH. Comprehensive visits are coded at level 5 and include comprehensive histories, extended HPI, extended ROS, complete ROS, and complete PFHS.

The Physical Examination and Reimbursement Decisions

The next key component is the physical examination. There are four levels of physical examination:

- Level 2 problem focused (brief or perform and document 1–5 elements identified by a bullet)
- Level 3 expanded problem (focused and brief or perform and document at least 6 elements identified by a bullet)
- Level 4 detailed (perform and document at least 2 elements identified by a bullet from each of six areas/systems or at least 12 elements identified by a bullet in two or more areas/systems)
- Level 5 comprehensive (perform all elements identified by a bullet and document at least two elements identified by a bullet from each of nine areas/systems)

There are specific documentation guidelines created by the American Medical Association (AMA) and the Centers for Medicare and Medicaid Services (CMS). There are two sets of documentation guidelines—1995 and 1997. The 1995 guidelines are body system focused and the 1997 is system area focused (Department of Health and Human Services, 2007).

The documentation guidelines determine the level of physical exam to be performed. There is a general multi-system examination and several specialty examinations options. The specialty examinations include: cardiology; hematology/oncology; musculoskeletal; neurology; ear, nose, and throat; genitourinary; psychiatry; respiratory; and skin.

If the provider documents an abnormal finding, an accompanying explanation is required. Normal and negative examination must be listed by organ or body system. Subjective without any documentation cannot be counted.

Medical Decision Making and Reimbursement

Medical decision making is the last key component. It takes into account the diagnosis, information required to make the diagnosis, and risks and complications associated with the diagnosis. The evaluation and management documentation guidelines describe four levels of medical decision making:

- Level 2 Straightforward
- Level 3 Low complexity
- Level 4 Moderate complexity
- Level 5 High Complexity

Factors such as number of diagnoses, comorbid conditions, data to be reviewed, number of management options, and risk of morbidity and mortality are considered in the level of medical decision making selected. The more risk involved in the patient's care, the greater the level of medical decision making.

How to Bill for a Visit

In order to bill for a visit, you must know which ICD-10 and CPT codes to use. In review, know where your feet are planted and use the specific location codes for where the care is provided. Decide if the patient is a new or established patient. Evaluate the level of history, physical examination, and medical decision making performed and the NP will have the tools to establish the codes for the visit. A new patient requires the level of history, examination, and medical decision making to be weighted equally. For example, if you have documented a level 4 history,

level 2 exam, and level 3 medical decision making, the visit is coded as a level 2 (99202). If this were an established patient, the highest two components out of the three are weighed for the visit. In the scenario just described, the level 4 history and level 3 medical decision making would be considered for billing purposes. The physical exam would be dropped. The visit will be coded as a level 3 (99213). Table 21-1 is a tool to assist the NP in accurately coding a visit by circling the amount of history, examination, and medical decision making performed for the visit. Documentation of these components occurs, selecting the column to the farthest right. Once all columns are filled, the visit can be billed. If it is a new patient, history, exam, and medical decision making are weighted equally. Look for the column with the circle to the farthest left. This is the level of service billed. If you have an established patient, the lowest level is thrown out and you bill to the next circle to the farthest left. This becomes the billed visit code.

Table 21-1	Documentation Guidelines 2015				
Documentation Grid for Patients					
New/Established	99211	99201/99212	99202*/99213	99203/99214	99204** 99205/99215
		Problem Focused	Expanded Problem Focused	Detailed	Comprehensive
History	Minimal	HPI 1–3 ROS none PFSH none	HPI 1–3 ROS 1 system PFSH none	HPI 4+ ROS 2–9 systems PFSH 1+	HPI 4+ ROS 10+ PFSH 3+
Physical Exam	Minimal	1–5 bullets	6–12 bullets	12–18 bullets 2 or more body systems or 2 bullets from 6 body systems	18 bullets 9+ organ systems
Decision-Making	Minimal	Straight-forward	* Moderate Comp Low Complexity 2+ minor or 1 stable + 1 acute OTC Tx	Moderate complexity 1+ chronic+ exacerb or 2+ stable + 1 new Rx mgmnt low-risk surg	** Moderate Comp High Complexity 1+ chronic + severe exacer Acute or chronic abrupt chg Rx/inc surg risk
Time	5 minutes	10 minutes	15 minutes	25 minutes	40 minutes

"""""" For new patient, all three: history, exam, and medical decision making

"""""" For established patient: need 2 of 3 components to base level of visit

How to Code:
1. Take credit for information documented in HX, PE, and Med-Dec to the farthest right.
2. Code the visit to the farthest left
   a. If a New patient, all three weigh the same and use the circle to the farthest left.
   b. If an Established patient, cross out the lowest, then take the next lowest unless they are both in the same column

Reproduced from Rapsilber, L.M, & Anderson, E.H. (2000). Understanding the Reimbursement Process. *Nurse Practitioner 25*(5), 36–56.

Coding Conundrums

There are coding situations that can be a challenge or a benefit if you know what they are and how to use them effectively. Coding by time, evaluation, and management, plus procedure, modifiers, shared evaluation and management, and "incident to" are examples that will be described in greater detail. Understanding these situations can make a difference in revenue for the practice, as well as avoiding legal pitfalls.

Coding by time is utilized when greater than 50% of the face-to-face time is spent discussing options with a patient, family member, or legal guardian. Little if any history or physical exam is performed. The visit is based upon the time spent with the patient, family member, or legal guardian. Nurse practitioners spend time teaching their patients about their disease or how to stay healthy or show them how to perform a task. All these can fall under coding by time. Documentation must support the time spent listed as a fraction (i.e., 35/40) and what was discussed. The amount of time corresponds to the code billed. Established patient codes 99213 equals 15 minutes, 99214 equals 25 minutes, and 99215 equals 40 minutes.

Evaluation and management, plus a procedure, occur when the same provider performs the evaluation and management, plus the procedure, on the same patient on the same day. A diabetic patient comes into the office for a follow-up visit and asks about a warty growth on his/her shoulder. It is a seborrheic keratosis and the NP performs cryosurgery on the lesion. The nurse practitioner bills a 99214 for the diabetic visit and codes for the cryosurgery one lesion. Since there is duplicity in work effort, there will be a modifier (25) placed on the office visit and the value will be decreased but the procedure will be reimbursed at 100 percent. Please be aware that an evaluation, management, and preventative visit in the same day may pose a problem. The patient has no co-pay for the preventative and will need to pay the co-pay for the evaluation and management part of the visit. This should be disclosed to the patient prior to the preventative visit.

Modifiers are a way to show that the evaluation and management code has changed. The service or procedure is altered. Modifiers can increase or decrease a value. It can indicate bilateral or multiple procedures. It can indicate additional work was performed in rendering the service. The two-digit modifier is always attached to the evaluation and management code. Most modifiers are used in the surgical arena.

Shared evaluation and management occurs when the nurse practitioner sees a patient in the hospital and documents the visit in the medical record. Later, the physician sees the patient and further documents this in the medical record. The visit from both providers can be billed as a shared visit and billed under the physician's NPI number. There must be clear separate documentation in the patient medical record. It does not mean the physician has to co-sign the nurse practitioners note. This is used for hospital billing and reimbursement purposes. This is different than "incident to" billing.

Incident to billing is used in the care of Medicare patients. The term "incident to" allows physicians to bill for various services provided in the office by health care personnel that is performed in "relation to" or "incident to" the care the physician provides (Goolsby, 2002). In this situation, the nurse practitioner bills for her services with the physician's NPI number. The visit is reimbursed at 100 percent, 15% more than billed under the nurse practitioner NPI number. This is problematic because the NP becomes visible in this method of billing and cannot show the income he or she is generating for the practice.

There are three major criteria that must be met by the practice before "incident to" billing can occur. The first criterion is that the nurse practitioner must be directly supervised by the physician. This is problematic because, in most states, nurse practitioners either practice autonomously or in collaboration with a physician. This stipulation means the physician must be available onsite to provide consultation to the NP. The physician cannot be in the hospital, on vacation, or out of the office. It does not mean the physician has to see the patient, but must be available for questions if the need arises. The second criterion for incident to billing to occur is that the physician must see the patient for the initial visit and develop the treatment plan. The nurse practitioner cannot see any new Medicare patients under the current guidelines. The last criterion is that the physician must have ongoing participation in the patient's care. The patient cannot have a new problem when they see the nurse practitioner. The physician cannot co-sign the nurse practitioner's documentation in this situation but must actually see the patient and modify the treatment plan or bill the service under the nurse practitioner's NPI number. The NP must be employed by the MD as well.

There are numerous problems with this type of billing for a nurse practitioner. The Office of the Inspector General is looking at the use of incident to and checking to see that the rules are being followed. Significant monetary penalties are being levied for violation of the rules. In addition, there are considerations subjecting the practice to an audit. Audit triggers include: billing non-covered services as covered, double billing, coding all visits at the same level, coding does not meet medical necessity, using incident to billing when the physician is not present in the office, waiving of co-pays and documentation not supportive of the level billed. NPs should check their state Nurse Practice Acts for reasons for loss of professional licensure, such as false reports, willful misrepresentation, submitting false statements, or other unprofessional conduct (Phillipsen, 2008). Table 21-2 shows the basic components of a compliance plan that should be instituted in each practice setting.

The nurse practitioner is responsible for what is billed during the patient encounter. The practice, physician, and billing staff is not. It is imperative the nurse practitioner understand the method to code

Table 21-2	Basic Components of a Compliance Plan

- Internal auditing system
- Policies and procedures specific to the practice
- Compliance officer in the practice to oversee and enforce the plan
- Education of all employees about the plan
- Prompt responses to any errors or offenses with corrective action
- Open communication

and bill for a patient visit properly to avoid an audit and to avoid fraudulent activity. Thus, it is fiscally prudent to have an understanding of this process.

Review Questions

1. It is important for the FNP to understand coding for all of the following reasons EXCEPT:
   A. Maintain fiscal responsibility.
   B. Calculate a raise.
   C. Add revenue to a practice.
   D. Decrease liability.

2. The CPT is known as which of the following?
   A. Common Physician Terminology
   B. Current Physical Terminology
   C. Current Procedural Terminology
   D. Common Procedural Terminology

3. Who can bill using the CPT?
   A. MD, PA, NP, RN
   B. MD, NP, MA
   C. MD, PA, NP, PT
   D. MD, PA, NP

4. What is NOT true of the CPT?
   A. Updated monthly
   B. Lists procedures and codes
   C. Has an appendix of coding examples
   D. Owned by the AMA

5. In 1997, President Bill Clinton signed the _____, which allows FNPs to be reimbursed.
   A. Balanced Bill Act
   B. Balanced Budget Act
   C. Balanced Budget Alliance
   D. Balanced Bill Alliance

6. The signed legislation mentioned in the previous question allows NPs to be reimbursed at what percentage?
   A. 65%
   B. 75%
   C. 85%
   D. 100%

7. The resource-based relative value scale replaced _____ as a method of reimbursement.
   A. fee for service
   B. cost balance
   C. bartering
   D. value-based

8. ICD (International Classification of Diseases) was developed by which of the following?
   A. HOW – Health Organization of the World
   B. HHS – Health and Human Services
   C. WOD – World Organization of Diseases
   D. WHO – World Health Organization

9. ICD provides all of the following EXCEPT:
   - A. Morbidity data.
   - B. Public health data.
   - C. World drug data.
   - D. Mortality data.

10. NPI stands for which of the following?
    - A. National Provider Number
    - B. National Provisionary Number
    - C. Numerical Provider Number
    - D. Numerical Physician Number

11. An FNP applies for a NPI number _____.
    - A. after graduating
    - B. after passing their certification exam
    - C. after being licensed
    - D. after getting their first job

12. An NPI costs how much?
    - A. $10
    - B. $50
    - C. $100
    - D. Free

13. The FNP must apply for a new NPI number if they change their practice to another state.
    - A. True
    - B. False

14. A provider number is _____.
    - A. the location where a service is rendered
    - B. linked with CPT
    - C. linked with ICD
    - D. linked with NPI
    - E. A, B, and C
    - F. B and C
    - G. A and D

15. What is medical necessity?
    - A. Reasonable and necessary
    - B. CPT and ICD
    - C. Determines payment
    - D. Defined by state governments
    - E. A and B
    - F. A and C

16. CMS stands for which of the following?
    - A. Centers for Medicare and Medicaid Services
    - B. Committee for Medicare Services
    - C. Center for Medicine Services
    - D. Center for Medicare and Medicaid States

17. The medical record should do all of the following EXCEPT:
    A. Be complete and legible.
    B. Reflect what was done and why it was done.
    C. Be signed by the provider.
    D. Be co-signed by the MD of the FNP notes.

18. What form must you sign in order to be credentialed on an insurance panel?
    A. Attestation form
    B. Regulatory form
    C. Affirmation form
    D. Declaratory form

19. An electronic health record should not _____.
    A. contain templates
    B. contain macros
    C. replace good documentation
    D. use cut and paste for all visits

20. All of the following are key components of documentation EXCEPT:
    A. Counseling.
    B. History.
    C. Medical decision making.
    D. Physical exam.

21. History includes which of the following?
    A. History of present illness
    B. Review of systems
    C. Past, Family, Social
    D. Financial

22. Medications are part of the past history.
    A. True
    B. False

23. A *new* patient is one who _____.
    A. has never been seen before in the office
    B. has not been seen in 5 years
    C. is a hospitalist referral
    D. A and B
    E. A and C

24. An *established* patient is one who is _____.
    A. seen by the FNP for the first time
    B. seen by the FNP in follow-up
    C. seen by the FNP for pre-op
    D. seen by the MD for a first visit

25. Practice authority is governed by the states. The three types of practice authority include which of the following?
    A. Full practice
    B. Reduced practice
    C. Limited practice
    D. Restricted practice

26. All of the following are true of Medicare EXCEPT:
    A. It is state-regulated.
    B. It is an entitlement for the elderly and disabled.
    C. It is for everyone starting at age 65.
    D. It is a federal program.

27. A collaborative agreement is between an FNP and an MD.
    A. True
    B. False

28. An FNP forgot to chart information in the EMR when she saw the patient two days ago. She should
    _____.
    A. know it cannot be added in after the fact
    B. put today's date on it and write that the omission was from the date of service and document it
    C. have IT override it so she can document what she omitted in that day's note
    D. add it when she sees the patient the next time.

29. There is a general multisystem examination and a single system examination form.
    A. True
    B. False

30. Which is NOT a single system examination?
    A. Cardiology
    B. Gastroenterology
    C. Musculoskeletal
    D. Psychiatry
    E. Dermatology

31. Medical decision making is based upon:
    A. Number of diagnoses.
    B. Number of treatment options.
    C. Data to be reviewed.
    D. Risk of morbidity and mortality.
    E. Level of history and physical exam.

32. Coding by time is used when greater than ___ of the visit is spent counseling or coordinating care.
    A. 40%
    B. 50%
    C. 75%
    D. 80%

33. Incident to billing is for Medicare patients.
    A. True
    B. False

34. Incident to billing is when the MD bills with the FNP provider number.
    A. True
    B. False

35. Incident to requires the MD to be in the office but not necessarily see the patient.
    A. True
    B. False

36. *Incident to* does not include which of the following?

    A. MD formulates treatment plan.

    B. MD signs FNP paycheck.

    C. Practice gets 100% reimbursement.

    D. Patient can have a new problem.

37. Medicare fraud is a costly problem. In a study published in 2010, how much revenue was billed fraudulently?

    A. Thousands

    B. Millions

    C. Billions

    D. Trillions

38. What can trigger an audit?

    A. Billing all visits using one code

    B. Collecting co-pays

    C. Billing non-covered services as covered

    D. Documentation does not support E&M billed

    E. CPT and ICD do not meet medical necessity

39. What is the most common established patient code billed?

    A. 99212

    B. 99213

    C. 99214

    D. 99215

40. What is the code for an initial office visit for a 13-year-old with comedopapular acne unresponsive to over-the-counter treatment?

    A. 99214

    B. 99211

    C. 99202

    D. 99204

41. What is the code for an office visit for a 32-year-old female established patient with new onset right lower quadrant pain?

    A. 99211

    B. 99202

    C. 99212

    D. 99214

42. What is the code for an office visit for a 60-year-old established patient with chronic hypertension on a multiple drug regimen who has come in for a blood pressure check?

    A. 99213

    B. 99204

    C. 99202

    D. 99215

43. What is the code for an initial evaluation of a 70-year-old patient with recent onset confusion?

    A. 99202

    B. 99203

    C. 99204

    D. 99205

44. What is the code for an office visit for an 82-year-old female established patient for a monthly B12 injection with a documented vitamin B12 deficiency?
    A. 99202
    B. 99211
    C. 99213
    D. 99203

45. What is the code for an initial office visit for a 42-year-old male on hypertensive medication, who is new to the area, has a diastolic pressure of 110, a history of recurrent renal calculi, episodic headaches, intermittent chest pain, and orthopnea?
    A. 99202
    B. 99203
    C. 99214
    D. 99215
    E. 99205

46.   What is the code for an office visit for a 50-year-old female established patient with insulin-dependent diabetes mellitus who has come in for monitoring?
    A. 99211
    B. 99212
    C. 99213
    D. 99214

47. What is the code for an initial office visit for a 33-year-old male with painless gross hematuria without cystoscopy?
    A. 99202
    B. 99203
    C. 99204
    D. 99205

48. What is the code for an office visit for a 10-year-old female established patient who has been swimming in a lake and has a one-day history of left ear pain with purulent discharge?
    A. 99211
    B. 99212
    C. 99213
    D. 99214

49. What is the code for an office visit for the evaluation of recent onset syncopal attacks in a 70-year-old female established patient?
    A. 99212
    B. 99213
    C. 99214
    D. 99215

50. The FNP is responsible for what is billed.
    A. True
    B. False

Answers and Rationales

1. B. Coding has nothing to do with a raise, which is part of the employment agreement.
2. C. It is published by the American Medical Association.
3. D. Only medical doctors, physician assistants, and nurse practitioners can bill for their services and be reimbursed.
4. A. The CPT is updated annually.
5. B. In 1997, President Clinton signed the Balanced Budget Act into law which allowed for reimbursement of nurse practitioner services.
6. C. The BBA of 1997 allowed for nurse practitioners to be reimbursed at 85% of the physician reimbursement rate.
7. A. The resource-based relative value scale replaced the fee for service method of reimbursement.
8. D. World Health Organization working with the United Nations. Started in 1860 when Florence Nightingale wanted to keep data on hospitals.
9. C. Classified diseases, symptoms, and injuries.
10. A. Unique identifier recognized through passage of the Health Insurance Portability and Accountability Act (HIPAA) in 1996.
11. B and C. You need a license in order to complete the application process for an NPI number with CMS.
12. D. There is no cost to apply for an NPI number.
13. B. The NPI number is yours only and travels with you wherever you practice.
14. G. The provider number is the location where a service is provided by the FNP.
15. E. CPT is what you are doing, while ICD is why you are doing it. This equals medical necessity. It does not guarantee payment.
16. A. See www.cms.gov.
17. D. Co-signature is not required by the MD for FNP documentation. The provider of record providing the service must sign the documentation.
18. A. The nurse practitioner will be required to complete an attestation form to verify that the information to the credentialing organization is correct.
19. D. The nurse practitioner must ensure that there is clear and accurate documentation at every visit.
20. A. Not a key component. Counseling is considered when coding by time.
21. D. It may be required for payment but has nothing to do with coding a visit.
22. A. Medications are being taken by a patient already, so they are considered part of the past medical history.
23. E. A new patient is new to the practice, has not been seen in three years, or has been referred by a hospitalist or other provider.
24. B. The FNP already has a relationship with the patient.
25. C. The practice authority map is located at www.aanp.org and is based upon the FNP's ability to diagnose, treat, and prescribe treatments under supervision (Restricted), collaboration (Reduced), or autonomously (Full).
26. A. Medicare is a federal program run by the federal government.
27. B. Depending upon the practice authority, the collaborative agreement can be with an MD or FNP.
28. B. This is the best way to handle an omission and the FNP should correct it as soon as it is known.
29. A. Single-system exam forms are for musculoskeletal, psychiatry, and cardiology, for example. More information can be found at www.cms.gov/medlearn.
30. B. Gastroenterology covers everything from the mouth to the anus, which is not a single system.

31. E. History and physical exam are the other two key components of evaluation and management coding.
32. B. This is used when the FNP is basing the visit on time and not the level of history, physical exam, or medical decision making.
33. A. Though it may happen with other insurance carriers, "incident to" is rooted in Medicare regulations.
34. B. "Incident to" billing is when the FNP bills with the MD NPI number.
35. A. The MD has to be available to the FNP for consultation or to answer questions.
36. D. The patient cannot have a new problem. If there is a new problem, the visit must be billed under the FNP NPI number.
37. C. $6.2 billion dollars was fraudulently billed. This is why, as part of the Affordable Care Act, Recovery Audit Contractors are hired to investigate fraudulent billing practices.
38. B. Co-pay is a monetary agreement between the insured and the insurance company.
39. B. This is based upon a study done by the Department of Health and Human Services and the Office of the Inspector General looking at claims from 2000–2010.
40. C. A new patient requires weighing history, physical exam, and medical decision making equally. A dermatology patient will have lower levels of visit codes. OTC treatment is not as risky as a prescription.
41. D. Abdominal pain requires a workup, and being female could be GYN, GI, or GU etiology.
42. A. An established patient with no change in medication.
43. C. The elderly require an extensive workup to determine etiology, because a change in mental status could be neuro, GU, or medication related.
44. B. B12 injections are given by an RN, which can be billed as a 99211.
45. E. This patient has many issues, requiring additional workup. Etiology can be cardiac, renal or respiratory.
46. C. An established patient with a stable condition and no treatment plan change.
47. B. A new patient requiring history, physical exam, and medical decision making weighed equally. The physical exam will keep the visit at 99203.
48. B. An established patient with localized body area and a problem-focused examination.
49. D. Any mental status change will require workup. Etiology can be neuro, cardiac, GU, or medication.
50. A. The provider of the service is responsible for what is documented and billed.

● ● ● **References**

Aalseth, P. (2006). *Medical coding: What it is and how it works*. Sudbury: Jones & Bartlett.

Classification of Diseases, Functioning, and Disability: International Classification of Diseases, Tenth Revision, Clinical Modification (ICD-10-CM). (2012 , October 4). Retrieved from Centers for Disease Control: http://www.cdc.gov/nchs/icd/icd10cm.htm

Contexo Media. (2015). International Classification of Diseases 10th Revision Clinical. Modification, ICD-10. *Contexo Media*, 1–703.

Contexo Media. (2015). Procedural Coding Expert Ultimate Guide to CPT Coding. *Contexo Media*, 1–33.

Contexo Media. (2015). The Complete Medial Office Handbook: Compliance, Policies, and Financial Information for the Physician Group, 1–653.

Control, C. f. (2011, October 11). *ICD-9-CM Official Guidelines for Coding and Reporting*. Retrieved from http://www.cdc.gov/nchs/data/icd9/icd9cm_guidelines_2011.pdf

Department of Health and Human Services. (2007). *Direct Billing and Payment for Non-Physician Practitioner Services*. Baltmore: Centers for Medicare & Medicaid Services.

Goodson, J. (2007). Unintended consequences of resource-based relative value scale reimbursement. *Journal of American Medical Association, 298*(19), 2308–2310.

Goolsby, M. (2002). *Nurse practitoner secrets: Questions and answers to reveal the secrets to successful NP practice*. Philadephia: Hanley & Belfus, Inc.

MedLearn Network. (2014). Evaluation and Management Services guidelines. *CMS*.

National Provider Identifier. (2012, October 30). Retrieved from National plan and provider enumeration system: https://nppes.cms.hhs.gov/NPPES/StaticForward .do?forward=static.npistart

Phillipsen, P. S. (2008). The most costly billing practices ever. *The Journal for Nurse Practitioners, 4*(10), 761–765.

Rapsilber, L. M., & Anderson, E. H. (2000). Understanding the Reimbursement Process. *Nurse Practitioner. 25,* 36–56.

Stanley, J. (2010). *Advanced practice nursing: Emphasizing common roles* (3rd ed.). Philadelphia: F.A. Davis.

The Coding Institute. (2007). Part B insider survival guide. *The Coding Institute,* 1.1–6.27.

What Is HCPCS? (2012). Retrieved from AAPC: Credentialing the business side of medicine: http://www.aapc .com/resources/medical-coding/hcpcs.aspx

22

Evidence-Based Practice Review for the Advanced Practice Nurse

Kerry A. Milner, DNSc, RN

To be competent, the family nurse practitioner (FNP) must understand the research process and use appropriate evidence when providing patient care. This chapter is a review of the scientific method and evidence-based practice for FNPs. At the end of this chapter, the FNP will be able to:

- Define the scientific method
- Define research literacy
- Define evidence-based practice (EBP)
- Describe the PICO method
- Match the level of evidence needed with the type of clinical question
- List free databases and the type of evidence they contain
- Identify the appropriate tools for critically appraising different types of evidence
- Define shared decision making
- List resources for patient and provider decision aids

Overview of the Scientific Method

Nurses conduct research to generate new knowledge that can be applied to patient populations, care processes, and health systems to improve the quality of care. Advanced practice nurses (APNs) are in a key position to help translate research into practice,

and they need research literacy skills to do this successfully. Research literacy is the ability to access, critically appraise, and interpret scientific literature from many disciplines (Nolan & Behi, 1996). Evidence-based practice incorporates several of these skills, however, and FNPs should be familiar with the basic steps of the research process and areas of potential bias so they can recognize quality research and apply it to practice.

Figure 22-1 displays the steps of the scientific method, also called the research process. Any research study starts with identifying a problem that is significant to that discipline. Next, the researcher reviews the literature and provides a summary of the background, rationale, and justification for studying the problem. The next step is to identify research questions that the study will answer and the hypotheses the researcher will test. The type of research question will impact the study design selection. Advance practice nurses must be knowledgeable about the types of study designs used to answer intervention, prognosis, diagnostic, etiology, and meaning questions. Any mismatch of the study question and the research design can cause bias and impact the results.

The next step in a research study is to describe the methods for data collection and analysis. Family nurse practitioners should be knowledgeable about the different types of measures used to collect data and the potential biases. For example, self-reported data is subject to recall bias, whereas biophysical

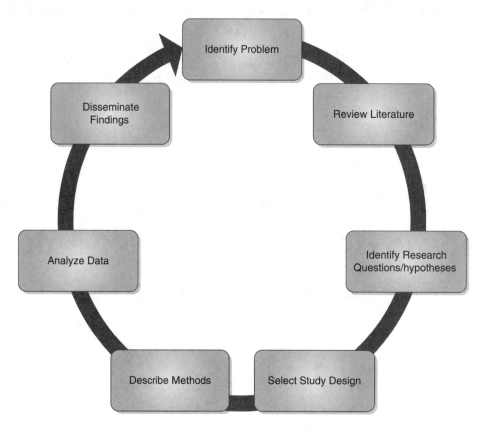

Figure 22-1 Steps in the Scientific Method

measures are not. Moreover, it is important for FNPs to understand basic statistics so they can assess if the data analysis plan is appropriate for the research question and level of measurement.

The second to last step in the research process is data analysis. This is where the researcher uses statistical techniques to analyze the data and draw conclusions from the sample and generalize it to the larger population. The FNP must decide if the findings from the study are clinically meaningful and relevant to their patients. The last step is to disseminate research findings by sharing with colleagues through presentations and publication.

In summary, FNPs must have basic research literacy skills which start with knowing the scientific method and areas of potential bias. Bias can occur at any of the steps in the research process. Research literacy is needed in order to interpret and critically appraise the evidence with confidence so that the APN can decide whether the evidence is valid and reliable and can be applied to practice.

Definition of Evidence-Based Practice

Evidence-based practice is defined as the use of best evidence, clinical data, clinical expertise, and patient values in care decisions. Moreover, EBP for the FNP

means keeping knowledge up to date, enhancing clinical judgment, and engaging in shared decision making with patients (Facchiano & Snyder, 2012). Evidence-based practice can foster lifelong learning, which is necessary given the rapid clinical advances and information overload occurring in health care. Advanced practice nurses must also think about the translation of existing evidence into clinical practice, with the goal of improving care processes and health system outcomes.

Steps in the Evidence-Based Practice Process

In nursing, EBP is comprised of six steps, as defined in the published literature by Bernadette Melnyk and her colleagues (Melnyk, Fineout-Overholt, Stillwell, & Williamson, 2010).

1. Create a clinical question.
2. Search the literature for evidence that is specific to the clinical question.
3. Critically appraise the evidence using appropriate tools.
4. Integrate the patient goals and values and clinician expertise into evidence-based decision making.

5. Evaluate outcomes relevant to the practice decision or change.
6. Disseminate the results.

EBP Step 1: Create a Clinical Question

Every day, busy FNPs are faced with clinical questions about the latest treatments, the precision of diagnostic tests, disease prognosis, risk factors, preventative measures, and more. It can be overwhelming to search for relevant evidence to answer these questions if the FNP doesn't have a well-defined clinical question. The PICO method can be used to develop a searchable clinical question. PICO is a mnemonic: P stands for population, patient, or problem; I stands for intervention or problem of interest; C stands for comparison, condition, or comparator; and O stands for outcome of interest (Facchiano & Snyder, 2012). Depending on the type of clinical question, the FNP may not need to use each letter in the PICO mnemonic. Table 22-1 describes the type of clinical question, the defining characteristics, and PICO example of each type.

EBP Step 2: Search for Evidence

Prior to searching for evidence, the FNP should identify the level of evidence needed to answer the clinical question. The level and quality of evidence are important to clinicians because they give them the confidence to make sound clinical decisions (Stillwell, Fineout-Overholt, Melnyk, & Williamson, 2010). Table 22-2 displays an evidence hierarchy and matches the level of evidence needed to answer various types of clinical questions. The FNP

in primary care practice may want to know the most effective exercise interventions for weight loss in people with osteoarthritis. The FNP should first identify the type of clinical question as a treatment question. Next, the FNP should know that the highest level of evidence (LOE=1) is the best evidence to answer this type of question. In this example, the FNP should start with searching for evidence using methods of meta-analysis/systematic reviews of single randomized control trials and move to level 2 evidence if appropriate evidence cannot be found.

There are several steps the FNP should follow when searching for evidence to answer a clinical question (Stillwell et al., 2010):

- Identify the type of PICO question (Table 22-1).
- Determine the level of evidence needed to answer the question (Table 22-2).
- Identify appropriate databases for the search (Table 22-3).
- Use keywords from the PICO question and relevant synonyms to search the databases (Table 22-4).
- Focus the search by doing the following:
  - Use the controlled language of the database (e.g., Medical Subject Headings, MeSH).
  - Search databases separately with each key term.
  - Use Boolean operators to combine individual searches within each database (e.g., AND).
  - Use search limits (e.g., English language, published last 5 years, adults)

Table 22-1	Clinical Questions and Corresponding PICO Examples	
Question Type	**Defining Characteristics**	**PICO Example**
Intervention	Treatment of chronic disease or illness	*In patients with valve replacements (P), what is the effect of self-management of warfarin (I) compared to provider management of warfarin (C) on INR levels (O)?*
Etiology or harm	Risk factors/causes for disease, disorder, or harm	*In patients with cardiac disease (P), does self-management of warfarin (I) increase risk for adverse events (stroke or bleed) (O)?*
Diagnosis	Act/process of identifying/determining the nature or cause of a disease or injury through evaluation	*For patients in need of mitral valve replacement (P), is heart catheterization (I) compared with heart echocardiography (C) more accurate in assessing valve damage (O)?*
Prognosis or prediction	Prediction of course of disease or treatment outcomes	*For breast cancer patients (P), does radiation treatment plus chemotherapy (I) compared to chemotherapy alone (C) increase risk of heart valve damage (O)?*
Meaning	How one experiences the phenomenon of interest	*What is it like for patients with valve replacements (P) to practice self-management of warfarin therapy (I)?*

Note: Depending on the question type, the FNP doesn't need to use all the letters to develop a solid searchable clinical question.

Table 22-2	Matching Level of Evidence with Clinical Question	
Level of Evidence	**Method/Design**	**Clinical Question**
1	Meta-analysis/systematic review of randomized control trials	Treatment Diagnosis
2	Single randomized control trial	Treatment Diagnosis
3A	Systematic review of observation studies	Prognosis or prediction Etiology or harm
3B	Single observational studies (cohort, cross-sectional, case-control)	Prognosis or prediction Etiology or harm
4A	Meta-synthesis of qualitative studies	Meaning
4B	Single qualitative study	Meaning
5A	Clinical practice guidelines	Identification of practice standards
5B	Expert opinion	Fact finding

Table 22-3	Free Databases the FNP Can Use to Access Various Types of Evidence	
Database	**Definition**	**Where to Find**
PubMed	Provides free access to MEDLINE and the National Library of Medicine database of indexed citations and original abstracts in medicine, nursing, and health care; search tutorials; evidence-based medical reviews (EBMR)	http://www.ncbi.nlm.nih.gov/pubmed
National Guideline Clearinghouse	A comprehensive free database of evidence-based clinical practice guidelines and related documents, an initiative of the Agency for Healthcare Research and Quality (AHRQ). Browse the database by condition or treatment/intervention.	http://www.guideline.gov/
Turning Research into Practice Database (TRIP)	A free meta-search engine for evidence-based health care topics; searches hundreds of evidence-based medicine and evidence-based nursing websites that contain synopses, clinical answers, textbook information, clinical calculators, systematic reviews, and guidelines.	http://www.tripdatabase.com/
Cochrane Database of Systematic Reviews (CDSR)	The leading resource for systematic reviews (SRs) in the world. Users can search for free and view abstracts and plain language summaries. Some SRs can be downloaded for free; others require a fee.	http://www.cochranelibrary.com/cochrane-database-of-systematic-reviews/index.html
Epocrates	Online or application provides for free the latest evidence on drug prescribing and safety information for thousands of brand, generic, and over-the-counter drugs. Can upgrade to Epocrates+ for a fee to access more evidence-based information.	https://online.epocrates.com/noFrame/

Table 22-3 displays several databases where FNPs can access different types of evidence for free via the Internet. PubMed can be searched for original studies using quantitative or qualitative research methodologies. The National Guideline Clearinghouse which is part of the Agency for Healthcare Research and Quality (AHRQ) houses clinical practices guidelines. The TRIP database allows the FNP to search for any type of evidence using regular search functions or the special PICO search or Trip rapid review functions. The PICO interface allows the FNP to input PICO keywords or synonyms and conduct a search. The TRIP rapid review allows FNPs to input the patient population and intervention, and then TRIP conducts a rapid analysis and synthesis of multiple research articles. The Cochrane Database of Systematic Reviews

Table 22-4	PICO Question, Keywords, and Synonym Template			
PICO Question: For elderly patients with dementia (P), how effective is a net enclosure bed (I) versus a sitter (C) in fall prevention (0)?				
	Keywords and Synonyms			
	P	**I**	**C**	**0**
Keyword	Elderly with dementia	Net enclosure bed	Sitter	Fall prevention
Synonyms	Older adults	Soma bed	1:1 observation	Patient safety
	Cognitively impaired adults	Posey bed	Continuous observer	Patient injury

houses five different types of reviews (intervention, diagnostic test accuracy, methodology, qualitative, and prognosis). Epocrates can be accessed online or through an app that gives up-to-date evidence-based information on thousands of drugs.

Table 22-4 is a template that can be used to organize the keywords and synonyms that will be used to search for evidence. It is possible that the keywords from the PICO question may not be representative of how they are indexed in the literature. For example, sitter is not a MeSH heading in PubMed, so it is wise to think of other synonyms. Another search strategy is to check the controlled language in the database you are searching to see if your keyword is indexed or indexed in a different manner. For more information on MeSH, see the PubMed tutorial at http://www.ncbi.nlm.nih.gov/mesh.

EBP Step 3: Critically Appraise the Evidence

In this step, the FNP conducts a critical appraisal of the relevant evidence found from the search. Critical appraisal can be defined as the systematic evaluation of evidence in order to establish that:

- The study addressed a clear, focused, clinical question
- Valid methods were used to answer the question
- The valid results of the study are important and applicable to clinical practice ("Critical Appraisal tools—CEBM," n.d.)

There are several tools that FNPs can use for critical appraisal, depending on the type of research design/method. Regardless of the tool selected for critical appraisal, common questions about the validity (trustworthiness) and reliability (consistency) of the data and applicability to the practice are the focus. Table 22-5 is an overview of typical research designs/methods and their associated critical appraisal questions. The FNP can use these questions to rapidly appraise the evidence and come to a conclusion about the validity and applicability of the results to practice.

Table 22-6 displays free popular tools that are used to critically appraise different types of evidence and to evaluate applicability of the evidence to practice. The John Hopkins Nursing Center for Evidence-Based Practice has easy to use research and non-research appraisal tools that come with detailed instructions for rating evidence level and quality. For example, if the APN wanted to critically appraise a quality improvement study, the JHNEBP non-research tool would be appropriate. If the APN wanted to critically appraise a systematic review the JHNEBP research tool would be appropriate. These tools can be accessed for free at the web address in the table. If the APN wanted to evaluate a clinical practice guideline from the National Guideline Clearinghouse, the appropriate tool to use would be the AGREE II. This tool has a companion guide that explains how to complete and score the tool. There is also online software called My AGREE PLUS where APNs can complete individual or group clinical practice guideline appraisals. In summary, critical appraisal tools help APNs with systematically evaluating the quality and strength of the evidence and applicability to practice.

Evidence synthesis is the last step in the critical appraisal process (Facchiano & Hoffman Snyder, 2012). This is where the APN decides to accept or reject the evidence. If the evidence does not answer the clinical question, then the APN continues to search for more evidence. If the evidence supports a practice change, the APN needs to determine how to integrate the evidence into practice.

EBP Step 4: The Integration of Evidence with Clinical Expertise and Patient Goals and Values in the Decision Making for Individual Patient Care

In this step, the FNP integrates evidence, usually from research, with clinical expertise and patient goals/values in decision making for individual patient care. The current focus in nursing education, and EBP is

Table 22-5	Type of Research Design/Method and Associated Critical Appraisal Questions
Research Design/Method	**General Critical Appraisal Questions**
Systematic Review/ Meta-Analysis	What focused clinical question does the review address? Were any important, relevant studies left out? Were the study selection criteria appropriate? Were the included studies evaluated using standard quality criteria that match the type of clinical question being asked (treatment, diagnostic, prognostic, etc.)? Were the results similar among the included studies? What were the results (e.g., Forrest plot)? Will the results help me care for patients?
Single Randomized Control Trial	Were subjects randomly assigned to an intervention and control group? Were groups similar at the study's start? Aside from the intervention, were the groups treated similarly? Were all the subjects enrolled accounted for? Were subjects analyzed in the groups they were assigned to (intention to treat analysis)? Were the subjects and investigators blinded to intervention allocation and outcome measures (this is more important if the measures are subjective)? How large was the intervention effect? How precise are the results (e.g., summary estimates relative risk, relative risk reduction, absolute risk reduction)? Will the results help me care for patients?
Observational (cross-sectional, cohort, case-control)	What focused clinical issue was addressed? Was the group (sample) recruited appropriately? Were the exposure, predictors, and outcome measures reliable and valid? Were there any confounding factors? Was the follow-up complete and long enough? Were the results plausible? Does other evidence support the results? How precise are the results? Will the results help me care for patients?
Diagnostic Accuracy Studies	Was the diagnostic test evaluated in an appropriate patient population? Where appropriate, were both the reference (gold) standard and index test done on all subjects? Was the application of both reference standard and index test applied to each subject independently and blindly? Are the sensitivity, specificity, and predictive values of the diagnostic test presented? Is the diagnostic test described in enough detail to allow for replication?

Data from Centre for Evidence-Based Medicine (CEBM). (2016). Critical appraisal tools. Retrieved from http://www.cebm.net/critical-appraisal/. Accessed May 9, 2015; STROBE. (2007). STROBE checklists. Retrieved from http://strobe-statement.org/index.php?id=available-checklists. Accessed May 12, 2015; Critical Appraisal Skills Programme (CASP). (2013). CASP Checklists. Retrieved from http://www.casp-uk.net/#!casp-tools-checklists/c18f8. Accessed May 12, 2015.

to use EBP steps 1 through 3 and clinical expertise when making patient care decisions; however, shared decision making is limited (Friesen-Storms, Bours, van der Weijden, & Beurskens, 2015). Shared decision making has been defined as "a process that aims to have the health care professional and the patient jointly arrive at a health care choice that is based on the best available research evidence, clinical expertise, and the values of the informed patient" (p. 395).

Essential elements of shared decision making as defined by Makoul & Clayman (2006) include:

- Define or explain the problem (both provider and patient)

- Present options (provider reviews options, and patient should raise options they know about)

- Discuss the pros and cons including benefits, risks, and costs (both provider and patient)

- Clarify the patient's values and preferences (provider)

- Discuss the patient's ability and self-efficacy to follow through on a plan of care (both provider and patient)

- Discuss the provider's knowledge and recommendations (both provider and patient)

Table 22-6	Free Tools for Critical Appraisal Based on Research Design or Evidence Type	
Tool	**Design**	**Where to Find**
JHNEBP Tools	The **J**ohn **H**opkins **N**ursing **E**vidence-**B**ased **P**ractice tools are two separate tools, one for critical appraisal of research evidence (e.g. systematic review, meta-analysis, randomized control trial) and the other for non-research evidence (e.g. literature review, quality improvement, expert opinion).	http://www.hopkinsmedicine.org/ institute_nursing/ebp/jhn_ebp .html
AGREE II	**A**ppraisal of **G**uidelines for **R**esearch and **E**valuation Instrument is a valid and reliable tool used to assess practice guideline quality, rigor, and completeness of recommendations.	http://www.agreetrust.org/
CEBM Tools	These **C**enter for **E**vidence-**B**ased **M**edicine tools are used for critical appraisal of different types of medical evidence and include helpful examples. Systematic Review Critical Appraisal Sheet Diagnosis Critical Appraisal Sheet Prognosis Critical Appraisal Sheet Therapy/RCT Critical Appraisal Sheet	http://www.cebm.net/ critical-appraisal/
CASP Tools	The **C**ritical **A**ppraisal **S**kills **P**rogramme has a set of 8 tools that can be used when critically appraising systematic reviews, randomized controlled trials, cohort studies, case-control studies, economic evaluations, diagnostic studies, qualitative studies, and clinical prediction rule.	http://www.casp-uk.net/ #!casp-tools-checklists/c18f8

- Check/clarify the patient's understanding throughout the process (both provider and patient)
- Make or explicitly defer the decision (patient may need to discuss with family or provider with other health care team members before reaching a decision)
- Arrange follow-up (both provider and patient)

Decision aids are helpful tools that FNPs and patients can use when there are multiple treatment options, options that have no clear advantage related to health outcomes, and options that have benefits and risks that patients value differently (Stacey et al., 2014). The aim of using decision aids is to improve the overall quality of provider/patient decisions. In an updated systematic review by Stacey and colleagues (2014), findings from high-quality evidence demonstrated that when patients used decision aids they improved their knowledge of options and felt more informed and clear about their values/preferences. Findings from moderate quality evidence demonstrated more accurate patient expectations of possible benefits and risks related to the options and more participation in decision making.

In Table 22-7, resources for accessing free decision aids for certain conditions or general health-related or social decisions are described. Both the

Ottawa Hospital Research Institute and Agency for Healthcare Research and Quality have decision aids that providers and patients can use to make difficult health care decisions. The International Patient Decision Aid Standards (IPDAS) Collaboration is a group of researchers, practitioners, and stakeholders that ensure that patient decision aids have reliable health information. Advanced practice nurses should be using decision aids with their patients as part of the EBP process.

EBP Step 5: Evaluate Outcomes Relevant to the Practice Decision or Change

In this step, the FNP should ask, *Were the best possible outcomes achieved from the practice decision?* Outcomes-based measurements may be care-related (effect of FNP interventions), patient-related (patient behaviors or actions), or performance-related (how FNPs perform their job) (Kleinpell, 2013). This step may also include self-evaluation, where the FNP assesses how well he/she is performing each step in EBP.

EBP Step 6: Disseminate the Results

This is the last step in the EBP process. Sharing EBP practice change results with others is a vital step that allows for local evidence to be used on a larger scale

Table 22-7	Decision Aid Resources	
Name	**Definition**	**Where to find**
Ottawa Hospital Research Institute	Patient Decision Aid Research Group was created in November 1995 to help patients and their health providers make difficult health care decisions. Houses over 500 decision aids for specific conditions or general health-related or social decision.	https://decisionaid.ohri.ca/
Agency for Healthcare Research and Quality (AHRQ)	Effective health care program includes interactive patient decision aids.	http://effectivehealthcare.ahrq.gov/
International Patient Decision Aid Standards (IPDAS) Collaboration	This is a collaboration that was formed to enhance the quality and effectiveness of patient decision aids by establishing a shared evidence-informed framework with a set of criteria for improving decision aid content, development, implementation, and evaluation.	http://ipdas.ohri.ca/

(Milner, 2014). There are several ways this can be done. The traditional way to share best practices is through poster or oral presentation at conferences and publication in practice journals. New ways of sharing best practices include Technology, Entertainment, Design (TED) Talks, blogs, podcasts, and twitter. The effectiveness of dissemination for these new modalities has yet to be tested; however, Harris (2013) found that Facebook and Twitter were effective for disseminating information to state health departments.

Summary

In this chapter, the basic components of the scientific method and evidence-based practice were reviewed. After reading this chapter, FNPs should be familiar with the steps in the scientific method and the link between research literacy and EBP. Many free tools and databases were described that FNPs can access via the Internet to support EBP and shared decision making.

Review Questions

1. The scientific method is best used for:
   A. Generating new knowledge to the advanced nursing practice.
   B. Answering practice questions.
   C. Evaluating the quality and strength of evidence.
   D. Evaluating methodological rigor.

2. Put the following steps of the scientific method in the order in which they are carried out.
   A. Select study design
   B. Analyze data
   C. Disseminate findings
   D. Describe methods
   E. Identify problem
   F. Identify research questions
   G. Review literature

3. Research literacy is defined as which of the following?
   A. The ability to access, critically appraise, and interpret scientific literature
   B. The ability to translate research findings into practice
   C. The ability to carry out a research study
   D. The ability to use best current evidence in practice

4. Evidence-based practice (EBP) includes the following (*choose all that apply*):
   A. EBP is a process used by advanced practice nurses to improve patient care.
   B. Shared decision making is used in the EBP process.
   C. EBP starts by forming a clinical question.
   D. The P in PICO stands for problem.
   E. All letters must be identified in the PICO mnemonic.

5. Put the following EBP steps in the order of which they are done:
   A. Disseminate the results
   B. Search for best current evidence
   C. Integrate patient goals and values, and clinical expertise
   D. Critically appraise the evidence
   E. Formulate a PICO question
   F. Evaluate the outcomes relevant to the practice change

6. What step would not be recommended when searching for evidence to answer a clinical question?
   A. Use controlled language of the database.
   B. Use keywords from a PICO question.
   C. Determine the level of evidence needed to answer the question.
   D. Search using multiple databases and keywords simultaneously.

7. What is the outcome in the following PICO question?
   In hospitalized patients on telemetry, does a nurse-led noise reduction program compared to standard nursing care improve patient satisfaction?
   A. Patients on telemetry
   B. Nurse-led noise reduction program
   C. Standard nursing care
   D. Patient satisfaction

8. What is the intervention in the following PICO question?

   In incarcerated females, does pedometer use plus portion control compared to pedometer use only decrease weight gain during the first 6 months?

   A. Incarcerated females
   B. Pedometer use plus portion control
   C. Pedometer use
   D. Weight gain

9. What is considered the highest level of evidence in an evidence hierarchy for intervention questions?

   A. Systematic review
   B. Meta-analysis
   C. Meta-synthesis
   D. Randomized control trial

10. What is considered the highest level of evidence in an evidence hierarchy for prognosis questions?

    A. Systematic review of randomized control trials
    B. Meta-analysis of randomized control trials
    C. A single randomized control trial
    D. Systematic review of observational studies

11. What is considered the highest level of evidence in an evidence hierarchy for meaning questions?

    A. Systematic review
    B. Meta-analysis
    C. Meta-synthesis
    D. Randomized control trial

12. Match the level of evidence (LOE) to the method/design and clinical question

LOE	Method/Design	Clinical Question
1	Systematic review of observation studies	Treatment
2	Meta-analysis of randomized control trials	Diagnosis
3A	Single randomized control trial	Prognosis or prediction
3B	Expert opinion	Etiology or harm
4A	Single qualitative study	Meaning
4B	Clinical practice guidelines	Identification of practice standard
5A	Meta-synthesis of qualitative studies	Fact finding
5B	Single observational study	

13. The following is what type of clinical question?

    For patients with a 75% blocked coronary artery, does medication therapy versus stent prevent occlusion?

    A. Intervention
    B. Etiology or harm
    C. Diagnostic
    D. Prognostic or prediction

14. National Guideline Clearinghouse is a free resource for accessing what type of evidence?

    A. Systematic reviews
    B. Meta-analysis
    C. Clinical trials
    D. Clinical practice guidelines

15. Epocrates is a free resource for accessing what type of information?
    A. Systematic reviews
    B. Drug prescribing and safety information
    C. Clinical trials
    D. Clinical practice guidelines

16. Select the database where the advanced practice nurse would find evidence-based synopses.
    A. National Guideline Clearinghouse
    B. Turning Research into Practice Database
    C. Cochrane Database of Systematic Reviews
    D. Epocrates

17. Which of the following can be used to critically appraise a quality improvement study?
    A. CONSORT
    B. SQUIRE
    C. PRISMA
    D. STROBE

18. Which of the following can be used to critically appraise a randomized control trial?
    A. CONSORT
    B. SQUIRE
    C. PRISMA
    D. STROBE

19. Which of the following elements does a shared decision include? (*choose all that apply*)
    A. Clarify patient values and preferences
    B. Present treatment options
    C. Discuss provider recommendations
    D. Discuss risks, benefits, and costs
    E. Clarify provider values and preferences

20. Resources for patient and provider decision aids can be found at which of the following?
    A. Ottawa Hospital Research Institute website
    B. National Guidelines Clearinghouse website
    C. Center for Evidence-Based Medicine website
    D. International Patient Decision Aid Standards website

21. The next 5 questions will be based on the following clinical scenario.

    Clinical Scenario: An adolescent boy comes to the primary care clinic for his yearly checkup. His blood-work shows an elevated total cholesterol level of 225 with a low-density lipoprotein (ldl) cholesterol level of 140. He has a family history of elevated cholesterol, so his mother requests medication to lower the cholesterol. However, the APN wants to try diet and exercise first.

    1. Write a focused clinical question in PICO format for this problem.
    2. Identify three sources of evidence that you would give you the most confidence in answering your PICO question.
    3. What type of research design would best answer your PICO question?
    4. Is using controlled language from the database compared to a keyword search likely to yield more or less articles?
    5. Your search yields two systematic reviews with meta-analyses. What tool will you select to critically appraise these articles?

Answers and Rationales

1. A. The scientific method is a formal, rigorous multi-step process designed to discover new knowledge or validate/refine existing knowledge. Researchers systematically identify a problem, review the literature, identify research questions, select a study design, describe study methods, collect data, analyze data, make conclusions that add to the existing knowledge base, and disseminate findings.

2. E, G, F, A, D, B, C. These seven steps of the scientific method create a systematic process of investigation and a formal method for obtaining data/knowledge.

3. A. The ability to translate research findings into practice is knowledge translation and is a critical step in the EBP process. The ability to carry out a research study is the job of researchers who have the appropriate formal training and education. The ability to use best current evidence in practice is a component of EBP.

4. A, B, C, D. It is not necessary to identify all letters in the PICO mnemonic. For example, a meaning question, "What is it like to be a professional athlete with type 1 diabetes?" would have a "P" for professional athlete and an "I" for type 1 diabetes.

5. E, B, D, C, F, A. The EBP process is a problem-solving approach to clinical practice that integrates the conscientious use of best evidence in combination with a clinician's expertise, as well as patient preferences and values to make decisions about the type of care that is provided. Resources should be considered in the decision-making process as well.

6. D. The clinician searches each database separately because the way in which each database organizes articles and the type of controlled language may be different. For example, MEDLINE and PubMed use MeSH, whereas CINAHL uses CINHAL headings.

7. D. The outcome is what the clinician wants to see happen after manipulating the independent variable. In this example, patients on telemetry is the population (P), nurse-led noise reduction program is the intervention (I), and standard nursing care is the comparison (C).

8. B. In the PICO mnemonic, examples of an intervention can be a treatment, procedure, or program. In this example, incarcerated females are the population (P), pedometer use is one of the two interventions being used (I), and weight gain is the outcome (O).

9. B. A meta-analysis is a method of analyzing statistically quantitative findings from multiple studies on the same topic to create new knowledge or validate existing knowledge. A systematic review is a type of literature review where the authors develop a specific protocol to systematically search for, critically appraise, and synthesize evidence from several studies on the same topic (Milner, 2014). A meta-synthesis is a method of analyzing qualitative findings from multiple studies on the same topic. A randomized control trial is a type of quantitative study design where subjects are either randomly selected from a population for the study or they are randomly assigned to the study, experimental, or control group.

10. D. Prognostic questions are best answered using observational study designs because the researcher is evaluating the course of a disease or treatment outcome over time and this cannot be accomplished using an experimental study design like a randomized control trial. Systematic review of randomized control trials, meta-analysis of randomized control trials, and single randomized control trials are considered the highest level of evidence needed for treatment or diagnosis questions.

11. C. Meaning questions are best answered using qualitative methods. A meta-synthesis is the highest level of evidence needed for answering meaning questions because it is a method of analyzing qualitative findings from multiple studies on the same topic. Systematic review of randomized control trials, meta-analysis of randomized control trials, and single randomized control trials are considered the highest level of evidence needed for treatment or diagnosis questions.

12. Answers:

    LOE 1, meta-analysis of randomized control trials, treatment and diagnosis

    LOE 2, single randomized control trials, treatment and diagnosis

    LOE 3A, systematic review of observational studies, prognosis, etiology

    LOE 3B, single observational study, prognosis, etiology

LOE 4A, meta-synthesis of qualitative studies, meaning

LOE 4B, single qualitative study, meaning

LOE 5A, clinical practice guidelines, identification of practice standard

LOE 5B, expert opinion, fact finding

See Table 22-2 Matching Level of Evidence with Clinical Question in the text.

13. D. This prediction question in PICO format will elicit a focused research for evidence that will aid in the treatment (medication versus stent) decision of a patient that has a 75% blockage in their coronary artery, with the goal of preventing a future outcome (occlusion).

14. D. To date, the National Guideline Clearinghouse is a free government-sponsored website where you will find clinical practice guidelines to guide practice. Systematic reviews can be found in PubMed or the Cochrane Database of Systematic Reviews. Epocrates online or the application provides free drug prescribing and safety information. Information on clinical trials can be found at https://www.clinicaltrials .gov/ct2/home.

15. B. Epocrates online or the application provides free drug prescribing and safety information. Systematic reviews can be found in PubMed or the Cochrane Database of Systematic Reviews. Information on clinical trials can be found at https://www.clinicaltrials.gov/ct2/home. The National Guideline Clearinghouse is a free government sponsored website where you will find clinical practice guidelines to guide practice.

16. B. The Turning Research into Practice (TRIP) database is a free meta-search engine where clinicians can find evidence-based synopses that are easy to understand and use in order to guide practice decisions. The National Guideline Clearinghouse is a free government-sponsored website where you will find clinical practice guidelines to guide practice. Systematic reviews can be found in the Cochrane Database of Systematic Reviews. Epocrates online or the application provides free drug prescribing and safety information.

17. B. CONSORT can be used to appraise single randomized control trials. PRISMA can be used to appraise systematic review and/or meta-analysis. STROBE can be used to appraise observational studies (e.g., cohort, cross-sectional, case-control).

18. A. SQUIRE can be used to appraise a quality improvement study. PRISMA can be used to appraise systematic reviews and/or meta-analysis. STROBE can be used to appraise observational studies (e.g., cohort, cross-sectional, case-control).

19. A, B, C, D, E. Shared decision making includes all the elements included in answers A–E.

20. A. The Ottawa Hospital Research Institute website has excellent resources for patient and provider decision aids, including the decision aids developed under the guidance of the Agency for Healthcare Research and Quality (AHRQ). The National Guideline Clearinghouse website has clinical practice guidelines only. The Center for Evidence-Based Medicine website has resources to support the search and critical appraisal processes associated with EBP. The International Patient Decision Aid Standards website has tools for assessing the quality of patient decision aids.

21. Answers:

   1. In adolescents with elevated total cholesterol and LDL cholesterol (P), does diet and exercise (I) compared to medication (C) reduce total cholesterol and LDL cholesterol (O)?

   2. Cochrane database of systematic reviews, PubMed, TRIP database

   3. Systematic review and meta-analysis of randomized control trials

   4. Using controlled language from the database is likely to yield more articles because it imposed uniformity and consistency in indexing the literature, and thus you should only end up with relevant literature.

   5. Use the PRISMA tool.

● ● ● **References**

CASP Tools & Checklists. (n.d.). Retrieved May 12, 2015, from http://www.casp-uk.net/#!casp-tools-checklists/c18f8

Critical Appraisal Tools—CEBM. (n.d.). Retrieved May 9, 2015, from http://www.cebm.net/critical-appraisal/

Facchiano, L., & Hoffman Snyder, C. (2012). Evidence-based practice for the busy nurse practitioner: Part three: Critical appraisal process. *Journal of the American Academy of Nurse Practitioners*, 24(12), 704–715. doi:10.1111/j.1745-7599.2012.00752.x

Facchiano, L., & Snyder, C. H. (2012). Evidence-based practice for the busy nurse practitioner: Part one: Relevance to clinical practice and clinical inquiry process. *Journal of the American Academy of Nurse Practitioners*, 24(10), 579–586. doi:10.1111/j.1745-7599.2012.00748.x

Friesen-Storms, J. H. H. M., Bours, G. J. J. W., van der Weijden, T., & Beurskens, A. J. H. M. (2015). Shared decision making in chronic care in the context of evidence-based practice in nursing. *International Journal of Nursing Studies*, 52(1), 393–402. doi:10.1016/j.ijnurstu.2014.06.012

Harris, J. K. (2013). The network of Web 2.0 connections among state health departments: New pathways for dissemination. *Journal of Public Health Management and Practice: JPHMP*. doi:10.1097/PHH.0b013e318268ae36

Kleinpell, R. M. (2013). *Outcome assessment in advanced practice nursing* (3rd ed.). Springer Publishing Company.

Makoul, G., & Clayman, M. L. (2006). An integrative model of shared decision making in medical encounters. *Patient Education and Counseling*, 60(3), 301–312. doi:10.1016/j.pec.2005.06.010

Melnyk, B. M., Fineout-Overholt, E., Stillwell, S. B., & Williamson, K. M. (2010). Evidence-based practice: Step by step: The seven steps of evidence-based practice. *The American Journal of Nursing*, 110(1), 51–53. doi:10.1097/01.NAJ.0000366056.06605.d2

Milner, K. A. (2014). 10 STEPS from EBP project to publication. *Nursing*, 44(11), 53–56. doi:10.1097/01.NURSE.0000454954.80525.8c

Nolan, M., & Behi, R. (1996). From methodology to method: The building blocks of research literacy. *The British Journal of Nursing*, 5(1), 54–57.

Price, B. (2010). Disseminating best practice through a Web log. *Nursing Standard: Official Newspaper of the Royal College of Nursing*, 24(29), 35–40.

Stacey, D., Légaré, F., Col, N. F., Bennett, C. L., Barry, M. J., Eden, K. B., . . . Wu, J. H. C. (2014). Decision aids for people facing health treatment or screening decisions. *The Cochrane Database of Systematic Reviews*, 1, CD001431. doi:10.1002/14651858.CD001431.pub4

Stillwell, S. B., Fineout-Overholt, E., Melnyk, B. M., & Williamson, K. M. (2010). Evidence-based practice, step by step: Searching for the evidence. *The American Journal of Nursing*, 110(5), 41–47. doi:10.1097/01.NAJ.0000372071.24134.7e

STROBE Statement: Available checklists. (n.d.). Retrieved May 12, 2015, from http://strobe-statement.org/index.php?id=available-checklists

Index

Page numbers followed by b, f, or t indicate material in boxes, figures, or tables, respectively.